CLINICAL MICROBIOLOGY AND INFECTIOUS DISEASE

VOLUME 2

VIROLOGY, MYCOLOGY, PARASITOLOGY, AND INFECTION CONTROL

Yevhen Tarasov and
Hanna Shevchuk

ALLIED
HEALTH
PRESS

Clinical Microbiology and Infectious Disease

Volume 2: Virology, Mycology, Parasitology, and Infection Control

Authors: **Yevhen Tarasov and Hanna Shevchuk**

Allied Health Press
4164 Lakeshore Road
Burlington ON L7L 1A4
Canada
www.alliedhealthpress.com
Email: orders@arclereducation.com

ISBN: 978-1-77956-811-3

ABOUT THE AUTHORS

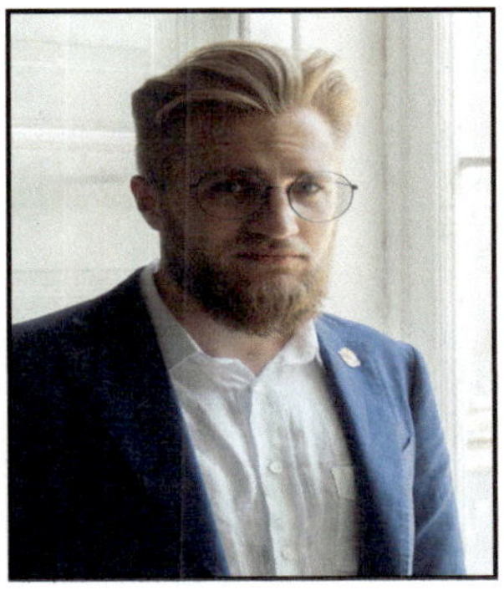

Yevhen Tarasov, MD, EuSpLM is a Senior Lecturer at the Department of General and Clinical Epidemiology and Biosafety with a course on Microbiology and Virology at Odesa National Medical University. Yevhen Tarasov received his MD in 2018 and got specialization in Medical Laboratory Science in 2019 with residency at The Filatov Institute of Eye Diseases and Tissue Therapy of the National Acadeny if Medical Science of Ukraine. He then joined the Department of General and Clinical Epidemiology and Biosafety with a course on Microbiology and Virology at Odesa National Medical University, Odesa, Ukraine as an assistant professor. His research interests include epidemiology and diagnostics of autoimmune diseases and allergy. He is a group leader of work group on Ukrainian adaptation of the the International Consensus on Antinuclear Antibody (ANA) Patterns (ICAP).

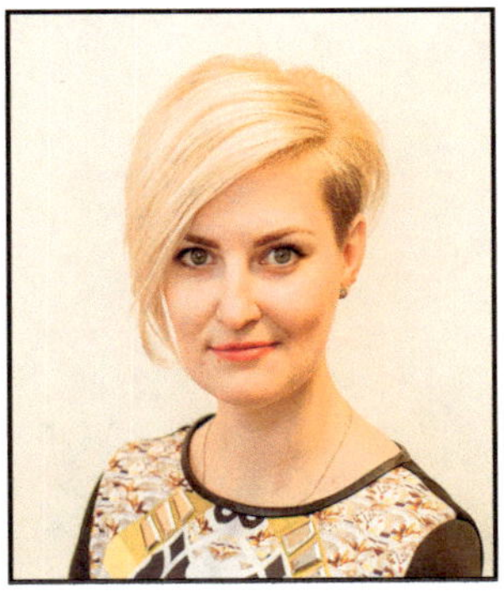

Hanna Shevchuk, PhD, is an Associate Professor and Head of Study at the Department of General and Clinical Epidemiology and Biosafety with a course in Microbiology and Virology at Odessa National Medical University (ONMedU), Ukraine. She also serves as a visiting lecturer at the International European University, Malta Campus. As. Prof. Shevchuk received her Master's degree in Microbiology and Virology from Odessa I.I. Mechnikov National University in 2005 and earned her PhD in Biological Sciences (specialty: molecular genetics) from the Institute of Food Biotechnology and Genomics of the National Academy of Sciences of Ukraine in 2012. Her academic journey includes positions ranging from laboratory assistant to researcher and faculty member at leading Ukrainian research institutes and universities. Her research interests focus on molecular genetics, microbiology, immunology, virology, epidemiology and innovative pedagogical practices in medical education. As. Prof. Shevchuk is an active member of the Society of Microbiologists of Ukraine named after S.M. Vynogradskyi, the Vavilov Society of Geneticists and Breeders of Ukraine and the Association of Clinical Chemistry and Laboratory Medicine of Ukraine. She has participated in international internships and seminars dedicated to modern challenges in higher medical education and is the author and co-author of scientific publications in microbiology, immunology, and pedagogy.

As. Prof. Shevchuk is recognized for her contributions to the development of educational programs and the implementation of advanced teaching methods, aiming to enhance the quality of training for specialists in medicine. In 2024, she was awarded the academic title of Associate Professor at Odessa National Medical University.

Brief Table of Contents

Detailed Table of Contents

CHAPTER 6

Hepatitis and Bloodborne Viruses 165

CHAPTER 7

Fungal Pathogens and Mycoses 195

CHAPTER 8

Protozoan Infections 227

CHAPTER 9

Helminthic Infections 261

CHAPTER 10

Central Nervous System Infections 291

LIST OF FIGURES

PREFACE

Clinical microbiology extends beyond the bacteria to encompass the vast world of viruses, fungi, and parasites that pose a significant threat to health. Viral pathogens, ranging from the innocuous common cold to the deadly hemorrhagic fevers, have an astonishing variety of structure, genetic makeup, and transmission modes. Fungal pathogens can infect mucosal and cutaneous surfaces or internal organs in immunocompromised individuals, while protozoa and helminths employ intricate life cycles for long-term vector and host infections. Collectively, these microorganisms contribute a significant percentage of acute and chronic disease burden worldwide, necessitating holistic laboratory methods and clinical management for detection, treatment, and prevention.

The last few decades have witnessed the emergence and resurgence of viral disease — driven by environmental transformation, global travel, and human encroachment into wildlife niches — with diseases such as SARS-CoV, influenza, and novel zoonoses commanding global attention. Advances in molecular diagnostics, high-throughput sequencing, and immunoassays have dramatically advanced the ability to identify viral pathogens rapidly, but challenges remain in resource-deprived settings where access to sophisticated platforms is low. Similarly, the identification of protozoal, fungal, and helminthic infections typically is a function of a combination of microscopy, culture, antigen detection, and serology, each with certain strengths and limitations to be balanced against clinical demand and facility capacity.

Clinical Microbiology and Infectious Disease — Volume 2: Virology, Mycology, Parasitology, and Infection Control blends fundamental principles and recent advances in virology, mycology, parasitology, and infection control. This book is aimed at guiding the reader through the biology of viral and nonviral pathogens, the laboratory approaches used to detect them, and the clinical relevance of these diseases. Case examples, methodological overviews, and evidence-based treatment guidelines add practical relevance, making the book a valuable read for both newcomers and veteran professionals in the field.

Chapter 1 presents an overview of fundamental virology principles, including virus structure and classification, replication cycles, and viral genetic diversity. It explains how these factors influence pathogenicity, host range, and detectability in the laboratory. Special consideration is given to the comparison between DNA viruses and RNA viruses, the significance of envelopes in viruses, and the mechanisms by which viruses infect, multiply within, and escape from host cells.

Chapter 2 deals with respiratory viruses such as influenza viruses, respiratory syncytial virus, adenoviruses, and coronaviruses. The chapter outlines clinical syndromes from mild upper respiratory infection to pneumonia, overviews specimen collection and rapid testing practices, and discusses antiviral therapy and vaccine strategies for influenza and other respiratory pathogens.

Chapter 3 covers gastrointestinal viruses, including rotaviruses, noroviruses, astroviruses, and enteric adenoviruses. It covers epidemiology and modes of transmission, highlights molecular panels in acute gastroenteritis, and covers supportive practices as well as emerging antiviral therapy on trial.

Chapter 4 discusses herpesviruses and oncogenic viruses, the biology and clinical disease of herpes simplex, varicella-zoster, cytomegalovirus, Epstein-Barr virus, and human herpesvirus-6, and papillomaviruses and hepatotropic oncogenic viruses. Laboratory diagnostic approaches such as PCR, serology, and viral load monitoring are covered, along with antiviral therapy and vaccine development.

Chapter 5 discusses emerging and re-emerging viral infections, with case studies of Ebola, Zika, chikungunya, and other viral diseases that have moved over geographical or species boundaries. It discusses surveillance systems, outbreak response systems, and the public health laboratory's role in the quick identification and containment of new viral threats.

Chapter 6 is a synopsis of hepatitis and bloodborne viruses, such as hepatitis A, B, C, D, and E viruses and the human immunodeficiency virus and other transfusion-transmissible agents. Diagnostic algorithms — serologic markers, molecular assays, and genotyping — and current antiviral regimens, prevention strategies, and global elimination goals are discussed in the chapter.

Chapter 7 covers fungal pathogens and mycoses, introducing yeasts, molds, and dimorphic fungi producing superficial, mucosal, and systemic infections. Topics include specimen processing for microscopy and culture, antigen and molecular tests, antifungal susceptibility testing, and antifungal pharmacology principles.

Chapter 8 deals with protozoal illnesses, which include amoebae, flagellates, sporozoans, and hemoflagellates such as *Plasmodium* species. The chapter highlights the identification according to morphology, antigen detection, nucleic acid amplification tests, and interpretation of serologic findings in the context of travel history and clinical presentation.

Chapter 9 discusses helminthic infections, outlining nematodes, cestodes, and trematodes parasitizing humans. It outlines stool examination techniques, concentration methods, serology, and molecular investigations in diagnosis and covers anthelmintic treatment schedules and control strategies in endemic regions.

Chapter 10 covers central nervous system infections such as viral, bacterial, fungal, and parasitic causes of meningitis and encephalitis. The chapter covers cerebrospinal fluid analysis, rapid multiplex PCR panels, and new biomarkers, alongside therapeutic for drugs such as herpesviruses, enteroviruses, and *Cryptococcus*.

Chapter 11 covers viral urethra and genital infections (e.g., herpes simplex) and bacterial, fungal, and parasitic urethra and genital infections (e.g., Trichomonas vaginalis). Diagnostic methods include culture, PCR, antigen tests, and microscopic examination, with mention of antimicrobial and antiviral treatments.

Chapter 12 addresses hospital-acquired infections (HAIs) and infection control practices. It addresses common nosocomial pathogens, including *Clostridioides difficile*, drug-resistant bacteria, and invasive fungal organisms, as well as surveillance concepts, environmental sampling, hand hygiene, and antimicrobial stewardship programs.

Chapter 13 concludes with vaccines and immunoprophylaxis, detailing vaccine development, mechanisms, and delivery of vaccines to prevent viral, bacterial, and parasitic infections. Topics include vaccine platforms (live-attenuated, inactivated, subunit, mRNA), cold chain logistics and management, herd immunity concepts, and vaccine deployment strategies in outbreak settings.

This textbook is intended for graduate students and medical students of microbiology, clinical laboratory scientists, infectious disease fellows, and practicing clinicians who need an integrated reference for viral, fungal, and parasitic infections. Public health practitioners, epidemiologists, and researchers will also find useful the extensive discussion of prevention and diagnosis platforms.

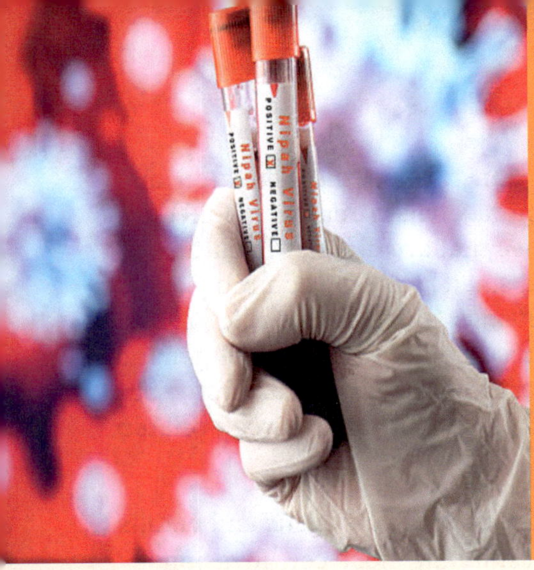

Chapter 1
INTRODUCTION TO VIROLOGY

Contents

Introduction

Virology is a fundamental branch in the domain of medical microbiology with particular reference to the biology, pathogenesis, and control of viruses. Virology is a science dealing with knowledge about virus structure, classification, and virus replication mechanisms. Viruses are single organisms; they consist of genetic material surrounded by a protein coat and are a challenge to traditional definitions of living organisms. Notably, their replication in host cells serves to highlight the intricate interactions between viruses and other biological systems. In medical microbiology, insight into such fundamental principles is imperative in designing diagnostic and treatment approaches against viral infections, which account significantly for human disease and health. Noted briefly, practical medical classes, i.e., "Practical Microbiology and Virology," illustrate different levels of agreement among students regarding their usefulness, suggesting a mismatch in bringing theoretical knowledge to practice (Ranjbarzadeh et al., 2014). Advances in virology have been facilitated by advanced technologies, particularly the breakthroughs of molecular diagnostics that have significantly transformed the detection and monitoring of viral pathogens. Amongst these technologies, polymerase chain reaction (PCR) has emerged as a valuable aid in the detection of viruses, especially those that are difficult to culture or lack an appropriate animal model. Human caliciviruses (HuCVs) and small round-structured viruses (SRSVs) are such instances that cannot be grown in laboratory settings (Butcher & Gould, 1997). The use of PCR-based methods in the diagnosis of viral infection also points to the use of genetic analysis in virology. Not only do these methods enhance our understanding of viral diversity, but they also enable the identification of isolated viral strains, which is crucial for outbreak-related epidemiological and public health responses.

Furthermore, the science of virology extends beyond the identification of pathogens and entails the examination of viral pathogenesis and host response. Understanding host cell invasion by viruses, immune evasion strategies, and disease-causing mechanisms is important for successful vaccine and antiviral drug design. This dynamic interaction between virus and host cell often dictates the clinical manifestations observed in patients. Also, the impact of viral diseases such as influenza, HIV/AIDS, and hepatitis on the host public health imposes a focus on carrying out sufficient research and surveillance in virology. Hence, using practical laboratory methods along with theoretical data is essential for future healthcare professionals. Admitting the significance of comprehensive education in virology, researching students' attitudes toward practical courses highlights the necessity of special educational measures of medical microbiology (Ranjbarzadeh et al., 2014).

Definition and scope of virology

Virology, a specialised branch of microbiology, predominantly concentrates on the study of viruses, encompassing their structure, classification, and the mechanisms they employ to infect host cells. It overlaps with fields such as genetics, molecular biology, and immunology to further understand the life and disease processes of viruses. The word virus itself embodies not only the etiological agent but also the nuances of its life cycle, including replication and mechanism of pathogenicity. The background of virology is significant as it emerged as a distinct branch of science in the early to mid-20th century, progressing from observation of viral pathogenicity to an examination encompassing virology methodology and theory. These advances highlight the field's dynamism and open the door to discussions of specific viral interactions in disease and human health (van Loon, 2002). Virology transcends fundamental research into medical microbiology practice. This includes the development of vaccines, antiviral drugs, and diagnostic techniques with a view to preventing viral infections. Research today puts a premium on technological innovation in vaccine manufacture and design, especially in response to emerging viral threats such as those represented by influenza. With the emerging complexity of viral strains, new solutions such as recombinant and reverse genetics technologies are needed to achieve optimal vaccine effectiveness (Cavicchi et al., 2012). Besides this, virology intersects with public health since knowledge of viral dynamics may be applied in the control of epidemics and pandemics, illustrating the crucial role that virologists can play in safeguarding public health. As virology expands, so also does it face the challenge of keeping pace with evolving viral threats, illustrating its ongoing relevance in the medical microbiology field. Virology is not only essential for understanding the complexity of viral infections but also for deciphering the effects of viral diseases on public health. Ongoing study into virulence factors has become a top priority in virology, driven by the need to map out and contain viral outbreaks that pose a significant threat to health. The interdisciplinary character of virology facilitates a multifaceted understanding of virus-host interactions and the formulation of therapeutic approaches to contend with viral pathogenesis. As virology changes with the times, its methodologies must be modified to find fit in the face of new threats, further underlining the need for ongoing research and development in this discipline. The interactive dynamics between virology and technology, and especially in accelerating the vaccine process, emphasize the role of being vigilant over surveillance and responding to viral epidemics as an integral responsibility of medical microbiology (van Loon, 2002; Cavicchi et al., 2012) (Figure 1.1).

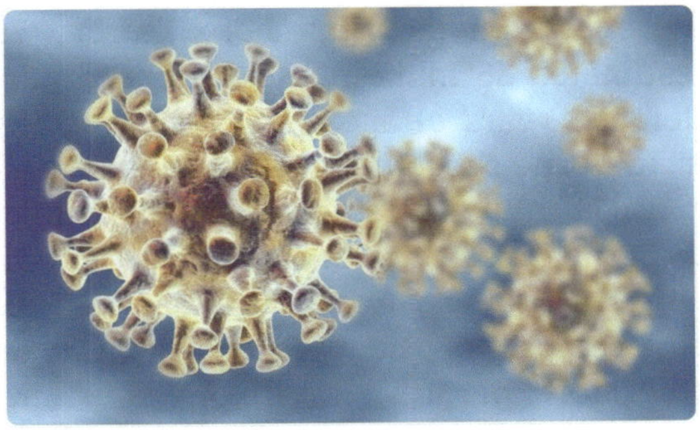

Figure 1.1. 3D illustration of a coronavirus particle, showing its characteristic spike proteins responsible for host cell attachment and viral entry.

Source: https://www.news-medical.net/image-handler/ts/20210317042002/ri/673/picture/2021/3/shutterstock_1625661736.jpg.

Historical context and development of virology

The history of virology is characterized by major milestones that have defined our knowledge of viral pathogens and their intricate interactions with hosts. The beginning of viruses came in the late 19th century with the understanding that infectious agents may be smaller than bacteria and could pass through porcelain filters. This was succeeded by the identification of the tobacco mosaic virus in 1892, which gave virology an early basis as an independent branch of science. Further advancements in the late 20th century, including the presence of electron microscopy and techniques of molecular biology, enabled scientists to view and work with viruses at the molecular level. These technological advances led the taxonomic designation and description of numerous viral species, ultimately giving rise to an orderly approach to virus taxonomy. The formation of the International Committee on Taxonomy of Viruses (ICTV) in 1966 was instrumental, establishing a systematic means of classifying viruses based on structural and genetic characteristics (Adams et al., 2017). The evolution of virology not only enriched our knowledge of viral diversity but also enabled effective strategic public health interventions. At the forefront are developments in vaccine technology, made possible by greater knowledge of viral pathogenesis and immunity. For instance, the successful cultivation of the polio vaccine in the middle of the 20th century was a remarkable feat in infectious disease control that saw the virtual eradication of a once-paralyzing disease that infected thousands.

Furthermore, the resurgence and re-emergence of arboviruses, as detailed in existing literature, highlight the continued challenges to the scientific community in the control of mosquito-borne diseases. Studies established that the prevalence of disease varies extensively across geographies, with determinants of ecological nature, such as climate and topography (Chrisafis, 2017). This evidence establishes the importance of history in virology, referring to the way past knowledge contributes to current actions against disease prevention and control. As virology continues to evolve, how history reveals itself related to current challenges is also established. Progress in recent years in awareness of global health, particularly in response to viral pandemics like HIV, Ebola, and SARS-CoV-2, has been underscored by the demand for robust virological research and effective public health policies. The ICTVs commitment to revising and reinforcing its resources is a reflection of a broader movement in virology that tries to engage with viral risk's evolving reality. Advanced online materials and public discussion facilitated by the ICTV assist in addressing the pressing challenges in virus classification and emerging viral diseases (Adams et al., 2017). With advancing science in the area of virology, it is also necessary that scientists and public health policymakers capitalize on existing expertise and create new methods for combatting viral pathogens effectively, predicting future pandemics and improving global health security (Figure 1.2).

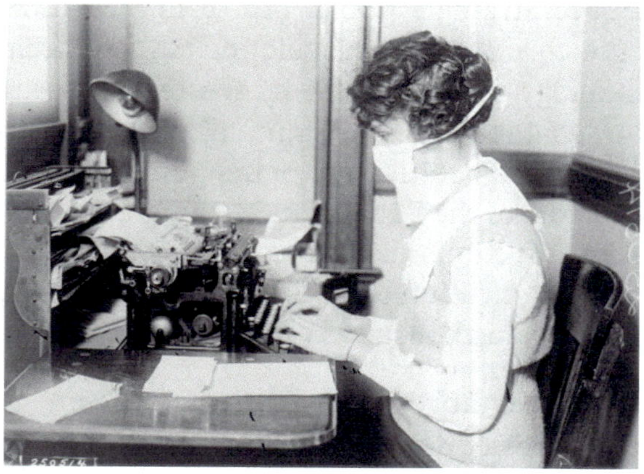

Figure 1.2. A woman working during the 1918–1919 influenza epidemic.

Source: https://upload.wikimedia.org/wikipedia/commons/9/9d/Influenza_Pandemic_Masked_Typist.jpg.

Importance of virology in medical microbiology

The virology is significant as a branch of the broader field of medical microbiology because it explains how viruses interfere with their hosts and bring about disease. Understanding this kind of information is crucial in developing effective therapy and prevention mechanisms. Viruses have a unique pattern of replication that gets in the way of cellular function and yields a wide array of pathophysiological effects. Therefore, virology as a science illuminates disease dynamics, specifically viral outbreaks. The data derived from studies in virology also assist in detecting potential viral pathogens in clinical specimens, ultimately resulting in early treatment and diagnosis. By describing the lifecycle of various viruses, virology not only contributes to the health care sector but also to public health policy aimed at curbing the spread of viral diseases. The worldwide infectious burden of viral diseases, particularly in vulnerable groups of individuals, highlights the need for research in virology. For instance, respiratory syncytial virus (RSV) is widespread in its effects on the health of children, with an estimated 33 million cases among children under five years of age, resulting in extreme morbidity and substantial healthcare costs (Jha et al., 2016). An understanding of epidemiology and pathogenesis of such viruses enables health practitioners to design effective public health campaigns and vaccination strategies. Furthermore, progress in virology is essential to the exploration of new antiviral medicines and vaccines as potential solutions to currently intractable viral illnesses. This virology application fills the gap between basic research and applied medical science and emphasizes its value in developing an overall strategy for minimizing viral hazard. Beyond its immediate usefulness in infectious illness, virology has a basic function to illuminate chronic illness secondary to viral infection. The link between severe infantile RSV bronchiolitis and subsequent respiratory sequelae like asthma is one such multifaceted interaction (Jha et al., 2016). This chronic effect highlights the role of virology not only in the care of acute infection but in the prevention of its chronic impact. Further, the quest for viral interactions within the immune system fosters our understanding of how viruses can exploit host defense and induce persistent infection or cancer. As medical microbiology progresses, the integration of virology into its core ensures a complete understanding of both acute and persistent health issues and paves the way for new diagnostic, therapeutic, and preventive measures.

1.1. Structure and Classification of Viruses

The viral anatomy is characterized by its very simple but diverse composition, which makes them successful in infecting a wide range of hosts, from animals and plants to bacteria. They possess in their core a genome either of DNA or RNA, single or double-stranded, with further classification based on their genetic material. This genome is housed in a protein shield called a capsid, which encloses viral nucleic acids when it is being transmitted to safeguard them. There are also some viruses with an outer lipid envelope originating from the host cell's membrane, which enhances the virus's ability to infect new cells. The distinction between non-enveloped and enveloped viruses is relatively clear-cut; non-enveloped viruses tend to be more resilient to environmental conditions, whereas enveloped viruses can utilize their lipid membranes to assist cell entry and assist in immune evasion (Cavicchi et al., 2012). Virus classification is a complex procedure that employs a range of criteria, including the type of nucleic acid, the presence of an envelope, and their reproductive mechanisms. The International Committee on Taxonomy of Viruses (ICTV) categorizes viruses into families, genera, and species based on these unique features. The classification system is of paramount importance in medical microbiology, as it dictates research paths and treatment strategies. Through the study of the arrangement and classification of viruses, scientists are able to craft targeted vaccines and therapies directed at certain viral families that have caused epidemics and pandemics, like with influenza (Cavicchi et al., 2012). Not only are viruses genetically diverse, but they are also diverse in their modes of transmission, which are responsible for their health effects in populations. A virus's mode of infection, its replication, and spread in populations are determined by its morphology. Enveloped viruses, for example, the human immunodeficiency virus (HIV), generally invade pathogens by the receptor-mediated endocytosis pathway, which is different from non-enveloped viruses like norovirus that even rely on direct cell lysis for the release of their progeny. An understanding of these mechanisms is essential to devise appropriate public health interventions and control measures, including those for managing outbreaks. Multiplication of research on viral structure and classification has driven innovation in vaccine research, with research continuing to improve the efficacy of response to emergent viral threats. This continued concern is paramount, given the background of previous influenza pandemics that require foresight in responding to viral infection globally (Orlova, 2012).

1.1.1. Basic components of viruses

A knowledge of viruses' simple structures is required for an appreciation of their role in medical microbiology. Viruses are really composed of genetic material in the form of DNA or RNA that is embedded in a protein shell known as a capsid. The capsid encapsulates the viral genome and protects it from damage, and is responsible for virus attachment to host cells. Some viruses, referred to as enveloped viruses, also possess an outer lipid bilayer from the host cell membrane, which also contributes to their infectivity and evasion of the host's immune system. Surprisingly, viruses are commonly grouped into various families and genera on the basis of these structural components, which reflects biological significance in the organization of their structure in facilitating viral replication and pathogenesis within a host organism. In virology, the concept of virulence and its objectification within scientific practices is of utmost significance. The history of the development of virology has revealed that the understanding of viruses as entities developed out of a rich interplay of diverse scientific methods and practices. Initially, viruses were not easy to classify due to their unusual characteristics, i.e., their cellularity and the requirement of a host cell in order to multiply. In time, the creation of a separate discipline of virology permitted researchers to grow and examine viruses in an orderly fashion, enabling them to make breakthroughs in diagnosing and treating virus-induced diseases. This finding emphasizes that the identification of viruses as purely biological entities was not an observation but a process that involved active scientific inquiry and interdisciplinarity across sciences (van Loon, 2002). In addition, the application of virology in public health and food safety is emphasized by the overlap with microbiological practices. For instance, the inactivation of food viruses by means of different methods, such as ozone treatment, demonstrates the practicability of our understanding in relation to viral components and their behavior. From the realization of viral structural make-up and their life cycles, researchers can explore new biocidal possibilities for virus transmission reduction in food items.

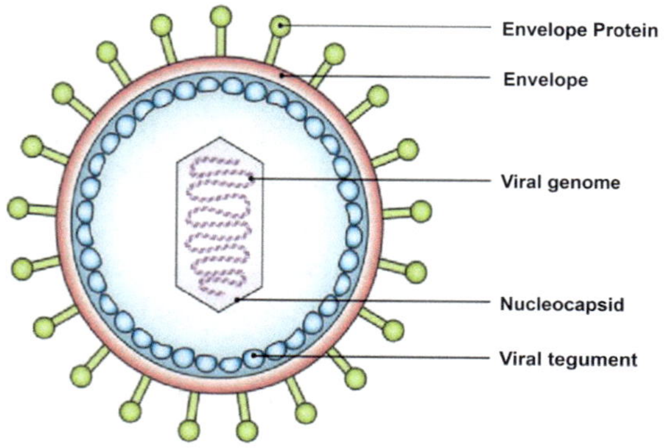

Figure 1.3. Basic structure of a virus.

Source: https://www.researchgate.net/profile/Olatunji-Kolawole-3/publication/340249925/figure/fig2/AS:874020920631297@1585394234735/Basic-structure-of-a-virus-Taylor-2019.png.

The translation of virological principles into practical applications demonstrates a vital link between laboratory research and real-world health problems. While pathogens like *E. coli* and *Salmonella enteritidis* continue to pose the main threat, efficient microbial control processes need to tap into extensive knowledge of the underlying viral structures and functionalities in a bid to enhance public health safety (Goudie et al., 2003) (Figure 1.3).

1.1.2. Classification systems for viruses

The viral classification schemes are essential in virology, especially in medical microbiology. They are essential in understanding the diversity and the complexity of viral pathogens. The International Committee on Taxonomy of Viruses (ICTV), established to offer order in viral classification, has significantly developed over the years to incorporate the growing awareness of virus diversity and improvements in characterization methods. As highlighted, the ICTV has initiated a dialogue with the virology community to address the problems facing virus taxonomy and enhance tools such as the ICTV Virus Taxonomy Report, which offers periodic revisions of viral classifications and serves as an important tool for researchers and health professionals alike (Adams et al., 2017). This careful system of classification not only facilitates communication between the scientific community but also informs the creation of targeted medical treatments. Acknowledging the complex character of viruses, classifications frequently respond to several different criteria, such as nucleic acid type, mode of replication, and physical structure. The system of viral classification has developed from a strictly morphological one to one incorporating genomic information, promoting a more subtle understanding of viral pathogens. This evolution points to the subtlety of objectifying viruses as agents in their own right in the field of virology. The course of virology's history reveals that the virulence of pathogens has been engineered by thorough laboratory procedures and a variety of research techniques. Therefore, the contemporary appreciation of viruses nowadays encompasses inter-disciplinary approaches that assist in condensing the complexity of the viral categories, in the long term, making them even more understandable to medical microbiology (van Loon, 2002). With the constantly evolving world of virology, there comes an increasing need for dynamic classification systems that can provide space for emerging new viruses as well as emerging strains. With the progress of molecular biology, new viral genomes are being unearthed at an unprecedented rate, necessitating regular updates and revisions to existing classification systems. The work of the ICTV remains pertinent in this context, as it has a systematic approach that not only allows for the accommodation of the organization of characterized viruses but also anticipates future breakthroughs in viral taxonomy. These classification efforts lead to easier research and diagnostics and, therefore, improved public health interventions for containing viral outbreaks. The integration of advancing methods and technological developments into existing systems of classification is a critical aspect of progressing the field, further emphasizing the importance of virus classification within the overall discipline of medical microbiology (Adams et al., 2017) (Figure 1.4).

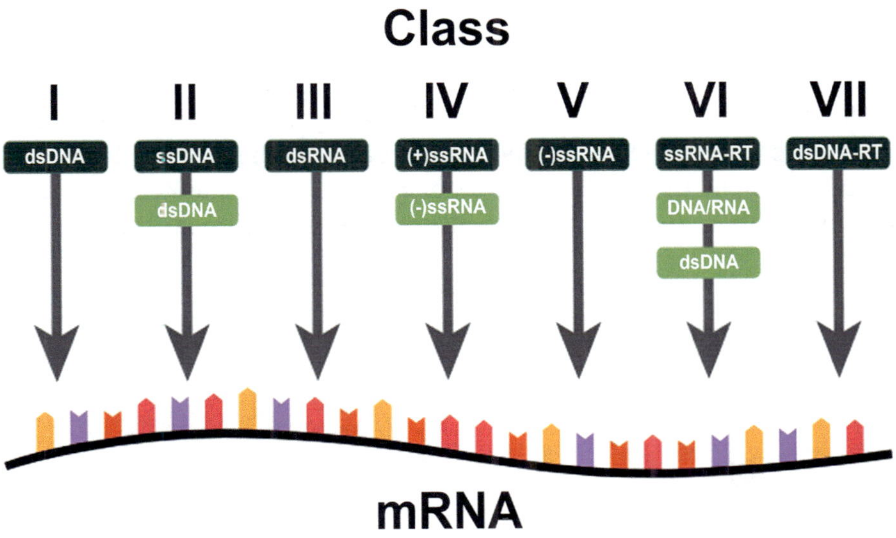

Figure 1.4. The Baltimore classification of viruses . The Baltimore classification system divides viruses into seven groups based on their genome structure and replication methods

Source: https://textimgs.s3.amazonaws.com/boundless-microbiology/rusbaltimoreclassification.svg#fixme.

1.1.3. Differences between DNA and RNA viruses

These distinctions between the DNA-using and the RNA-using viruses are central to how they replicate, mutate, and are pathogenic generally. DNA viruses, both double-stranded (dsDNA) or single-stranded (ssDNA), are genetically more stable with their more accurate replication mechanisms that involve DNA polymerases. This stability allows DNA viruses to hold onto their genomes for extended periods, in that their rate of mutation is slower than in RNA viruses. Conversely, RNA viruses composed of single-stranded RNA (ssRNA) or double-stranded RNA (dsRNA) mutate at a much higher rate because of the inaccuracy of RNA-dependent RNA polymerases. Such changes in genetic material necessarily affect each virus's interaction with host cells and the immune system's response, demonstrating the different evolutionary pressures working on viral actions in the medical microbiological world. In addition to mutation and replication, DNA and RNA viruses also differ in their general strategies for hijacking host cell equipment. DNA viruses typically enter the host cell nucleus, where they utilize the host mechanisms of DNA transcription and replication to produce viral constituents. The mechanism often involves the incorporation of viral DNA into the host genome, leading to latency or oncogenic changes. In contrast, RNA viruses favor replication in the cytoplasm, utilize the host's ribosomes to quickly produce viral proteins, and can utilize complex mechanisms to evade immune detection. This difference of emphasis highlights theflexibility in utilizing host cell mechanisms to successfully replicate. As explained in research, differences in such kind of viruses significantly influence public health interventions and treatment strategies of specific types of viral infections, like respiratory viruses and viruses causing foodborne illness (Goudie et al., 2003). Moreover, the clinical uses of such differences cannot be exaggerated, particularly in virology and medical microbiology. The rate of mutations in RNA viruses makes them adapt rapidly, and they become difficult to treat and control as a result. The emergence of new coronaviruses and flu strains, for instance, is an example of how RNA viruses can flip rapidly according to environmental pressures, which is hard to vaccinate against. Conversely, DNA viruses such as human papillomavirus have been demonstrated to persist for long durations, which in turn causes chronic infections and related malignancies, highlighting their long-term status in human health. It is essential to comprehend the molecular basis of these groups of viruses, which has been specifically brought out by the large body of research that has taken place over the years, to devise effective preventive and therapeutic interventions in clinical practice (van Loon, 2002) (Figure 1.5).

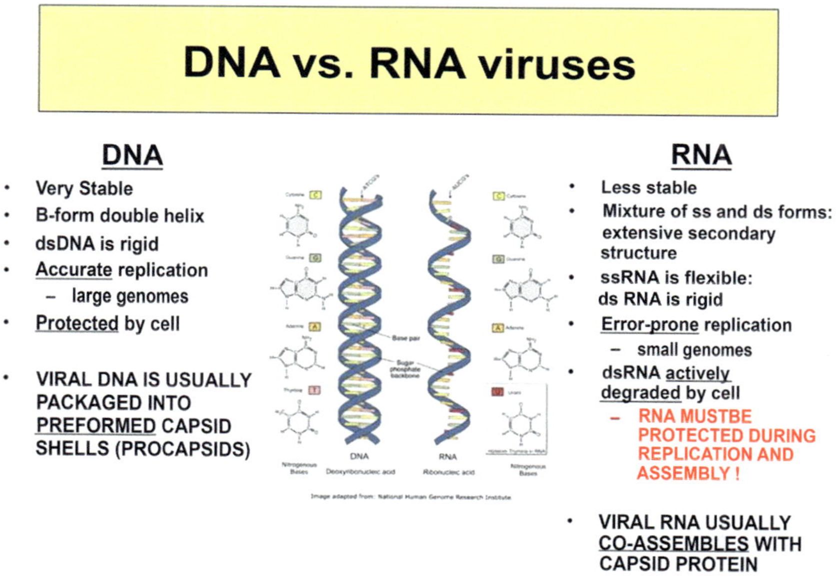

Figure 1.5. DNA versus RNA viruses.

Source: https://slideplayer.com/slide/3864327/13/images/4/DNA+vs.+RNA+viruses+DNA+RNA+Very+stable+B-form+double+helix.jpg.

1.2. Viral Replication and Life Cycle

The viral replication cycle and process are intricate, with a sequence of well-delineated steps that ultimately result in the formation of new viral particles. The initial step is that viruses must bind and enter their host cells, a step that is highly dependent on the interaction between viral surface proteins and specific cellular receptors. Upon entry into the host cell, the viral genome is deposited in the cytoplasm, where it hijacks the host's cellular machinery for replication. This involves the transcription of viral RNA and protein synthesis and serves to emphasize the reliance of the virus upon host cellular processes to manufacture new viral components. Each successful replication results in the production of new viral particles that are then discharged to infect new cells, repeating the cycle of viral life and re-emphasizing the parasitic nature of the organisms according to the contemporary view of viruses as molecular organisms (Claudiu, 2009). Beyond the simple biology, the significance of the viral life cycle extends far into the field of medical microbiology. Viral infections have the tendency to take over existing cellular mechanisms and, therefore, become refractory to inhibition by conventional antimicrobial therapy. The advancement in antiviral therapy is thus directed towards interfering with specific steps of viral replication in order to inhibit infection. For instance, interference of the attachment step using neutralizing antibodies can hinder viral entry, while antiviral drugs can interfere with viral polymerases to hinder replication. Besides, a thorough comprehension of viral replication mechanisms informs vaccine construction, with the differences within such processes holding the key to leading scientists into preventing viral outbreaks beforehand. This information is vital in viral disease control, particularly in cases where fast mutation gives rise to new strains of viruses with the capability of evading existing schemes of therapy (Goudie et al., 2003). Recent research continues to uncover the beauty of viral evolution as well as its effects on public health. The fusion hypothesis, where viruses may have originated from parasitic cellular life, revolutionizes viral biology. In addition to this perspective, this enriches the discourse concerning the significance of viruses in cellular evolution and also highlights the relevance of continued research into their life cycles. Because there are parasites that go through evolutionary processes to become viral, such an evolutionary process exemplifies the dynamic relationship between viruses and host organisms, illuminating mechanisms of viral emergence and virulence. As additional evidence becomes supportive of this model, scientists are challenged to explore the phylogenetic relationships between viruses and cellular life, ultimately offering the potential for new therapeutic applications and furthering our knowledge of viral impact in the greater context of life (Claudiu, 2009) (Figure 1.6).

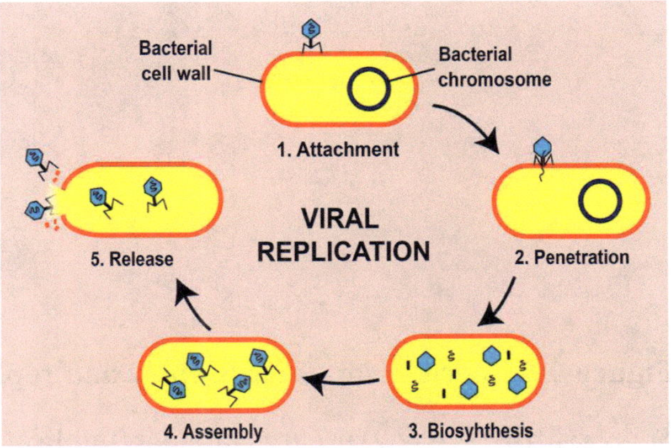

Figure 1.6. Diagram showing the viral replication cycle.

Source: https://teachmephysiology.com/wp-content/uploads/2023/07/Viral_replication.png.webp.

1.2.1. Mechanisms of viral entry into host cells

Understanding the entry mechanisms of viruses into host cells is crucial to the broader field of virology and its applications in medical microbiology. Viruses generally use specific mechanisms to hijack the machinery of the host cell to initiate the infection process. One such familiar mechanism is viral surface protein-host cell receptor interaction. Interaction has a tendency to define the host specificity of a virus. For instance, viral surface proteins bind to host cell receptors, either directly entering the cell by endocytosis or fusing with the cell membrane. Different viruses utilize variations of the same mechanisms, a testament to the advanced evolutionary processes that control host-pathogen interactions. These mechanisms illustrate the delicate balance between viral infectiousness and the hosts' immune defense mechanisms, potentially leading to therapeutic intervention. Endocytosis is an important process by which the majority of viruses enter host cells. Endocytosis encompasses many forms, including macropinocytosis and clathrin-mediated endocytosis, which are involved in the uptake of external material.

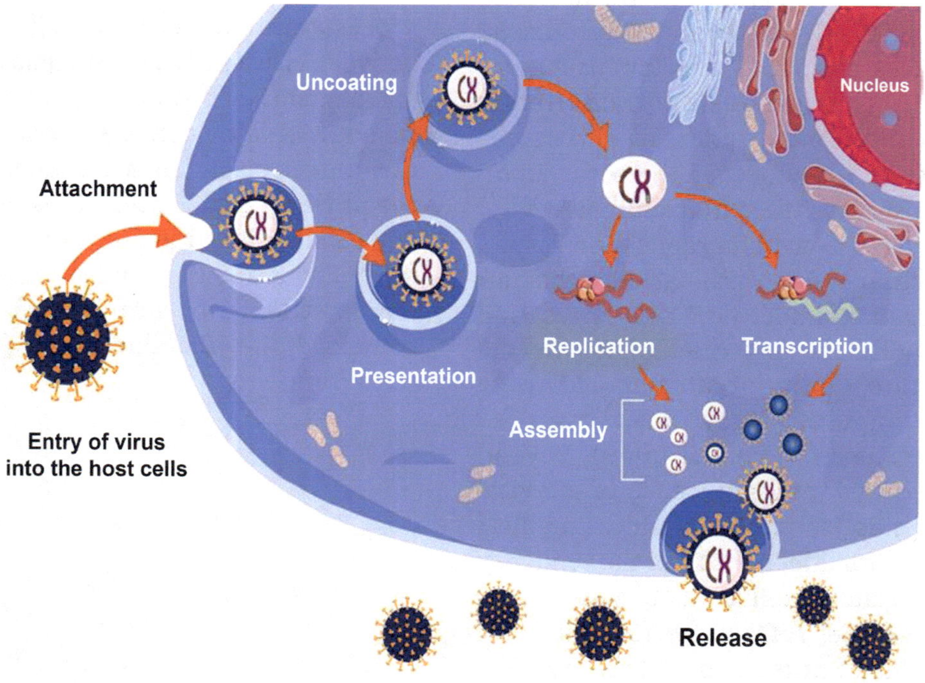

Figure 1.7. Mechanism of virus entry and replication in host cells.

Source: https://www.researchgate.net/publication/343804004/figure/fig1/AS:11431281212024262@1702524990492/Mechanism-of-virus-entry-and-replication-in-host-cells.tif.

The virus initially binds to cellular surface receptors, leading to the viral particle being internalized into an endosomal compartment. Upon entry, the endosomal acidic pH may induce conformational changes of viral proteins that allow the release of viral nucleic acid to the cytoplasm. The efficacy of this entry pathway varies among virus families, with some viruses, such as influenza and HIV, demonstrating great proficiency in using the endocytic pathway. Understanding these entry modes further directs the development of antiviral drugs that can disrupt these critical early stages of infection. The study of viral entry mechanisms is carried into the clinical realm, particularly targeting treatment-resistant viruses. As in the example of HIV, which has been a source of such immense challenge in effective treatment due to its ability to evade the immune system and gain drug resistance, new approaches are necessary (Dwivedi & Shrivastava, 2011). Researchers are already studying approaches such as RNA interference (RNAi) to suppress viral replication by specifically killing viral RNA or preventing viral proteins essential for entry. Advances in nanotechnology also provide promising means to advance drug delivery systems with high specificity for targeting viral entry. With further innovation in these therapeutic modalities, public health issues resulting from viral infections are easily addressed, minimizing their impacts on global health systems (Dwivedi & Shrivastava, 2011). All of these collaborations underscore the importance of investigating mechanisms of viral entry in developing new medical interventions (Figure 1.7).

1.2.2. Stages of viral replication

The process of viral replication is a complex, multi-step phenomenon that is crucial for viral propagation within host cells. The first steps in this process of replication involve attachment and entry. Viruses exploit certain host cell surface receptors to facilitate attachment before entering the cell membrane. This is critical because the virus must be able to successfully counteract host defensive mechanisms to establish infection. Once inside, the viral genome is uncoating, releasing genetic material into the cytoplasm of the host cell, an event critical for effective viral replication. These phases are important to comprehend in medical microbiology because they shed light on possible targets of therapy for antiviral treatment.

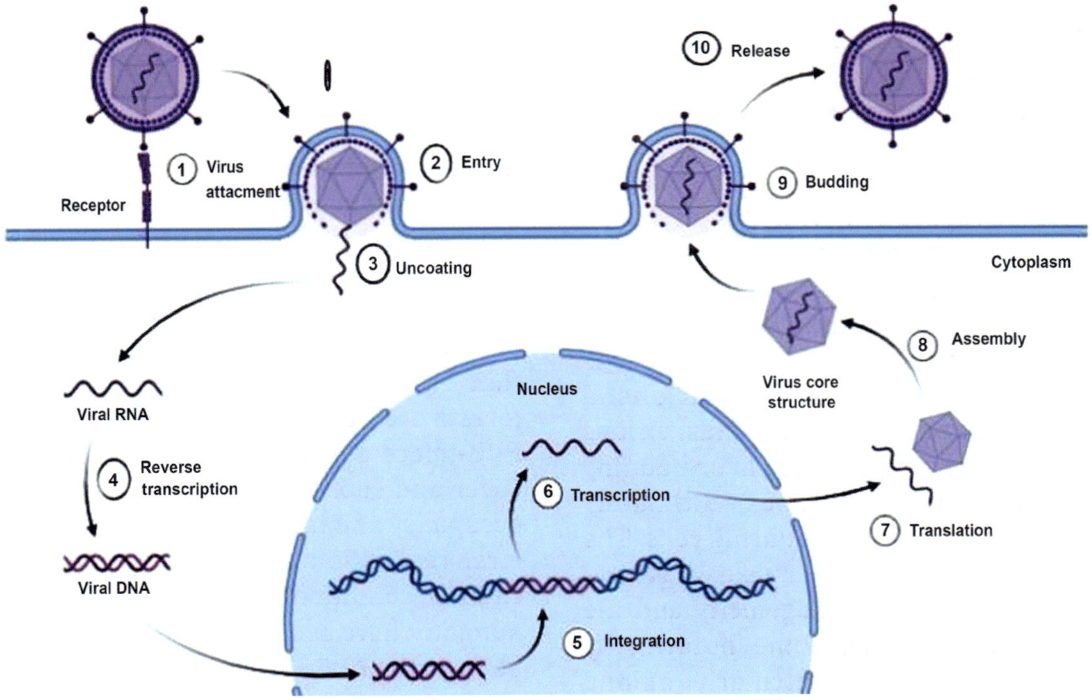

Figure 1.8. Diagram of viral replication process.

Source: https://www.researchgate.net/publication/348869255/figure/fig2/AS:986086943764480@1612112856637/Diagram-of-viral-replication-process-BioRendercom-Coronavirus-Replication-Cycle-2020a.jpg.

Future research can be grounded on these findings to enhance our comprehension of viral entry processes and find innovative means of interfering with them, particularly with regard to managing significant pathogens (Goudie et al., 2003). Following the uncoating process, the cycle of viral replication proceeds with the steps of transcription and translation. Within this period, the viral genome, whether DNA or RNA, takes over the machinery of the host to produce viral proteins and replicate its own genetic information. This takeover is necessary since it allows the virus to produce structural proteins necessary for forming new virions. The intricate process of interaction between host and viral structures during these processes reveals weaknesses that can be exploited for therapeutic advancement. Notably, the majority of viruses have evolved means of evading host immune responses during this period, enhancing their replication efficiency. It will aid researchers in the development of vaccines and antiviral drugs that target particular processes and inhibit the virus's ability to propagate (Cumberworth et al., 2017). The final stages of viral replication include assembly and release, which complete the process of replication with the formation of new virions capable of infecting other host cells. The newly synthesised viral components are brought together within the host cell to form complete viral particles. The assembly is an exact coordination between available viral proteins and host cell machinery. Thus, virions are released either by lysis of cells or budding from host cellular membranes, ultimately spreading infection to neighbouuring cells. The efficiency of such release mechanisms is critical in controlling the virus pathogenicity and the host's immune response. Some noteworthy research in this area, particularly among flaviviruses, has revealed how the viruses can take over the host cellular mechanisms to optimize their replication and evade immune detection, offering insight into potential antiviral targets (Goudie et al., 2003; Cumberworth et al., 2017) (Figure 1.8).

1.2.3. Factors influencing viral life cycles

Identification of viral life cycle determinants is crucial in the understanding of viral pathogenesis and viral transmission patterns. Various internal and external determinants are pivotal in controlling how viruses replicate, survive, and spread within host populations. Of these, host availability and population dynamics play a critical role in determining virus prevalence. For example, studies have shown that zoonotic viruses such as the Puumala virus (PUU) have spatio-temporal patterns closely associated with host populations, e.g., bank voles (*Clethrionomys glareolus*), which have large population oscillations. In highly endemic areas of *Nephropathia epidemica*, high bank vole populations enhance PUU transmission to humans, especially in autumn when human activity in contaminated habitats is increased. This dynamic relationship highlights the extent to which ecological and environmental components greatly control viral life cycles to become valuable considerations in medical microbiology (Olsson, 2003). Environmental components also greatly control viral life cycles independent of host dynamics. The nature of the habitat that promotes host populations can enhance the circulation and persistence of viruses. For example, studies have revealed that characteristics such as old-growth wet forests are accompanied by larger numbers of PUU-infected bank voles. The presence of dense cover and substrate for cover supports rodent occupancy and therefore enables the habitat for viral replication and transmission. Moreover, climatic conditions, including temperature and humidity, have been discovered to influence host behavior and viral persistence in the external environment. Thus, a comprehension of the insidious interactions among the environmental determinants and viral epidemiology remains critical to predicting outbreaks and establishing successful control measures in public health programs (Goudie et al., 2003). Further, the viral genome itself harbors variations that can influence a virus's adaptability and efficacy in the life cycle. Mutation rates and the possibility for genetic reassortment to lead to the creation of novel strains able to access alternative ecological niches or circumvent host defensive mechanisms are a topic in viral evolution that requires ongoing monitoring of viral populations, especially against changing environmental conditions or host dynamics that may maximize transmission. The complex interplay between viral genomes and environmental forces embodies the uniquely multidisciplinary nature of viral life cycles. Lastly, understanding these dynamics provides invaluable insights for the development of strategies to combat viral infections and the understanding of virus-host interactions within the scope of medical microbiology (Olsson, 2003).

1.3. Pathogenesis of Viral Infections

The pathogenesis of viral infections is defined by an active interaction between the virus and the host immune response. Initial infection often occurs at mucous surfaces, where viruses exploit epithelial cells to enter. After entering, viruses appropriate the host's cell machinery to replicate and assemble new virions. Cell loss or impairment may follow, leading eventually to tissue damage and inflammation. For example, epithelial cell loss can be extremely massive in respiratory viruses, compromising airway epithelial integrity and promoting secondary bacterial infection. These occurrences are extremely significant as they dictate the disease outcome and the hosts' immune response, which can be extremely varied among populations according to the differential impact of genetic and environmental determinants. Immune evasion is the hallmark of viral pathogenesis. The majority of viruses have evolved mechanisms to counteract the immune response of the host, thereby enabling sustained infection and transmission. Such mechanisms include suppression of host antiviral response, regulation of major histocompatibility complex (MHC) expression, and modulation of apoptotic pathways. For instance, certain viruses code for proteins that function to inhibit interferon signaling, which is crucial for antiviral response. These avoidance mechanisms not only allow viral persistence but also maximize pathology through chronic inflammation, potentially leading to disease progression. The chronic activation of immune responses, in turn, creates a permissive environment for secondary infections and complications, reflecting the exquisite balance between viral replication and host defense. The long-term consequences of viral infection are likely to cascade into chronic disease. For example, infections caused by certain viruses, such as hepatitis B and C, are associated with the etiology of chronic liver disease and hepatocellular carcinoma. These chronic outcomes are due to persistent viral replication, immune-mediated liver damage, and accumulation of genetic mutations induced by the viral genome. At large, viral pathogenesis and chronic disease entwine each other by emphasizing the imperative of ongoing research aimed at discovering viral mechanisms of pathogenesis. This is crucial for structuring effective vaccines and therapeutic interventions able to counteract the impact of viral infection on public health, as recent research into viral constituents and how they interact within host systems has shown (Goudie et al., 2003; Generalov, 2016).

1.3.1. Mechanisms of viral pathogenicity

Understanding viral pathogenicity mechanisms is necessary for the advancement of medical microbiology and specifically for designing effective treatments and prevention strategies. Viruses have multiple mechanisms to invade host cells, take over cellular functions, and evade host defenses. Some viruses can modify host cell signal pathways that favor their replication while also repressing the host defense mechanisms. Such manipulation can lead to cellular apoptosis, necrosis, or other pathophysiologic mechanisms leading to disease. Elucidation of these mechanisms can identify targets for antiviral drugs that counter these viral strategies, once again emphasizing the importance of knowledge about viral pathogenicity in medical virology. The immune response is exaggerated in viral pathogenicity, as Flavivirus group viruses have developed intricate mechanisms for evading host defenses. There have been recent findings showing how flaviviruses, such as dengue and Zika, have mechanisms to exploit type I interferon pathways, which are a critical component of the host immune system, against them.

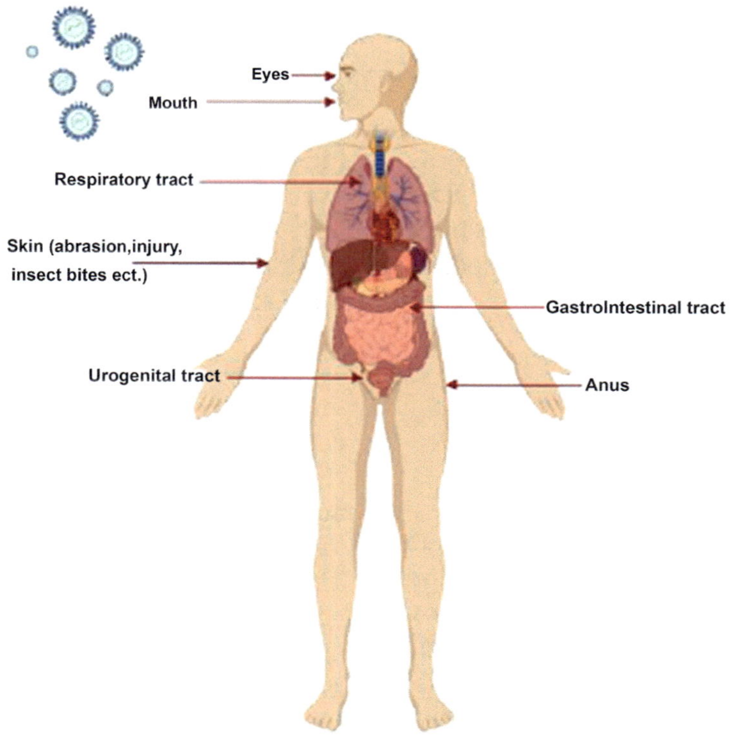

Figure 1.9. Typical sites of virus entry into the body: The first steps of viral infection are determined by the site at which the virus implants into the body. This subsequently dictates the mechanisms of viral pathogenesis.

Source: https://upload.wikimedia.org/wikipedia/commons/thumb/2/29/Typical_sites_of_virus_entry_into_the_body.png/800px-Typical_sites_of_virus_entry_into_the_body.png.

Through these avenues, flaviviruses can inhibit the antiviral activity of interferons and support productive infection and increased virulence. The two-way interaction between virus and host immune system demonstrates the complexity of viral pathogenesis and the importance of thorough studies to uncover new treatment modalities. Aside from the basics of science, knowledge about these interactions can be applied to design clinical practice and public health planning to avert viral infections and consequently the burden on healthcare systems (Cumberworth et al., 2017). Aside from immune evasion mechanisms, some viruses have also developed mechanisms that directly influence cellular processes, which further enable them to survive and reproduce in the host. For example, viral protein-host cell pathway interaction can be responsible for dysregulation of critical cellular processes in a manner that facilitates a viral replication-permissive status. Among foodborne pathogens, enterovirus subgroup viruses, among others, have been shown to utilize such strategies as described from studies on their resistance to some biocidal chemicals used for food safety (Goudie et al., 2003). The intricate viral pathogenic processes make it challenging for researchers to establish infection control and treatment strategies. Through the study of these mechanisms, researchers will be able to comprehend better the lifecycle of the virus and advance on complete interventions to intervene against the viral infections affecting public health (Figure 1.9).

1.3.2. Host immune response to viral infections

The viral infection's host immune response is a complex interplay between innate and adaptive immunity that works together to detect and eliminate the pathogen. Upon the entry of the virus, the innate immune response is triggered, primarily by pattern recognition receptors (PRRs) that detect virus components. This results in type I interferons (IFNs) and other cytokine induction, which serves to make an antiviral environment in adjacent cells. Also, activation of natural killer (NK) cells and phagocytic cells contributes to the prompt response against viral pathogens. Viruses, however, have developed subtle mechanisms for evading these defenses, such as downregulation of PRR signalling cascades and blockade of interferon responses. These interactions play a central role in the creation of efficient treatments against viral infections, particularly with the focus on emerging and re-emerging viruses that potentially impact human health significantly, as seen in recent virological research. Adaptive immunity is also responsible for modulating the host response to viral infections through T and B lymphocyte activation. The activation of CD8+ cytotoxic T cells is a vital element of cellular immunity, as these cells are tasked with directly killing infected cells by viruses. At the same time, CD4+ helper T cells ensure the activation and proliferation of B cells, which secrete virus-specific antibodies. The antibodies neutralize the viruses and block their binding and entry into host cells. These adaptive immune reactions have been neutralized by some viruses, e.g., Flavivirus genus viruses, through mechanisms evolved within the virus. For instance, they may disrupt the interferon-triggered host signalling pathways in order to evade immune surveillance and impair the effectiveness of the host's antibody response.

These adaptations underscore the necessity for ongoing research into virus-host interactions because this knowledge can be utilized for vaccine identification and therapeutic host immune system targeting as a means of enhancing the host immune response (Cumberworth et al., 2017). Despite the innate and adaptive immune responses, certain viral infections can lead to significant morbidity and mortality and reflect deficiencies in host defenses. The issue is in the ability of some viruses to take over the immune response of the host and develop long-term infections. As is the case with findings in ongoing research, even when it comes to foodborne pathogens, such as those that have been covered in microbial research, conditions and environments can facilitate exposure to infections (Goudie et al., 2003). This shows the intricate interplay between the virulence factors of the pathogen and the immunological environment of the hosts. Control of this complexity warrants a multidisciplinary approach that includes immunology, microbiology, and virology, revealing the possibility of new therapeutic strategies. With the knowledge of these dynamics, researchers will be able to better predict viral behaviour and design better regimens for therapy that can stimulate the host immune response, thus bettering patient outcomes in viral infections (Figure 1.10)

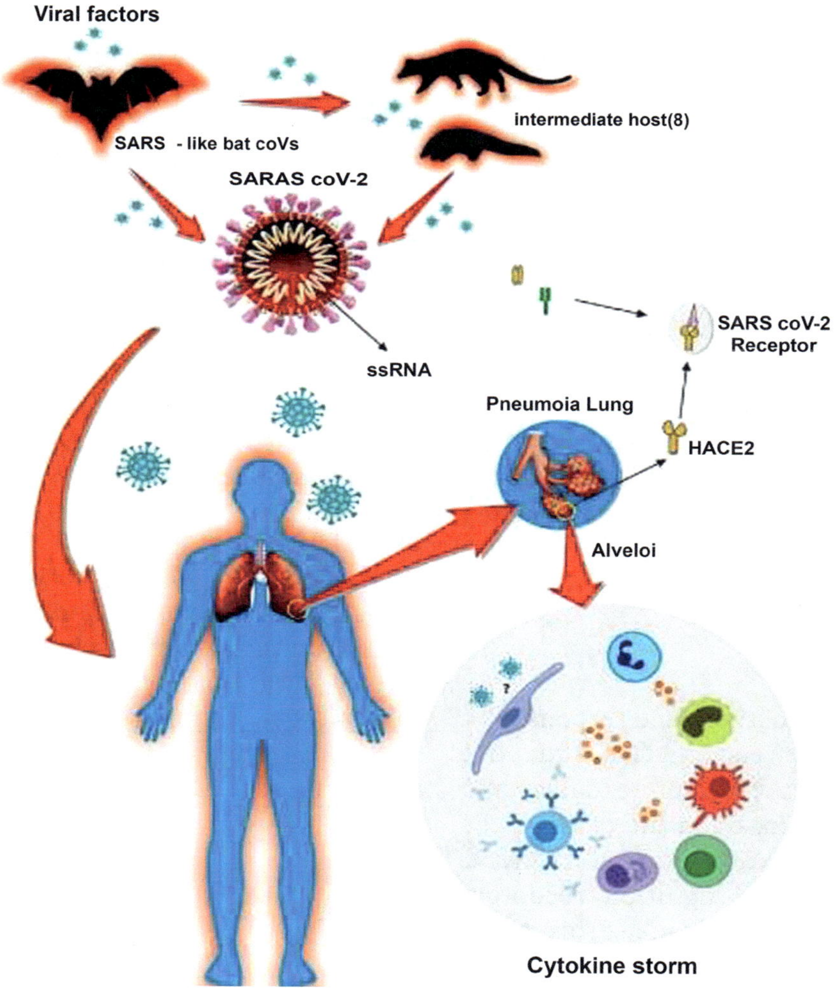

Figure 1.10. Proposed host immune response during SARS-CoV-2 infection.

Source: https://www.researchgate.net/profile/Adel-Elmaghrabi/publication/342889750/figure/fig1/AS:912806652174336@1594641473184/Proposed-host-immune-response-during-SARS-Cov-2-infection.jpg.

1.3.3. Examples of diseases caused by viruses

The viral disease spectrum is broad and encompasses a variety of infective agents that are the source of significant morbidity and mortality in the world. A prime example is the Human Immunodeficiency Virus (HIV) that leads to acquired immunodeficiency syndrome (AIDS). The virus attacks the body's immune system in a systematic manner, lowering the body's resistance to infections and malignancies. Patients with progressive HIV may develop opportunistic infections that are features of the disease progression. Furthermore, Hepatitis B and Hepatitis C viruses generate liver diseases such as cirrhosis and hepatocellular carcinoma that present a significant burden to health systems globally. These types of viral pathogens showcase not just the complexity of the interactions between viruses in human hosts but also the various implications they present to public health that require large-scale research in areas such as the development of vaccines and drug interventions. The second concerning viral disease is the influenza virus, which is a principal cause of recurrent seasonal epidemics and sporadic pandemics. According to whether it is type A, B, or C, influenza has special challenges in terms of transmissibility and virulence. Seasonal influenza resulting from the annual epidemic can lead to severe respiratory illness, with considerable hospitalization and mortality, particularly among risk groups. The ephemeral nature of the influenza virus, coupled with its ability to mutate by antigenic shift and drift, complicates the development of effective vaccines. This implies there needs to be continuous surveillance to monitor prevailing strains and modify vaccination strategies accordingly. The dynamics of influenza underscore the importance of virology to interpret patterns of transmission and develop effective means to mitigate its effect on the public health infrastructure globally. Furthermore, viruses such as norovirus and rotavirus have the viral pathogenesis of gastroenteritis that causes acute gastrointestinal illness in millions of individuals worldwide. Norovirus, in particular, is notoriously famous for high infectivity, particularly in such closed settings as cruise ships and nursing homes, where it induces outbreaks of debilitating the entire population. Rotavirus, on the other hand, has been a predominant cause of severe diarrhoea in children. Vaccination campaigns have lowered the rate of rotavirus disease substantially, illustrating the value of virology to preventive medicine. The challenge posed by such viruses emphasizes the demand for effective diagnostic methods and surveillance systems for disease control in preventing outbreaks. Indeed, progress in molecular techniques, as shown in the detection of human caliciviruses, plays a critical role in our response to such viral threats (Butcher & Gould, 1997; Goudie et al., 2003) (Figure 1.11).

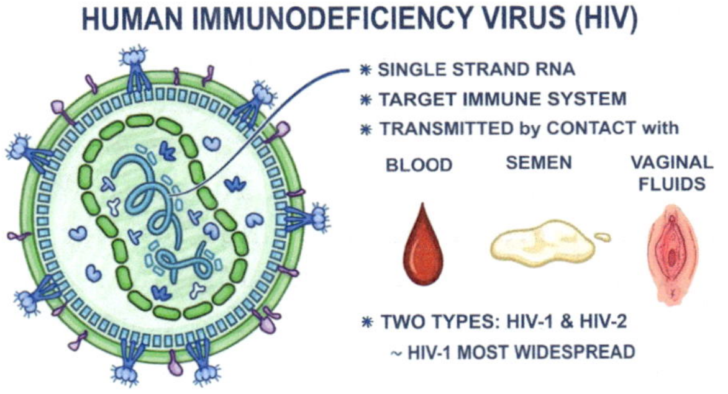

Figure 1.11. Human immunodeficiency virus (HIV).

Source: https://www.osmosis.org/_next/image?url=https%3A%2F%2Fd16qt3wv6xm098.cloudfront.net%2FZ4KjyynnSsSQvX1XlQ5Tc_NwRhSeEFMm%2F_.jpg&w=3840&q=75.

1.4. Diagnostic Techniques in Virology

The advent of molecular diagnostics has revolutionized the field of virology, offering unprecedented sensitivity and specificity in virus detection. Techniques such as polymerase chain reaction (PCR) and reverse transcription PCR (RT-PCR) allow for the amplification of viral nucleic acids, making it possible to identify viruses even at low concentrations. This capacity is especially valuable in infection monitoring like respiratory syncytial virus (RSV), which infects millions of children annually and contributes to high morbidity and mortality (Jha et al., 2016). Besides, these molecular techniques are not just limited to virus detection but can also provide information on viral load and strain variation, thereby contributing to treatment monitoring and epidemiological studies. With advancing technology, these technologies continue to fine-tune our understanding of viral infections, emphasizing the critical role of precise diagnostic techniques in successful medical microbiology. In addition to molecular methods, serological tests remain crucial for the diagnosis of viral infections through the detection of antibodies produced as an immune response to a virus. Enzyme-linked immunosorbent assay (ELISA) and Western blot are two such serological tests that are commonly applied in the clinic. These approaches are particularly important for the diagnosis of infections where viral loads may be below the sensitivity of molecular tests or for monitoring immune response after vaccination. Serological tests can also help identify previous infection, which is important in measuring population immunity and epidemiologic trends. Historical development of such diagnostic methods indicates the convergent progress of clinical virology and immunology, as indicated by landmark research in feline leukaemia virus (FeLV) that laid the groundwork for the discovery of new viral pathogens and the function of antibody response in controlling viral infections (Anderson et al., 2013). Emerging technologies such as next-generation sequencing (NGS) are establishing a new standard for diagnostic virology. NGS makes the complete analysis of viral genomes possible and illuminates genetic diversity and patterns of evolution of viruses within populations. The technique has been of invaluably great assistance in ascertaining the origin of outbreaks, as in cases of viral epidemics where frequent rates of mutation render response to public health issues. The ability to quickly sequence and analyzes viral DNA or RNA from clinical specimens provides diagnostic capabilities far superior to conventional methods. In addition, NGS can help determine co-infections and evaluate the effectiveness of therapeutic interventions across time. As these advanced diagnostic instruments become increasingly woven into general clinical practice, they hold the promise to better enable us to fight viral disease, ultimately benefiting the patient and guiding public health efforts in virology.

1.4.1. Traditional methods of virus detection

Traditional viral detection technologies have played a crucial role in the diagnosis of viral infections for decades, particularly before molecular technology. A few of the oldest and simplest detection techniques are tissue culture tests, where viruses are identified from the patient's sample by inoculating the susceptible cell lines. In this technique, one observes cytopathic effects as infected cells by the virus will change their shape. While tissue culture remains a cornerstone of viral diagnosis, it is often cumbersome and time-consuming and requires specialized facilities. Moreover, it is not applicable for all viruses, particularly those refractory to *in vitro* culture. The intrinsic limitations of the traditional culture methods have stimulated the continued desire for faster and more sensitive methods of detection, further underlining the utility of the integration of these traditional methods with the newer molecular technologies to further extend diagnostic capabilities. Serological assays represent yet another of the common techniques employed in virus detection. Serological assays utilize the antibody specificity, and antibodies might be used to identify virus-linked antigens in patient specimens. Enzyme-linked immunosorbent assays (ELISAs) and hemagglutination inhibition tests have been effectively used to determine antibodies elicited after viral infections. For instance, serological testing has been used to screen for diseases such as hepatitis and human immunodeficiency virus (HIV). Nevertheless, serological assays suffer the limitation that they are based on the host immune response, which may be dormant in early infection. This lag can lead to false negatives in immunocompromised patients. Despite these challenges, serological methods remain valuable in epidemiology studies, providing cues toward population immunity as well as prevalence of infection with the passage of time. Increasingly, integrating conventional methods with new technology has been necessary in clinical virology. For instance, integration of conventional culture methods with PCR diagnostics can enhance the sensitivity as well as the specificity of virus detection. Traditional methods, though stereotypically described as old-fashioned at times, continue to be powerful and effective in validating newer molecular assays. The interplay between the traditional and novel approaches not only ensures efficient detection and surveillance of viral pathogens within populations but also validates knowledge about viral epidemiology.

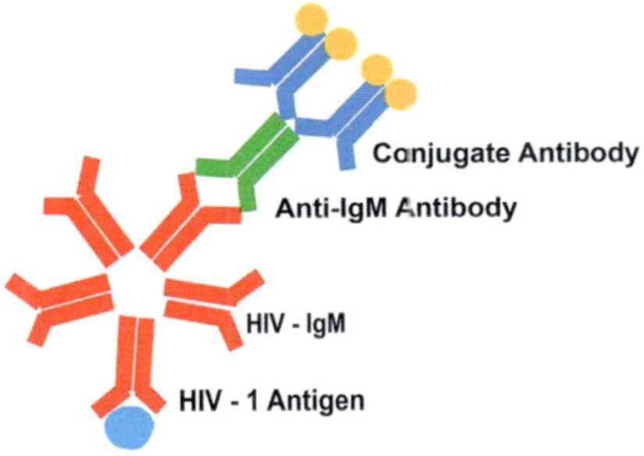

Figure 1.12. Enzyme-linked immunosorbent assay (ELISA) method for detecting anti-HIV1 IgM antibody captured by membrane-bound recombinant gp41.

Source: https://www.researchgate.net/publication/281340996/figure/fig7/AS:669650295734279@1536668480363/Enzyme-linked-immunosorbent-assay-ELISA-method-for-detecting-anti-HIV1-IgM-antibody.jpg.

As medical microbiology evolves, upkeep and improvement of established procedures become of utmost importance, particularly in contexts such as emerging viral threats where capacity for swift response is paramount. Important, research has portrayed the importance of maintaining a balanced diagnostic arsenal, balancing the strengths of traditional and modern approaches to deal with changing clinical challenges, as attested through present assessments of various pathogens and their corresponding diagnostics (Goudie et al., 2003; Jha et al., 2016) (Figure 1.12).

1.4.2. Molecular techniques for viral diagnosis

Molecular approaches have revolutionized the diagnosis of viruses by significantly enhancing their speed and specificity in identifying pathogens at the clinic. Traditional diagnoses by viral cultures and serological analyses are generally insensitive and take several days to yield results. Molecular approaches, e.g., polymerase chain reaction (PCR) and next-generation sequencing (NGS), facilitate rapid detection of viral nucleic acids with fast clinical decision-making. This change is of particular significance in the case of infections such as the respiratory syncytial virus (RSV), which exhibits a high incidence rate across the world, particularly among young children and the elderly. Utilization of these molecular devices has transformed viral diagnostics, allowing for real-time detection and therapy of viral infections, thereby reducing the morbidity and mortality attached to such infections (Jha et al., 2016). In addition to PCR and NGS, new molecular techniques like RT-PCR and *in situ* hybridization are progressively playing key roles in viral diagnosis. These procedures not only allow for the detection of viral RNA but also allow for the study of the distribution of viruses in tissues. More advanced techniques, such as quantitative PCR (qPCR), enable viral load measurement, which is essential in monitoring disease progression and antiviral treatment efficacy. Utilization of the molecular technologies in diagnostics is underscored by their ability to provide critical information regarding the extent of disease and outbreak risk. While molecular diagnostics continue to be developed, they hold the promise of enhanced surveillance and control of outbreaks, securing their role in the management of public health problems related to viral infections (van Loon, 2002). Theoretical design of the use of molecular techniques in virology is also brought about by a better understanding of pathogen virulence and its significance in the field of medical microbiology. Virology history as a discipline has brought to the fore the need for interdisciplinary approaches to understanding viral behaviors and interactions with host systems as a whole. Growth is part of a broader trend in scientific research, in which objectification of viruses in the laboratory setting has paved the way for novel approaches towards viral classification and diagnostics. With the convergence of various technological and methodological advances, researchers are in a position to extend their understanding of viral pathogenesis and improve diagnostic protocols. Hence, the ongoing evolution of molecular methods will not only advance the discipline of virology but will also provide for the development of targeted therapies and vaccines, ultimately resulting in the diminution of the impact of viral diseases globally (Jha et al., 2016) (Figure 1.13).

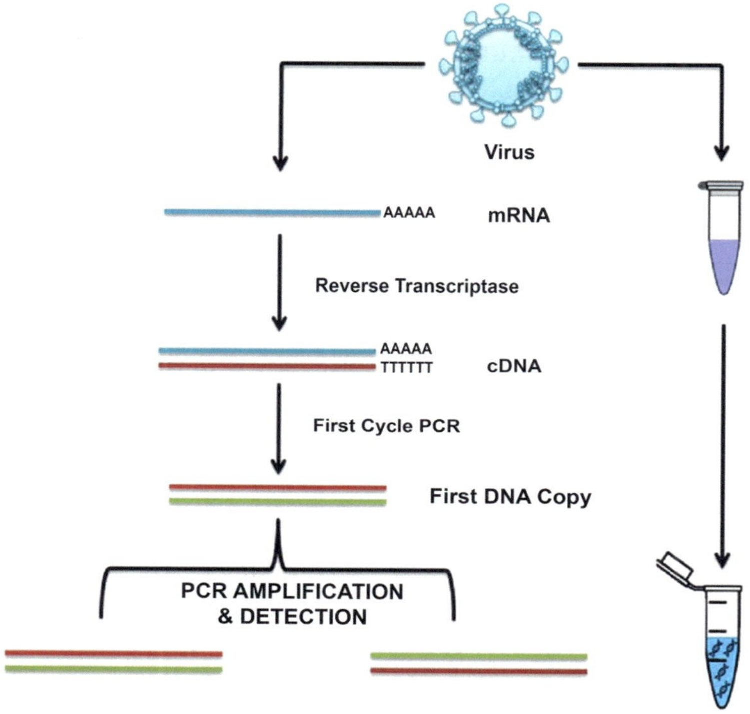

Figure 1.13. Graphical illustration of RT-PCR.

Source: https://www.researchgate.net/profile/Fakhar-Khan-6/publication/343407421/figure/fig2/AS:921968421392386@1596825809346/Graphical-illustration-of-RT-PCR.png.

1.4.3. Serological assays and their applications

The use of serological tests in clinical diagnostics is an essential aspect of medical microbiology, particularly when considering viral infections. The tests are designed to detect specific antibodies in serum from a patient and thus can reveal previous infection and present immune response. For instance, the development of enzyme immunoassays (EIA) greatly enhanced the capability to diagnose such infections as RSV and influenza by detecting virus-specific antibodies. The traditional approaches focus on single-analyte formats, although the shift towards multiplex microarray immunoassays (MAIA) enhances the capability for testing multiple viral infections simultaneously with a more comprehensive assessment of a patient's immune status. This modification not only makes diagnosis easier but also facilitates large-scale serosurveillance in populations and, therefore, public health surveillance and response systems, particularly in young children who are highly susceptible to severe viral infection (Kazakova, 2019). Apart from increasing diagnostic effectiveness, serological tests are also vital in determining vaccine effectiveness. The research on antibodies formed post-vaccination provides vital information in terms of the immunity of the population against specific viral infections. The employment of serological assays such as the multiplex microarray immunoassay has been proven to have a good correlation with the conventional ones, therefore validating its application in the lab and clinic. For example, studies through the MAIA have enabled the detection of IgG and IgM antibodies against various strains of influenza, proving its functionality in monitoring immunity in pediatric and adult populations. Enhanced capability in this regard is vital in conducting epidemiological research, tracking the spread of viruses, as well as setting up vaccination programs to address emerging public health issues effectively (Kazakova, 2019). Secondly, other sampling techniques are being designed in collaboration with serological technologies for optimizing participant compliance as well as accessibility to immunization programs. For instance, antibody detection from oral fluid would provide a non-invasive technique with the potential to improve subject recruitment in long-term studies. The development of assays like the IgG antibody capture enzyme-linked immunosorbent assay (GACELISA) for detecting antibodies specific to mumps is a case in point. These methods have demonstrated 100% sensitivity and specificity compared with the traditional serum-based assays, and they signal the potential for non-invasive samples in expanding serological surveillance to more individuals. Some limitations persist, however, such as the lower antibody concentration in saliva, which needs to be improved in assay sensitivity. Research into the application of recombinant antigens and emerging technologies like immuno-polymerase chain reaction (I-PCR) may aid future advancement in improving the performance of serological tests in the laboratory and clinical environments.

1.5. Treatment and Prevention of Viral Infections

Prevention and cure of viral infections are essential features of clinical management and public health in the context of medical microbiology. Advances in the knowledge of viral pathogenesis have led to new directions in disease control resulting from viral infection. Prevention is of crucial significance for most viral infections, with notable examples being respiratory syncytial virus (RSV) and human immunodeficiency virus (HIV). For RSV, doctors apply supportive treatment methods since there are no highly effective antiviral medications. Palivizumab has become a licensed preventive method for certain high-risk infants and illustrates the necessity of targeted prophylaxis among high-risk populations, particularly in light of the widespread morbidity of RSV among children and the elderly (Jha et al., 2016). The ongoing development of vaccines and antiviral medications underscores the continually changing character of antiviral therapeutics, where emphasis lies in reducing the burden of disease and mortality. HIV adds a complicating factor in treating and preventing it in the context of its persistent high rates of prevalence, particularly where southern Africa is concerned. The efficacy of antiretroviral treatment (ART) as prevention, or treatment as prevention (TasP), is a measure that can lower transmission of the virus. A Botswana community-based trial demonstrates the multifaceted intervention required to eliminate the HIV epidemic. The trial consolidates ART with other forms of prevention, underlining the necessity of HIV testing, male circumcision, and clinical linkage to achieve complete protection. Through the use of viral phylogenetics, researchers can illuminate the dynamics of transmission as well as quantify the effects of interventions, thereby adopting the data-driven approach in public health interventions (Essex et al., 2014). This dual prevention strategy is vital in preventing the ongoing epidemic. Bearing in mind its biologic viral infection context, the landscape of biologic agents is constantly evolving with each step in new antiviral drugs and global vaccination strategies. Of note, the genomics revolution has provided the tools to create vaccines that have the potential to induce robust immune responses with little likelihood of disease enhancement. The biggest challenge is to develop effective and safe therapeutic regimens for all viral diseases, including those without approved therapy. As public health systems adapt to these challenges, education, access to preventive interventions, and advances in molecular diagnostics will be the pillars. This holistic approach not only seeks to suppress current health problems but also seeks to induce resilience against future viral infections so that it may create enhanced global health.

1.5.1. Antiviral therapies and their mechanisms

The discovery of antiviral drugs is a milestone in the field of medical microbiology, particularly against viral diseases that are hazardous to health. Antivirals act by inhibiting particular stages in the viral life cycle, preventing replication, and lowering disease severity. For example, nucleoside analogues are specifically designed to interfere with viral genome replication through the mechanism of appearing natural nucleotides that induce termination of viral DNA or RNA synthesis. This effect is most pronounced in the treatment of chronic viral infections such as hepatitis B, where drug resistance may complicate therapeutic strategies. Through an appreciation of the mechanisms of action of these antivirals, clinicians will be able to adapt therapeutic regimens to maximize patient gain and minimize the effect of viral disease in the population. In the case of respiratory syncytial virus (RSV), with concomitant high morbidity in susceptible populations, antiviral availability is restricted, necessitating a focus on research on new drugs. Current management is primarily focused on supportive therapy, and passive immunity may be provided with the monoclonal antibody palivizumab for high-risk infants. Despite these limitations, active research in new antiviral drugs promises the discovery of new drugs that will selectively block RSV entry or replication. Pathophysiologic understanding of RSV-induced bronchiolitis, characterized by overwhelming airway inflammation, directs the design of targeted immunomodulatory therapy that can complement existing treatment paradigms. With every improving leap in knowledge of viral mechanisms, the hope of developing effective antiviral treatments for RSV and other viruses becomes increasingly a reality, making the urgency of continued research more imperative (Jha et al., 2016). The complexity of viral infection, particularly chronic viral infections like hepatitis B, increases the need to monitor antiviral resistance increasingly. As the strains of the virus mutate and accumulate mutations, as in the case of the hepatitis B virus reverse transcriptase, treatment effectiveness can be severely compromised, and early virus characterization is thus important to guide therapy. It has been proven that drug-naive patients themselves harbor naturally occurring resistance mutations, which further complicates treatment. The identification of such mutations before the initiation of antiviral therapy allows clinicians to tailor treatment, preventing the possibility of selecting for resistance. This advanced approach demonstrates the critical fusion of virology and clinical microbiology, requiring personalized treatment protocols honouring the adaptive potential of viruses and the requirement for continued monitoring of antiviral effectiveness (Mahabadi et al., 2013) (Figure 1.14).

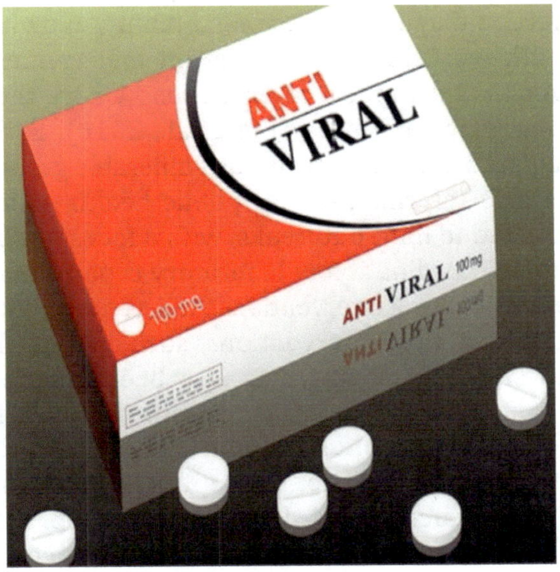

Figure 1.14. Antiviral medication.

Source: https://www.eehealth.org/-/media/images/modules/blog/posts/2021/06/hd-life-covid-antiviral-medication.jpg?h=499&w=750&hash=77E351993CAEB6CDA4FEF99E14A3D9B9.

1.5.2. Vaccination strategies against viral diseases

The increasing rate of viral infection worldwide has necessitated consideration of effective vaccination strategies. Vaccination is a significant means of inducing immunity against specific pathogens and, therefore, curtailing the spread of viruses and protecting populations, particularly vulnerable groups such as children and the elderly. Vaccines can be categorized into various forms, including live-attenuated, inactivated, and subunit vaccines, each with varying immunological properties and advantages. For instance, live-attenuated vaccines tend to induce strong immune responses and long-term immunity, while inactivated vaccines offer a safer option, particularly for high-risk groups. With the ever-changing viral pathogens, it is still crucial to develop these vaccination techniques to combat public health conditions (Goudie et al., 2003). Advances in the technology of vaccines in the recent past underscore the importance of developing vaccines against widespread viral diseases well known for their high morbidity and mortality. Recombinant DNA vaccines and mRNA technology have transformed the landscape, the best example being how vaccines against COVID-19 were rolled out at lightning speed with unprecedented effectiveness within a very short period of time. These technologies arguably not only enhance immunity but also allow for the facilitation of rapid vaccine adaptation to new variants. Also, as in the case of respiratory syncytial virus (RSV) infections, which manifest in millions of cases among young children, the invention of new vaccines is of utmost significance (Jha et al., 2016). As such strategies keep evolving, they have the potential to minimize the extent of the complications of viral infections and bring better health outcomes. Enforcement of vaccination interventions is also made more difficult by factors such as vaccine hesitancy, unequal access, and variations in public health policy. These all point to the need for intensive education campaigns to boost awareness regarding the impact and safety of vaccines. It is important to ensure sufficient knowledge on the preventive capacity of vaccines among individuals for the success of herd immunity, which is essential for curbing the spread of viral infections. Coordination among governments, health workers, and society is central to overcoming barriers to immunization and guaranteeing equitable access, particularly in settings that are scarce of resources. The success of immunization programs depends not just on the scientific achievement in vaccine development but also on the social obligation to establish a culture of health and prevention (Goudie et al., 2003) (Figure 1.15).

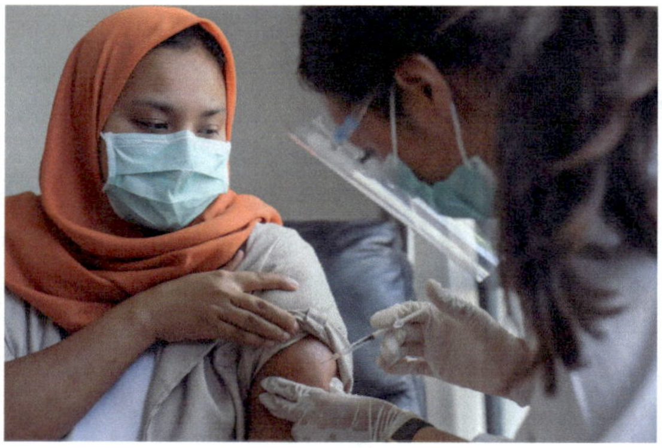

Figure 1.15. Vaccination against viral diseases.

Source: https://www.bread.org/wp-content/uploads/2024/03/iStock-1320262755-scaled.jpg.

1.5.3. Public health measures for virus control

Public health intervention is a key aspect in viral infection prevention, which is, through the introduction of vaccine programs. Apart from personal protection, vaccination also provides herd immunity, reducing the aggregate prevalence of infectious diseases in a population. For example, vaccines for influenza offer significantly reduced transmission of the virus, thus inhibiting the associated morbidity and mortality rates. The biggest challenge right now is the virus antigenic drift potential, for which yearly updates of vaccine strains are required. Research has shown that A/H3N2 evolves more quickly than other influenza lineages and is the cause of yearly variations in immunity needed for effective deployment of vaccines (Bedford et al., 2013). Consequently, public health facilities have to continuously monitor prevalent virus strains to optimize vaccination drives, highlighting the intersection of virology and public health policy in combating infectious diseases. Aside from vaccination, diagnostic testing is a cornerstone of virus control and public health interventions. Rapid and accurate viral infection detection guarantees timely intervention, and transmission levels are reduced. The invention of molecular diagnostic tests has revolutionized our ability to diagnose complex viral infections such as respiratory syncytial virus (RSV), a very dangerous virus for children and susceptible populations. With the estimated 33 million cases annually in children under the age of five years, effective diagnostics become a reality, allowing health workers to offer relevant management options and support interventions where they are urgently required (Jha et al., 2016). Early diagnosis not only safeguards vulnerable groups but also informs broader public health policy intended to limit outbreaks, with a focus on the critical coordination of laboratory capacity and epidemiological interventions. Adherence to non-pharmaceutical interventions, such as hygiene and social distancing, has also been effective in containing virus transmission, particularly in pandemic contexts. Non-pharmaceutical interventions restrict susceptible hosts and hence reduce the pace of infection spread. Populations that embrace measures such as mask-wearing, regular handwashing, and reducing social gatherings display decreased levels of virus transmission during outbreaks. They complement vaccination drives, affirming the need for a multifaceted strategy towards public health. The viral evolution-public health dichotomy calls for a dynamic countermeasure. Therefore, the public health authorities have to remain proactive, reconstructing procedures based on the evolving landscape of viral diseases so that the control of outbreaks remains scientifically sound and methodologically robust.

1.6. Emerging Viruses and Global Health

Emergence of new viruses represents a very severe risk to global human health, particularly given how they intersect with changing environmental and social trends. Generally speaking, zoonotic viruses originating from animal reservoirs are the most concerning since they can so readily conform to human hosts. The epidemiology of NE, for instance, provides an example of the synergy between changing environmental conditions and viral transmission. Studies from northern Sweden indicate that the Puumala virus (PUU), the causative agent of NE, also has a strong correlation with its primary host population peak, the bank vole. When these small rodents thrive under certain environmental conditions, such as mature moist forests, human risk for exposure increases with the peak vole populations, especially during autumn (Olsson, 2003). Such interactions must be clarified for the development of effective prevention measures against emerging viral diseases. The environmental determinants' role in oscillating emergence of viruses highlights interdisciplinary work in virology and environmental science. Apart from epidemiology patterns, demographic factors also have a remarkable role to play in understanding the spread of emerging diseases. Findings from Swedish research show that NE disproportionately affects middle-aged men, which suggests that some lifestyle aspects, such as outdoor recreation near rodent nests, have a tendency to subject these men to increased infection risk. The above underscores the necessity of considering demographic data while assessing risks from new viruses. Public education among high-risk groups can be important in mitigating the impact of these infections and is central to an international health response strategy (Grecco et al., 2018). International cooperation and integrated health systems are most valuable in addressing the challenges brought about by emergent viruses. The interconnectedness of the world on a global level means that viral outbreaks do not become localized but have the potential to become pandemics worldwide. Surveillance systems must be designed to capture not only traditional virology markers but also ecological and demographic indicators that are used to input into risk assessment models. Awareness and preparedness programs in communities for regional outbreaks are especially germane. For instance, integrating veterinary and environmental health surveillance can pick up early warning signs of viral emergence in wildlife populations to facilitate proactive risk management for human health. Within this dynamic landscape of new viral threats, collective efforts are required to safeguard public health and narrative resilience (Olsson, 2003).

1.6.1. Factors contributing to the emergence of new viruses

The emergence of new viruses increasingly relies on various ecological and anthropogenic processes that generate good conditions for viral evolution and transmission. One such process is the phenomenon of zoonotic spillover, during which viruses are transferred from animal reservoirs to humans. Such an event typically occurs as a result of increased human incursion into wildlife habitats, thereby increasing interspecific contacts. As an example, the transmission dynamics of canine parvovirus (CPV) illustrate how interspecies interactions enable viruses to accommodate novel hosts. The evolutionary histories of CPV, which has become highly differentiated genically in Europe and South America, illustrate how migrations and local adaptation result in new viral strains. With these types of interactions, viruses develop and mutate, and they can become competent for novel functions, posing a public health threat in several populations, hence demonstrating the relationship between ecological perturbation and viral emergence. Antigenic evolution is also a cause of the emergence of new viruses, as shown by the ongoing mutation of influenza viruses. These viruses make use of processes like antigenic drift, which allows them to evade host immunity created from earlier strains. The rapid evolution in influenza lineages, particularly A/H3N2, demonstrates the virus's ability to produce mutant forms less recognisable by the immune system. This antigenic drift is central to determining the effectiveness of existing vaccines, as the genetic variation introduced by mutation could lead to great differences between vaccine and circulating strains. Through modelling such antigenic and genetic patterns, researchers have gained insights into the changes over time in viral strains, which is important to understand the dynamics of rates of viral infection and transmission across populations and to implement efficacious public health interventions, including vaccination policies, as highlighted by Bedford et al. (2013). In addition, global warming, urbanization, and globalization facilitate the geographic diffusion of viruses. Climate change redistributes the hosts' and vectors' habitat and range of migration, which can lead to novel interactions that cause the emergence of viruses. For instance, rising temperatures may expand the range of certain zoonoses, such as those spread by mosquitoes and ticks, a process likely to expose viruses to new human populations that were otherwise isolated. Ongoing spread of viral strains, as characterized in studies of populations of canine parvovirus, reveals the manner in which waves of viral genomic material travel across continents, combining indigenous strains with strains from remote locations, as described by Grecco et al. (2018). Such interdependence highlights the need for global surveillance and coordinated public health efforts to monitor and respond to emerging viral threats, which have multifaceted environmental and social determinants (Figure 1.16).

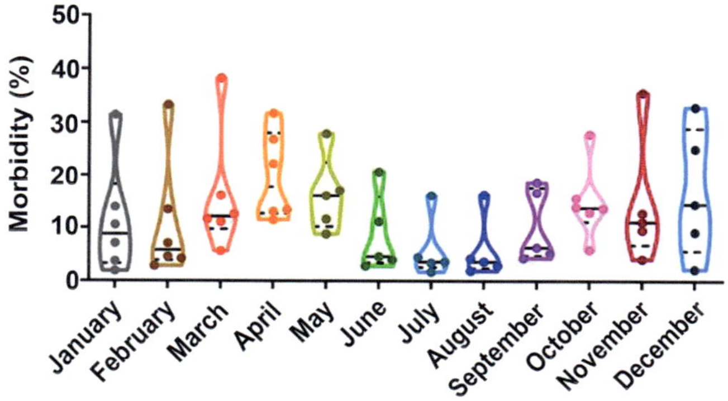

Figure 1.16. Monthly correlation analysis of canine parvovirus (CPV) infections in China.

Source: https://www.researchgate.net/publication/339383394/figure/fig3/AS:11431281241655916@1715185322446/Monthly-correlation-analysis-of-canine-parvovirus-CPV-infections-in-China.tif.

1.6.2. Case studies of recent viral outbreaks

The emergence of viral infections like hand, foot, and mouth disease (HFMD) has become a public health concern, particularly in the densely populated regions of the Asia Pacific. While the condition is typically mild, it is primarily caused by the human enteroviruses and could lead to serious neurological and cardiopulmonary outcomes, particularly in vulnerable populations. Studies indicate that while HFMD transmission in the developing world is more faeco-oral, in developed nations it is respiratory droplet, hence more difficult to prevent. The geographical predominance of virulent outbreaks in the Asia Pacific could be attributed to factors such as environmental hygiene, as well as the genetic susceptibility of host populations. This model of epidemiology points to the extreme need for careful surveillance because the rapid transformation and genetic reassortment of the virus can create a volatile epidemic, necessitating a thorough disease surveillance and control regimen (Goudie et al., 2003). Recent case studies have focused on the alarming potential of viral pathogens to change and persist in diverse environments, becoming serious public health issues. For instance, research on inactivation processes for viruses has established the efficacy of ozone as a biocidal agent in inactivating common foodborne pathogens, such as *Campylobacter jejuni* and *Salmonella enteritidis*. Research indicates that variations in treatment conditions, such as the population size and temperature, can significantly affect the efficacy of ozone in inactivating the hazards. This relevance extends beyond food safety; the ability to contain viral epidemics, especially in disease-intensive situations, can be crucial to averting large-scale epidemics. Understanding of the interaction of these pathogens in their surroundings is critical to the implementation of effective strategies to mitigate risk discussed in such case studies (Goudie et al., 2003). Furthermore, the relationship between viral persistence and environmental conditions reinforces the challenges of viral outbreak control with globalization. Enterovirus outbreaks become more adversely facilitated in areas of low sanitation and health facilities, allowing for prolonged survival and transmission of the pathogens. The emergence of new viral species complicates vaccine development due to their rapid genetic evolution and the fact that the diseases they cause are mild, leading to underreporting and insufficient public health responses. As in the HFMD example, identification of genetic recombination and monitoring emerging epidemics are paramount in preparation for effective public health interventions. Expanded studies are essential to assess treatment options, for instance, the efficacy of intravenous immunoglobulin in extreme complications, and potentially lead to more targeted and effective interventions against viral infection epidemics (Lau et al., 2010) (Figure 1.17).

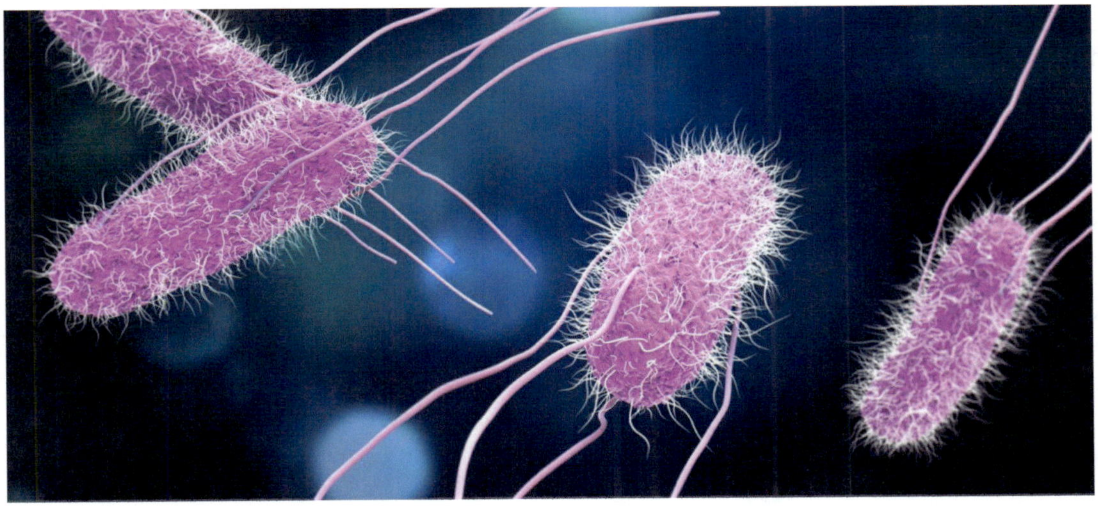

Figure 1.17. *Salmonella enterica.*

Source: https://cdn-dblhd.nitrocdn.com/baaZZsBRyWsSkxvRjeuJnYOHtwzeoEKd/assets/images/optimized/rev-95552f6/microbe-investigations.com/wp-content/uploads/elementor/thumbs/Salmonella-Enterica-qyn0kjeycjhbzea47298yx8ixprvfqh4cgryknd5ew.jpg.

1.6.3. The role of global surveillance in virology

Surveillance across the world plays a core role in virology, particularly in monitoring and understanding viral epidemics around the globe. Through the systematic collection and analysis of information on viral infections, health authorities can trace patterns of transmission and potential hotspots for emerging viral outbreaks. Such surveillance plays a key role in infectious disease control and timely public health response. The use of genomic information in surveillance networks enables scientists to track mutations and viral evolution, providing them with useful knowledge on how viruses evolve and spread. Surveillance like this empowers health authorities to implement efficient vaccination campaigns and allocate resources in an effective manner, saving lives and reducing healthcare costs in the long term. In the case of respiratory viruses, and particularly the influenza virus, global surveillance becomes significant. Influenza viruses exhibit antigenic drift and cause periodic epidemics and sporadic pandemics. Surveillance work is focused on tracking these antigenic shifts to predict upcoming outbreaks and direct vaccine development protocols. By applying techniques such as the hemagglutination inhibition (HI) assay, researchers are able to create antigenic maps that demarcate the ongoing development of influenza strains. Recent studies highlight dynamic patterns of antigenic drift of viral lineages that show ongoing surveillance can significantly aid us towards learning about viral behavior and associated epidemiological patterns (Bedford et al., 2013). Such information is the cornerstone of unleashing preemptive measures to address influenza's impacts worldwide. Global surveillance is not exclusive to influenza; it applies to many viral pathogens, especially in high-burden disease areas. For example, global monitoring of HPV and HIV infection in sub-Saharan Africa indicates robust correlations with increasing cervical cancer incidence. Another area that is gaining momentum as research is the interaction between viral infections and cervicovaginal microbiota, since dysbiosis may raise cancer threats among vulnerable populations (Angeletti et al., 2020). By uncovering such interactions through extensive surveillance, public health action may feed into specific interventions against viral persistence and associated diseases. In essence, global surveillance is the backbone of virology in medical microbiology that offers us the data on which to base intelligent, successful public health policies.

SUMMARY

In concluding an investigation of general virology in medical microbiology, there is a necessity to acknowledge the evolutionary process that has hit virology since its origin as a scientific branch. Growth in the discipline of virology was marked by spectacular advances in the knowledge of the virulence of pathogens that had led to the objective characterization of viruses. This process was more than mere accumulation of facts; it was the complicated process of objectification, in which virulence ideas were actively constructed and produced by various scientific practices. As theoried in the objectification of the virus discussion, the science of virology was an outcome of decades of fragmented investigation, reshaping methods and technologies to achieve a coherent idea of viral agents (Van Loon, 2002). This foundation guides contemporary virology and its integration with medical microbiology. Furthermore, the ongoing evolution of virology underscores the synergy between scientific progress and technology. The International Committee on Taxonomy of Viruses (ICTV) has played a focal role in the organization and classification of viral diversity, a basis for future research and clinical applications. Reflecting on the ICTV's history over the past half-century, there is one thing that stands out: a commitment to staying up to speed with technology and streamlining communication between virologists. Today's endeavors supported by grants, aimed at pushing online resources and facilitating debate, represent an innovative approach to meeting challenges in virus taxonomy and characterization (Adams et al., 2017). Such collaborative efforts are central to appreciating the complexities of viral diseases, emphasizing an integrated plan that is crucial in medical microbiology. In conclusion, the crux of this discussion reaffirms that general virology is an integral component of medical microbiology, very integrated with scientific information and advances in public health. As our body of knowledge on viruses continues to develop and increase, implications for medical science increase in depth. The complex interaction between scientific question, technological innovation, and appropriate application serves to illustrate the need for ongoing research and interdisciplinarity. Acceptance of the context of history and contemporary developments in virology serves to better appreciate its critical role in combating global health challenges. Lastly, the history of virology is every bit a history of scientific achievement as it is one of collective responsibility for protecting the health of the public against viral disease.

The science of virology, understood in the context of medical microbiology, points to the progression of viruses from their early speculative studies to where they are now. It began with speculative studies without a common framework, which made it more difficult to understand in terms of pathogen virulence. But technological and methodological refinements over the years have facilitated the objectification of viruses so that it is easier to study them holistically. This evolution was not a linear process but rather was characterized by a complex combination of the various scientific disciplines that contributed to the creation of virology as a distinct field. The establishment of the so-called "virology-assemblage" in the first half of the 1950s was a turning-point, as it allowed for joint progress of knowledge and techniques, ultimately providing scientists with the possibility to handle viruses in a state of coherence previously impossible (van Loon, 2002). The significance of human cytomegalovirus (HCMV) also bears witness to the crossroads of virology and medical microbiology. HCMV exemplifies the inherent viral pathology complexity because it can be harbored for a lifetime in the host with potentially life-threatening reactivation in those belonging to high-risk groups, such as congenitally infected neonates or immunocompromised hosts. Resistance to antiviral drugs, coupled with the fact that there are no effective vaccines, is perhaps the greatest challenge in the management of HCMV infection. This is also exacerbated by HCMV's ability to evolve quickly through immune evasion mechanisms that render therapy challenging. The study on the genetic composition and evolutionary patterns of HCMV illustrates how recombination leads to immense genetic variability, making it challenging to treat and reinforcing the need for revolutionary methods in vaccine development (Lassalle et al., 2016). Briefly, viral dynamics in medical microbiology demonstrate the intricate interaction between virus adaptation and host immune response. The ability of viruses such as HCMV to adapt and diversify quickly by homologous recombination poses formidable challenges for clinical management and antiviral drug discovery. As stressed, the hyper-variable regions of the viral genome responsible for coding proteins essential in immune evasion not only offer a survival mechanism but also reveal the ongoing arms race between viruses and host immunity. By continuing to explore these evolutionary patterns, medical microbiology is in a position to further our understanding of virus-host interactions, which will ultimately drive treatments and vaccines toward solutions tailored to combat the ever-evolving threats viral pathogens pose (Lassalle et al., 2016).

CLOSER LOOK

DNA VERSUS RNA VIRUS REPLICATION

Replication by viruses is a complex process that differs significantly for DNA and RNA viruses due to their constituent genetic material. They both completely rely on host cells for replication, but the process is distinct depending on how their genomes are read and transcribed. Identification of such differences is most critical in designing specific antiviral treatments and vaccines. DNA viruses tend to replicate in the host cell nucleus, utilizing the DNA-dependent DNA polymerases of the host.

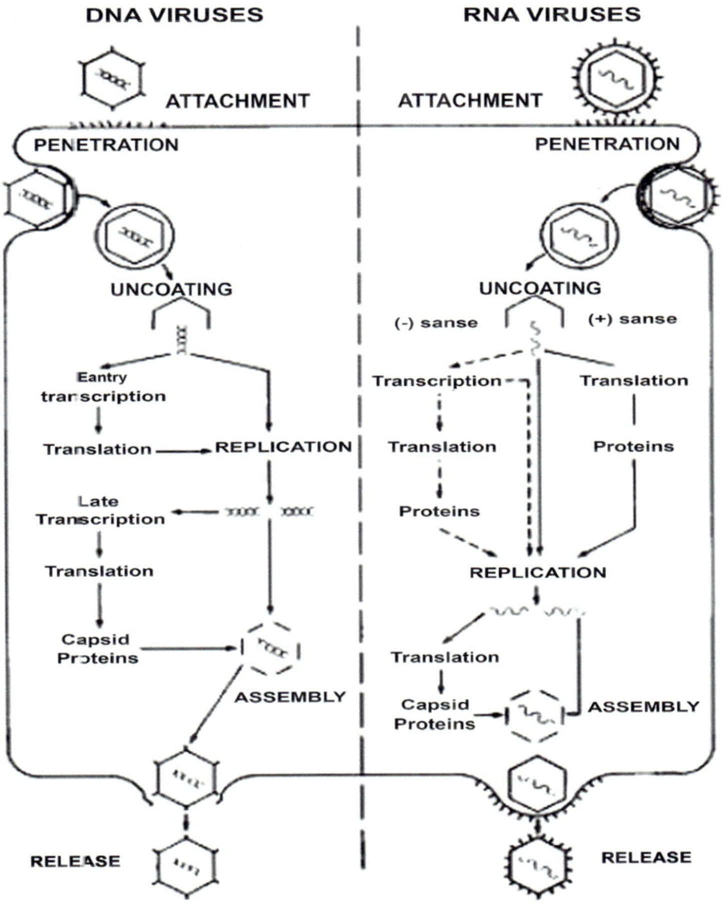

Figure 1.18. Comparative diagram of DNA and RNA virus replication cycles, detailing the steps from attachment and penetration to uncoating, replication, protein synthesis, assembly, and release of new viral particles.

Source: http://www.oculist.net/downaton502/prof/ebook/duanes/pages/v8/ch085/001f.html.

Most DNA viruses follow the molecular biology central dogma, where the DNA is initially transcribed to produce mRNA that is then translated into proteins. A few DNA viruses, including adenoviruses and herpesviruses, use host RNA polymerase II for transcribing their genes. Others, such as the poxviruses, are produced entirely in the cytoplasm and have their own transcriptional machinery since the host transcriptional enzymes reside in the nucleus. DNA viruses, in general, have more stable genomes due to the proofreading function of the DNA polymerases, so they have lower mutation rates than RNA viruses. This genome stability often allows for longer-term immunity and makes the DNA viruses more suitable vaccine candidates (Figure 1.18).

On the other hand, RNA viruses primarily replicate in the cytoplasm and have to code for their own RNA-dependent RNA polymerase because cells in host organisms do not possess enzymes that are able to replicate RNA from an RNA template. RNA viruses are also categorized according to the polarity of the genome. Positive-sense RNA viruses (e.g., poliovirus, dengue virus) contain genomes that can be used directly as mRNA and translated by host ribosomes as soon as they enter the cell. Negative-sense RNA viruses (e.g., influenza virus, rabies virus) must first be transcribed into complementary positive-sense RNA, then translated. Such viruses must contain their own RNA polymerase within the virion. Double-stranded RNA viruses, like rotaviruses, also require their own polymerases and more complicated replication.

A fascinating case is the retroviruses (e.g., HIV), RNA viruses that encode from a DNA intermediate. They use reverse transcriptase to write out their RNA genome into DNA that becomes part of the host genome. New viral RNA and protein are then produced from this integrated form by host machinery.

Because RNA-dependent RNA polymerases lack proofreading ability, RNA viruses have mutation rates much greater than DNA viruses. This rapid evolution enables them to evolve and change quickly in new hosts or evade immune attacks but also makes them prone to the generation of defective mutants. This high mutation rate is one of the greatest challenges in controlling RNA viruses such as influenza, HIV, and SARS-CoV-2 because it can lead to constant emergence of new strains.

REFERENCES

1. Trevor Bedford Marc A Suchard Philippe Lemey Gytis Dudas Victoria Gregory Alan J Hay John W McCauley Colin A Russel l Derek J Smith Andrew Rambaut (2014) Integrating influenza antigenic dynamics with molecular evolution eLife 3:e01914.
2. https://doi.org/10.7554/eLife.01914(accessed on 16th July 2025).
3. Mahabadi, M., Norouzi, M., Alavian, S. M., Samimirad, K., Azad, T. M., Saberfar, E., Mahmoodi, M., Ramezani, F., Karimzadeh, H., Malekzadeh, R., Montazeri, G., Nejatizadeh, A., Ziaee, M., Abedi, F., Ataei, B., Yaran, M., Sayad, B., Hossein Somi, M., Sarizadeh, G., Sanei-Moghaddam, I., ... Jazayeri, S. M. (2013). Drug-related mutational patterns in hepatitis B virus (HBV) reverse transcriptase proteins from Iranian treatment-naïve chronic HBV patients. *Hepatitis monthly*, *13*(1), e6712. https://doi.org/10.5812/hepatmon.6712(accessed on 16th July 2025).
4. Adams, M. J., Lefkowitz, E. J., King, A. M., Harrach, B., Harrison, R. L., Knowles, N. J., Kropinski, A. M., Krupovic, M., Kuhn, J. H., Mushegian, A. R., Nibert, M. L., Sabanadzovic, S., Sanfaçon, H., Siddell, S. G., Simmonds, P., Varsani, A., Zerbini, F. M., Orton, R. J., Smith, D. B., Gorbalenya, A. E., ... Davison, A. J. (2017). 50 years of the International Committee on Taxonomy of Viruses: progress and prospects. *Archives of virology*, *162*(5), 1441–1446. https://doi.org/10.1007/s00705-016-3215-y (accessed on 16th July 2025).
5. Grecco, S., Iraola, G., Decaro, N., Alfieri, A., Alfieri, A., Gallo Calderón, M., da Silva, A. P., Name, D., Aldaz, J., Calleros, L., Marandino, A., Tomás, G., Maya, L., Francia, L., Panzera, Y., & Pérez, R. (2018). Inter- and intracontinental migrations and local differentiation have shaped the contemporary epidemiological landscape of canine parvovirus in South America. *Virus evolution*, *4*(1), vey011. https://doi.org/10.1093/ve/vey011(accessed on 16th July 2025).
6. Goudie, A. C., Olateju, F., Anderson, J. G., Rowan, N., & MacGregor, S. J. (2003). *Inactivation of pathogens on food and contact surfaces using ozone as a biocidal agent.* Poster session presented at Society for General Microbiology – 152nd Meeting – –, University of Edinburgh. (accessed on 16th July 2025).
7. Anderson, M. J., Benveniste, R. E., Willett, B. J., Brown, S. A., et al. (2013). *Feline leukemia virus: Half a century since its discovery.* https://core.ac.uk/download/9400690.pdf (accessed on 16th July 2025).
8. Angeletti, P. C., Kahesa, C., Klein, C., Mwalselage, J., et al. (2020). *How the cervical microbiota contributes to cervical cancer risk in Sub-Saharan Africa.* https://core.ac.uk/download/287614750.pdf (accessed on 16th July 2025).
9. Lassalle, F., Depledge, D. P., Reeves, M. B., Brown, A. C., Christiansen, M. T., Tutill, H. J., Williams, R. J., Einer-Jensen, K., Holdstock, J., Atkinson, C., Brown, J. R., van Loenen, F. B., Clark, D. A., Griffiths, P. D., Verjans, G. M. G. M., Schutten, M., Milne, R. S. B., Balloux, F., & Breuer, J. (2016). Islands of linkage in an ocean of pervasive recombination reveals two-speed evolution of human cytomegalovirus genomes. *Virus evolution*, *2*(1), vew017. https://doi.org/10.1093/ve/vew017(accessed on 16th July 2025).
10. Bandea, C. I. (2009). *The origin and evolution of viruses as molecular organisms.* https://core.ac.uk/download/pdf/288872.pdf (accessed on 16th July 2025).
11. Jon R. Cavicchi, Stanley P. Kowalski, et al, "Patent Landscape of Influenza A Virus Prophylactic Vaccines and Related Technologies" (2012).(accessed on 16th July 2025).

12. Butcher, S. A., & Gould, E. A. (1997). *Production of positive controls for calicivirus-specific PCR using recombinant baculovirus technology*. https://core.ac.uk/download/11020756.pdf (accessed on 16th July 2025).

13. Chrisafis, G. C. (2017). *Historical Patterns of Arboviral Seroprevalence Across Africa and Asia*. https://core.ac.uk/download/84397690.pdf (accessed on 16th July 2025).

14. Cumberworth, S. L., Clark, J. J., Kohl, A., & Donald, C. L. (2017). Inhibition of type I interferon induction and signalling by mosquito-borne flaviviruses. *Cellular microbiology*, *19*(5), e12737. https://doi.org/10.1111/cmi.12737 (accessed on 16th July 2025).

15. Dwivedi, L., & Shrivastava, M. (2011). *Anti-HIV Therapy: Pipeline Approaches and Future Directions*. https://core.ac.uk/download/pdf/289772.pdf (accessed on 16th July 2025).

16. Essex, M. (2014). *140 Reversing the epidemic of HIV-1C in Southern Africa with treatment as prevention*. https://core.ac.uk/download/28951260.pdf (accessed on 16th July 2025).

17. Jha, A., Jarvis, H., Fraser, C., & Openshaw, P. J. M. (2016). Respiratory Syncytial Virus. In D. S. Hui (Eds.) et. al., *SARS, MERS and other Viral Lung Infections*. European Respiratory Society. (accessed on 16th July 2025).

18. Generalov, I. I. Instructions for laboratory training in Special Microbiology and Virology for students of Faculty of Dentistry / I. I. Generalov, A. V. Frolova ; Ministry of Health Care of the Republic of Belarus, Vitebsk State Medical University, Dep. of Clinical Microbiology. - Vitebsk : [VSMU], 2016. - 32 p. (accessed on 16th July 2025).

19. Kazakova, A. (2019). *Multiplex diagnostics: Development of serological dual-mode multiplex microarray immunoassay and analysis of influenza and respiratory syncytial virus disease burden in early childhood*. https://core.ac.uk/download/275894270.pdf (accessed on 16th July 2025).

20. Kinney, A. L. (2007). *National scientific facilities and their science impact on non-biomedical research*. http://arxiv.org/abs/0705.1797 (accessed on 16th July 2025).

21. Lau, S. K. P., Wong, S. S. Y., Yip, C. C. Y., Yuen, K. Y., et al. (2010). *Human Enterovirus 71 and Hand, Foot and Mouth Disease*. https://core.ac.uk/download/37950461.pdf (accessed on 16th July 2025).

22. McKie, A. (2003). *Immunity surveillance of mumps and rubella: Improved methods for the detection of virus-specific antibody*. hsttps://core.ac.uk/download/9657304.pdf (accessed on 16th July 2025).

23. Olsson, G. E. (2003). *Nephropathia epidemica and Puumala virus occurrence in relation to bank vole (Clethrionomys glareolus) dynamics and environmental factors in northern Sweden*. https://core.ac.uk/download/11694648.pdf (accessed on 16th July 2025).

24. Orlova, E. (2012). *Bacteriophages and Their Structural Organization*. https://core.ac.uk/download/19509491.pdf (accessed on 16th July 2025).

25. Salek Ranjbarzadeh, F., Rasi Marzabadi, L., Roshangar, L., Karimi Shoar, M., & Piri, R. (2014). *Medical students' view about the effects of practical courses on learning the general theoretical concepts of basic medical sciences*. https://core.ac.uk/download/pdf/27043736.pdf (accessed on 16th July 2025).

26. van Loon, J. (2002). A Contagious Living Fluid. *Theory, Culture & Society*, *19*(5-6), 107-124. https://doi.org/10.1177/026327602761899174 (Original work published 2002)

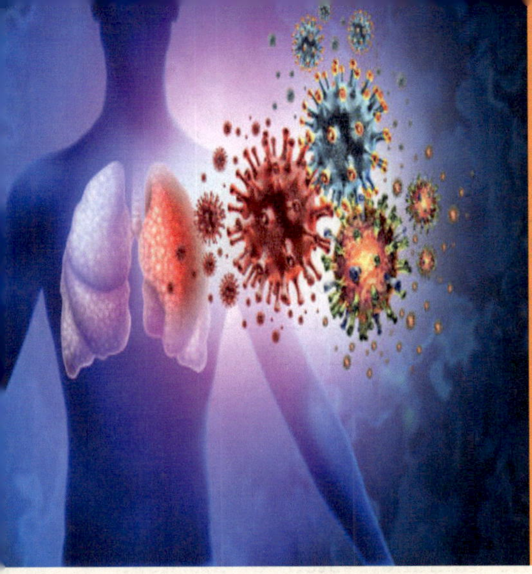

Chapter 2
RESPIRATORY VIRUSES

Contents

Introduction

The significance of respiratory viruses in public health should not be underestimated since they are responsible for a wide spectrum of conditions that affect individuals globally. The viruses, including influenza, coronaviruses, and respiratory syncytial virus, are both seasonal and pandemic threats. Respiratory viruses are spread primarily by respiratory droplets expelled upon sneezing and coughing, which makes enclosed areas high-risk settings. As highlighted in research for the large-scale mass assemblies, such as the Hajj, the medical risks of outbreaks dramatically increase, and stringent medical measures and vaccinations for involved participants are required (Al-Tawfiq & Memish, 2019). Identifying mechanisms of viral transmission and infection is crucial for formulating appropriate public health interventions to mitigate the impact of these pathogens. In addition to their immediate impacts on human health, respiratory viruses also have profound and long-term effects on healthcare systems and economies. Seasonal influenza alone causes high morbidity and is responsible for tens of thousands of hospitalizations and deaths each year in the United States. Furthermore, the emergence and spread of new respiratory viruses can cause mass panic and disruptions to daily life, as witnessed in recent epidemics of coronaviruses. The interspecies jumping ability and adaptability of viruses add an element of complication, as seen during the case of H7N7 avian influenza outbreak that jumped between birds and humans (de Jong et al., 2009). Thus, it requires a multidisciplinary approach, encompassing epidemiology, virology, and public health policy, to address the respiratory virus threat. Public information and education are also vital components of battling respiratory viruses. Public outreach, public communication, and vaccination campaigns can significantly reduce the transmission rate. Education on simple preventative hygiene measures, such as cough hygiene and hand washing, can empower the public to protect themselves and others. Ongoing research into vaccine development and antiviral medication is also essential in staying a step ahead of these adaptive viruses. As every new respiratory virus develops, vigilance and collaboration between healthcare professionals, researchers, and legislators become ever more important. This step not only aims to minimize the prevalence of respiratory infection but also aims to strengthen public health overall against new viruses.

Definition of Respiratory Viruses

Respiratory viruses constitute a broad group of viral pathogens with their major target being the respiratory tract and causing an array of diseases ranging from minor colds to fatal pneumonia. Respiratory viruses are broadly classified into two categories: pandemic and seasonal strains. Seasonal respiratory viruses, such as influenza and respiratory syncytial virus (RSV), follow predictable patterns and are typically associated with the particular season of the year. Conversely, pandemic strains can occur without warning and are a serious public health issue. Their mode of transmission is primarily through respiratory droplets or soiled surfaces, making them highly infectious and a likely source of widespread outbreaks. Ongoing mutation of these viruses requires ongoing observation and research to understand their behaviour and impact, particularly on vulnerable groups like infants and the elderly.

Clinical presentation of respiratory viral infections varies significantly with the virus in question and the immune system of the host. The presentation involves symptoms such as cough, throat soreness, fever, and, in some cases, respiratory difficulty. RSV has been identified to be a leading cause of bronchiolitis in children, with evidence revealing its dominance in epidemic peaks in some months, especially during colder months (Cangiano et al., 2016). Similarly, influenza viruses are renowned for their capacity to transmit disease, as is manifested from current surveillance studies in tropical settings, which have recorded several instances of influenza-like illness and matching viral strains (Forshey et al., 2010) (Figure 2.1).

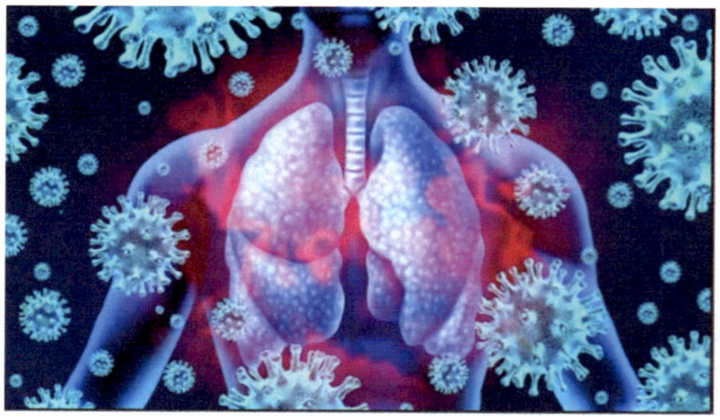

Figure 2.1. Respiratory viruses.

Source: https://images.theconversation.com/files/477255/original/file-20220802-23-r6z7fj.jpg?ixlib=rb-4.1.0&rect=0%2C0%2C2297%2C1292&q=20&auto=format&w=320&fit=clip&dpr=2&usm=12&cs=strip.

Significantly, such clinical presentations are of crucial significance to the health workers in establishing diagnostic and management leads for respiratory infections. Furthermore, the range of respiratory viruses expands into mechanisms through which they result in disease, and co-infection possibilities. Where there are multiple viral pathogens sharing a single host, the clinical scenario is made more complex and patient outcomes compromised. For example, children with bronchiolitis commonly present in co-infection with other respiratory viruses that cause varying clinical severity and requirement for specific therapies based on some viral detections (Cangiano et al., 2016). Similarly, studies identify that host factors such as age and environmental factors have a critical role to play in susceptibility and response to respiratory viruses (Forshey et al., 2010). This multivalence of respiratory viruses establishes the significance of stringent public health interventions, including surveillance, prevention, and education, to counteract the public health burden of these infections globally.

Importance of Studying Respiratory Viruses

Accurate information regarding respiratory viruses is crucial to public health, particularly after pandemics have shown how fast these pathogens can spread. Research on respiratory viruses allows researchers to identify trends of transmission, virulence, and host interaction that are indispensable in the creation of proper prevention strategies. The global impact of viruses such as influenza, SARS-CoV-2, and respiratory syncytial virus (RSV) shows that creative approaches must be taken to counter their impact. As viral transmission leads to high morbidity and mortality, especially among vulnerable populations, scientists must study the dynamics involved to develop useful solutions. Identification of the distinct characteristics of respiratory viruses can lead to more effective public health interventions, thus reducing the burden on the healthcare system and improving the health outcomes of the populations affected. Moreover, technological innovation is expanding our ability to study respiratory viruses at the molecular level. For instance, clinical metagenomic next-generation sequencing (mNGS) has begun to revolutionize the practice of diagnostics by allowing analysis of microbial and host genetic material simultaneously. This new approach enhances respiratory virus detection, co-infection, and viral evolution knowledge. Clinicians can personalize treatment approaches better and develop more targeted therapies through mNGS to take care of each patient's needs. Apart from challenges in clinical laboratory use of mNGS, its advantage in patient care and outcomes in public health makes it an essential resource in the study of respiratory viruses (Chiu et al., 2019).

Continuous investment in the technologies will likely continue to provide significant information that can guide treatment protocols and response plans in outbreaks. The collaboration among researchers, public health professionals, and clinical practitioners is crucial in overcoming barriers to successful research translation into practice. Unmet research and clinical needs should be highlighted in guiding future research activities in respiratory viruses (Deeks et al., 2013). Through the fostering of interdisciplinary interactions, the scientific community can accelerate the chain from basic research to clinical utility such that findings on respiratory viruses are delivered to a population that most acutely requires them. As the viral menace continues to reconfigure the landscape, it is more important than ever to remain vigilant when researching respiratory viruses. Participating in this research can allow societies to anticipate, prevent, and manage outbreaks before they worsen, preserving public health and safeguarding vulnerable segments of the population.

2.1. Types of Respiratory Viruses

Respiratory viruses come in numerous different forms, each with distinct characteristics and public health implications. The most prevalent are the influenza viruses, which are divided into type A and type B. Influenza A viruses are distinguished by their capacities to mutate and reassort, resulting in seasonal epidemics and sporadic pandemics. In contrast, influenza B primarily results in seasonal epidemics, with each lineage generating a different epidemiological pattern. Current studies highlight the predominance of influenza B in certain populations, particularly children, and illustrate the evolving epidemiology of influenza illness over time. Notably, from 2010 to 2016, influenza B viruses regularly surpassed influenza A in certain flu seasons, making them more significant in respiratory virus spread and warranting constant vigilance (Alicino et al., 2018).

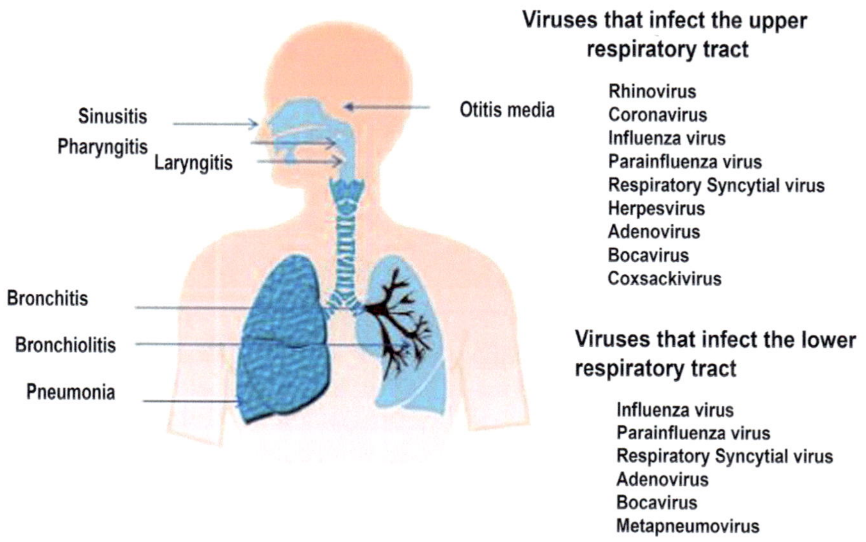

Figure 2.2. The respiratory tract and the main syndromes caused by viral infections.

Source: https://www.intechopen.com/chapters/42375.

Yet another prominent family of respiratory viruses is coronaviruses, which represent a heterogeneous group of viruses that have been implicated in producing mild colds to fatal respiratory syndromes. Historically, coronaviruses such as HCoV-229E and HCoV-OC43 have long been linked with seasonal respiratory disease. However, the identification of Middle East Respiratory Syndrome Coronavirus (MERS-CoV) and SARS-CoV-2 has reoriented public health response to respiratory infection. These emerging strains hint at the possible virulence and transmission dynamics of coronaviruses, particularly in crowded environments like the Hajj pilgrimage. Systematic review cited influenza, rhinovirus, and parainfluenza as common viruses among pilgrims, accentuating the increased risk of respiratory virus acquisition at such massive gatherings (Al-Tawfiq et al., 2018). Rhinoviruses, other than influenza and coronaviruses, also play an important role in respiratory disease, particularly in children. Rhinoviruses, being major causative agents of the common cold, are highly infectious and result in quick infections. They act best in temperate temperatures and therefore are active predominantly during the fall and spring seasons. There has also been a keen interest in the emergence of non-polio enteroviruses since they induce respiratory infections as well as have the potential to induce widespread outbreaks. The continuous occurrence of various respiratory viruses, along with their capacity to evolve and affect several populations, also underscores the importance of exhaustive surveillance and vaccination strategies to stem their influence on public health. As the developing picture of respiratory viruses poses a challenge, it becomes important to understand their types, patterns of transmission, and epidemiological significance (Figure 2.2).

2.1.1. Influenza Viruses

Influenza viruses are a significant public health concern due to their capacity to cause seasonal epidemics and the rare pandemics. They constitute a genus of viruses belonging to the Orthomyxoviridae family that is primarily divided into four types: A, B, C, and D. Influenza A and B infect the majority of humans, with type A viruses further divided depending on their hemagglutinin and neuraminidase proteins. Seasonal epidemics of influenza every year induce massive morbidity and mortality, for which the importance of immunization and public health surveillance cannot be overstressed.

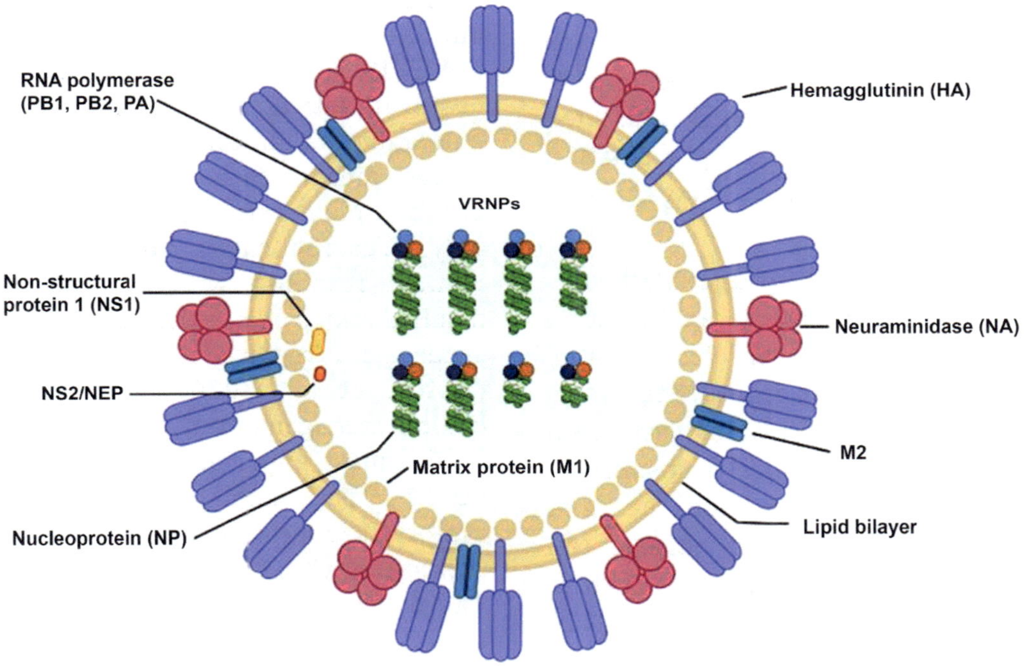

Figure 2.3. The structure of influenza A virus.

Source: https://en.wikipedia.org/wiki/Influenza_A_virus#/media/File:Viruses-12-00504-g001.webp.

The continuous alteration of the influenza virus through antigenic drift and shift renders it challenging to acquire permanent immunity. Surveillance programs and studies continue to be important in tracking changes in the virus, an aspect that is critical in the development of effective vaccines and therapeutic treatments for influenza (Al-Tawfiq et al., 2018). The impacts of influenza viruses do not stop at the individual, with the virus having implications on healthcare systems and economies as a whole. Respiratory viruses, most notably the influenza virus, cause a wide spectrum of complications that range from mild respiratory disease to severe pneumonia and aggravation of chronic illness. Influenza has a severe effect on at-risk populations like the elderly, young children, and those who have pre-existing medical conditions. Medical professionals must be wary in diagnosing influenza because early detection is vital to the administration of appropriate antiviral treatment as well as the prevention of complications. Preventive interventions, including mass immunization campaigns and health education, are central to the containment of the impact of influenza in epidemic periods. Increasing evidence of the role of viral respiratory infections in causing morbidity and mortality makes targeted intervention in management and prevention a must, particularly in high-risk settings (Fisher et al., 2012) (Figure 2.3).

Further, understanding the Pathways through which influenza viruses are transmitted is crucial in establishing efficient control measures. The Hajj annual pilgrimage that brings together millions in close proximity, presents a case study for respiratory viral transmission within overcrowding. Evidence indicates that influenza and other respiratory viruses can be transmitted among pilgrims, and further studies and monitoring of health are necessary to protect this group. Evidence has revealed that respiratory viruses like influenza, rhinovirus, and parainfluenza are most commonly detected among Hajj pilgrims, making it critical to raise awareness about the risk of outbreaks at mass gatherings. The preventive measures against it include health authorities implementing rigorous screening and instituting prevention interventions, such as vaccination campaigns among pilgrims prior to undertaking the journey. These preventive steps are particularly significant in reducing the spread of influenza viruses in densely populated places, ultimately resulting in better public health (Al-Tawfiq et al., 2018).

2.1.2. Coronaviruses

Coronaviruses are a diverse group of viruses known to be implicated in respiratory infections in humans, ranging from mild illness to fatal illness. They are classified into four broad genera: alpha, beta, gamma, and delta coronaviruses, the former two primarily infecting animals. Beta-coronaviruses, particularly SARS-CoV, MERS-CoV, and recently SARS-CoV-2, have garnered immense attention since they are implicated in severe respiratory syndromes. The SARS-CoV-2 outbreak, which has caused the COVID-19 pandemic, has amplified international health initiatives towards understanding and mitigating the impacts of such viral infections. Disease mechanisms induced by coronaviruses are complex, with common roles of not only virus replication but also intense host immune response, with resulting deleterious manifestations like acute respiratory distress syndrome, as reported by some clinical evidence (Ansari et al., 2020). Understanding the clinical management of coronavirus infections is of utmost importance, especially since the COVID-19 pandemic. Management of respiratory symptoms is varied and ranges from supportive therapy, antiviral therapy to immunomodulators. There has been some recent evidence that certain anti-rheumatic agents and antimalarials have been reported to exhibit potential in inhibiting viral replication or ameliorating the cytokine storm that can occur in severe COVID-19 (Ansari et al., 2020). In addition, the exigency for specialty treatment protocols arises from the observation of coronaviruses ability to create hyper-inflammatory responses. As the global medical fraternity continues to study possibilities of treatment, gathering evidence and following up on patients are crucial elements in refining our way of treating these infections. As countries grapple with coronaviruses' persistent challenges, risk reduction strategies have played a pivotal role in inhibiting their persistence. Systematic analysis of interventions that have been implemented worldwide shows a collection of interventions, including mobility control measures, distancing, and hygiene practices, aimed at minimizing transmission. Although the quantitative effect of certain measures has yet to be fully appraised, early experience is that a multiple-track approach combining voluntary and compulsory measures yields the most successful result in managing outbreaks. The lessons learned in COVID-19 have enhanced our understanding of respiratory viruses overall and underscored the value of readiness and flexible responses to future public health emergencies. Such ongoing evaluations are critical to guide actions that safeguard global health, particularly against new viral threats (Figure 2.4).

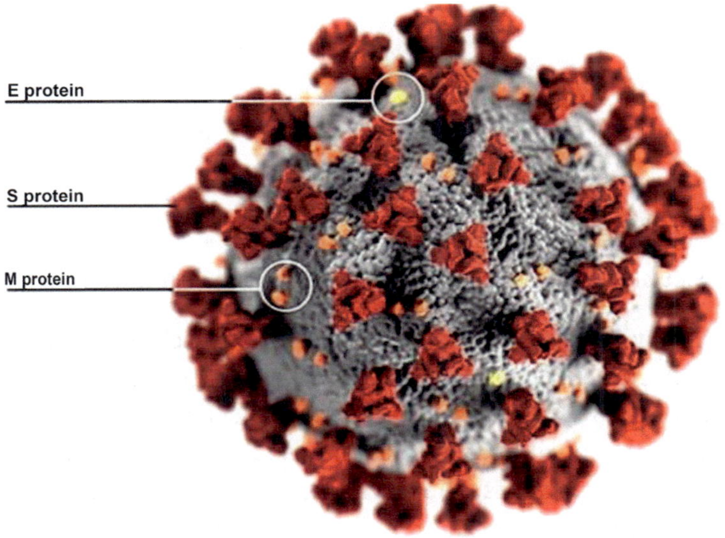

Figure 2.4. Coronaviruses.

Source: https://www.news-medical.net/image-handler/picture/2020/3/%40227498_web.jpg.

2.1.3. Rhinoviruses

Rhinoviruses within the family Picornaviridae are among the most frequent causes of respiratory illness all over the world. Though commonly associated with the common cold, their impact does not end there with minor illnesses. A three-year, large-scale study in Kilifi, Kenya, pediatric surveillance identified a high rate of human rhinoviruses (HRV) among children with various respiratory symptoms. Of the 441 real-time reverse transcriptase polymerase chain reaction (RT-PCR) detected positive samples, 47% were HRV-A, 5% were HRV-B, and 48% were HRV-C. The study highlighted the co-circulation of virus types and pointed to the absence of a well-defined seasonal pattern, which emphasizes the need for continuous surveillance and epidemiological understanding of HRVs across different geographical areas (Onyango et al., 2012). Rhinoviruses have also been noted for their severity beyond their common syndrome of the cold, particularly in compromised hosts. Even if classically regarded as etiologic agents of mild upper respiratory illness, they are increasingly well recognized to cause pneumonia and other severe respiratory illnesses, particularly in immunocompromised individuals and the elderly. A study notes that certain viral pathogens, like HRVs, are increasingly being held responsible for pneumonia in vulnerable adults and suggests that HRVs are likely to produce severe respiratory illness under specific conditions. With evolving literature, information on mechanisms and clinical features of rhinovirus infection becomes pertinent to the development of targeted intervention strategies (Cesario, 2012) (Figure 2.5).

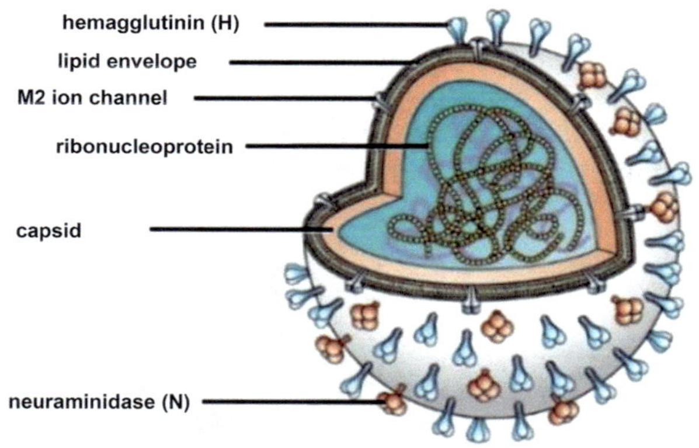

Figure 2.5. Anatomy of rhinovirus.

Source: https://vitrosens.com/what-is-rhinovirus-how-does-the-rhinovirus-test-kit-work/.

The complexity of rhinovirus infections is not just in their clinical symptomatology, but also in molecular diversity and epidemiological patterns. One of the fascinating aspects of the HRV classification is its division into a number of different species and subtypes that have unique epidemiological behaviors and clinical impacts. For instance, while HRV-A and HRV-C are frequently isolated from outpatients and inpatients, the correlation between some species and severity of respiratory disease is still a matter of investigation. The phenomenon described above underlines the need for intense genomic surveillance and strain monitoring, particularly during epidemic periods, to better understand the role of rhinoviruses as etiological agents of respiratory morbidity and to identify potential therapeutic targets in the course of infection (Onyango et al., 2012) (Figure 2.6).

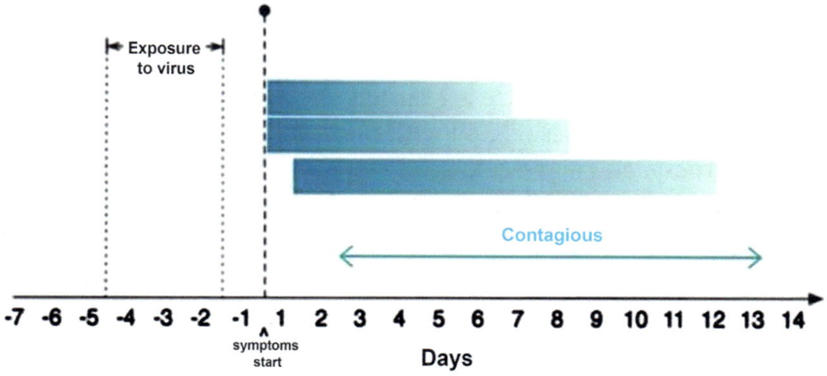

Figure 2.6. Timeline of a rhinovirus infection.

Source: https://vitrosens.com/what-is-rhinovirus-how-does-the-rhinovirus-test-kit-work/.

2.2. Transmission and Spread

Understanding of transmission and dissemination of the respiratory viruses is critical to stemming their impact on public health. Respiratory viruses such as the coronaviruses are transmitted primarily through respiratory droplets when an individual infected by them coughs, sneezes, or even speaks. These droplets fall either directly into the mucous membranes of another person or become deposited on surfaces, where they last for various periods, influenced by environmental conditions. The infectivity of these viruses outside a host is greatly influenced by factors like temperature and humidity. Data has proposed an empirical model to categorize coronaviruses based on their transmission pattern in relation to the structural characteristics of their viral shells. This grouping guides public health action to reduce the spread of such pathogens during outbreaks with a focus on tailoring responses to different viral behavior (Goh et al., 2012). In addition to transmission by droplets, the role of built environments in respiratory virus transmission has become increasingly significant, particularly for the COVID-19 pandemic. New studies highlight how indoor spaces, such as the workplace, schools, and hospitals, can facilitate the spread of pathogens through environmental routes. Filtration systems, ventilation quality, and surface material are significant factors in determining the persistence and viability of viruses like SARS-CoV-2 in the indoor environment. Through a discussion of microbial exchanges occurring within these spaces, authorities suggest simple interventions to avoid transmission risks. Building managers and owners are encouraged to implement improved sanitation practices and improve indoor air quality in order to minimize the chances of viral transmission between building occupants, illustrating the synergy of environmental control and infectious disease prevention (Dietz et al., 2020). The extremely dynamic character of respiratory virus transmission continues to highlight the importance of public understanding of and adherence to health standards. Effective communication measures are paramount in enlightening the public on the risks associated with respiratory viruses and on steps people can take to avoid spread, such as vaccination, wearing masks, and proper use of hygiene. Following these recommendations can help significantly in lowering transmission chances. Ongoing variation of respiratory viruses also presents challenges for vaccine production and efficiency, something that needs perpetual checking and studies. By a more sensitive understanding of transmission dynamics and promoting collaborative efforts among public health professionals, scientists, and communities, society can reinforce its immunity to the threats posed by respiratory viruses and ultimately protect public health and safety.

2.2.1. Modes of Transmission

It is essential to understand the transmission modes of respiratory viruses to implement effective public health interventions and policy designs. Coronaviruses and Nipah virus spread through different modes, such as direct contact, droplets, and fomites. Transmission dynamics are based mainly on the structural attributes of the virus and stability in the environment. Interestingly enough, much of the coronavirus behavior has been rationalized to some degree by studying their intrinsic disorder within viral proteins. This involves viral transmission patterns being influenced by the disorder distribution in the membrane (M) and nucleocapsid (N) proteins. By categorizing different strains based on these characteristics, researchers can more accurately forecast their transmission behavior, which is critical for predicting public health response during an outbreak (Goh et al., 2012). The Nipah virus is a notable example of the variability of modes of transmission across strains with attendant implications for virulence and for outbreak management. Initially linked to zoonotic spread from infected pigs, the Nipah virus later manifested human-to-human modes of transmission that facilitated its spread during epidemics. Interestingly, the correlational study on the intrinsically disordered N protein across several different strains illustrates an enhanced correlation between disorder degrees and case-fatality ratios (CFR). This revelation illustrates the need to examine genetic and structural considerations together when transmission modes are taken into account. The novel differential in the mode of transmission, especially between the Malaysian and Bangladeshi strains, highlights the need for differential epidemiological responses that are sensitive to the peculiarities of the virus in question (Goh et al., 2020) (Figure 2.7).

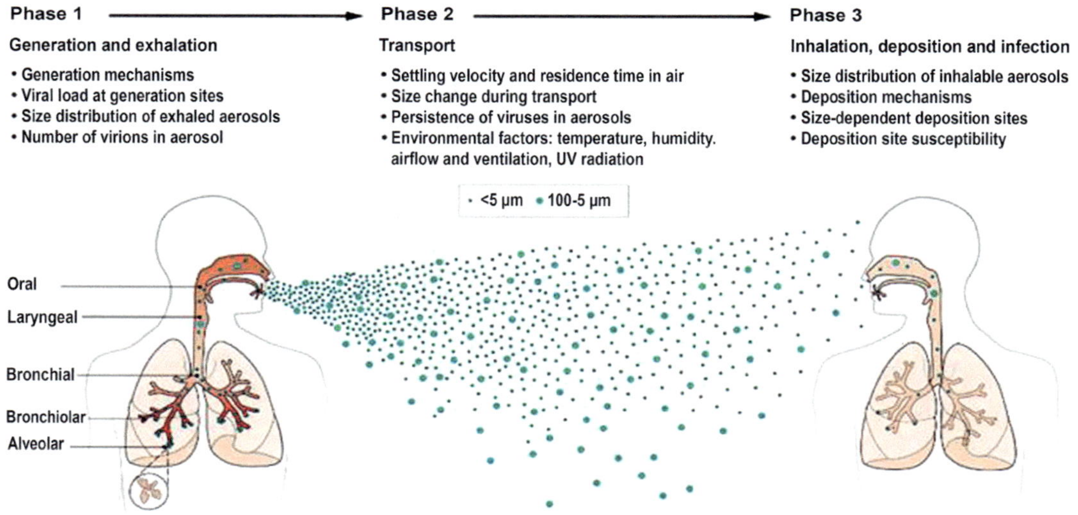

Figure 2.7. Phases involved in airborne transmission of respiratory viruses.

Source: https://www.science.org/doi/10.1126/science.abd9149.

Further, explanation of the intrinsic disorder of viral proteins may offer hints into paths of possible vaccine development and strategies for outbreak control. Through the illumination of the connection between modes of transmission and differences in structural characteristics, scientists can plan specific interventions aimed at influencing viral transmission. This intrinsic disorder profiling may offer new insights into what respiratory viruses' behavior is like across hosts and environments. Classifying viruses according to their transmissibility can also streamline diagnostic tests and enhance vaccine research. These works show how complex viral behavior is, but also how genomic, structural, and epidemiological factors become entangled in shaping the natural history of respiratory viruses (Goh et al., 2012, 2020).

2.2.2. Environmental Factors Influencing Spread

The relationship between environmental conditions and respiratory virus transmission dynamics has been of increasing scholarly interest. Environmental conditions, notably temperature and humidity, play a very important role in the survival and transmission of such pathogens. Research indicates that respiratory viruses, including influenza and coronaviruses, exhibit higher transmission frequency during winter seasons when congestion indoors is more prevalent. Moreover, studies indicate that low humidity enhances viral particle aerosolization, hence increasing the risk of infection in susceptible populations. Climatic conditions can augment these factors, which suggests that it is significant to understand environmental factors to predict viral epidemicity as well as implement specific public health interventions. Moreover, one should not underestimate the role of wild and migratory birds in transmitting respiratory illnesses. While there is limited documentation of direct virus transmission from birds to humans, these bird species can act as reservoir hosts for various pathogens, e.g., influenza A virus, and thereby make the epidemiology of respiratory disease complicated. Wild birds are also capable of carrying viruses over long distances, hence initiating pathogen entry into new geographic locations. The potential for viral mutations as they travel through different environments can lead to the potential for creating strains that become more infectious or more virulent in human populations. Understanding these pathways is essential for epidemiologists to disentangle the complexities of respiratory virus epidemics (Tsiodras et al., 2008). Climate change also has the effect of hastening the spread and outbreak of respiratory viruses, as climatic and temperature changes may enhance the ambient conditions that promote viral replication. In this case, climatic variation is directly linked with altering public health situations, impacting the spread and virulence of respiratory pathogens. Evidence indicates that the rise in mean global temperatures has been associated with the re-emergence of diseases previously contained, and this has revealed a need for adaptive responses in healthcare systems worldwide. Public health institutions must anticipate the issues environmental changes present, which influence the epidemiology of respiratory viruses and necessitate an overhaul of existing policies and strategies on health to counter their effects on vulnerable populations (Petruzelli, 2020) (Figure 2.8).

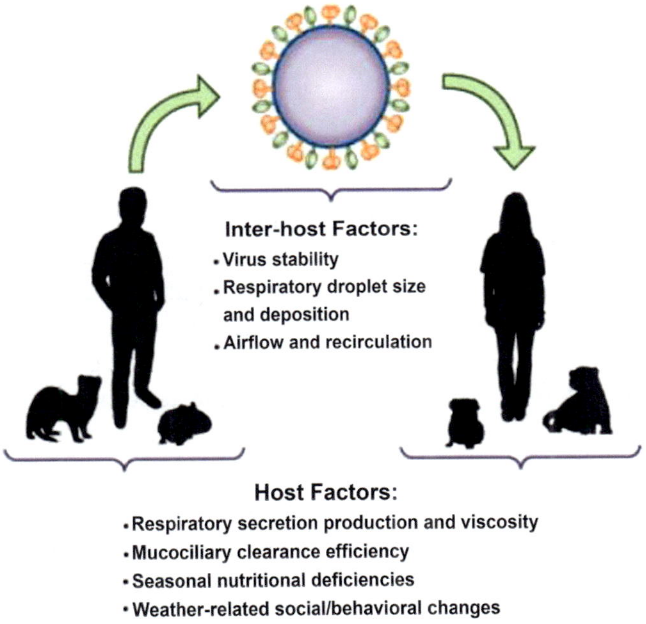

Figure 2.8. Environmental modulation of respiratory virus transmission.

Source: https://ars.els-cdn.com/content/image/1-s2.0-S1879625711001891-gr1.jpg.

2.2.3. Role of Human Behavior in Transmission

Human behavior has a major impact on the dynamics of respiratory virus transmission, which is largely attributable to social interactions enabling the transmission of infection. Who decides to engage in specific high-risk behaviors, such as close-contact events or who does not observe preventive measures, has serious implications for public health. For instance, when there are outbreaks of respiratory virus, behavioral variables such as violated social distancing or inappropriate use of masks can expedite transmission rates. Furthermore, psychological and social factors including individual risk perceptions, personal experiences, and perceived vulnerability, play important roles in shaping people's reactions to public health advice. Psychological and behavioral responses can directly impact the success of interventions designed to reduce transmission, hence the importance of public health interventions incorporating the psychological and social dimensions of human behavior alongside the biological pathways of transmission. The partnership type theory, particularly in sexually active persons, helps explain the interaction between relationship dynamics and compliance with preventive interventions for respiratory viruses. Participants in partnerships characterized by low-risk behavior are less likely to use preventive health measures than individuals in higher-risk partnerships, according to research. This behavior differential suggests that the social setting of personal relationships, characterized by trust and intimacy, can affect not only people's choices to engage in unsafe activities but also compliance with public health programs. A positive case in HIV prevention illustrates this condition: men who have sex with men (MSM) with more than one partner presented improved PrEP adherence according to their awareness of ongoing risk (Moore et al., 2017). This is a universal rule that can be applied to respiratory viruses, where open communication of risk within social relationships can stimulate guideline compliance. Environmental circumstances also coincide with human behavior in the respiratory virus transmission, specifically public space and the built environment. Indications show that the prevalence of respiratory viruses such as SARS-CoV-2 can be tremendously reduced by understanding how human behavior is intertwined with environmental circumstances. For example, indoor ventilation measures can reduce the virus transmission, but such success is greatly based on human behavior and dress code while meeting and social interactions (Dietz et al., 2020). Public choice of building users in relation to hygiene and social interaction can redesign the transmission pathways, implying that the public must be educated regarding their role while in public (Dietz et al., 2020). Therefore, it is important to address the behavioral dimensions of individuals and groups in order to achieve multi-faceted pandemic preparedness and response plans that seek to stem respiratory virus transmission.

2.3. Symptoms and Clinical Manifestations

The manifestation of the signs in respiratory viruses is a critical aspect of research, particularly with regard to their complexity and impact on health outcomes. Illnesses caused by viruses from influenza, coronaviruses, and rhinoviruses have the tendency to cause convergent clinical presentations that complicate differential diagnosis and treatment. Common symptoms that typically form the spectrum of the acute respiratory disease include fever, cough, sore throat, and fatigue. Most notably, during the COVID-19 pandemic, other presentations were observed, including loss of taste or smell, reported to occur even among patients with mild disease. These broad-based symptoms underscore the importance of increased awareness and clinical vigilance, especially in the context of new viral strains and varying pathogenic spectra of respiratory viruses with the potential to cause both mild illness and life-threatening complications (Vonck et al., 2020). Furthermore, the interaction between co-infections and respiratory viruses also plays a very significant role in increasing the severity of disease. For example, co-infections are very common in infants, particularly those under the age of six months, where co-infections with *Bordetella pertussis* alongside respiratory viruses tend to complicate the clinical picture.

Research indicates that even if viral co-infections in patients with pertussis do not always exacerbate clinical presentations, there are notable demographic variations between infected infants. Infants infected with *B. pertussis* only are reported to be younger and less frequently breastfed compared to those infected with viral co-infections, and this may suggest that immunologic factors are largely responsible for the severity of disease (Agricola et al., 2017). Understanding these dynamics can bring about improved patient management and targeted therapeutic strategies. Lastly, the clinical manifestations of respiratory viruses can extend beyond the respiratory tract to involve neurological and other systemic symptoms.

More recent evidence implies that COVID-19 itself is defined by a variety of neurological manifestations such as alterations in consciousness, cranial nerve dysfunction, and autoimmune sequelae. These presentations not only indicate the virus neurotropism but also suggest that systemic presentation could be due to direct viral invasion as well as indirect mechanisms like inflammatory reactions. With the growing realization of the effects of SARS-CoV-2 on various organ systems, clinicians must be alert to such a possibility, realizing that worsening of patients could be due to these complex clinical presentations. This underscores the need for an integrative perspective on the etiology of respiratory virus symptoms and the potential long-term impact on the health of the patients (Vonck et al., 2020).

2.3.1. Common Symptoms Associated with Respiratory Viruses

The symptoms witnessed with respiratory viruses are likely to present predominantly in the upper and lower respiratory tracts and, as such, produce diverse clinical presentations. The most frequent upper respiratory manifestations include nasal stuffiness, nasal discharge, sore throat, and cough, which typically accompany viral infections such as rhinovirus and parainfluenza. The symptoms are more acute in nature and range from mild to severe and, as such, present many to the hospital. Lower respiratory symptoms, such as wheeze and dyspnea, indicate potential lower airway involvement, particularly in vulnerable populations. As stated, early viral infections correlated with augmented neutrophilic inflammation and bacterial pathogens in infected patients, demonstrating the intricacies of the immune response elicited by respiratory viruses (Davis et al., 2019). It is necessary to understand the spectrum of these symptoms for appropriate diagnosis and treatment, especially in populations like infants with underlying disease. A problem with the treatment of respiratory viral infections is overlapping symptoms with bacterial infections, and therefore, clinical distinction is difficult. For instance, a productive cough and chest pain could be caused by pneumonia, which is typically bacterial, but there are similar symptoms arising from an infection that is viral. In an infant cohort study of cystic fibrosis, previous viral infections were highly correlated with elevated neutrophil counts in bronchoalveolar lavage, illustrating the effect of exacerbation of underlying pulmonary status due to infections (Deschamp et al., 2015) (Figure 2.9).

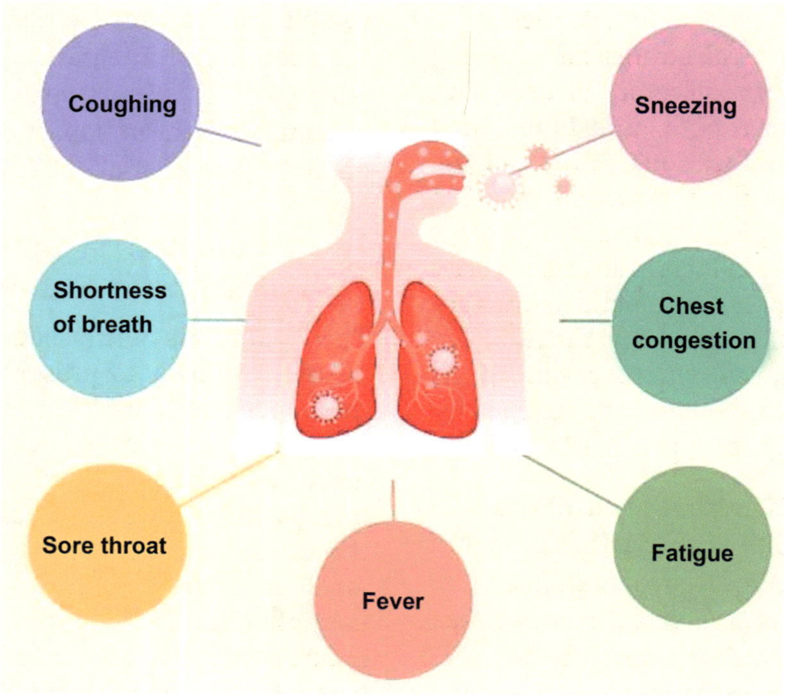

Figure 2.9. Respiratory infection symptoms.

Source: https://continentalhospitals.com/uploads/mceu_76758755211707805028591.jpg.

These complicating factors underscore the need for thorough clinical assessment and diagnostic laboratory analysis, e.g., viral swabs, upon presenting with respiratory illness. Identification of the specific virus can trigger more targeted treatment regimens, reducing unnecessary antibiotic use, which is typically applied in respiratory-related issues. The onset and duration of symptoms can also vary depending on the specific respiratory virus. For instance, influenza will more frequently present with more serious systemic symptoms such as fever and myalgias, along with respiratory distress, while rhinovirus infections may predominantly present with mild features. This distinction has extremely significant implications for public health since, although influenza can lead to significantly greater morbidity and mortality, particularly among high-risk persons such as the elderly and those with chronic underlying medical conditions, infections with rhinovirus may only lead to minimal presentation. The interplay among initial viral infections and the development of inflammation in the lungs, particularly among infants, as identified in various studies, underscores the importance of prevention and early intervention measures (Davis et al., 2019). Knowledge of such distinctions informs public health programs to prevent the transmission and impact of respiratory viruses among populations.

2.3.2. Severe Cases and Complications

Severe infections of respiratory viruses are common among vulnerable populations, including the elderly and those with comorbid disease. In these patients, influenza virus and RSV infections can cause severe complications, including viral pneumonia and bronchitis. The interaction between the host immune status and the virulence of the virus tends to determine disease progression.

Above all, viral pneumonia, characterized by lung inflammation and consolidation, can establish itself and infect rapidly in immunocompromised and chronically ill patients to cause life-threatening conditions. With the population aging and increasing numbers of immunocompromised cases reported, the incidence of severe respiratory viral illnesses as well as their complications becomes increasingly common, leading healthcare professionals to concentrate on early detection and intervention strategies to prevent adverse outcomes (Cesario, 2012) (Figure 2.10).

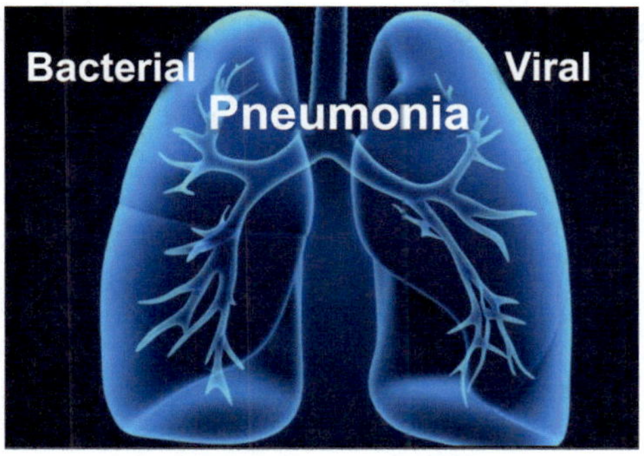

Figure 2.10. Bacterial pneumonia.

Source: https://i.ytimg.com/vi/eJppC_W_LnQ/maxresdefault.jpg.

Their mortality and morbidity are underlined by their capacity to cause an abrupt worsening of patients' conditions. RSV is one such example that predominantly affects infants and the elderly and is typified by its capacity to cause worsening of already compromised respiratory states and result in acute conditions such as bronchiolitis and pneumonia. A high number of children with acute respiratory infection admitted to the hospital experience comorbidities, making treatment and outcome even more challenging. Hospitalization is tremendously elevated among infants younger than three months old, particularly those with hypoxemia, which indicates an urgent need for close monitoring and supportive care during outbreaks. Severe infections entail serious implications, indicating the necessity of understanding the epidemiology patterns and determinants of risk associated with respiratory viruses, since they have wide-ranging implications on public health in addition to clinical practice (Bakir et al., 2014). Effective management of severe cases of respiratory viral infections depends on immediate employment of curative and preventative measures. Antiviral medication treatment early on may be helpful in certain viral infections, though such treatments are not applicable across all pathogens. For RSV, for example, preventative measures, including application of monoclonal antibodies to high-risk infants, demonstrate a reduction in the prevalence of severe disease. Also, the role of vaccination in preventing complications caused by influenza cannot be overstated, as annual campaigns for vaccination contribute significantly to reducing hospitalizations and deaths due to severe respiratory illnesses. By enhancing our understanding of the complexities surrounding severe infection and complications of respiratory viruses, we shall be in a position to prepare health systems better for efficient responding during outbreaks and enhance patient care in intensive care units (Cesario, 2012).

2.3.3. Differences in Symptoms Among Various Viruses

Dissimilarity in the manifestations of various respiratory viruses is of significant significance in diagnosis and therapeutic interventions. The influenza viruses, for example, exhibit a sudden onset of high temperature, chills, and muscle aches, which can progress rapidly to more acute respiratory features such as cough and dyspnea. In contrast, the rhinoviruses cause primarily mild symptoms such as a runny nose, sore throat, and sneezing. This heterogeneity in symptomatology will most commonly lead to misdiagnosis, particularly at peak flu season when influenza and rhinoviruses co-circulate.

Furthermore, fever is a distinguishing symptom of influenza, whereas lack of fever typically signifies infection by the rhinoviruses. Therefore, it is essential for clinicians to become well-informed about these nuances of symptom profiles to be in a position to differentiate between respiratory viral infections and to undergo appropriate and timely treatment, thereby improving patient outcomes. Additionally, the subtype and lineage of respiratory viruses may influence the severity and nature of symptoms presented by infected individuals. Studies on influenza B viruses, i.e., the B/Victoria and B/Yamagata lineages, determined that symptoms were significantly different across age groups. B/Victoria virus infected a younger population, commonly found in the community, while B/Yamagata viruses tended to have a greater incidence in hospitalized patients with evidence of more severe disease. Infection symptoms that could be displayed by B/Yamagata might include longer respiratory distress and complications in patients who are hospitalized, as opposed to the more benign community-based B/Victoria infections. These findings underscore the necessity for continuous surveillance and awareness of lineage-specific patterns in order to effectively manage viral infections and formulate suitably designed vaccination programs because the differential symptoms have an impact on treatment and vaccine compositions (Alicino et al., 2018) (Figure 2.11).

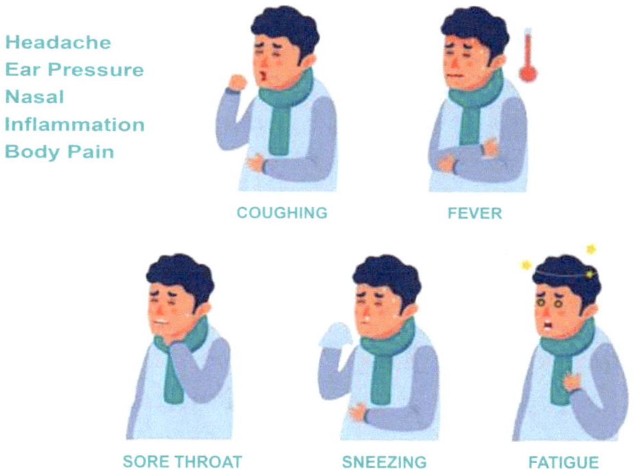

Figure 2.11. Symptoms of rhinovirus infection.

Source: https://vitrosens.com/what-is-rhinovirus-how-does-the-rhinovirus-test-kit-work/.

Moreover, the cross-talk between specific respiratory viruses and host immune reactions might lead to varied levels of lung damage and symptom presentations. Investigations on severe acute respiratory syndrome (SARS) and the 2009 H1N1 influenza pandemic highlighted that individual viral infections could induce heterogeneous inflammatory responses, which significantly influence clinical outcomes. For example, while H1N1 might cause severe acute lung injury after robust immune responses, the underlying mechanisms of epithelial and endothelial damage remain complicated and not well understood. The presentation of such diseases might be variable, with H1N1 causing extreme amounts of respiratory distress and inflammation. Less severe respiratory signs and systemic manifestations might be seen with other viruses. It is important to understand such intricate processes to develop focused therapies that will be able to abrogate lung injury and promote recovery from respiratory viral infections, increasing the standard of care in practice (Hendrickson & Matthay, 2013).

2.4. Diagnosis of Respiratory Viral Infections

Diagnosis of respiratory viral infections is crucial in guiding effective treatment and management options. Physicians employ an array of diagnostic modalities, from the conventional to emerging molecular technologies. Polymerase chain reaction (PCR) has gained popularity due to its specificity and sensitivity for the identification of viral nucleic acids. The test facilitates the identification of several respiratory viruses, such as influenza, respiratory syncytial virus, and adenovirus. But PCR interpretation is made difficult by remaining viral RNA from previous infections that can generate false positives. In sub-Saharan Africa and elsewhere, the diagnostic approach that is presently available is evolving. The conventional cultural methods tend to be inadequate since isolation of fastidious viruses in clinical specimens has been problematic, indicating the necessity for more advanced testing methods capable of differentiating viral from bacterial etiology with accuracy (Ho, 2014). The increased appreciation of respiratory viruses as the main generators of respiratory disease, particularly among vulnerable groups, confirms the need for accurate diagnosis. Viral pneumonia has been described to differ in prevalence and etiology considerably between different geographic regions, particularly in sub-Saharan Africa, where co-morbid conditions complicate diagnosis and treatment. Its sophisticated understanding can inform public health programs that would de-intensify these diseases. An integration of epidemiological information with clinical presentation enables distinguishing viral from bacterial infections, hence better management of the patient. As highlighted in studies of Hajj pilgrim respiratory infections, immediate data gathering and monitoring are essential to understand patterns of viral transmission and guide preventive interventions (Al-Tawfiq et al., 2018). International collaboration to create standardized diagnostic protocols is required by this. New technologies hold the key to transforming respiratory virus diagnosis by enabling swift and accurate identification. Point-of-care testing, using next-generation sequencing, promises near-real-time surveillance of outbreaks and deeper insight into viral evolution. Future advances in molecular diagnostics have the potential to create improved outbreak preparedness and response plans. Global access to these technologies in resource-poor settings is also needed, where conventional diagnostic methods may be suboptimal. By utilizing widespread surveillance and accepting multi-modal diagnostic approaches, health systems can enhance their capacity to effectively treat respiratory viral infections. This is particularly imperative as the epidemiology of respiratory viruses continues to change internationally due to human action, environmental factors, and the interaction of viral genetics, necessitating flexible, creative diagnostic response within the health system (Ho, 2014).

2.4.1. Laboratory Testing Methods

Evaluation of laboratory testing methods for respiratory viruses is important in the accurate diagnosis of infection. Recent studies show that multiplex reverse transcriptase polymerase chain reaction (RT-PCR) is the optimal method due to its good sensitivity and specificity. In research conducted on older adults with respiratory tract infections (RTI), RT-PCR using the Luminex xTAG Respiral Viral Panel detected 100% of positive samples compared to other diagnostic tests. For instance, standard cultures and rapid tests produced significantly lower detection rates, reinforcing the necessity for new methods in clinical settings (She et al., 2010). Given that respiratory viruses are bound to be prevalent, accurate testing is of the essence for effective management, control, and treatment of the infections, particularly in risk groups such as the elderly. The laboratory testing serves more than just diagnosis; it affects clinical decision-making and public health measures. The evidence shows that elderly patients' losses contain smaller titers of respiratory viruses and need to be tested using assays capable of detecting even minute levels of viral RNA with precision. Because standard techniques such as direct fluorescent antibody testing and rapid antigen testing were not very effective in detecting viruses among the elderly, RT-PCR has become critical. This is particularly critical in the event of respiratory virus outbreaks, as early treatment can significantly lower morbidity and mortality levels. In addition, extensive testing in asymptomatic carriers can support understanding of virus transmission dynamics and vaccination policy and public policy in the midst of national and global health crises, such as those certified as a pandemic by agencies like the World Health Organization (Relich & Abbott, 2018) (Figure 2.12).

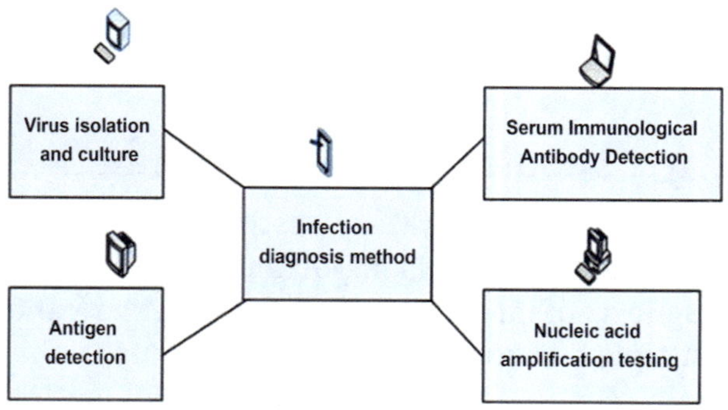

Figure 2.12. Laboratory diagnostic methods for respiratory viral infections.

Source: https://www.researchgate.net/figure/Laboratory-diagnostic-methods-for-respiratory-viral-infections_fig2_363887373.

Laboratory diagnosis methods for respiratory viruses have significant implications for both clinical practice and epidemiology. The established efficacy of RT-PCR, particularly in discriminating infection among elderly individuals, underscores the imperative for ongoing research and adaptation of testing regimes. Physicians must stay current with the merits and liabilities of alternative tests in order to refine their diagnostic strategy according to current best evidence. Although respiratory viral infections continue to pose a public health threat, improved laboratory techniques need to be developed and utilized in order to adequately monitor and control them. Thus, the continuous evaluation of test modalities will not only increase the diagnostic accuracy but also enhance the resilience of global health facilities against future epidemics of respiratory viruses.

2.4.2. Clinical Evaluation Techniques

Clinically diagnosing respiratory viruses requires a multidisciplinary solution that employs numerous varied diagnostic techniques to allow for enhanced accuracy and speed. Of these techniques, molecular testing, particularly reverse transcription polymerase chain reaction (RT-PCR), has become the gold standard due to high specificity and sensitivity. These procedures can detect viral RNA within hours, something important for effective infection control and containment strategies. Rapid and precise diagnoses are particularly significant in outbreaks, such as the outbreak of the 2019-nCoV virus, where early treatment can be a dramatic game-changer for transmission patterns and health status. Greater emphasis on rapid diagnosis capacity underlines the significance of current research and development in techniques able to deliver precise results in high-pressure situations, thereby facilitating public health action and patient care schemes (Du et al., 2020) (Figure 2.13).

Under clinical sample examination of patients with respiratory infections, the choice of diagnostic test used plays a major role in confirming viral pathogens. Comparative studies on various laboratory tests reveal striking differences in their detection capacity. Multiplex

RT-PCR testing, for instance, utilizes advanced diagnostic technology that provides a very high detection rate and has the capacity to detect multiple respiratory viruses simultaneously. This is particularly useful in populations such as older individuals, who may have atypical viral loads, thereby complicating the diagnosis. Tests showed that standard methods such as rapid antigen tests and viral cultures were significantly less effective in detecting viral infections in this age group, indicating that high-sensitivity tests such as RT-PCR would be needed.

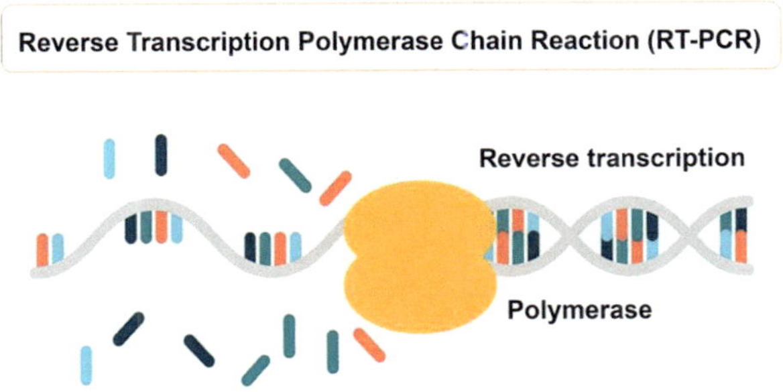

Figure 2.13. Reverse transcription polymerase chain reaction (RT-PCR).

Source: https://external-content.duckduckgo.com/iu/?u=https%3A%2F%2Fmicrobiologynotes.org%2Fwp-content%2Fuploads%2F2021%2F03%2FReverse-transcription-polymerase-chain-reaction-RT-PCR.jpg&f=1&nofb=1&ipt=5c0dd8063e3dae9a52c3eabaf1001f98ac87ba09729fb01e00dc1756e187ed83.

This shift in take-up of techniques reflects the evolving scenario of viral diagnosis in clinical practice (She et al., 2010). Moreover, the use of such clinical evaluation techniques not only enhances the knowledge regarding respiratory viruses but also facilitates increased therapeutic interventions and patient management. Through the use of an integrated diagnostic testing approach, healthcare workers can ascertain the etiological reason for respiratory disease more efficiently. This is critical in guiding appropriate disinfectant treatment regimens, reducing unnecessary antibiotic use, and improving the overall patient outcome. Harmonization of clinical routines with next-generation diagnostic methods emphasizes the need for ongoing interdisciplinary research, which will drive the development of next-generation assays for effectively responding to future respiratory viruses. Consequently, the focus on clinical assessment techniques reflects a core aspect of public health policy aimed at diminishing the impact of viral respiratory infections on global people's health (She et al., 2010).

2.4.3. Challenges in Accurate Diagnosis

Accurate diagnosis of respiratory viruses is a complex issue that has a significant impact on patient outcomes as well as public health administration. One of the major difficulties lies in overlapping symptoms common to most respiratory infections, which tend to confuse medical professionals. Respiratory viruses like influenza, RSV, and coronaviruses often present similar clinical features such as fever, cough, and exhaustion. This symptom overlap can lead to misdiagnosis or inappropriate delays in effective treatment, complicating outbreak control and potentially exacerbating the severity of disease among at-risk groups. Moreover, the dynamic evolutionary nature of respiratory viruses complicates diagnosis further, as newly arising strains have differential pathogenic profiles, so diagnostic pathways have to be able to match the pace of change in viral epidemiology. Technology improvements in diagnostic tools, such as clinical metagenomic next-generation sequencing (mNGS), possess the potential for higher accuracy but bring with them their own challenges. Though mNGS makes it possible to analyze the microbial and host genomic materials in detail and facilitates an expedient diagnosis of a number of pathogens simultaneously, its use in the clinical setting is fraught with difficulties. Aspects such as high costs, technical ability requirements, and the need for standardization procedures remain the current restraints to large-scale uptake in clinical laboratories. Further, an excess of data generated with the aid of mNGS overwhelms physicians, especially if pertinent results are not well prioritized. Such challenges must be addressed for the mNGS to realize its full potential in the accurate diagnosis of respiratory viruses, which will ultimately lead to enhanced patient care and outcomes (Chiu et al., 2019) (Figure 2.14).

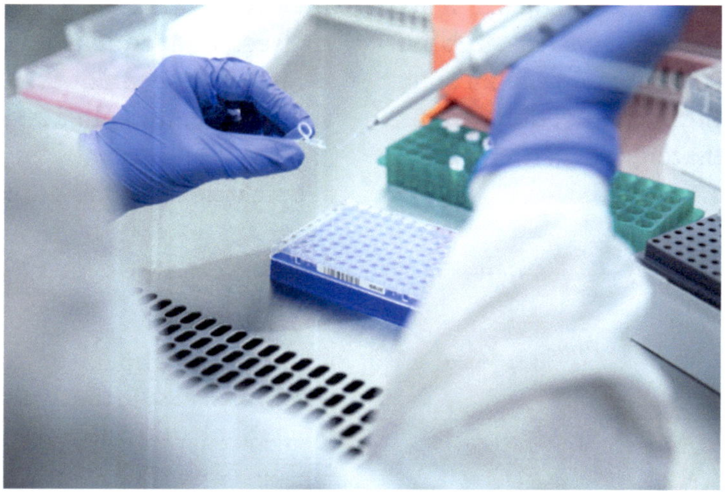

Figure 2.14. Accurate diagnosis of respiratory viruses.

Source: https://external-content.duckduckgo.com/iu/?u=https%3A%2F%2Fwww.infectiousdiseaseadvisor.com%2Fwp-content%2Fuploads%2Fsites%2F16%2F2024%2F08%2FCOVID.Lab_.Testing_G_1327475879.jpg&f=1&nofb=1&ipt=ae686a6ce8696566c1a28d48305baf4ca7ec62832840c4f310701707ca633b9a.

Also, the unexpected emergence of pandemics, as evidenced by the global COVID-19 pandemic, has prompted the demand for advanced diagnostic methods. While health practitioners within the public health field are trying to contain outbreaks, prompt identification of causes is imperative; however, existing diagnostic systems do not keep pace with increased demand. Furthermore, disparities in the availability of advanced diagnostic equipment across different health systems can exacerbate diagnostic hurdles. Restricted resource availability in poor nations may lead to reliance on less sensitive conventional methods, thus underestimating the prevalence and patterns of viruses and actual transmission. An effort to develop and distribute low-cost, accurate diagnostic methods that can rapidly adapt to future respiratory viruses must, thus, be made to efficiently track and contain all populations during the occurrence of new infectious epidemics (Al-Tawfiq & Memish, 2014).

2.5. Treatment and Management

Management of respiratory viruses is multidisciplinary, particularly in high-risk populations such as children with malignancies or recipients of hematopoietic stem cell transplants. Bacterial and fungal infections have long been the focus of attention. The recent recrudescence of viral pathogens as important causes of illness mandates that management be reconsidered. In the absence of a number of effective antiviral drugs, prevention is paramount. This involves severe pre-exposure and post-exposure prophylaxis as well as the initiation of antiviral suppressive therapeutic regimens. An intense infection control policy tailored to the needs of such patients can effectively counteract the harmful effects of viral infections, eventually resulting in enhancing patient outcomes and reducing morbidity and mortality due to such pathogens (Fisher et al., 2012). Advances in diagnostic technology are key to effective management and treatment of respiratory viruses. Clinical metagenomic next-generation sequencing (mNGS) is a significant innovation in the rapid and precise detection of viral pathogens. The comprehensive analysis of microbial and host genetic material enables the early diagnosis of respiratory viruses, which can lead to timely and appropriate therapeutic interventions. mNGS is not only helpful in diagnosing infectious diseases, but also in informing antimicrobial resistance patterns and microbiome to clinicians to make it even more accurate in treatment. The application of mNGS in clinical laboratories has challenges, though, and that should be addressed in order to maximize the potential impact of mNGS in patient care. Successful incorporation of mNGS into standard diagnostic regimens implies that physicians can quickly counter respiratory viral infections with targeted management strategies (Chiu et al., 2019). Effective treatment of respiratory viruses must also involve supportive care interventions to alleviate symptoms and facilitate recovery. Patients tend to have fever, cough, and fatigue, which can play a huge role in their quality of life. Supportive management methods such as hydration, rest, and symptomatic relief with antipyretics and analgesics are essential components of the management. Furthermore, treatment such as oxygen therapy can be initiated in patients with severe respiratory distress to ensure adequate oxygenation while avoiding complications. With the altered epidemiology of viral respiratory infections, it is of utmost importance that treating clinicians remain vigilant and adaptable in the management of these conditions. By combining antiviral interventions with firm supportive care, healthcare systems can provide comprehensive management for patients presented with the issue of respiratory viruses and ultimately improve outcomes and foster resilience in the healthcare community.

2.5.1. Antiviral Medications

Antiviral medications are of critical relevance in the therapy of respiratory viral infections, particularly those caused by influenza viruses. Unlike antibiotics that act against bacterial infections, antivirals are specifically employed to inhibit virus replication in the host. In the context of respiratory viruses such as influenza, medications oseltamivir and zanamivir can do well to reduce the duration and also minimize the severity of the symptoms if administered early in the course of illness. This antiviral therapy is most beneficial in high-risk groups, including the elderly and patients with co-morbid conditions. A proper use of antivirals at the right time will prevent complications, thereby minimizing hospitalization and death from severe cases of influenza. Moreover, ongoing research continues to be devoted to finding newer antiviral agents that are specifically directed against the viral mechanism for greater effectiveness against new mutant resistant strains. The complex interplay between viral infections and the immune system mandates a nuanced strategy towards antiviral therapy. For instance, while antivirals are known to suppress symptoms and reduce viral loads, their success is generally reliant on early diagnosis and treatment. As highlighted by studies comparing rapid viral diagnosis testing, the inclusion of such tests in clinics can inform therapeutic antiviral prescribing and thus enhance patient outcomes (Bang et al., 2019) (Figure 2.15).

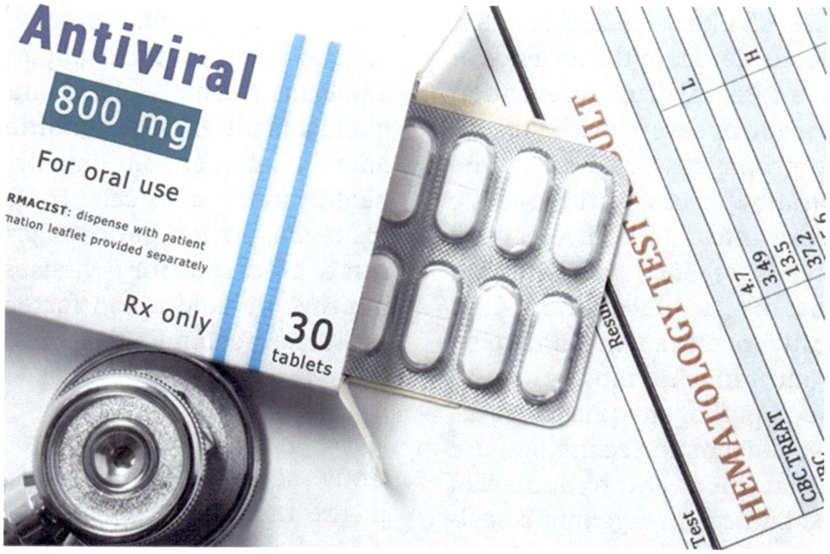

Figure 2.15. Antiviral medications play a critical role in managing respiratory viral infections.

Source: https://www.eehealth.org/-/media/images/modules/blog/posts/2021/06/hd-life-covid-antiviral-medication.jpg.

Quick diagnosis permits physicians to distinguish between viral and bacterial infections, reducing the improper prescription of antibiotics, which is critical in the fight against antibiotic resistance. Hence, the utilization of fast diagnostic tools, accompanied by effective antiviral therapies, is a multi-pronged response to counter respiratory viruses and optimize patient treatment. Despite the benefits that antiviral medication provides, barriers to its accessibility and resistance occurrence persist. Unavailability of certain antiviral drugs, coupled with resistant viral strains, poses unique challenges to effective treatment. An example is the observation by the Centers for Disease Control and Prevention that resistance patterns of antiviral drugs are seasonal- and region-dependent, necessitating ongoing monitoring. Furthermore, patient adherence to ordered antiviral regimens also impacts the outcome of treatment. To ensure optimal use of antiviral drugs, there is an urgent need for public health intervention that informs people about the symptoms of respiratory viruses and the importance of early treatment. By working discreetly through these constraints, a more robust infrastructure for antiviral application can be established, which will, in turn, improve public health responses to respiratory viral infection outbreaks.

2.5.2. Supportive Care Strategies

Supportive care management plays a key role in the treatment of respiratory viruses, particularly in viral infections that result in mild to severe manifestations. Symptomatic relief, maintenance of respiratory status, and complication prevention are the primary objectives of supportive care. For instance, in acute viral pneumonia, protective ventilation of the lung has been identified as necessary. Even more so, when the condition is associated with acute lung injury (ALI) (Hendrickson & Matthay, 2013). The approach seeks to minimize ventilator-induced lung injury via the use of decreased tidal volumes and optimization of oxygenation without exacerbating the underlying compromised respiratory condition. Supportive treatment is also comprised of hydration, nutritional support, and application of antipyretics, all of which contribute to enhancing patient comfort and convalescence. Proper implementation of such interventions can enhance the body's native resistance to viral infections, particularly if lung defenses have been compromised by the virus. In spite of the emphasis on care that is supportive, therapy for respiratory viral infections often has physicians resorting to antibiotic treatment. This is particularly so in the developing world, where physicians prescribe antibiotics hoping they will prevent the evolution into more severe acute respiratory infections (ARI). Nonetheless, a trial that evaluated the effectiveness of ampicillin with supportive care failed to find any significant increase in recovery rates among children with mild ARI (Frerichs et al., 1991). These results underscore the importance of prioritizing supportive care over unnecessary antibiotic prescription since overuse can lead to increasing antibiotic resistance without providing any clinically important gain. Therefore, healthcare workers need to understand the distinction between viral and bacterial infections, with more focus on support interventions that positively contribute to the recovery of the patient and less focus on drug-based treatments that are of little benefit in viral infections. The role of the supportive care approach extends beyond symptom management; it has a direct impact on the overall health care approach to managing viral respiratory infections. Education of patients and caregivers regarding the importance of supportive care can significantly enhance patient participation and compliance with treatment. Prevention of dehydration and nutritional support, as well as symptomatic management, not only improves recovery but also decreases the risk of developing secondary complications that are associated with viral infections (Hendrickson & Matthay, 2013). Furthermore, community-oriented programs aimed at supportive care resources, such as self-care ability and detection of warning signs of disease deterioration, can reinforce health outcomes even further. Encouraging an integrated knowledge of supportive care helps healthcare systems prepare individuals better to deal with the complexities of respiratory viruses in a productive way, leading to improved individual and public health responses to viral epidemics.

2.5.3. Public Health Interventions

Public health interventions play a major role in safeguarding against the impact of respiratory viruses, especially in vulnerable populations such as children. One of the best examples is vitamin D supplementation, which has been increasingly in the spotlight for its ability to enhance immune function and reduce the burden of upper respiratory tract infections (URTIs). Research indicates that a high proportion of children in North America are inadequately vitamin D, particularly during winter, and this is associated with higher rates of respiratory disease and asthma complications (Maguire et al., 2014). Through randomized controlled trials to assess the effectiveness of various doses of vitamin D, health practitioners and policymakers aim to establish the most effective regimens of supplementation that can prevent viral infections and lower the expenditure on healthcare for these common conditions among young children. Interventions focusing on hygiene practices also play a significant role in preventing the spread of respiratory viruses. Education initiatives focusing on the importance of hand washing and respiratory hygiene have proven to be effective interventions in reducing infection levels. Such interventions are particularly relevant in settings such as schools and daycare facilities, where the viruses quickly disseminate among children. More insight into the role of disgust in pathogen avoidance can also help in such endeavors, as higher disgust sensitivity individuals have been noted to have more preventive behaviors against getting sick (De Barra et al., 2014). Such blending of psychological insight and education may thus help towards a more holistic public health approach towards reducing the burden of respiratory infections. Finally, mass vaccination campaigns against respiratory viruses are a key public health intervention. Vaccines have been a key factor in preventing outbreaks of infections such as influenza, which constitutes a major threat to both adults and children. Implementing mass vaccination campaigns, along with public education regarding the use of immunization, can reliably improve vaccination coverage. Moreover, immunizing at-risk groups, i.e., children and older adults, ensures that the most susceptible populations receive the benefits of vaccination. Therefore, ongoing funding for vaccine research and public health initiatives is important in the continued fight against respiratory viruses. Through vaccination for building group immunity and coupling it with nutrition and behavioral health interventions, public health leaders can drastically inhibit the transmission and impact of respiratory infections.

2.6. Prevention Strategies

Prevention measures for respiratory viruses have advanced by leaps and bounds, with the focus primarily on both vaccination and novel therapeutic approaches. Vaccination has provided the cornerstone of viral infection prevention for hundreds of years, enabling herd immunity to be achieved and morbidity and mortality due to respiratory viruses to be significantly reduced. However, some viruses are not candidates for vaccine development due to various reasons, such as genetic variability or safety. This limitation has steered research towards other methods of prevention, which include the innovative method referred to as Biochemical Prevention and Treatment, to leverage monoclonal antibodies for this purpose and possibly other protein-based therapies to block viral entry and replication. Such advances are likely to transform our response to respiratory viruses, particularly in those at risk who cannot be vaccinated safely, thereby enhancing overall public health (Fang et al., 2004). Understanding the environmental and socio-economic determinants of the transmission of respiratory viruses is of immense benefit in making comprehensive prevention strategies. The majority of pandemics-causing viruses, as noted, are animal-derived and could be initiated by environmental changes, human behavior, and global travel. This calls for the establishment of more effective surveillance systems based on the use of modern technologies for the identification of potential zoonotic agents prior to their jumping to the human population. Interventions can then be focused based on data gathering and analysis of points of intersection between animal and human health.

In addition, such interventions allow for dynamic risk assessments that are sensitive to emerging data, thereby aiming efforts to prevent viruses most likely to cause the highest risk to human health (Morse et al., 2012). Such proactive initiatives are critical not only for stemming outbreaks but also for establishing a model for long-term public health resiliency. In addition, public health education and public participation are critical to the effectiveness of prevention strategies against respiratory viruses. By building an educated population, health authorities can provide a basis for ensuring recommended behaviors such as hand hygiene, mask wearing, and getting vaccinated when available are practiced. These behavioral changes are especially important during epidemics, as they have the potential to lower transmission levels significantly. Educational efforts focusing on the role of personal responsibility and collective action have the potential to empower people to take an active role in their health and in that of the community. Along with advancements in medical treatments, such an extensive initiative can better control the impact of respiratory viruses and enable societies to resist future infections, ultimately leading to lesser health care spending and improved quality of life for individuals across the globe (Figure 2.16).

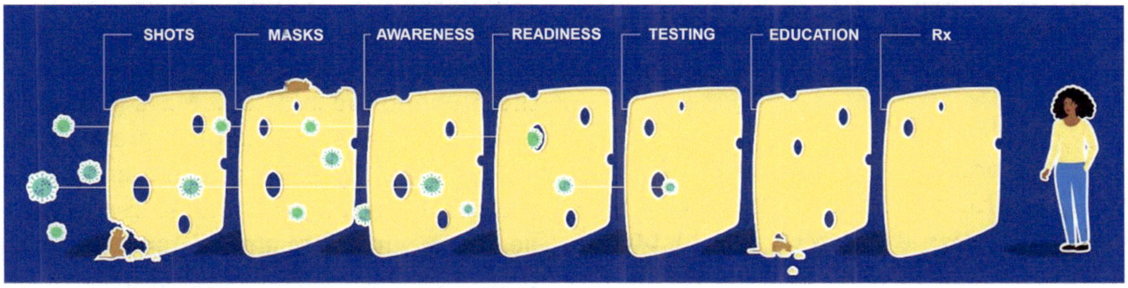

Figure 2.16. Smarter steps for respiratory viruses prevention.

Source: https://www.cdph.ca.gov/Programs/CID/DCDC/PublishingImages/COVID-19/SMARTER_Graphic.png.

2.6.1. Vaccination Programs

Vaccination programs are significant components in the management of respiratory viruses, particularly in the prevention of outbreaks of diseases such as influenza. Using particular vaccination approaches, public health officials can substantially curtail both morbidity and mortality rates for the disease. A comprehensive knowledge of viral infectious dynamics allows stakeholders to efficiently assign priorities to vaccination programs. Current evidence suggests that mortality-based strategies are optimal when transmission rates are high and the most susceptible are given priority. Conversely, in moderately transmissible strains, morbidity-based strategies addressing broader, high-prevalence groups could prove more effective. These considerations highlight the importance of adaptive vaccination campaigns that account for real-time epidemiology, which is important in curbing respiratory virus transmission in outbreak settings (Bansal et al., 2006). Economic implications of vaccination schemes extend beyond public health benefits to the extent that they also pose important financial implications. Its cost-benefit relationship using widespread vaccination as a measure with respect to respiratory viruses can surpass the economic cost of probable outbreaks. For instance, the moral of Aujeszky's disease in swine that early vaccination significantly puts the brake on virus transmission and safeguards productivity is the necessity of intervention in early stages. Studies show that early vaccination covering more than 75% of a susceptible population minimizes the negative economic effects following an outbreak, which is also the case with human respiratory virus scenarios. This illustrative model illustrates the manner in which vaccine investment not only sustains health but also sustains economic stability in outbreak-affected communities (Colomer et al., 2020). In addition, immunization campaigns can enable herd immunity, hence covering even the population that cannot be vaccinated on medical grounds. This principle is central to public health policy, especially in the face of respiratory viruses that can infect many. Through enough vaccination coverage, populations are able to reduce the transmission rates of the viruses significantly, ultimately safeguarding the most susceptible. Nevertheless, this comes at the cost of active participation in public health initiatives to enhance vaccination among the population. It is essential to educate people about the safety and efficacy of vaccines to encourage the population's participation, especially during mass vaccination campaigns. In this manner, vaccinations become not only personal protection but also mass protection from the dissemination of respiratory epidemics, highlighting the need to maintain continued efforts in public health immunization programs (Bansal et al., 2006).

2.6.2. Hygiene Practices

Proper hygiene practices are necessary in order to prevent respiratory viruses from spreading. Such viruses, if they are very severe in their illness, usually spread through respiratory droplets that are released when an individual sneezes, coughs, or speaks. In such a group setting, particularly with schools or daycares, the likelihood of an outbreak is higher in case no good hygiene practices are followed. Encouraging frequent handwashing and hand sanitizer usage has become a core infection control strategy. These practices effectively lower the levels of viral pathogens on surfaces and the skin, hence the chances of spreading infections. Apart from that, routine cleaning practices, particularly for the high-touch sites, must be exercised by the schools because such routines greatly contribute to maintaining the healthy environment for the children who are susceptible to severe respiratory illnesses (Fisher et al., 2012). Apart from hand washing, respiratory hygiene practices play a vital role in averting the risk of respiratory viral infections. Sneezing or coughing onto an elbow or tissue, and not the hands, is a vital preventive measure. People can restrict droplet transmission by making such acts a habit, thus protecting peers and vulnerable individuals. Public campaigns to educate individuals regarding the importance of respiratory hygiene can trigger a shift in cultural hygiene attitudes, resulting in increased accountability while in shared settings. Because evidence indicates that respiratory viruses have the potential to produce great morbidity as well as health expenditures, implementing these hygiene practices is all the more necessary. Such preventive measures are not just capable of protecting individuals but also can limit healthcare system burdens over the most infectious months (Marcone et al., 2015). Finally, the incorporation of hygiene practices into routine public health policy is required in order to diminish the impact of respiratory viruses, particularly given their economic burden. Mass immunization campaigns and adequate hygiene education can significantly enhance community resilience against respiratory infections. In regions where health resources are limited, targeted campaigns that encourage raising individuals' awareness of correct hygiene procedures can prove to be of significant assistance. For instance, in middle-income countries, the understanding of the prevalence of respiratory disease can allow health authorities to target interventions to enhance hygiene and, in doing so, reduce infection rates and associated hospitalizations (Marcone et al., 2015). By employing hygiene interventions within a comprehensive public health strategy, we may establish an effective multi-component approach both to forestall and control respiratory virus outbreaks among the population.

2.6.3. Public Awareness Campaigns

Public awareness campaigns play a central role in preventing and controlling respiratory viruses, especially during the era of disinformation when public health crises are compounded. By educating members of the community about what such viruses are, how they are transmitted, and how they can be countered, public awareness campaigns can significantly contribute to community awareness. For instance, a study done in Shaikh Zayed Medical College revealed that while medical students were found to have sufficient knowledge on swine flu transmission and etiological agents, there were knowledge gaps in the areas of vaccination and prevention (Bakhtawar et al., 2020). Reducing such knowledge gaps with accurate awareness campaigns may assist in generating more vigilant populations, likely to take preventive actions against respiratory diseases. Effective public awareness campaigns typically employ several strategies to reach out to various groups, framing messages in a way that will resonate with the target group. In respiratory viruses, outreach programs have utilized clinics, schools, and social media platforms to disseminate key information. Intervention by education has been found to effectively change the attitude of patients towards antibiotic use, resulting in improved knowledge on the appropriate use of antibiotics (Bell et al., 2019). These findings suggest that similar action could be applied in respiratory virus education, where knowledge content can enable individuals to identify symptoms, receive appropriate medical care, and perform preventative health behaviors. In addition, success in public education campaigns for respiratory viruses relies on multidisciplinary collaboration between healthcare professionals, educators, and community leaders. By facilitating collaboration between these stakeholders, campaigns can leverage mixed expertise to disseminate unified and credible messages. The above scenario of antibiotic awareness illustrates that while patient-focused education could enhance knowledge and attitudes, the addition of clinician education enhances the effect of such programs (Bell et al., 2019). This synergy is evident particularly when looking at respiratory viruses, where timely and accurate information can lead to reduced rates of transmission and improved health outcomes in the community, ultimately lessening the impact of respiratory infections.

SUMMARY

The research on respiratory viruses indicates that such pathogens have a huge impact on public health and must be under constant surveillance and research. The emergence of new strains such as the respiratory syncytial virus (RSV) BA genotype demonstrates the dynamic nature of viral evolution and the difficulty it poses in disease control. Above all, the emergence of new group B viruses in Kenya raises critical questions about viral persistence and transmissibility and therefore necessitates close observation for the purpose of informing public health interventions. Such emergence of respiratory viruses underscores the importance of adaptive research tools for understanding the pathogens and implementing timely interventions to curb their impact on human health, particularly in vulnerable populations. Additionally, having regard to the ramifications of respiratory viruses extends beyond human illness, as with animals, for example, horses. Underestimated viral pathogens can cause severe respiratory distress and disease in equines, which, in turn, also pose threats to animal welfare and agricultural productivity. The findings of research showing the prevalence of gamma herpesviruses in symptomatic horses reveal an urgent need for robust diagnostic protocols to accurately detect and trace such infections. Incorporating these into larger surveillance activities could enhance our preparedness to respond to potential respiratory disease outbreaks across species, as much for the health of equines as it is for protecting public health interests. Lastly, the response to the multifaceted problem generated by respiratory viruses requires an integrative approach that bridges data from different health arenas. National and global networks for surveillance, in addition to interdisciplinary research studies, have to be prioritized so that the risk factors of respiratory pathogens may be overcome. For instance, findings of the study on the endemicity of some viruses in human beings as well as horses can be utilized in formulating specific vaccination and treatment strategies. By our advocacy for collaborative research linking human and animal health, we can enhance our capability to address the changing epidemiology of respiratory viruses and respond appropriately, making an effective public health response with a focus on prevention and early detection.

Respiratory viruses are a wide variety of pathogens with significant implications for public health. Of significant note are the influenza viruses, respiratory syncytial virus (RSV), and coronaviruses that induce acute respiratory illness in different age groups. Understanding their characteristics and modes of transmission is crucial. For instance, influenza viruses are capable of antigenic shift and drift, such that vaccine preparation and effectiveness become difficult. Besides, respiratory syncytial virus is particularly prevalent in infants and toddlers, with a propensity to develop bronchiolitis and pneumonia. The prevalence of coronaviruses, i.e., SARS-CoV-2, has brought preparedness and response to respiratory viruses into focus, as well as how quickly they can evolve and impact society worldwide. Due to biotechnological progress, the potential for vaccine manufacture against respiratory viruses has been considerably enhanced. A notable example is the use of Newcastle disease virus (NDV) as a mammalian species vaccine vector, which possesses unique benefits. NDV is highly efficient in causing immunity without being virulent in mammals, and hence poses very minimal risk. Studies have indicated that NDV-based vaccines given intramuscularly are efficient enough to provide total protection against a broad spectrum of viral infections, including Rift Valley fever virus (RVFV). This technology is an indicator of growing trends towards the application of new platforms for vaccine delivery, which calls for research in the optimization of immune responses in species in respiratory infections (Harmsen et al., 2011). Efficacy of vaccines by age is a major consideration in the management of respiratory viruses. Studies on the efficacy of trivalent seasonal influenza vaccines show considerable variation by age groups. For example, immunization in children below five years of age revealed 87% efficacy, while in higher age groups it was significantly lower, highlighting the vulnerability of young age groups to influenza infection. The residual protection in younger children who received the monovalent 2009 pandemic influenza vaccine also highlights the ongoing role of immunization strategies in securing population health. Continuing surveillance and targeted vaccination measures should be used to address the burden of circulating respiratory viruses, particularly among child populations with high morbidity and mortality (Smyth et al., 2013).

CLOSER LOOK

RESPIRATORY SYNCYTIAL VIRUS (RSV)

Respiratory syncytial virus (RSV) is an extremely infectious and prevalent virus that predominantly infects the respiratory tract, particularly in infants, young children, older individuals, and those with compromised immunity. RSV belongs to the family Paramyxoviridae within the genus Orthopneumovirus. It is a negative-sense, single-stranded RNA virus with an enveloped structure. RSV is one of the important causative pathogens of lower respiratory tract infections (LRTIs) such as bronchiolitis and pneumonia in children under the age of five years all over the world.

RSV is transmitted mainly by respiratory droplets, direct contact with infected secretions, or infected surfaces. Following inhalation, the virus infects epithelial cells lining the upper and lower airways. The F (fusion) protein facilitates viral fusion with the host cell membrane and also leads to syncytia formation — multinucleated giant cells formed through the fusion of infected cells. This causes sloughing of epithelial cells, inflammation, airway obstruction, and mucus production, particularly in small airways, to wreak havoc on infants' and toddlers' breathing (Figure 2.17).

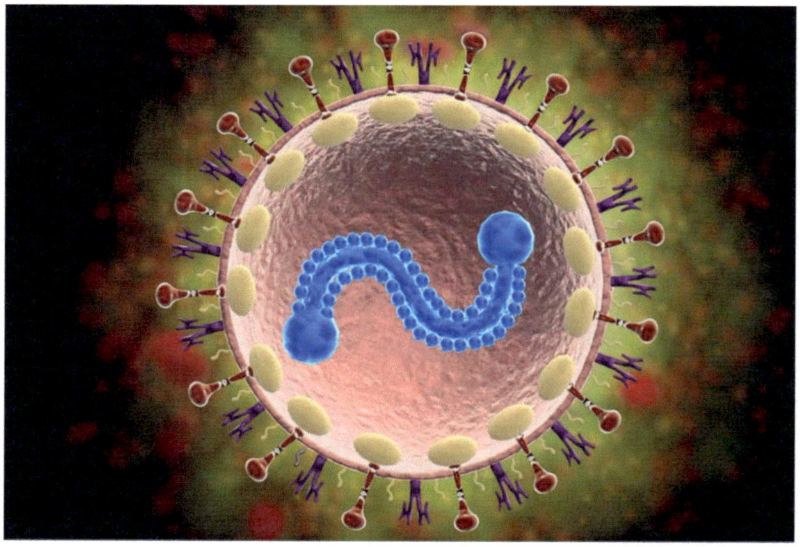

Figure 2.17. 3D illustration of the respiratory syncytial virus (RSV), showing its lipid envelope, surface glycoproteins, and helical RNA genome.

Source: https://hospitalsmagazine.com/wp-content/uploads/2023/05/respiratory.synctial.virus_G_594382057-1-scaled-1.jpg.

Clinically, RSV infection starts symptomatically in a very similar manner to an ordinary cold: sore throat, fever, cough, and runny nose. In more serious cases, particularly in infants and vulnerable groups, it leads to pneumonia and bronchiolitis, causing wheeze, respiratory distress, hypoxia, and intolerance to feeds. RSV is also increasingly being recognized as the cause of severe lower respiratory illness in older adults, leading to hospitalization and death, as with influenza.

RSV can be identified through nasopharyngeal swab testing with detection by rapid antigen test, RT-PCR, or viral culture. RT-PCR is the most sensitive and specific, especially during outbreaks of RSV or in the hospital setting.

Treatment of RSV is largely supportive, taking care of hydration, oxygenation, and the need for mechanical ventilation in serious cases. Specific antiviral drugs are not routinely available for use against RSV, but ribavirin has been employed in carefully selected high-risk patients with uncertain benefit. Prevention of RSV is therefore essential, particularly in high-risk individuals. Palivizumab, a monoclonal antibody to the RSV F protein, is given as a prophylactic to high-risk infants such as premature infants or those with congenital heart disease, but is expensive and needs to be given monthly during RSV season.

There have been recent advances in RSV prevention in the form of new long-acting monoclonal antibodies and maternal vaccines that can immunize infants through passive immunity. These innovations, combined with continued surveillance and infection control measures, are key to reducing the total burden of RSV globally.

REFERENCES

1. Relich, R. F., & Abbott, A. N. (2018). Syndromic and Point-of-Care Molecular Testing. *Advances in Molecular Pathology*, *1*(1), 97–113. https://doi.org/10.1016/j.yamp.2018.07.007(accessed on 16th July 2025).
2. Onyango, C. O., Welch, S. R., Munywoki, P. K., Agoti, C. N., Bett, A., Ngama, M., Myers, R., Cane, P. A., & Nokes, D. J. (2012). Molecular epidemiology of human rhinovirus infections in Kilifi, coastal Kenya. *Journal of medical virology*, *84*(5), 823–831. https://doi.org/10.1002/jmv.23251(accessed on 16th July 2025).
3. Agoti, C. N., Cane, P., Gitahi, C. W., Medley, G., et al. (2013). *Identification of group B respiratory syncytial viruses that lack the 60-nucleotide duplication after six consecutive epidemics of total BA dominance at coastal Kenya*. https://core.ac.uk/download/18327344.pdf (accessed on 16th July 2025).
4. Agricola, E., Buttinelli, G., Campagna, I., Carsetti, R., et al. (2017). *Infants hospitalized for Bordetella pertussis infection commonly have respiratory viral coinfections*. https://core.ac.uk/download/98349327.pdf (accessed on 16th July 2025).
5. Forshey, B. M., Laguna-Torres, V. A., Vilcarromero, S., Bazan, I., Rocha, C., Morrison, A. C., Stoddard, S. T., Alegre, Y., Gomez, J., Scott, T. W., & Kochel, T. J. (2010). Epidemiology of influenza-like illness in the Amazon Basin of Peru, 2008-2009. *Influenza and other respiratory viruses*, *4*(4), 235–243. https://doi.org/10.1111/j.1750-2659.2010.00139.x(accessed on 16th July 2025).
6. Fisher, B. T., Alexander, S., Dvorak, C. C., Zaoutis, T. E., Zerr, D. M., & Sung, L. (2012). Epidemiology and potential preventative measures for viral infections in children with malignancy and those undergoing hematopoietic cell transplantation. *Pediatric blood & cancer*, *59*(1), 11–15. https://doi.org/10.1002/pbc.23417(accessed on 16th July 2025).
7. Alicino, C., Ansaldi, F., Calamusa, G., Canepa, P., Colomba, G. M. E., Orsi, A., et al. (2018). *Trends of influenza B during the 2010–2016 seasons in 2 regions of north and south Italy: The impact of the vaccine mismatch on influenza immunization strategy*. https://core.ac.uk/download/287859184.pdf (accessed on 16th July 2025).
8. Al-Tawfiq, J. A., & Memish, Z. A. (2014). Emerging respiratory viral infections: MERS-CoV and influenza. *The Lancet. Respiratory medicine*, *2*(1), 23–25. https://doi.org/10.1016/S2213-2600(13)70255-8(accessed on 16th July 2025).
9. Al-Tawfiq, J. A., & Memish, Z. A. (2019). The Hajj 2019 Vaccine Requirements and Possible New Challenges. *Journal of epidemiology and global health*, *9*(3), 147–152. https://doi.org/10.2991/jegh.k.190705.001f (accessed on 16th July 2025).
10. Al-Tawfiq, J. A., Benkouiten, S., & Memish, Z. A. (2018). *A systematic review of emerging respiratory viruses at the Hajj and possible coinfection with Streptococcus pneumoniae*. https://core.ac.uk/download/322846904.pdf (accessed on 16th July 2025).
11. Amory, H., Broux, B., Deprez, P., Frippiat, T., et al. (2016). *Prevalence of respiratory pathogens in nasal swabs from horses with acute respiratory disease in Belgium*. https://core.ac.uk/download/74662608.pdf (accessed on 16th July 2025).
12. Ansari, A. A., Ceribelli, A., De Santis, M., Gershwin, M. E., et al. (2020). *Recommendations for coronavirus infection in rheumatic diseases treated with biologic therapy*. https://core.ac.uk/

download/323069262.pdf (accessed on 16th July 2025).

13. Cangiano, G., Nenna, R., Frassanito, A., Evangelisti, M., Nicolai, A., Scagnolari, C., Pierangeli, A., Antonelli, G., Papoff, P., Petrarca, L., Capocaccia, P., Moretti, C., & Midulla, F. (2016). Bronchiolitis: Analysis of 10 consecutive epidemic seasons. *Pediatric pulmonology*, *51*(12), 1330–1335. https://doi.org/10.1002/ppul.23476(accessed on 16th July 2025).

14. Harmsen, M. M., Antonis, A. F., Moormann, R. J., & Kortekaas, J. (2011). Parenteral vaccination of mammalian livestock with Newcastle disease virus-based vector vaccines offers optimal efficacy and safety. *Bioengineered bugs*, *2*(1), 58–62. https://doi.org/10.4161/bbug.2.1.13349(accessed on 16th July 2025).

15. Marcone, D. N., Durand, L. O., Azziz-Baumgartner, E., Vidaurreta, S., Ekstrom, J., Carballal, G., & Echavarria, M. (2015). Incidence of viral respiratory infections in a prospective cohort of outpatient and hospitalized children aged ≤5 years and its associated cost in Buenos Aires, Argentina. *BMC infectious diseases*, *15*, 447. https://doi.org/10.1186/s12879-015-1213-4(accessed on 16th July 2025).

16. Bakhtawar, M. (Haq, M. U.), Iftikhar, S. (S.), Rizwan, M., et al. (2020). Awareness of swine flu among the medical students of Shaikh Zayed Medical College Rahim Yar Khan. https://media.neliti.com/media/publications/302010-awareness-of-swine-flu-among-the-medical-8b23412a.pdf (accessed on 16th July 2025).

17. Bakir, J., Castellano, V., Gentile, Á., Grobaporto, A., et al. (2014). Respiratory syncytial virus: Clinical and epidemiological pattern in pediatric patients admitted to a children's hospital between 2000 and 2013. https://core.ac.uk/download/159292401.pdf (accessed on 16th July 2025).

18. Bang, H., Hon, S., May, L., Mooso, M., et al. (2019). Rapid multiplex testing for upper respiratory pathogens in the emergency department: A randomized controlled trial. https://core.ac.uk/download/323070651.pdf (accessed on 16th July 2025).

19. Tsiodras, S., Kelesidis, T., Kelesidis, I., Bauchinger, U., & Falagas, M. E. (2008). Human infections associated with wild birds. *The Journal of infection*, *56*(2), 83–98. https://doi.org/10.1016/j.jinf.2007.11.001(accessed on 16th July 2025).

20. Bell, R. A., Burstein, V. R., Kravitz, R. L., May, F. P., et al. (2019). Communication interventions to promote the public's awareness of antibiotics: A systematic review. https://core.ac.uk/download/323070637.pdf (accessed on 16th July 2025).

21. Maguire, J. L., Birken, C. S., Loeb, M. B., Mamdani, M., Thorpe, K., Hoch, J. S., Mazzulli, T., Borkhoff, C. M., Macarthur, C., Parkin, P. C., & TARGet Kids! Collaboration (2014). DO IT Trial: vitamin D Outcomes and Interventions in Toddlers - a TARGet Kids! randomized controlled trial. *BMC pediatrics*, *14*, 37. https://doi.org/10.1186/1471-2431-14-37(accessed on 16th July 2025).

22. Vonck, K., Garrez, I., De Herdt, V., Hemelsoet, D., Laureys, G., Raedt, R., & Boon, P. (2020). Neurological manifestations and neuro-invasive mechanisms of the severe acute respiratory syndrome coronavirus type 2. *European journal of neurology*, *27*(8), 1578–1587. https://doi.org/10.1111/ene.14329(accessed on 16th July 2025).

23. Bruinen de Bruin, Y., Clevestig, P., Colosio, C., Goulart, M., et al. (2020). Initial impacts of global risk mitigation measures taken during the combatting of the COVID-19 pandemic. https://core.ac.uk/download/305118327.pdf (accessed on 16th July 2025).

24. She, R. C., Polage, C. R., Caram, L. B., Taggart, E. W., Hymas, W. C., Woods, C. W., Schmader, K., & Petti, C. A. (2010). Performance of diagnostic tests to detect respiratory viruses in older adults. *Diagnostic microbiology and infectious disease*, *67*(3), 246–250. https://doi.org/10.1016/j.diagmicrobio.2010.02.020(accessed on 16th July 2025).

25. Morse, S. S., Mazet, J. A., Woolhouse, M., Parrish, C. R., Carroll, D., Karesh, W. B., Zambrana-Torrelio, C., Lipkin, W. I., & Daszak, P. (2012). Prediction and prevention of the next pandemic zoonosis. *Lancet (London, England)*, *380*(9857), 1956–1965. https://doi.org/10.1016/S0140-6736(12)61684-5(accessed on 16th July 2025).

26. Centers for Disease Control and Prevention (CDC). (2025). CDC influenza division technical key points: February 16, 2018. https://core.ac.uk/download/154402140.pdf (accessed on 16th July 2025).

27. Cesario, T. C. (2012). Viruses Associated with Pneumonia in Adults. https://core.ac.uk/download/323075396.pdf (accessed on 16th July 2025).

28. Chiu, C. Y., & Miller, S. A. (2019). Clinical Metagenomics. https://core.ac.uk/download/323062552.pdf (accessed on 16th July 2025).

29. Dietz, L., Horve, P. F., Coil, D. A., Fretz, M., Eisen, J. A., & Van Den Wymelenberg, K. (2020). 2019 Novel Coronavirus (COVID-19) Pandemic: Built Environment Considerations To Reduce Transmission. *mSystems*, *5*(2), e00245-20. https://doi.org/10.1128/mSystems.00245-20(accessed on 16th July 2025).

30. Colomer, M. À. (M. À.), Fraile Sauce, L. J., & Margalida, A. (2020). Vaccination is a suitable tool in the control of Aujeszky's disease outbreaks in pigs using a population dynamics P systems model. https://core.ac.uk/download/323287755.pdf (accessed on 16th July 2025).

31. Deeks, S., Drosten, C., Picker, L., Subbarao, K., et al. (2013). Roadblocks to Translational Challenges on Viral Pathogenesis. https://core.ac.uk/download/323073673.pdf (accessed on 16th July 2025).

32. Du, L., Jiang, S., Ojcius, D. M., Pan, H., et al. (2020). Measures for diagnosing and treating infections by a novel coronavirus responsible for a pneumonia outbreak originating in Wuhan, China. https://core.ac.uk/download/323063844.pdf (accessed on 16th July 2025).

33. Goh, G. K., Dunker, A. K., Foster, J. A., & Uversky, V. N. (2020). Nipah shell disorder, modes of infection, and virulence. *Microbial pathogenesis*, *141*, 103976. https://doi.org/10.1016/j.micpath.2020.103976(accessed on 16th July 2025).

34. Goh, G. K., Dunker, A. K., & Uversky, V. N. (2012). Understanding Viral Transmission Behavior via Protein Intrinsic Disorder Prediction: Coronaviruses. *Journal of pathogens*, *2012*, 738590. https://doi.org/10.1155/2012/738590(accessed on 16th July 2025).

35. Fang, F., Le Calvez, H., & Yu, M. (2004). Biochemical prevention and treatment of viral infections – A new paradigm in medicine for infectious diseases. https://core.ac.uk/download/pdf/3550099.pdf (accessed on 16th July 2025).

36. Frerichs, R. R., Reingold, A. L., & Sutrisna, B. (1991). Randomized, controlled trial of effectiveness of ampicillin in mild acute respiratory infections in Indonesian children. https://core.ac.uk/download/323081106.pdf (accessed on 16th July 2025).

37. Hendrickson, C. M., & Matthay, M. A. (2013). Viral pathogens and acute lung injury: Investigations inspired by the SARS epidemic and the 2009 H1N1 influenza pandemic. https://core.ac.uk/download/323072736.pdf (accessed on 16th July 2025).

38. Ho, A. (2014). Viral pneumonia in adults and older children in sub-Saharan Africa — Epidemiology, aetiology, diagnosis and management. https://core.ac.uk/download/151170258.pdf (accessed on 16th July 2025).

39. de Barra, M., Islam, M. S., & Curtis, V. (2014). Disgust sensitivity is not associated with health in a rural Bangladeshi sample. *PloS one*, *9*(6), e100444. https://doi.org/10.1371/journal.pone.0100444 (accessed on 16th July 2025).

40. Moore, D., Ellorin, E., Blumenthal, J., Corado, K., Hoenigl, M., Dube, M., et al. (2017). Recent HIV risk behavior and partnership type predict PrEP adherence in men who have sex with men. https://core.ac.uk/download/294625910.pdf (accessed on 16th July 2025).

41. Deschamp, A. R., Hatch, J. E., Slaven, J. E., Gebregziabher, N., Storch, G., Hall, G. L., Stick, S., Ranganathan, S., Ferkol, T. W., & Davis, S. D. (2019). Early respiratory viral infections in infants with cystic fibrosis. *Journal of cystic fibrosis : official journal of the European Cystic Fibrosis Society*, *18*(6), 844–850. https://doi.org/10.1016/j.jcf.2019.02.004(accessed on 16th July 2025).

42. Petruzelli, N. (2020). The influence of climate change on disease and public health. https://core.ac.uk/download/322826252.pdf (accessed on 16th July 2025).

43. Bansal, S., Pourbohloul, B., & Meyers, L. A. (2006). A comparative analysis of influenza vaccination programs. *PLoS medicine*, *3*(10), e387. https://doi.org/10.1371/journal.pmed.0030387 (accessed on 16th July 2025).

44. Smyth, B., Kearns, C., Moore, C., Robertson, C., Castilla, J., Fleming, D. M., et al. (2013). *Age-specific vaccine effectiveness of seasonal 2010/2011 and pandemic influenza A(H1N1) 2009 vaccines in preventing influenza in the United Kingdom*. https://core.ac.uk/download/9558257.pdf (accessed on 16th July 2025).

45. de Jong, M. C., Stegeman, A., van der Goot, J., & Koch, G. (2009). Intra- and interspecies transmission of H7N7 highly pathogenic avian influenza virus during the avian influenza epidemic in The Netherlands in 2003. *Revue scientifique et technique (International Office of Epizootics)*, *28*(1), 333–340. https://doi.org/10.20506/rst.28.1.1859(accessed on 16th July 2025).

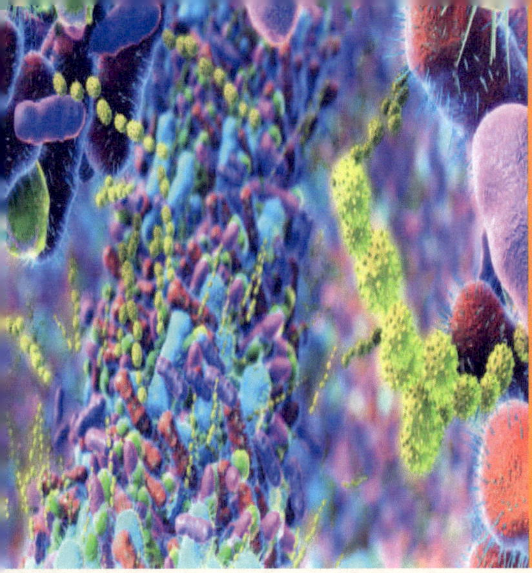

Chapter 3

GASTROINTESTINAL VIRUSES

Contents

Introduction

The role of gastrointestinal viruses in human health has emerged significantly in the past few years, particularly regarding their role in symptomatic disease as well as in broader public health concerns. Gastrointestinal viruses like noroviruses and rotaviruses cause a large morbidity and mortality burden worldwide, particularly in the most susceptible groups of the population, i.e., infants, old people, and immunocompromised individuals. The quick transmission of these viruses underscores the requirement for effective public health intervention for prevention and control. With advances in diagnostic techniques, it has now been established that viral infections are significant determinants of gastrointestinal disease that challenge the earlier concepts based largely on bacterial and fungal etiology. This paradigm shift demands keen insights into viral pathogenesis and the mechanisms through which these pathogens disrupt gut health and hence defines the imperative for continuous research and intervention measures in this area (Fisher et al., 2012). Additionally, the effect of viral infections extends beyond short-term gastrointestinal disease, often resulting in long-term health consequences and healthcare expenditures. The persistence and prevalence of gastrointestinal viruses are of particular concern in health facilities and crowded environments since their outbreaks can have catastrophic effects. Viral pathogens may also complicate clinical patient care, particularly among patients who are already predisposed to infection due to pre-existing health conditions. Thus, it is necessary to explore the epidemiology of such infections, find out about the transmission patterns of these, and try to identify the causes responsible for their emergence and re-emergence. Particularly noteworthy, rising evidence of viral co-infection with other pathogens makes the clinical picture still more complicated, so there is a need for an integrative strategy in approaching viral as well as non-viral causative factors of gastrointestinal illnesses (Kijlstra et al., 2003). Against this background of shared issues, the development of specifically targeted prevention techniques and therapies is a priority. Current research emphasizes not only the necessity of the importance of vaccination against individual viruses such as rotaviruses, but also the necessity of strict infection control that can effectively curtail the risk of outbreaks. Enhanced surveillance and diagnostic practices are central to the early detection of viral pathogens, enabling clinicians to implement effective treatment modalities. Furthermore, ongoing research into newer antiviral drugs and treatment regimens is essential to neutralize the pathogenic effects of enteric viruses. These initiatives will contribute positively by interdisciplinary interaction, encompassing design for virology, public health, and clinical practice to build a better understanding of how to control gastrointestinal viral diseases. Overall, knowledge acquisition for the intricate nature of gastrointestinal viruses is crucial for protecting public health as well as enhancing patient outcomes in a more epoch time when these pathogens represent significant challenges (Fisher et al., 2012).

Definition of Gastrointestinal Viruses

The family of gastrointestinal viruses represents a heterogeneous collection of viral pathogens which are etiological agents of gastrointestinal infections. They infect the intestinal tract mainly and produce diarrhea, vomiting, and abdominal pain. The most prevalent gastrointestinal viruses are norovirus, rotavirus, adenovirus, and astrovirus, each having specific features in the mode of spread, infectivity, and epidemiology. For instance, norovirus is notorious to spread rapidly and is among the most frequent causes of viral gastroenteritis outbreaks in mass gatherings such as on cruise ships and in schools. Being aware of what gastrointestinal viruses are is significant to public health surveillance and intervention since outbreaks may be important indicators of viral transmission patterns in populations. With their considerable contribution to acute gastroenteritis, this family of viruses remains a considerable problem in the study of infectious diseases. The study of how gastrointestinal viruses interact with the host can shed light on the potential mechanisms behind various disorders, including autoimmune disease. Present research suggests that gastrointestinal viruses are capable of stimulating immune responses that may contribute to the causation of disease like myalgic encephalomyelitis/chronic fatigue syndrome (Fisher et al., 2012) (Figure 3.1).

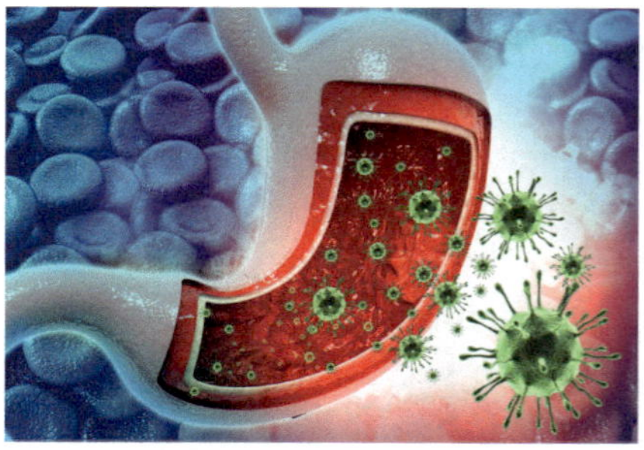

Figure 3.1. Viral gastroenteritis.

Source: https://cdn.apollohospitals.com/health-library-prod/2021/08/Viral-Gastroenteritis-scaled.jpg.

Gastrointestinal viruses can also be infectious agents that trigger or exacerbate autoimmune mechanisms, causing prolonged immune-associated symptoms among infected individuals, according to new research. This connection underlines the importance of looking into the virome in the gastrointestinal tract since it has the ability to reveal new correlations between viral infections and chronic conditions. The possible link between viral infection and autoimmune phenomenon serves to emphasize the need for continued research in the field of gastrointestinal viruses, both to aid diagnostics and aid treatments in patients suffering from these complex conditions (Navaneetharaja et al., 2016). Aside from their obvious health impact, gastrointestinal viruses may have further implications when understanding neurological disease. There is evidence to suggest that environmental factors and infectious agents, such as viruses, can interact with genetic predispositions to determine the occurrence of disorders like autism. Although the mechanisms involved are yet to be fully understood, there is some evidence to suggest a possible role for gastrointestinal health and neurodevelopmental disorders, possibly mediated by the gut-brain axis. The CHARGE study, for instance, is examining the interaction between environmental and genetic exposures, i.e., viral infection, to inform on risk factors for autism and other developmental delays. By broadening the definition of the gastrointestinal viruses to encompass their systemic effect, the scientists better understand the complexity of the viral pathogens as well as their role in human health, providing an opportunity for more effective prevention and treatment strategies (Croen et al., 2006).

Importance of Studying Gastrointestinal Viruses

Scientific research into viral gastroenteritis is vital to outline its significant impacts on public health and disease prevention. Norovirus and other viruses are a primary cause of gastroenteritis globally and have provided notable morbidity and mortality, particularly in vulnerable individuals such as children and the elderly. By studying the epidemiology and transmission patterns of gastrointestinal viruses, scientists are able to determine high-risk populations and track outbreak trends, which is invaluable to launching efficient public health interventions. Additionally, thorough research can be used to guide vaccination practices, enhancing the general health status of communities. Given that gastrointestinal viruses are likely to spread rapidly in dense populations, the awareness of their spread and transmission can contribute significantly towards devising targeted interventions, thereby weakening their effects on public health. Secondly, gastrointestinal virus research enhances the comprehension of the gut microbiome and the consequential health implications. The microbial ecology of the gastrointestinal tract is in a delicate equilibrium such that dysbiosis can be caused by upsets like infection by gastrointestinal viruses. This dysbiosis also has profound effects on many body processes, including digestion and immunity, so it is worth learning how viral infection disturbs the balance. Contrary to what might be expected, gastrointestinal viruses are also capable of impacting gut microbiota composition, which can establish an infection-balance cycle. By combining partnerships with studies of interactions between such viruses and gut microbiome dynamics, researchers can unravel clues, hopefully translated into therapeutic advances for gastrointestinal disease and more, addressing important medical needs currently faced in clinics (Cacciotti et al., 2016). In addition, the global health significance of gastrointestinal viruses necessitates that research and intervention become multi-disciplinary in its strategy. Zoonotic diseases, overall, present serious challenges, in particular in the low- and middle-income nations with potentially limited resources to address such health threats. Trans-sectoral, cross-disciplinary, and cross-border collaborations can enhance our intelligence and action against such viral diseases. For instance, studies with health policy and systems concepts can identify feasible study themes that focus on optimal prevention and control strategies, particularly in low-resource settings (Sekar et al., 2011). In doing so, this method also ensures that the outcomes are generalizable across diverse populations and settings, thereby promoting fairness in health solutions. Working with the complexity of gastrointestinal viruses not only moves forward scholarly understanding but also enhances the efforts towards constructing a healthier world society, addressing the immediacy and importance of this research field.

3.1. Types of Gastrointestinal Viruses

The gastrointestinal viruses are diverse, specifically encompassing the noroviruses, rotaviruses, and adenoviruses. Noroviruses are among the leading viral causes of gastroenteritis, notably within close quarters such as on cruise ships and in nursing homes. Prevalent and highly contagious, norovirus infections precipitate abrupt inflammation of the stomach and intestines, which appears in the form of vomiting, diarrhea, and abdominal cramps. On the other hand, rotaviruses are largely seen in infants and young children with severe diarrhea that can have consequent dehydration and hospitalization. Rotavirus is largely prevented by vaccination in the majority of regions, showing the efficacy of public health measures. Adenoviruses, though less commonly associated with gastrointestinal disease, affect children and adults alike and can present in a variety of presentations from respiratory disease and conjunctivitis to gastrointestinal upset. All these viruses underscore the need for constant vigilance in public health activity. The structural characteristics and modes of transmission of these viruses of the gastrointestinal tract yield critical details about their persistence and implications for public health. Noroviruses, for instance, possess a robust protein coat that enables them to survive rough environmental conditions, a property that makes transmission easy for them to achieve. They are transmitted by contaminated food and water and by direct contact with infected people or surfaces. Rotaviruses are transmitted primarily by the fecal-oral route, most commonly by contaminated hands or surfaces, so cleanliness and hand washing are crucial in controlling outbreaks. Adenoviruses, while capable of causing gastrointestinal disease, are more famously recognized to cause disease in the respiratory and ocular systems, presenting a range of presentations. As there is constant evolution of the epidemiology of these viruses, understanding their transmission patterns and structural features is paramount in the planning of effective prevention strategies.

The impact of gastrointestinal viruses is not just on individual health but also on higher-level public health infrastructure and healthcare expenditure. Outbreaks of viral gastroenteritis can overwhelm healthcare systems with increased hospitalization and emergency department visits, primarily among high-risk populations such as the elderly and immunocompromised individuals. Furthermore, the economic burden of such diseases is considerable, going well beyond the expense of healthcare to the loss of productivity. Novel therapeutic approaches such as phage therapy are under investigation for their potential to treat bacterial co-infections complicating viral gastroenteritis, according to research. Such developments underscore the interconnected nature of viral and bacterial illness in gastrointestinal disease, necessitating a unified treatment and prevention strategy. With scientists continuing to identify the complexities of such viruses, it is increasingly recognized that overall measures are important in protecting public health and curbing the devastating impacts of gastrointestinal viruses on society (Banu et al., 2016; Lin et al., 2017).

3.1.1. Norovirus

As a novel case in the category of gastrointestinal viruses, Norovirus stands out on account of its high infectivity and public health impact. Set to induce acute gastroenteritis, Norovirus can induce vomiting, diarrhea, and abdominal cramps and develops between 12 and 48 hours of exposure. It is of greatest significance that it is responsible for causing a huge percentage of viral gastroenteritis worldwide, particularly in settings such as cruise ships, schools, and hospitals. The virus's survival under varied environmental conditions, coupled with its low infectious dose, renders control difficult. Failure to cope with outbreak management has led to the need for research to understand the virus's epidemiology and the mutational patterns, which are crucial for effective public health intervention. With the growing impact of Norovirus, prevention and control in an integrated manner is the need of the hour to minimize its extensive effects on the health systems, particularly among vulnerable populations. The cost of Norovirus outbreaks extends far beyond direct healthcare expenditure and is more of a societal burden. In developed nations, gastrointestinal viruses like Norovirus are expected to bear considerable healthcare expenses due to hospitalization, outpatient care, and lost productivity of infected individuals (Figure 3.2).

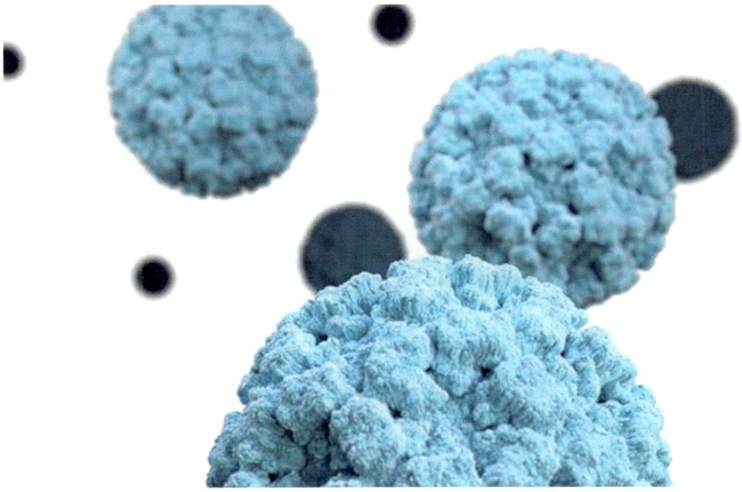

Figure 3.2. Norovirus.

Source: https://external-content.duckduckgo.com/iu/?u=https%3A%2F%2Fwww.cdc.gov%2Fnorovirus%2Fimages%2Fnorovirus-virions.jpg&f=1&nofb=1&ipt=129af773168e1a66f4317bbc7cb171f0580507f9233ce2cb49e4e7bd9f149838.

To this picture are added the indirect costs of school and daycare closures, along with decreased workforce productivity, which amplifies the monetary effect of such outbreaks. A noteworthy study on infectious intestinal disease noted that, while some cases are advanced, there is systematic under-reporting that remains a prevalent concern when determining the true burden of Norovirus and its impact on public health budgets (Gauci et al., 2006). These gaps in data underscore the necessity for expanded surveillance and investigation to aid in better-informed outbreak response efforts and prompt policymakers to the critical importance of prevention activities. Furthermore, intervention against Norovirus consists of implementing effective infection control practices and public health programs tailored for high-risk groups.

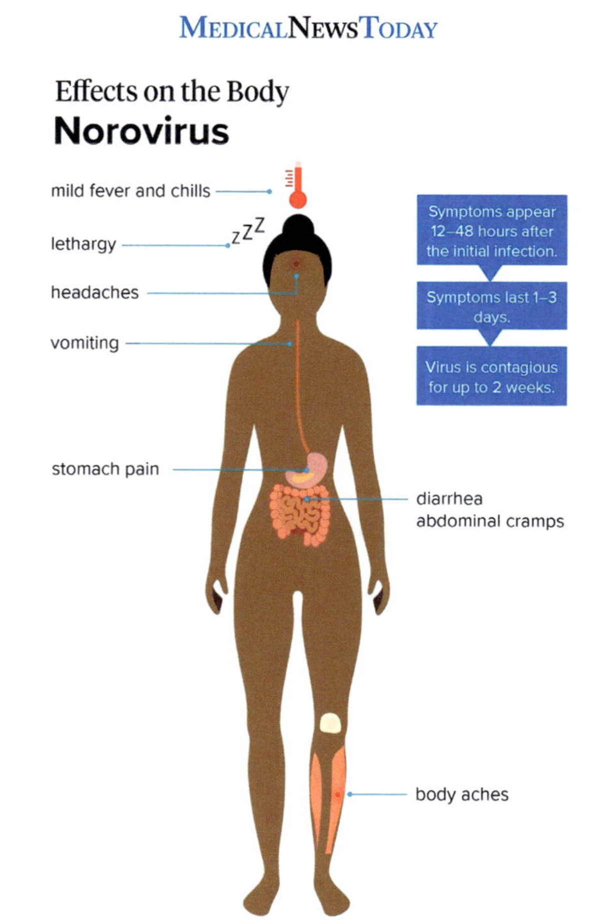

Figure 3.3. Effects of norovirus on the body.

Source: https://i0.wp.com/post.medicalnewstoday.com/wp-content/uploads/sites/3/2020/02/Effects-on-the-Body-Norovirus_ver4.jpg?w=1155&h=4830.

The lack of effective antiviral therapies against Norovirus also underscores the importance of prevention activities, particularly in high-density settings. Prevention is intensive hand hygiene, food safety, and rapid response to outbreaks to prevent transmission. Evidence indicates that intensive infection control strategies can reduce the undesirable effects of viral infections in vulnerable groups, such as pediatric cancer patients (Fisher et al., 2012). Hence, an interrelated plan of education, community effort, and improved healthcare protocols is required in the battle against the spread of Norovirus, minimizing its health impacts along with economic impacts, and ultimately maximizing the entire response to gastrointestinal viruses in public health systems (Figure 3.3).

3.1.2. Rotavirus

The significance of rotavirus in gastrointestinal viruses is underscored by its contribution as the worldwide leading cause of hospitalization and severe diarrhea in infants and young children. The virus is highly contagious and has a single target site in the intestinal tract, which leads to immense fluid loss and dehydration.

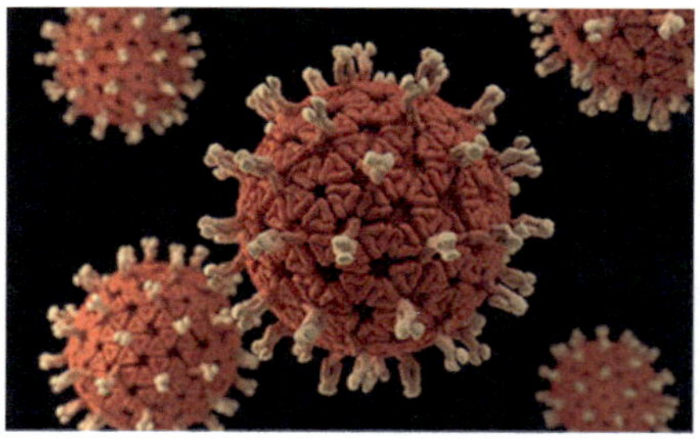

Figure 3.4. Anatomy of rotavirus.

Source: https://external-content.duckduckgo.com/iu/?u=https%3A%2F%2Fwww.ecdc.europa.eu%2Fsites%2Fdefault%2Ffiles%2Fstyles%2Fis_full%2Fpublic%2Fimages%2FRotavirus_H.jpg%3Fitok%3D507vmnMd&f=1&nofb=1&ipt=46a09823f2f6ab145e7b68717da413615094f0bea39c23a6b0e6729e7b8a30db.

This is potentially life-threatening in susceptible populations. In third-world nations, rotavirus diarrhea is also exacerbated by restricted access to medical treatment and undernutrition, complicating recovery. Effective prevention strategies have been pivotal to reducing hospitalization. Vaccine programs have been successful in reducing rotavirus-related morbidity and mortality, pointing towards the influence of preventive healthcare to combat infectious diseases like rotavirus (Fisher et al., 2012) (Figure 3.4).

In addition, the economic burden of rotavirus infections cannot be underrated because it is equivalent to substantial healthcare spending associated with the management of life-threatening diarrheal illnesses among children. The spending entails not only hospitalization but also long-term morbidity that may affect the growth and development of a child. Even in the developed world, despite improved sanitation and hygiene practices that have reduced the incidence of rotavirus infections, outbreaks do still occur and constant surveillance and prevention efforts are needed. The social consequences extend beyond healthcare costs, considering that lost productivity among caregivers and diversion of public health expenditures to treat these infections can strain healthcare systems. Hence, the focus on rotavirus must include prevention and care measures in its totality, considering its deep influence on worldwide health (Gauci et al., 2006). Infectious intestinal disease (IID), with rotavirus being among the leading causes, is a collection of disorders with varying rates of severity. IID prevention and control, along with rotavirus infections, are crucial in curtailing overall morbidity and mortality due to gastrointestinal disorders. Early treatment and early detection are critical in the prevention of the adverse effects of rotavirus infections, particularly as symptoms would rapidly deteriorate from light to severe. Enhanced public health promotion for universal vaccination against rotavirus and public campaigns on the right hygiene protocols can effectively reduce the transmission rates. These combined approaches are crucial to controlling the place of rotavirus in IID, thereby improving the health outcomes of such groups and confirming the value of ongoing vigilance in managing gastrointestinal viruses (Fisher et al., 2012) (Figure 3.5).

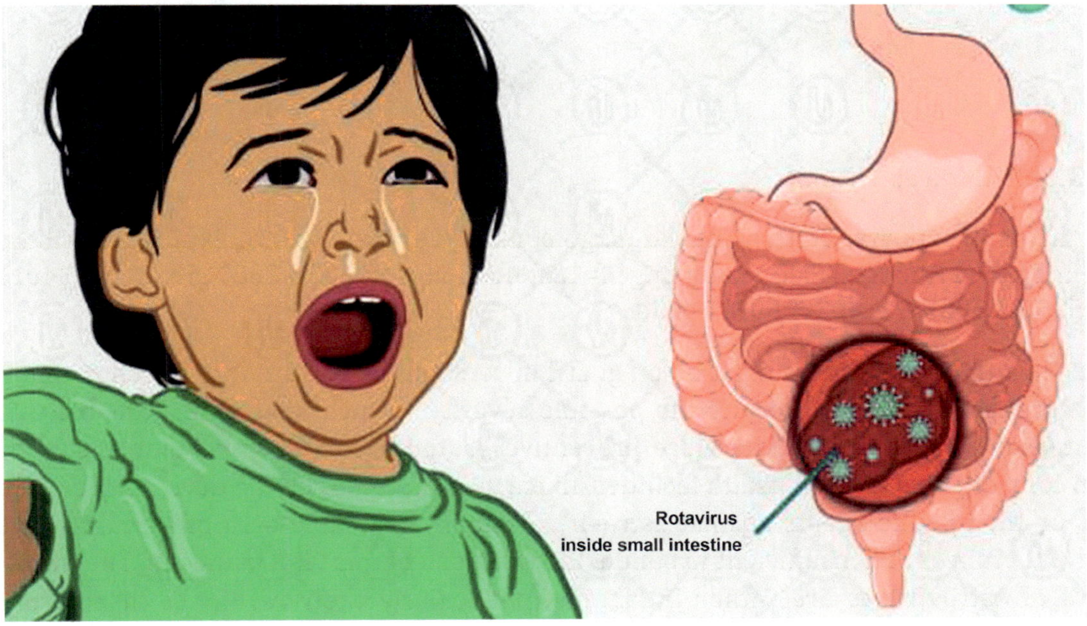

Figure 3.5. Rotavirus infection in children.

Source: https://www.myupchar.com/en/disease/rotavirus.

3.1.3. Astrovirus

Astroviruses are a family of non-enveloped RNA viruses that occupy a significant position in the causation of gastrointestinal disease, particularly in immunocompromised hosts and infants. Astroviruses are most frequently associated with mild to moderate gastroenteritis and are characterized by symptoms such as vomiting, diarrhea, and abdominal cramping. The epidemiology of astrovirus infection reveals that they predominantly occur in outbreak mode, particularly in the presence of closed or semi-closed settings like daycare centers and nursing homes. This underscores their potential for rapid spread and points to the importance of understanding their pathogenic processes. Improved diagnostic techniques have enabled medical professionals to identify astrovirus infections with greater ease, and this is crucial since viral gastroenteritis can mimic bacterial and parasitic infections in clinical presentation, making diagnosis and treatment more challenging. Apart from acute gastroenteritis, the clinical significance of astrovirus infections is elsewhere. In the immunocompromised host, such as cancer patients undergoing chemotherapy or those infected with HIV/AIDS, astroviruses can result in severe and long-lasting gastroenteritis that may lead to significant morbidity and, sometimes, mortality.

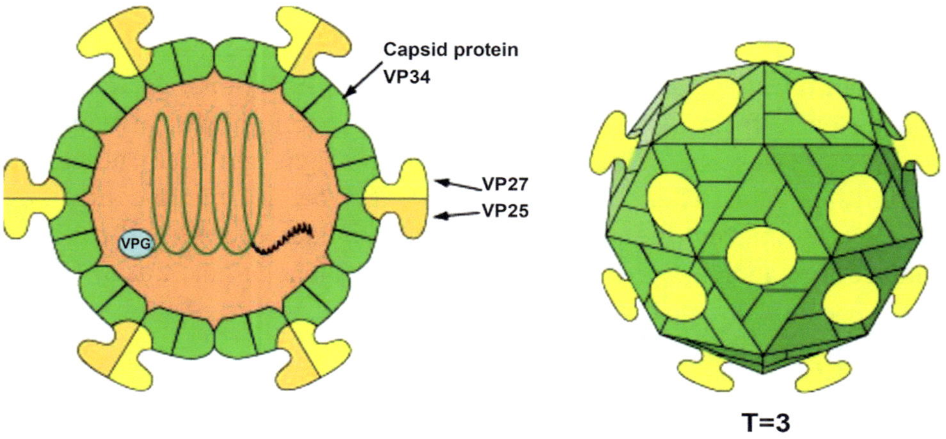

Figure 3.6. Astrovirus virion.

Source: https://external-content.duckduckgo.com/iu/?u=http%3A%2F%2Feducation.expasy.org%2Fimages%2FAstroviridae_virion.png&f=1&nofb=1&ipt=f4b010f8887c5b81ab1c34c1e4a70b1b8b5150550e305573cce98079901d4edd.

Thus, healthcare providers must be on guard in screening for astrovirus infection among such high-risk groups of patients. Despite the possible severity of such infections, available therapy is still limited and effective, and therefore preventive protocols are so important, including strict infection control procedures in health facilities. In particular, studies on the development of valuable vaccines or therapeutic agents against astrovirus remain a valuable area of research, given that supportive therapy is still insufficient to handle the workload of this viral pathogen. The transmission dynamics of astroviruses are rather intriguing, particularly their resilience in environmental situations, to gives them the ability to survive diverse environments. It has been found by studies that astroviruses may remain infectious on unclean surfaces, further person-to-person spreading. Astroviruses are shed from the feces, which indicates the need for hygienic and sanitary practices for preventing outbreaks. Health education campaigns on hand hygiene and food protection can go a long way in containing the transmission of astrovirus, especially in public areas. Such preventive methods are most needed in the aftermath of the new astrovirus strains, which are proving difficult for traditional diagnostic and treatment paradigms. There is a need for an interrelated strategy to enhance surveillance, increase diagnosis, and alleviate astrovirus as a principal gastroenteritis virus (Fisher et al., 2012; Nelsen, 2022) (Figure 3.6).

3.2. Transmission and Infection

The transmission of gastrointestinal viruses is often through the fecal-oral route, making proper sanitation and hygiene practices important in controlling outbreaks. Contaminated food and water are primary vectors through which norovirus and rotavirus spread within populations easily. The virus particles can survive on surfaces and in the environment for a prolonged period, facilitating transmission through indirect routes by contact with contaminated surfaces or objects. In addition, human behavior, such as social contact and food preparation, is also critical to virus spread. Public health interventions to decelerate transmission, such as hand hygiene and food handling practices, have also lowered infection rates significantly. Understanding transmission mechanisms enables health care personnel to use specific interventions capable of mitigating the risks from gastrointestinal viruses and, in so doing, protect vulnerable groups, mainly children and old people, who are at increased risk of severe outcomes. Infection with gastrointestinal viruses can lead to a spectrum of clinical presentation ranging from mild gastroenteritis to intractable diarrhea and, in a minority of cases, admission to hospital. Upon entering the host, these viruses utilize the intestinal mucosa to establish infection, and they damage cells and induce inflammation. Kinetics of immune response are an important consideration; however, certain gastrointestinal viruses circumvent the host's immune system to ensure long-term infection along with increased morbidity. The conditions of immunodeficiencies, induced by other infectious agents, also worsen the situation with infections since these conditions can predispose the patients to more serious forms of gastrointestinal virus infections. For example, in immunocompromised patients, normal responses to infections are affected, potentially resulting in opportunistic infections with other microorganisms, which may add to the health problems suffered by such individuals. Hence, full comprehension of mechanisms of infection can help in establishing effective therapeutic strategies tailored to heterogeneous patient groups (Sykes, 2010).

The host factors of gastrointestinal viral infections are key to comprehending how such pathogens adapt to their environment. Some cell receptors and glycan modifications, for example, sialic acids (Sias), play a great role in the host's susceptibility to viral infection. Sia variations regulate the virus's ability to adhere to host cells, modify the virus's tropism, and affect the process of infection. An example is the presence of 9-O-acetylated Sias in some animal tissues, showing how the modification can redefine pathogen-host interactions and affect viral transmission and outcomes of infection in different host species (Wasik et al., 2017). This heterogeneity in receptor expression not only contributes to the susceptibility of the host to gastrointestinal viruses but also threatens current approaches to vaccine development and therapeutic regimens. Thus, ongoing studies of the complex interactions between host factors and viral pathogens are essential for illuminating the dynamics of transmission and enhancing public health responses to outbreaks of gastrointestinal viruses.

3.2.1. Modes of Transmission

Understanding gastrointestinal viruses' modes of transmission is critical so that they can be controlled and outbreaks minimized. They, such as norovirus and rotavirus, are significantly transmitted through the fecal-oral pathway, with food, water, or surfaces serving as vectors for infection. Transmission patterns might be complex, with different environmental vectors or human contact. Of special interest are outbreaks in group settings such as schools, cruise ships, and nursing homes due to the density of the population and shared facilities. This necessitates strict hygiene practices, including hand washing and sanitation protocols, to break the chain of infection. The multiplicity of such pathways puts emphasis on constant public health education regarding preventive steps that prevent contact with contaminated material and thus the frequency of gastrointestinal infection. Direct person-to-person transmission is another significant method of transmission of such viruses, apart from the fecal-oral route. When an infected individual engages in activities that involve close contact, e.g., caregiving or communal feeding, they can directly pass virions to susceptible hosts. In addition, viral particles persist on surfaces, and thus indirect transmission by way of contaminated fomites is feasible. It is for this reason that cleanliness has to be maintained within shared living spaces since surfaces such as kitchen countertops and bathroom components may harbor infectious agents. The immune and behavioral patterns among individuals also influence susceptibility to the viruses and suggest that host factors are implicated in the transmission dynamics. Interventions to enhance community awareness regarding direct and indirect routes of transmission are essential in averting outbreaks of gastrointestinal viruses (Figure 3.7).

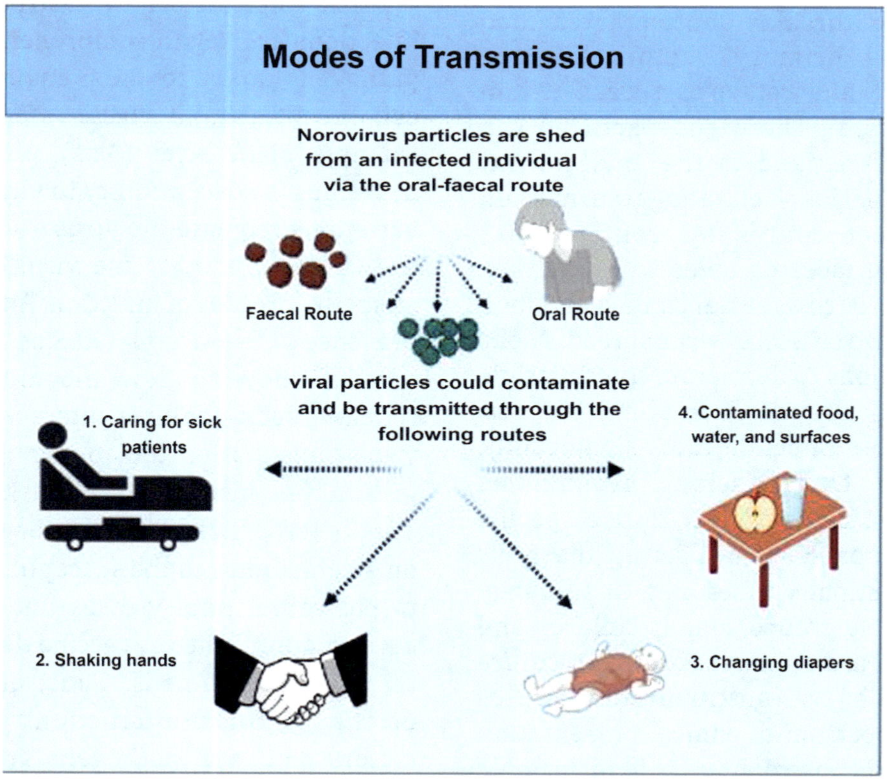

Figure 3.7. Transmission modes of NoV reported by the CDC.

Source: https://www.mdpi.com/1999-4915/14/12/2811.

Of particular interest are recent research studies on viral transmission mechanisms that point to the complexity of dynamics in gastrointestinal viruses. For instance, research on coronaviruses has illuminated other mechanisms that involve hybrid spreading mechanisms for HIV-1, which accommodate cell-free as well as cell-to-cell modes of transmission. Such research enables modelers to model the dynamics of viruses and infer possible transmission routes with more precision, thereby providing a foundation for intervention measures. In deciphering such complicated schemes of interaction, there can be new ways in which vaccine production and therapeutic treatment can be optimized. Keeping this in consideration, further research into the unique patterns of gastrointestinal virus transmission remains relevant in the field of epidemiology, as it informs public health policy and enables more effective responses to viral epidemics (Goh et al., 2012; Zhang et al., 2015).

3.2.2. Risk Factors for Infection

The increasing incidence of gastrointestinal viruses is often accounted for by more than one risk factor that amplifies the likelihood of infection. Included in these risk factors is the immunocompromised status of patients, particularly among cohorts such as pediatric cancer patients and hematopoietic stem cell transplant recipients. Research indicates that while healthcare providers have traditionally focused efforts on bacterial and fungal infections in these groups, viral pathogens are increasingly identified as primary causes of morbidity and mortality.

The complex relationship between immunocompromised status and viral exposure emphasizes the importance of prevention efforts in these vulnerable populations. Since there are few antiviral treatments with established efficacy, preventive measures such as pre-exposure prophylaxis and strict infection control practices are central to avoiding the risk of viral infection, requiring integrated approaches to healthcare in avoiding these declining health outcomes (Fisher et al., 2012). A further significant risk factor for gastrointestinal infection is the consumption of contaminated water. Impeccably treated drinking water carries little risk; however, poorly treated or contaminated water sources introduce profound vulnerabilities. Viral waterborne ingestion, especially for the purposes of hepatitis A, hepatitis E, and viral gastroenteritis, illuminates the natural affinity between water safety and public health. Community health interventions would target the integrity of water distribution systems to prevent post-treatment contamination because this is the main factor in viral transmission upon system failure. Surveillance for routine bacterial indicators can also prove an efficient measure in protection against potential viral contamination and thereby enable alleviation of gastrointestinal virus burden (Cartwright, 1997). Furthermore, environmental and socio-economic determinants also play an important role in shaping the risk environment for gastrointestinal infections. Poor sanitation, limited access to health care, and high population density are all conditions that can lead to the transmission of viral pathogens. In low-income communities, limited resources further increase susceptibility to infection, resulting in a higher incidence of gastrointestinal disease. Public health interventions to promote sanitation, enhance hygiene education, and ensure access to pure water are vital steps in preventing these risk factors. In addition, close attention when monitoring outbreaks and initiating instant response mechanisms can reduce the spread of infections within communities. Therefore, understanding the multi-factorial function played by risk factors in gastrointestinal viruses is imperative in designing effective public health measures to contain infections, along with overall community well-being.

3.2.3. Incubation Periods and Symptoms

It is valuable to know of the incubation periods and presentation of gastrointestinal viruses to manage and diagnose them appropriately. The incubation period varies widely among different viral pathogens. Norovirus infection, for instance, has an incubation period of 24 to 48 hours and therefore usually develops symptoms one to two days after exposure. Rotavirus can have symptoms for a bit longer after infection.

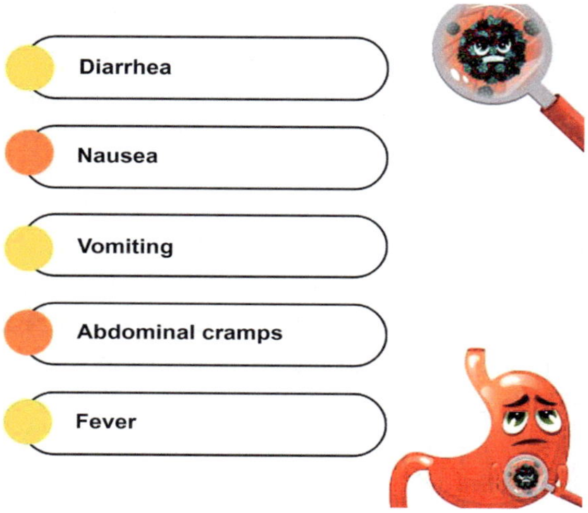

Figure 3.8. Symptoms of viral gastroenteritis.

Source: https://continentalhospitals.com/uploads/mceu_60677228111700556725682.jpg.

This variation is likely to impact the ability of public health officials to trace disease sources, as the incubation period may be prolonged, posing a risk of widespread transmission before detection of the virus. Proper knowledge of these timeframes enables clinicians to detect and isolate outbreaks, thus reducing viral gastroenteritis-related morbidity. Nausea, vomiting, diarrhea, and stomach cramps are common symptoms of viral gastroenteritis. The symptoms range from mild to severe and can have a notable effect on patients' hydration and nutrition status. The illness course takes one to three days, but this takes longer in certain groups, such as infants, the elderly, or immunocompromised (Figure 3.8).

The clinical picture is often that of an acute onset of symptoms, and this makes diagnosis all the harder in that such symptoms may be imitative of other gastrointestinal pathology. The precipitous course from exposure to symptomology underlines the highly infectious nature of such viruses and serves to emphasize the imperative for rapid response protocols in clinical settings and public health practice to control and contain such outbreaks effectively. Gastrointestinal viruses have been found to have complex pathology and symptomatology through the research conducted on them.

For example, the severity of the symptoms may be a function of the level of the immune response and the viral load. In most individuals, they recover uneventfully, but in vulnerable persons, the symptoms are very severe. Studies into these viral diseases have shown the variability of the ways that interaction between virus and host immune responses can happen; e.g., certain viruses are capable of initiating an exaggerated immune response, leading to increased inflammation and damage to the gut epithelial barrier. Such understanding is in accordance with findings obtained from the study of other viral pathogens, i.e., those for the respiratory tract, which have corresponding patterns of immune system activation (Hendrickson & Matthay, 2013 Adu-Gyamfi, 2019). The patterns could prove useful to develop targeted therapeutic strategies toward mitigating symptoms and improving patient outcomes.

3.3. Diagnosis of Gastrointestinal Viral Infections

Diagnosis of viral gastrointestinal infections is primarily clinical presentation, epidemiology, and advanced laboratory techniques. The process begins in most cases with a detailed history of the patient and the symptoms, trying to differentiate viral from bacterial or parasitic causes. Diarrhea, vomiting, and abdominal pain are non-specific symptoms that can be caused by many etiologic agents and hence the initial diagnosis becomes tricky. Because viral gastroenteritis is usually self-limiting, physicians must weigh the benefits of laboratory diagnosis against symptom severity and duration. Accurate diagnosis not only helps confirm the viral etiology but also guides public health efforts at containing outbreaks, especially in community settings like schools and nursing homes. Laboratory diagnosis has been revolutionized, with traditional technologies like enzyme immunosorbent assays (EIAs) being complemented by molecular technologies.

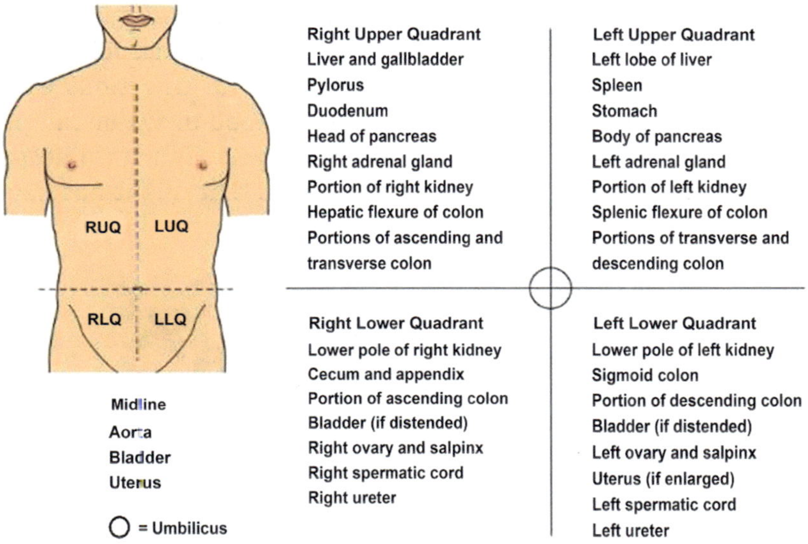

Figure 3.9. Diagnostic test for gastrointestinal system.

Source: https://external-content.duckduckgo.com/iu/?u=https%3A%2F%2Fimage1.slideserve.com%2F2211695%2Fdiagnostic-tests-l.jpg&f=1&nofb=1&ipt=c7d136af285f33d97e14bbf552e9c370170c386d6b725fa3db7ad252da6d713b.

The use of real-time polymerase chain reaction (RT-PCR) allows for the rapid and specific detection of viral nucleic acids with superior sensitivity and specificity compared to traditional culture. Moreover, the addition of clinical metagenomic next-generation sequencing (mNGS) has ushered in a new era of diagnosing gastrointestinal infection. This new technology enables global microbial pathogen analysis in a single assay, with critical information relating to mixed or co-infections that may clinically manifest. Thus, the use of such emerging technologies represents a new era in gastrointestinal viral infection diagnosis, with better accuracy and timeliness in patient care. In addressing the challenge of viral infection diagnosis, laboratories are faced with issues of standardization of tests, cost and turnaround time. While molecular tests like RT-PCR are greatly sought after in terms of specificity, they are resource-demanding and therefore present issues of accessibility to smaller health facilities or for low-resource communities. Further, the transition to mNGS, even though highly sought after, requires training and infrastructure development so that it can be maximally utilized for its clinical applications. Despite these challenges, the ongoing refinement of test procedures continues to educate and refine our control and knowledge of viral gastrointestinal diseases. By a circumvention of such challenges, healthcare providers can make timely diagnosis and facilitate appropriate intervention, thus relieving the burden of such common but ignored viral pathogens on public health services (Relich & Abbott, 2018; Chiu & Miller, 2019) (Figure 3.9).

3.3.1. Clinical Evaluation and History

During clinical evaluation of patients with gastrointestinal symptomatology, careful history-taking is crucial for accurate diagnosis and management. Interviewing the patients should begin with questioning on the onset, duration, and severity of symptoms and associated signs such as fever or weight loss, which may point towards viral gastroenteritis or infectious etiology. Also, a keen inquiry of recent travel, diet, and contact with contaminated food or water can provide clues about the etiologic source. In immunocompromised individuals, especially with illnesses such as AIDS, it is more complex because there are more possible pathogens that might not have induced disease in immunocompetent individuals.

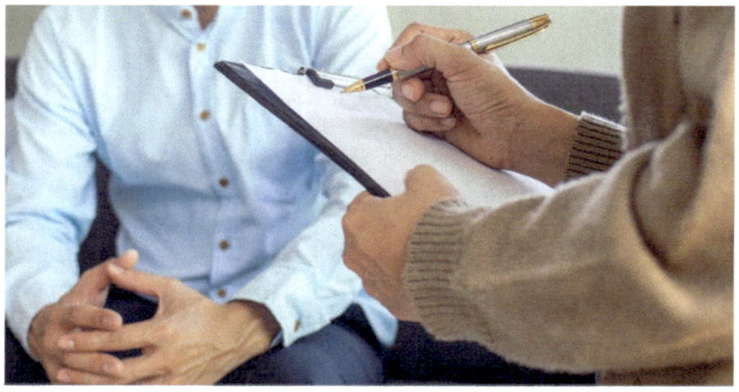

Figure 3.10. Clinical interviews help diagnose gastrointestinal symptoms.

Source: https://external-content.duckduckgo.com/iu/?u=https%3A%2F%2Fbvpsychsolutions.com%2Fwp-content%2Fuploads%2F2023%2F08%2F4-2.jpg&f=1&nofb=1&ipt=86d1dabaa1699d4ea3d4d5cc169fddb82d0bc5bb8225c66ad120521d8496f926.

Differential diagnosis must consider unusual viral pathogens and co-infection, and this requires a subtle understanding of virus pathophysiology and patient susceptibility (Cello & Day, 2009). Confirmatory tests are typically in the middle after a thorough clinical history. For suspected viral gastroenteritis, stool is tested for discrete pathogens to determine the determination of treatment course. Enzyme-linked immunosorbent assays (ELISA), polymerase chain reaction (PCR) tests, and viral cultures diagnose gastrointestinal viruses such as norovirus and rotavirus. Additionally, in patients with persistent gastrointestinal symptoms or those who have been resistant to initial therapy, searching for inflammatory or autoimmune disease may be essential. Past studies have highlighted the potential of viral infections to trigger autoimmune responses, underlining the importance of understanding the interface between viral pathogenesis and host immunity

(Navaneetharaja et al., 2016). Finally, the importance of a multidisciplinary approach to the clinical evaluation of gastrointestinal viruses cannot be overstated. Multidisciplinary coordination of work between various experts, including gastroenterologists, infectious disease specialists, and immunologists, is required to counter the many-sided manifestations of viral infection and its implications. In particular, complicated-case patients, like those with AIDS diarrhea, require multidisciplinary coordination in treatment management and diagnosis. Multidisciplinary coordination of efforts enables practitioners not only to treat the acute viral illness but also to manage the related health problems encountered by patients. By considering the various aspects of the patient's current presentation and health history, clinicians can devise a more customized and effective management plan, ultimately leading to better patient outcomes in the field of gastrointestinal well-being (Cello & Day, 2009) (Figure 3.10).

3.3.2. Laboratory Testing Methods

The scientific environment of laboratory diagnostic testing methods for gastrointestinal viruses has undergone a significant change to emphasize the importance of rapid and accurate diagnostic techniques toward guiding proper patient management. Among them, polymerase chain reaction (PCR) has emerged as a cornerstone due to its sensitivity and specificity for the detection of viral nucleic acids. PCR facilitates the identification of pathogens such as norovirus and rotavirus that are common causes of gastroenteritis. In addition, multiplex PCR progress allows for the detection of many viruses simultaneously, decreasing diagnostic procedures and strengthening epidemiological surveillance. As the global burden of gastrointestinal infections poses significant public health issues, the diagnostic techniques that accelerate and improve the accuracy of the diagnosis are required in clinical settings. Not only do these advances facilitate targeted therapy, but they also play a role in outbreak investigations, ultimately resulting in improved patient outcomes and control of the disease. Serological testing represents the second critical component in gastrointestinal viral diagnosis, providing essential data in the form of antibody detection (Figure 3.11).

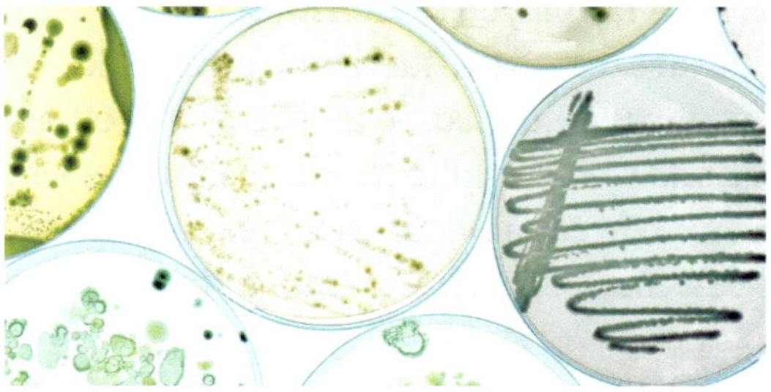

Figure 3.11. Laboratory testing methods for gastrointestinal viruses.

Source: https://external-content.duckduckgo.com/iu/?u=https%3A%2F%2Fclpmag.com%2Fwp-content%2Fuploads%2F2023%2F04%2Fbateria-media-dish-1280x640.jpg&f=1&nofb=1&ipt=2563e38cb354ebdcfc5ebcb93f0f484e628ffcf070be64cf6b4434fe21253ee3.

Enzyme-linked immunosorbent assays (ELISAs) are commonly employed for this use, enabling the detection of specific antibodies in patient specimens and thus for the assessment of viral infections. The assays have been of valuable assistance in understanding immune responses against viruses such as hepatitis A and enteric adenoviruses. Serological methods can also assist epidemiologic studies to assess levels of population immunity and the prevalence of viral infections within communities. The ability of public health interventions to be tailored to the specific context of viral disease is enhanced by serological data, which emphasizes the holism of what is required in laboratory diagnosis. Consequently, the complementary application of serological analysis with molecular techniques further facilitates a better understanding of gastrointestinal viruses. It is only in recent years that advancements in next-generation sequencing (NGS) have revolutionized the identification and characterization of gastrointestinal viruses, as well as permitting extensive characterization of viral genomes. NGS offers unparalleled depth and resolution, allowing scientists to detect novel strains and track viral evolution in real time. NGS has played a decisive role in explaining the nature of multi-factorial outbreaks, as it allows for whole virome analysis as well as co-infections that complicate clinical presentation. NGS is also capable of uncovering mutations that can influence viral pathogenicity and drug resistance.

The combination of NGS and traditional laboratory methods raises surveillance capacity and provides beneficial information for vaccine design and public health. By filling the gap between research and application, such cutting-edge methods emphasize the significance of laboratory testing in the understanding and management of gastrointestinal viruses, further making it imperative in contemporary diagnostics.

3.3.3. Differential Diagnosis

Differential diagnosis is a crucial component of clinical practice, especially when confronted with gastrointestinal virus infections. Healthcare professionals must consider a range of potential causes that present with the same set of symptoms, such as diarrhea, vomiting, and abdominal cramps. For gastrointestinal viruses, the presentation can be mimicked by bacterial or protozoal causes. For instance, the severity of clinical signs may vary extensively across species, primarily in ruminants, as neonatal and juvenile population research has noted. Furthermore, it is important to identify the specific viral agent since it will determine the patients treatment and public health concern, particularly if zoonotic infections are considered, thus it is important to have extended and careful differential diagnosis protocols (Heller & Chigerwe, 2018). In diagnosing a patient with viral gastrointestinal infection, an extensive history and physical examination are essential components of the differential. Precipitants of the disease, like contact with infective agents, travel history in the last week, or consumption of contaminated food, need to be considered. A case from Uruguay reflected the significance of environmental history, where a child developed symptoms following a trip to a beach contaminated with a toxic algal bloom. The ensuing hospitalization and the diagnosis of acute liver failure reinforce the importance of considering not just viral pathogens but also their potential interactions with environmental toxins like microcystins (Andrinilo et al., 2017). This case shows that the spectrum of differential diagnosis is broader than infectious causes and extends to environmental determinants, which may complicate gastrointestinal illnesses. Lastly, the differential diagnosis of the gastrointestinal viruses requires an integrative process that combines clinical experience and modern laboratory methods. Diagnostic tools like serological tests and advanced methods like liquid chromatography, electrospray ionization high-resolution mass spectrometry can be applied to identify specific pathogens or their derivatives. Identification is important because it has implications for management as well as accounting for the need for public health interventions. Understanding the nuances of different gastrointestinal pathogens, such as their symptomology, allows for targeted management interventions and helps ease overall treatment that can be provided to patients suffering from these complex ailments. A thoughtful differential diagnosis is thus critical in managing gastrointestinal viruses effectively in the overall framework of infectious disease management.

3.4. Treatment Options

Management of gastrointestinal viruses often needs a multi-faceted approach tailored to the individual virus and the patient's clinical picture. In most cases, treatment can be divided into symptomatic treatment and antiviral treatment against a specific virus. Symptomatic treatment typically includes rehydration and electrolyte replacement, which is necessary in patients with significant diarrhea or vomiting.

This approach limits dehydration risk, particularly in vulnerable populations such as the elderly and children. Immunocompromised patients, such as HIV/AIDS, are an additional challenge as viral gastroenteritis has the potential to be complicated by pre-existing illnesses. Highly active antiretroviral therapy is a cornerstone of treatment for these patients, with adjunct treatment potentially needed to control concomitant gastrointestinal symptoms (Cello & Day, 2009). Antiviral drug therapy targeted for certain viral pathogens causing infection of the gastrointestinal tract has emerged as a significant treatment protocol.

For example, medications like nitazoxanide have been designated for the treatment of cryptosporidiosis, which may occur in association with viral infections among immunocompromised individuals. Early treatment with antivirals decreases the severity and duration of the illness significantly. Aside from that, the recent advancements in molecular diagnostics enable clinicians to identify specific pathogens quickly, therefore permitting more specific treatment modalities. There remain certain infections that are difficult to treat due to the emergence of resistant strains or atypical presentations. Thus, ongoing research and clinical investigation must be conducted in order to develop new antiviral agents and evaluate their effectiveness against gastrointestinal viruses (Cello & Day, 2009) (Figure 3.12).

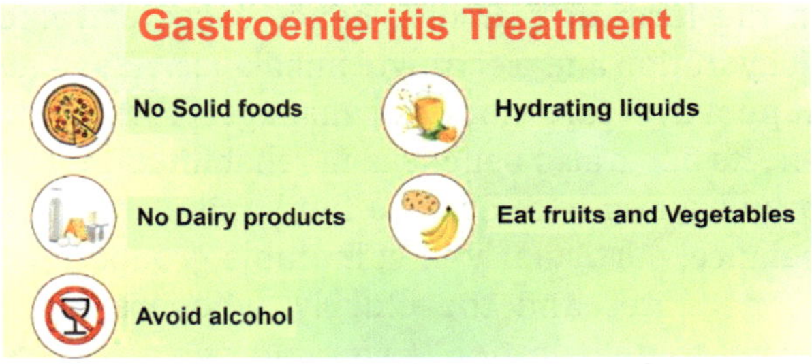

Figure 3.12. Gastroenteritis treatment option.

Source: https://external-content.duckduckgo.com/iu/?u=https%3A%2F%2Fwww.jaipurgastro.com%2Fwp-content%2Fuploads%2F2020%2F01%2FTreatment.jpg&f=1&nofb=1&ipt=b07fff8e7bec132ccea6b21def9cec58435f256c7b6b3f1cd2d7daae6c8a60e5.

Apart from pharmacological management, non-pharmacological methods are also essential in the treatment of gastrointestinal viruses. These include prevention measures, such as sanitation, hygiene, and immunization where available. The role of sanitation in public health cannot be overstated, especially in developing nations where clean water and improved sanitation are not readily available. Research has shown that source separating sewers could optimize nutrient recycling while limiting pathogens exposure. Education interventions with a focus on hygiene are also linked to a significant reduction in the prevalence of gastroenteritis in the population. By integrating both these measures, medical professionals can optimize viral gastroenteritis-affected patient outcomes and contribute to public health against gastrointestinal viruses as a whole.

3.4.1. Supportive Care and Hydration

The management of gastrointestinal viral infections needs an integrative approach, and supportive care and hydration are major components. As viral pathogens cause significant gastrointestinal distress, symptoms manifest in the form of diarrhea, hence cause extreme dehydration and electrolyte imbalance. Adequate supportive care not only manages these side effects but is also beneficial in rehabilitation. The primary aim is to achieve fluid and electrolyte balance, particularly in vulnerable groups such as neonates and the elderly, who are more prone to dehydration. Favorable outcomes are contingent on early interventions that can avert further complications such as endotoxemia or sepsis, indicating the importance of effective supportive care strategies in the management of gastrointestinal viruses (Heller & Chigerwe, 2018). Hydration must be tailored according to the severity of illness and overall condition of the patient. For patients with mild to moderate dehydration, oral rehydration solutions (ORS) prove to be very effective. These consist of balanced electrolytes and carbohydrates that enhance water absorption in the intestine. In severe dehydration, parenteral fluid therapy can be a consideration, with the immediate replenishment of fluids and electrolytes directly into the circulation. Apart from fluid resuscitation, adequate nutrition management is also important, particularly in children, where the risk of growth and development is implicated. Adequate hydration through ORS facilitates prevention of complications as well as the provision of body resources to enable the body to adequately counteract the viral infection with an immune response (West, 1997). Consequences of supportive care extend beyond the acute management of fluid; they involve a global plan for patient recovery. Supportive care protocols may include antiemetic medication, pain management strategies, and continuous monitoring of vital parameters and laboratory tests to monitor patient improvement. Furthermore, patient and caregiver teaching about recognizing dehydration and adherence to therapeutic interventions can benefit recovery. By sensitization and preemptive care, healthcare workers can best reduce the gastrointestinal virus burden among populations. Supportive care and hydration at its essence reiterate an extremely crucial intersection of patient education and clinical practice that forms the nucleus in managing the complexities of gastrointestinal viral illnesses (Heller & Chigerwe, 2018) (Figure 3.13).

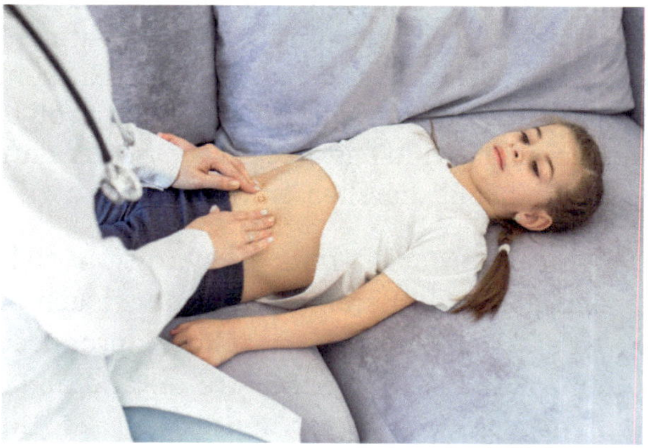

Figure 3.13. Supportive care for gastrointestinal viral infections.

Source: https://www.ankurahospitals.com/wp-content/uploads/2024/09/pediatric-gastrointestinal-infections.jpeg.

3.4.2. Antiviral Medications

Antiviral medications are of central importance in treating viral illnesses that infect the gastrointestinal tract. In contrast to antibiotics, whose purpose is to inhibit bacterial infections, antivirals are focused on inhibiting virus replication and have the potential to abate symptoms expressed by such infections as norovirus and rotavirus. Those viruses infecting the gastrointestinal system can pose the possibility of morbidity, especially in susceptible hosts such as the young, old, and immunocompromised host. By decreasing viral load and shortening the course of illness, antiviral medications not only enhance patient outcomes but also decrease transmission risk in communities. Their efficacy typically depends on early administration following symptom onset, making early diagnosis and intervention critical in the treatment of viral gastroenteritis.

In addition to conventional antiviral drugs, new therapy research has expanded the treatment modalities for gastrointestinal viruses. Nitazoxanide and favipiravir are among the drugs that have been promising in preclinical and clinical studies and suggesting that novel antivirals may be more efficacious against resistant viral strains. Furthermore, research still investigates the adjunctive use of drugs such as probiotics and immunomodulators that may enhance the antiviral effects synergistically or otherwise enhance colonic health upon infection. The initial evidence supports that such combinations would not only suppress the gastrointestinal symptoms but also rectify normal colonic flora that is altered in the pathogenesis of viral infections. Although promising, data available must pass through rigorous clinical trials to establish their precise roles in antiviral therapy regimens, as per the limitations of the literature (Kilgore & Najm, 2010) (Figure 3.14).

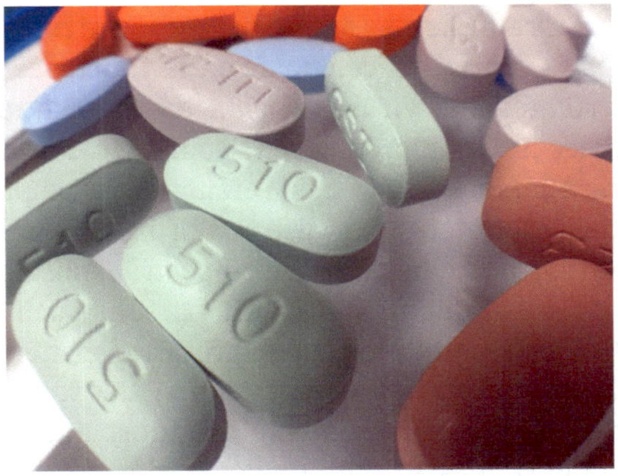

Figure 3.14. Antiviral medication stops gastrointestinal viruses.

Source: https://upload.wikimedia.org/wikipedia/commons/3/36/Antiretroviral_Drugs_to_Treat_HIV_Infection_%2831793869534%29.jpg.

The difficulty of adequately controlling gastrointestinal viral infections with antiviral drugs is exacerbated by the continuously changing nature of the viruses. Resistance may ensue, and some antiviral drugs become less effective with time, a factor that requires constant monitoring and research.

Changing therapeutic approaches in response to local epidemiology and virus mutation is important for achieving the best possible outcomes for patients. Furthermore, public health interventions to boost vaccination and hygiene practices are essential supplements to antiviral medication control strategies in controlling gastroenteritis outbreaks of viral origin. Ultimately, an interdisciplinary effort combining pharmaceuticals, preventive care, and patient education will prove to be essential in combating the gastrointestinal viral disease burden across multigroup populations (Azher et al., 2017).

3.4.3. Role of Probiotics

The role of probiotics in the context of gastrointestinal viruses is gaining more and more popularity due to their potential to enhance gut health and boost immune response. Probiotics are live microorganisms that, when the right dose is administered, confer beneficial health effects on the host, particularly the gastrointestinal tract. Evidence points towards their role in inhibiting the growth of pathogenic bacteria and biofilm formation, thus inducing gastrointestinal infections.

By provoking the immune system and modulating inflammatory responses, probiotics are able to help manage and decrease viral infections in the gastrointestinal tract. It is all the more relevant with the rising instances of gastroenteritis and other viral infections that disrupt gut homeostasis. Indeed, probiotics also have potential fields of application for the enhancement of gastrointestinal resistance to various viral pathogens, as aligned with the ongoing research into their biotherapeutic potential in the field of medicine (Sullano & Florez, 2020). In addition, communications between the gut microbiota and gastrointestinal tract viruses emphasize the necessity of maintaining a balanced microbial community. Research has indicated that dysbiosis, or microbial imbalance of gut microbiota, can potentially weaken the body's defense system and make it susceptible to viral infections. Probiotics as strategic mediators can restore microbial balance and fortify gut barriers and thus potentially alleviate the severity of gastrointestinal viruses. Next-generation probiotics with diverse bacterial strains can potentially enhance therapeutic efficacy. These emerging probiotics can promote attachment within the gastrointestinal tract and increase a widespread immune response. The scientific community is continuing to investigate these associations, prioritizing well-designed clinical trials to substantiate the role of these microorganisms in preventing viral infections (Hage et al., 2017). The existing knowledge of probiotics as part of viral gastroenteritis prevention and treatment paradigms is still evolving. With more research, it would seem that personalized approaches, which are tailored for unique gut microbiota patterns, may be most effective in augmenting the efficacy of probiotic therapy. This is in concordance with modern biotherapeutic interventions that rely on gut microbiome manipulation through dietary alterations, prebiotic intake, and diverse probiotics. The addition of probiotics to routine treatment protocols has the potential to reduce the duration and severity of viral gastrointestinal infections as well as improve overall digestive health. Therefore, a comprehensive review of the role played by probiotics as an inhibitor of intestinal viruses not only enhances our understanding of their biological functions but perhaps shifts our strategy of treating viral infections in the gut, ushering in a new age of prophylactic healthcare practices (Sullano & Florez, 2020).

3.5. Prevention Strategies

Prevention measures are particularly significant in the field of gastrointestinal viruses, where forestalling the health consequences of such infections is paramount. Multipronged prevention measures, ranging from immunization to strict standards of hygiene, need to be adopted to limit the transmission of norovirus and rotavirus. Vaccination has proven to be effective, particularly among children, because vaccines have been found to significantly reduce the incidence of viral gastroenteritis. But with very limited antiviral treatment options, preventive measures are once again the focus, including care provider and healthcare worker education on effective practice to minimize the risk of infection. Adherent hand hygiene, especially in settings such as schools and daycare centers, can limit transmission of these organisms and is paramount in controlling outbreaks. Therefore, raising awareness of preventive steps is crucial to controlling the incidence of gastrointestinal viruses within the population. Further, isolation protocol and contact tracing are critical components of the overall prevention plan against gastrointestinal viruses. During outbreaks, isolating infected patients stops transmission, particularly among vulnerable persons such as the elderly and immunocompromised patients. Contact tracing allows health authorities to track and inform individuals who are most likely to have been infected with the virus, thus allowing timely intervention. Proactive intervention is particularly important in healthcare facilities, where the potential for nosocomial infection is heightened. Through the use of these methods in addition to environmental disinfection protocols, viral loads borne by shared surfaces can be significantly decreased. Merging these interventions with community health programs provides a comprehensive thrust for reducing the effects of gastrointestinal viruses, as promoted in best practice infection prevention studies across various facilities (Fisher et al., 2012). As the tide continues to shift with gastrointestinal viruses, ongoing examinations of new ways of prevention are paramount. New discoveries of antiviral drugs and new vaccine formulations are some of the research areas that are being given significant scientific attention. Apart from this, public awareness programs demanding food safety and correct handling procedures while food preparation can also be an important prevention measure. Improved surveillance systems and reporting schemes can also be useful in the identification of outbreaks early and in allowing swift response measures. Pooling results from studies of different types can yield insight into viral transmission processes and host response and aid in the development of targeted intervention design. A continually dynamic preventive approach will thus be essential in combating the challenge of gastrointestinal viruses and, ultimately, influencing public health (Kijlstra et al., 2003) (Figure 3.15).

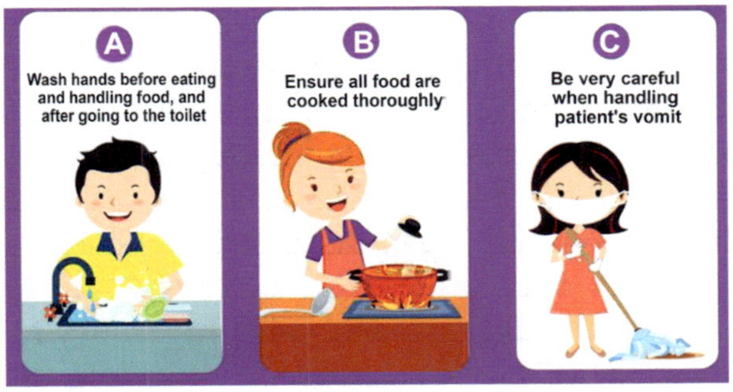

Figure 3.15. Prevent viral gastroenteritis.

Source: https://external-content.duckduckgo.com/iu/?u=https%3A%2F%2Fwww.chshb.gov.tw%2Fsites%2Fdefault%2Ffiles%2Finline-images%2F55ecdd49-b65c-4655-a4b2-08e9c458939a_0.jpg&f=1&nofb=1&ipt=fa9a6a71567e1d1a239c4cf3fb3a49e6b957555a583409396b43017566ab26dd.

3.5.1. Hygiene Practices

The importance of adhering to proper hygiene practices in curtailing the transmission of gastrointestinal viruses cannot be overemphasized. The disease-causing organisms may readily transmit in the community and in hospitals, leading to significant morbidity and, in some situations, death, particularly among vulnerable populations such as immunocompromised individuals. Strong infection control is of paramount significance in the prevention of viral diseases, as highlighted by recent data that show traditional bacterial and fungal infections have been usurped by viruses in specific patient populations. Thus, it is important to develop unique hygiene protocols, pre-exposure and post-exposure prophylaxis, in lessening the disease burden of gastrointestinal viruses and in preserving public health (Fisher et al., 2012). Hand hygiene plays a critical role in the prevention of transmission of gastrointestinal viruses. Evidence shows that the hands are significant vehicles for disease-causing factors and are responsible for the spread of diverse diseases like foodborne disease and nosocomial infection. The practice of hand hygiene, in which the hands are cleaned thoroughly using water and soap or disinfectants, has been shown to reduce the microbial load significantly. In studies that compared various hand wash brands, results indicated that all brands tested were found to have antibacterial properties, particularly against common pathogens like *Staphylococcus aureus* and *Escherichia coli*. In particular, the efficacy of hand hygiene is assessed based on the correct technique and handwashing agents' concentration, indicating that adherence to advised practice, i.e., washing between five and ten minutes, plays an important role in maximizing protection from gastrointestinal viruses (Akande et al., 2013). The role of hygiene measures extends beyond independent actions to encompass broader community health interventions. Educational campaigns in schools, the workplace, and health facilities that promote hand hygiene can greatly raise awareness of the need for proper hygiene practices, especially during outbreaks of gastrointestinal viruses. Integrating hygiene education into policy at the public health level encourages behavioral change that has a drastic effect on infection rates within populations. Establishing usable sanitation facilities, such as adequate handwashing stations and antibacterial products, also enhances community resistance to viral infection. Lastly, a complex system that combines individual responsibility with collaborative action will be able to empower communities to effectively combat the spread of gastrointestinal viruses and maintain public health objectives (Fisher et al., 2012).

3.5.2. Vaccination Efforts

Vaccination efforts are crucial in the war against gastrointestinal viruses, particularly among vulnerable populations such as children and immunocompromised individuals. Vaccine effectiveness in preventing infection by viruses cannot be overstated since it does a lot to reduce the morbidity and mortality rates of such pathogens. Some of the advances in vaccine research in recent years have focused on the creation of vaccines for gastrointestinal viruses such as rotavirus and norovirus, which are notorious for causing serious gastroenteritis. Vaccination campaigns on a large scale try to increase herd immunity, thereby vaccinating not only the vaccinated but also unvaccinated members who cannot be vaccinated due to medical reasons. The efficacy of such campaigns has been evident in the substantial decline in hospitalizations and their associated healthcare costs due to these viral diseases. As much as the vaccination campaign has been enhanced, challenges remain, particularly when placed in the context of viral diversity and the emergence of new strains that are capable of evading existing immunity. Continuous guard is called for as gastrointestinal viruses undergo evolution and mutation and pose a challenge to the efficacy of existing vaccines. In addition, the development and implementation of vaccine strategies need to be devised to overcome the distinctive epidemiological patterns of these viruses in given locations. For instance, determinants such as socioeconomic status and healthcare access may influence vaccination coverage rates, necessitating public health services supporting the provision and education for vaccines. As more is learned through new research on the mechanisms of resistance and immunity by gastrointestinal viruses, vaccination guidelines must be revised accordingly in a bid to maximize their delivery and promotion of universal protection. Furthermore, immunization campaigns can be synergized with other preventive measures such as improved sanitation and hygiene practices to enhance the payoffs of immunization against gastrointestinal viruses. This multi-faceted intervention is particularly important in settings where outbreaks are impending, such as nursing homes and childcare centers. Vaccination alone cannot entirely prevent people from getting infected; hence, infection control measures are vital to the prevention and management of viral spread. For instance, in target populations with specific vulnerabilities, e.g., recipients of organ transplants or cancer treatment, targeted vaccination in addition to meticulous infection control measures can significantly reduce the incidence of complications arising from viral infection. As has been discussed, "a balanced approach that utilizes all of these can be effective at reducing the negative impact of viral infection" (Fisher et al., 2012). Ultimately, the interface between vaccination campaigns and integrative public health efforts is required for effectively countering the danger represented by gastrointestinal viruses.

3.5.3. Public Health Initiatives

Public health initiatives play a crucial role in curbing the impact of gastrointestinal viruses, which pose threats to public health globally. Surveillance and reporting mechanisms are integral parts of efficient public health programs in order to detect and trace such viruses. As indicated, infectious intestinal diseases (IID) result in considerable morbidity and mortality, particularly in industrialized nations where viruses are the major cause of illness. Underreporting of IID, particularly from nations like Malta, emphasizes the need for intensified surveillance in terms of population-based studies. These programs are set to provide holistic data that can be applied in decision-making and resource allocation, resulting in improved health outcomes. Integration of these systems is crucial in understanding the epidemiology of gastrointestinal viruses and responding promptly to outbreaks, hence protecting public health effectively (Gauci et al., 2006). Education and community awareness are some of the most important components of public health programs aimed at controlling gastrointestinal viruses. Health literacy enables individuals to recognize symptoms, become knowledgeable about transmission modes, and adopt preventive measures such as practicing good hygiene and safe food handling. All media can be exploited by public health campaigns to inform individuals about gastrointestinal viruses, particularly in communities that are prone to outbreaks. In Indonesia, for example, collaboration between local health authorities and research centers has enabled training and outreach programs that have enhanced the awareness of zoonotic infections and their impact on the health of humans. Through addressing particular health problems in society, public programs for health programs are able to enhance collective effort in the reduction of gastrointestinal virus spread. Participation from stakeholders in different sectors also adds to the effectiveness of the programs (Molia et al., 2012). Investment in research and development is also an integral part of the public health initiatives towards the prevention of gastrointestinal viruses. Consistency in researching the dynamics and ecology of virus transmission enables the development of effective vaccines and treatment strategies. Academic organizations, government health agencies, and international collaboration enables common knowledge and innovation in solution development to fight viruses. Studies such as those described in Indonesia to combat rabies and wildlife disease illustrate the importance of multidisciplinary approaches to prevent emerging infectious diseases. By prioritizing research toward the major mechanisms of transmission of gastrointestinal viruses, public health initiatives can design evidence-based interventions that effectively reduce disease prevalence. Lastly, coordinated focus on research not only stimulates real-time outbreak interventions but also underlines longer-term preventative measures (Molia et al., 2012).

SUMMARY

The study of gastrointestinal viruses helps to highlight their food security and public health significance. Norovirus and rotavirus are leading gastroenteritis pathogens and cause serious challenges to healthcare systems worldwide. That they are highly transmissible implies that effective surveillance and management procedures must be in place to limit outbreaks. It is also essential to comprehend their transmission behavior and host interaction for the sake of formulating effective preventive measures. Enhanced diagnostic techniques and ongoing research into viral infection epidemiology can provide important insights into their persistence and ability to adapt and eventually influence public health policy. The significance of research into gastrointestinal virus infection extends beyond direct clinical utility and recognizes the importance of adopting a more comprehensive approach to viral control that takes sociocultural factors and global health policy into account. Secondly, the descriptions of the molecular mechanisms through which gastrointestinal viruses interact with the host cells present possibilities for novel therapeutic intervention. The factor of glycan modifications, emphasized in the context of microbial interactions, reveals a sophisticated interaction between viral pathogenicity and host susceptibility. Research has indicated that variations in sialic acids on the host cell surfaces significantly influence virus tropisms as well as infection outcome (Wasik et al., 2017). Therefore, modulation of these interactions can pave the way for new antiviral treatments. Second, a multi-disciplinary strategy involving contributions from virology, immunology, and epidemiology will be required to decipher the complexity of these infections. Effective vaccines and treatments can only be achieved through targeted research interventions, thus reducing the burden of gastrointestinal viral diseases globally. Finally, facing the challenges posed by gastrointestinal viruses will demand collaboration between researchers, clinicians, and policymakers. Effectively curtailing the impact of these pathogens relies on the implementation of evidence-based public health interventions that promote sanitary and hygiene behaviors within populations. The recognition of high-risk groups, such as infants and toddlers and immunocompromised subjects who are most affected by the health impact of gastrointestinal virus infections is necessary. Education campaigns can empower individuals to adopt preventive behavior, thereby preventing transmission rates. In addition, ongoing research into the health impacts associated with organic and conventional modes of farming reveals interconnections between agriculture and the transmission of gastrointestinal viruses (Kijlstra et al., 2003). Not only does this integrated approach concentrate on ongoing research, but it also calls for a paradigm shift in the study of gastrointestinal viruses as well as their far-reaching impacts on global healthcare.

In looking into the role of gastrointestinal viruses, a common thread is that they contribute to deranging gut microbiota and overall health. The human gastrointestinal tract contains an intricate ecosystem of microorganism, and disturbances in balance can lead to severe disease, including infection and other gastrointestinal diseases. Existing studies indicate the efficacy of fecal microbiota transplantation (FMT) in the treatment of conditions such as recurrent *Clostridium difficile* infection (rCDI). As a new treatment, its possibilities are attracting attention, and scientists continue to seek its applications in other gastrointestinal disorders. With the restitution of healthy microbiota, FMT promises relief not only from rCDI but in treating broader gastrointestinal disease. The significance of this research presents therapeutic potential for viral-associated gastrointestinal illness and underscores the need to know more about host-microorganism dynamics in disease formation (Rub et al., 2019). Gastrointestinal viruses have increased in occurrence, triggering efforts toward establishing environmental and genetic origins for such infections. Etiologic research indicates that genetic susceptibility may be a significant consideration as an interaction with extrinsic factors, where a complex interplay determines the individual's susceptibility. Such support for interaction is furnished by epidemiologic studies, which place particular focus on environmental aspects like viral exposure in particular windows of development. Furthermore, disparities in host reactions to viral infections of the gastrointestinal tract indicate that individualized treatment and preventive strategies might be necessary. By studying these intricate relationships, researchers can more effectively determine how viral spread in the gastrointestinal tract influences health at a population level (Croen et al., 2006). Significantly, future research, including that with the CHARGE study, aims to make a general study of the interaction between gastrointestinal viruses, genetic susceptibility, and environmental exposure. Through exploration of a wide variety of chemical and biological factors, researchers seek the mechanism of viral illness and associated health consequences. This longitudinal investigation is most likely to yield significant information regarding numerous variables influencing gastrointestinal health and disease. In addition, the multi-factorial design of this investigation will enable greater knowledge of phenotypic variability between infected individuals, thus enabling more targeted interventions. With continued exploration of these intricate dynamics, its implications for public health policy and clinical practice will become increasingly important, ultimately determining our approach to gastrointestinal viruses and improving outcomes for afflicted populations (Croen et al., 2006).

CLOSER LOOK

VIRUS-HOST INTERACTIONS IN THE GASTROINTESTINAL (GI) TRACT

The GI tract is a highly diverse and dynamic environment where viruses interact with host cells, immune response, and gut microbiota. Many viruses infect the GI tract as the primary site of infection or as an entry point. The interactions can generate asymptomatic colonization, gastrointestinal disease confined to the site, or systemic infection. Enteral viruses such as rotavirus, norovirus, adenovirus, astrovirus, and enteroviruses are prevalent pathogens that utilize the GI tract as a means of infecting, replicating, and spreading (Figure 3.16).

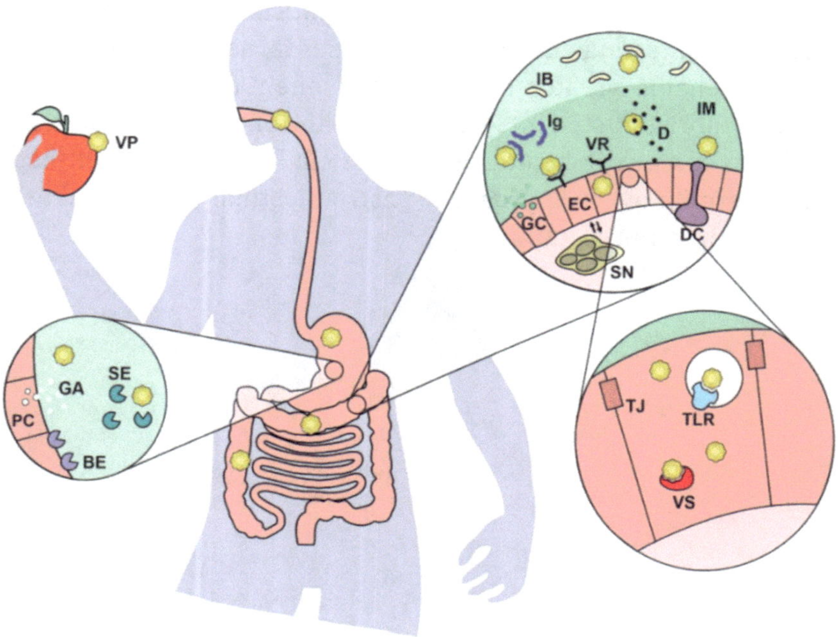

Figure 3.16. Schematic illustration of the gastrointestinal tract showing the pathway of ingested viral particles (VP), their interaction with gut-associated immune cells, and potential mechanisms of viral entry, replication, and immune recognition.

Source: https://www.mdpi.com/ijms/ijms-22-04734/article_deploy/html/images/ijms-22-04734-g001.png.

The first critical event in virus-host interaction is viral entry, typically via the fecal-oral route. Viruses must survive the conditions of hostility in the stomach, including acidic pH, digestive enzymes, and bile salts, prior to invading and infecting small or large intestine epithelial cells. Stable capsids have evolved among most enteric viruses to protect them from being killed in this hostile environment. Once they have entered the intestine, they bind to specific receptors on intestinal epithelial cells, for example, histo-blood group antigens (HBGAs) in noroviruses or integrins and gangliosides for rotaviruses.

Infecting the host, viruses hijack the cellular machinery of the host to make copies of themselves, typically causing damage to the intestinal epithelium. For example, rotavirus infection leads to the destruction of enterocytes in the small intestine, with subsequent malabsorption, disrupted fluid and electrolyte balance, and diarrhea. Some viruses, such as enteroviruses, can penetrate into the gut epithelium and into the bloodstream, leading to systemic infections of the nervous system or other organs.

The immune system plays a part in controlling viral infection of the GI tract. The mucosal immune system, secretory IgA antibodies, innate immune cells, and pattern recognition receptors like Toll-like receptors (TLRs) recognize viral constituents and initiate responses to limit infection. Interferons and cytokines are also generated to inhibit viral replication and draw immune cells. But the majority of viruses have developed mechanisms of immune evasion, such as preventing interferon signaling or avoiding recognition through altering viral surface antigens.

One key but often underemphasized component of virus-host interactions in the intestine is the gut microbiota. Commensal bacteria have the potential to regulate viral infectivity through a variety of mechanisms. Certain viruses employ bacterial structures, such as lipopolysaccharides (LPS), to facilitate stability or augment attachment to host cells. Conversely, a healthy microbiota can enhance mucosal immunity and limit viral infection. Disruption of the microbiome by antibiotics or illness can increase susceptibility to viral gastroenteritis.

Apart from causing disease, some viruses produce persistent infections in the GI tract, especially in immunocompromised hosts. Persistent infections can be able to induce chronic inflammation, delayed healing, or sequelae like malnutrition and growth retardation in children.

REFERENCES

1. Relich, R. F., & Abbott, A. N. (2018). Syndromic and Point-of-Care Molecular Testing. *Advances in Molecular Pathology, 1*(1), 97–113. https://doi.org/10.1016/j.yamp.2018.07.007 (accessed on 16th July 2025).
2. Navaneetharaja, N., Griffiths, V., Wileman, T., & Carding, S. R. (2016). A Role for the Intestinal Microbiota and Virome in Myalgic Encephalomyelitis/Chronic Fatigue Syndrome (ME/CFS)?. *Journal of clinical medicine, 5*(6), 55. https://doi.org/10.3390/jcm5060055(accessed on 16th July 2025).
3. Adu-Gyamfi, S. (2019). *Ebola hemorrhagic Fever in Africa: A Necessary Highlight.* https://core.ac.uk/download/480549437.pdf (accessed on 16th July 2025).
4. Akande, V. A., Dahunsi, S. O., & Oranusi, S. U. (2013). *Assessment of microbial quality and antibacterial activity of commonly used hand washes.* https://core.ac.uk/download/18295288.pdf (accessed on 16th July 2025).
5. Alexander, K. A., Bagirova, M., Blackburn, J. K., Carlson, C., et al. (2019). *The global distribution of Bacillus anthracis and associated anthrax risk to humans, livestock and wildlife.* https://core.ac.uk/download/287623894.pdf (accessed on 16th July 2025).
6. Fisher, B. T., Alexander, S., Dvorak, C. C., Zaoutis, T. E., Zerr, D. M., & Sung, L. (2012). Epidemiology and potential preventative measures for viral infections in children with malignancy and those undergoing hematopoietic cell transplantation. *Pediatric blood & cancer, 59*(1), 11–15. https://doi.org/10.1002/pbc.23417(accessed on 16th July 2025).
7. Andrinolo, D., Caixach, J., Cavalieri, M. L., D'Agostino, M., et al. (2017). *Recreational exposure during algal bloom in Carrasco beach, Uruguay: A liver failure case report.* https://core.ac.uk/download/159292906.pdf (accessed on 16th July 2025).
8. Azher, T. N., Huang, A. J. W., Stuart, P. M., Tajfirouz, M., et al. (2017). *Herpes simplex keratitis: Challenges in diagnosis and clinical management.* https://core.ac.uk/download/129069102.pdf (accessed on 16th July 2025).
9. Banu, P., Constantin, V. D., Nistor, M. F., Popa, D., et al. (2016). *Perforated small intestine in a patient with T-cell lymphoma: A rare cause of peritonitis.* https://core.ac.uk/download/144552420.pdf (accessed on 16th July 2025).
10. Borchardt, M. A., Kieke, B. A., Lambertini, E., Loge, F. J., et al. (2012). *Viruses in nondisinfected drinking water from municipal wells and community incidence of acute gastrointestinal illness.* https://core.ac.uk/download/323070050.pdf (accessed on 16th July 2025).
11. Zhang, C., Zhou, S., Groppelli, E., Pellegrino, P., Williams, I., Borrow, P., Chain, B. M., & Jolly, C. (2015). Hybrid spreading mechanisms and T cell activation shape the dynamics of HIV-1 infection. *PLoS computational biology, 11*(4), e1004179. https://doi.org/10.1371/journal.pcbi.1004179(accessed on 16th July 2025).
12. Sophie Molia (CIRAD), Nicolas Gaidet (CIRAD), Hervé Bourhy (Institut Pasteur) (2012). *Mission to Indonesia to participate to the 1st Indonesia-France Seminar in Medicine & Public Health and investigate potential collaborations on animal health: 2nd–9th of November 2012.* http://agritrop.cirad.fr/567354/1/document_567354.pdf (accessed on 16th July 2025).
13. Cacciotti, F., Cicerone, C., Corazziari, E. S., Gagliardi, L., et al. (2016). *Eubiosis and dysbiosis:*

The two sides of the microbiota. https://core.ac.uk/download/54532058.pdf (accessed on 16th July 2025).

14. Cartwright, R. Y. (1997). *Viruses and Drinking Water.* https://core.ac.uk/download/11020755.pdf (accessed on 16th July 2025).

15. Cello, J. P., & Day, L. W. (2009). Idiopathic AIDS enteropathy and treatment of gastrointestinal opportunistic pathogens. *Gastroenterology, 136*(6), 1952–1965. https://doi.org/10.1053/j.gastro.2008.12.073(accessed on 16th July 2025).

16. Heller, M. C., & Chigerwe, M. (2018). Diagnosis and Treatment of Infectious Enteritis in Neonatal and Juvenile Ruminants. *The Veterinary clinics of North America. Food animal practice, 34*(1), 101–117. https://doi.org/10.1016/j.cvfa.2017.08.001 (accessed on 16th July 2025).

17. Chiu, C. Y., & Miller, S. A. (2019). *Clinical Metagenomics.* https://core.ac.uk/download/323062552.pdf (accessed on 16th July 2025).

18. Croen, L. A., Hansen, R., Hertz-Picciotto, I., Jones, C., et al. (2006). *The CHARGE study: An epidemiologic investigation of genetic and environmental factors contributing to autism.* https://core.ac.uk/download/323070787.pdf (accessed on 16th July 2025).

19. Goh, G. K., Dunker, A. K., & Uversky, V. N. (2012). Understanding Viral Transmission Behavior via Protein Intrinsic Disorder Prediction: Coronaviruses. *Journal of pathogens, 2012*, 738590. https://doi.org/10.1155/2012/738590(accessed on 16th July 2025).

20. Egozcue Rubí, J. J., Goloshchapov, O. V., Olekhnovich, E. I., Sidorenko, A. A., et al. (2019). *Long-term impact of fecal transplantation in healthy volunteers.* https://core.ac.uk/download/294830713.pdf (accessed on 16th July 2025).

21. Kijlstra, Aize; Groot, Maria; Roest, van der, Joop; Kasteel, Daniella and Eijck, Ineke (2003) Analysis of black holes in our knowledge concerning animal health in the organic food production chain. Wageningen UR , Animal Sciences Group.(accessed on 16th July 2025).

22. El Hage, R., Hernandez Sanabria, E., & Van de Wiele, T. (2017). *Emerging trends in 'smart probiotics': Functional consideration for the development of novel health and industrial applications.* https://core.ac.uk/download/147045642.pdf (accessed on 16th July 2025).

23. Florez, K., & Sullano, C. (2020). *Probiotic Biotherapy: Discussing its Influential Role in Oral Health.* https://core.ac.uk/download/322936745.pdf (accessed on 16th July 2025).

24. Gauci, C., Gilles, H. M., Mamo, J., O'Brien, S. F., et al. (2006). *Infectious intestinal disease: Do we know it all?* https://core.ac.uk/download/46602090.pdf (accessed on 16th July 2025).

25. Hendrickson, C. M., & Matthay, M. A. (2013). *Viral pathogens and acute lung injury: Investigations inspired by the SARS epidemic and the 2009 H1N1 influenza pandemic.* https://core.ac.uk/download/323072736.pdf (accessed on 16th July 2025).

26. Sekar, N., Shah, N. K., Abbas, S. S., Kakkar, M., & Roadmap to Combat Zoonoses in India Initiative (2011). Research options for controlling zoonotic disease in India, 2010-2015. *PloS one, 6*(2), e17120. https://doi.org/10.1371/journal.pone.0017120 (accessed on 16th July 2025).

27. Kilgore, D., & Najm, W. (2010). *Common Respiratory Diseases.* https://core.ac.uk/download/323075715.pdf (accessed on 16th July 2025).

28. Lin, D. M., Koskella, B., & Lin, H. C. (2017). Phage therapy: An alternative to antibiotics in the age of multi-drug resistance. *World journal of gastrointestinal pharmacology and*

therapeutics, *8*(3), 162–173. https://doi.org/10.4292/wjgpt.v8.i3.162(accessed on 16th July 2025).

29. Nelsen, A. (2022). *Emerging Respiratory Viral Pathogens*. https://core.ac.uk/download/552445500.pdf (accessed on 16th July 2025).
30. Nordin, A. (2007). *Ammonia-Based Sanitation Technology*. https://core.ac.uk/download/11695241.pdf (accessed on 16th July 2025).
31. Sykes, J. (2010). *Immunodeficiencies Caused by Infectious Diseases*. https://core.ac.uk/download/323070119.pdf (accessed on 16th July 2025).
32. Wasik, B. R., Barnard, K. N., Ossiboff, R. J., Khedri, Z., Feng, K. H., Yu, H., Chen, X., Perez, D. R., Varki, A., & Parrish, C. R. (2017). Distribution of O-Acetylated Sialic Acids among Target Host Tissues for Influenza Virus. *mSphere*, *2*(5), e00379-16. https://doi.org/10.1128/mSphere.00379-16(accessed on 16th July 2025).
33. West, N. J. (1997). *Prevention and Treatment of Hemorrhagic Cystitis*. https://deepblue.lib.umich.edu/bitstream/2027.42/90047/1/j.1875-9114.1997.tb03745.x.pdf (accessed on 16th July 2025).

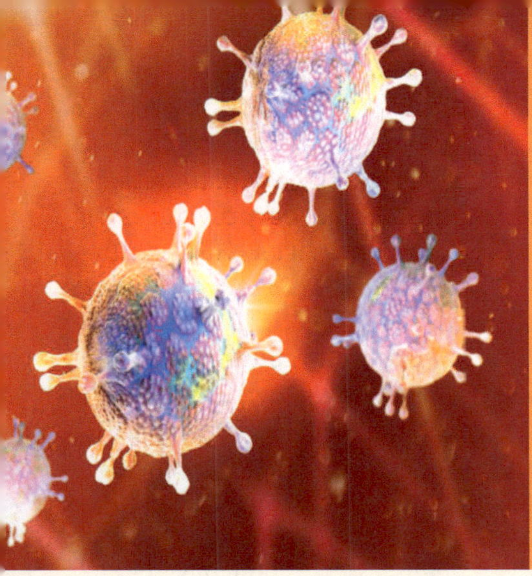

Chapter 4

HERPESVIRUSES AND ONCOGENIC VIRUSES

Contents

Introduction

The intricate relationship between herpesviruses and oncogenic viruses has been of scientific concern, particularly in the investigation of cancer etiology. Herpesviruses form a large group of agents whose etiological roles have been very well defined through their ability to establish lifelong infections within their hosts, which typically remain latent until reactivation. Several members of this group, including Epstein-Barr virus (EBV) and *Kaposi sarcoma*-associated herpesvirus (KSHV), have been implicated in a variety of malignancies, thus forming significant public health concerns. The degree of intricacy in mechanisms of viral replication and latency adds yet another layer of complexity, necessitating detailed scrutiny of the molecular pathways through which these viruses can cause oncogenesis. This kind of scrutiny is necessary both for the disentanglement of cancer pathophysiology as well as the generation of targeted therapies. Recent studies have proven the capacity of oncogenic viruses to modulate host cell milieus to their advantage, particularly in the form of metabolic reprogramming. It is not an off-target effect but a critical component of the life cycle of the virus, aiding viral replication and survival in host cells. Research describing the role of metabolic hijacking by such viruses has been of interest, as such an association may provide insight into targets to cure cancer. For instance, oncogenic viruses modulate tumor metabolism via viral proteins that disrupt host pathways, as is discussed in recent reviews. This interaction between viral infection and host metabolism underpins the need to proceed with more mechanistic research to explain such interactions and better understand oncogenesis caused by viruses (Thaker et al., 2019). Particularly within the area of central nervous system tumors, the relationship between chronic viral infections like herpesvirus-induced infections and tumorigenesis has come to represent an area of intense investigation. These tumors significantly affect morbidity and mortality rates and consequently necessitate further understanding of their basic mechanisms. Although the precise role of viral infections in neuro-oncogenesis remains controversial, there is certain evidence of a possible neuro-oncomodulatory activity exerted by these agents. Evidence shows varying detection frequencies of polyomavirus and herpesvirus between tumor subtypes, and these suggest difficulties in making final causal relationships. The controversies raise the need for systematic, well-planned studies to address such uncertainties. With advancing knowledge, knowledge on the mechanisms by which the viruses increase cancer development will be pivotal in developing effective prevention as well as treatment strategies (Saddawi-Konefka & Crawford, 2010).

Definition of Herpesviruses

Herpesviruses are a heterogeneous collection of double-stranded DNA viruses characterized by their ability to establish long-term latency in the host. Over a hundred different species of such pathogens exist and are classified into three subfamilies based on their characteristics and mechanisms of pathogenicity: the alpha, beta, and gamma subfamilies. Alpha herpesviruses, which include herpes simplex virus (HSV) and varicella-zoster virus (VZV), are neurotropic and highly suited to the induction of acute infection and latent infection in neural tissues. Beta herpesviruses, like cytomegalovirus (CMV), infect cells of more than one lineage, e.g., lymphocytes and epithelial cells, and produce serious morbidity in immunocompromised individuals. Gamma herpesviruses, including EBV and *Kaposi sarcoma*-associated herpesvirus (KSHV), are most notably linked with oncogenesis, hence highlighting the importance of categorizing this complex virus family within the broader domain of infectious disease and cancer research. Herpesviruses' morphology is at the core of their virulence and infectivity. They have an icosahedral capsid containing their viral genome, which in turn is covered by a lipid coat derived from the host cell membrane. This unique morphology not only allows access to host cells by receptor-mediated endocytosis but also allows the virus to inject its genome into the nucleus, the beginning of the cycle of replication. During virion assembly, a crucial component known as the portal-vertex plays a significant role, acting as a portal through which the viral genome moves in and out of the capsid. Recent advances in cryo-electron microscopy have revealed this delicate structure with significant insight into its composition and function (Bhella et al., 2018). Such knowledge is paramount to the understanding of herpesvirus biology that has the potential to impact therapeutic management to combat infections and their associated malignancies. The oncogenic activity of some herpesviruses also underscores the need to revisit their definitions and classification in the field of virology. For example, Marek's disease virus (MDV), which has in the past been considered a gammaherpesvirus, has itself been re-assessed based on its phylogenetic connection to neurotropic alphaherpesviruses (Brunovskis & Velicer, 1995) (Figure 4.1).

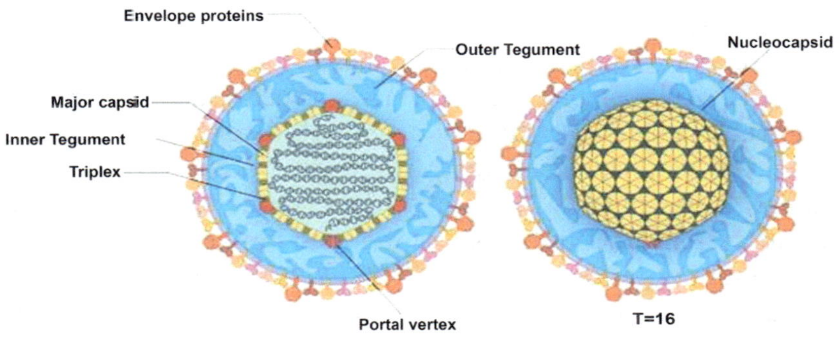

Figure 4.1. The structure of herpesviruses.

Source: https://www.cusabio.com/infectious-diseases/herpesviruses.html?srsltid=AfmBOoqqX-f00aqj0l4LGvkGkFAWEZIBNy6eaN68zrBCWia3H6f1iBUb.

Most importantly, MDV has also been linked to lymphomagenesis in birds, and the serious implications for animal disease and productivity are undeniable. Furthermore, EBV is perhaps most famous for causing numerous cancers, including Hodgkin's lymphoma and nasopharyngeal carcinoma, and underscores the central intersection of herpesvirology and oncogenesis. These definitions are not only academic in nature; they have a profound effect on research priorities, preventive practices, and treatment interventions as the scientific community struggles to untangle the intricate webs of relationships among these viruses and the illnesses they produce.

Overview of Oncogenic Viruses

The oncogenic viral landscape is densely inhabited by numerous viral families, with herpesviruses being unique in their immense contribution towards the causation of cancer. Oncogenic viruses are those that have the ability to cause tumor formation in the infected host, either by direct oncogenicity or by having an effect on host cellular mechanisms. Among the herpesviruses, EBV and *KSHV* are of special interest. Both viruses persist life-long in the human host and both participate in causing different malignancies, including Burkitt's lymphoma and *Kaposi's sarcoma*, respectively. Both increase their oncogenic potential through the ability to control host cell signaling pathways, illustrating the complex interaction between viral proteins and cellular regulatory machinery. The molecular mechanisms of viral oncogenesis have generated enormous research attention, particularly the mechanism by which such viruses suppress the immune response and facilitate the process of tumor development. For example, EBV encodes several latent proteins that can disrupt normal cellular function and lead to cancerous cell growth and survival. KSHV also exploits different mechanisms, including the synthesis of viral microRNAs, for altering host gene expression and causing oncogenesis. The exploration of viral proteomes by large-scale proteomic approaches has unveiled the intricate network of interactions between these viruses and the host, validating the identification of potential therapeutic targets. As stated, the understanding of such viral interactions significantly facilitates the discovery of novel therapies to manage the malignancies induced by these chronic infections (Baquero-Perez et al., 2014). Moreover, the oncogenic function of microRNAs is more apparent, as demonstrated by several herpesviruses. Specifically, the presence of microRNA clusters in herpesviruses' genomes, such as Marek's disease virus and infectious laryngotracheitis virus, signifies their evolutionary selection for the regulation of host cell pathways. The conservation of some microRNA sequences, coupled with their capacity to target key cellular processes, suggests a complex tumorigenesis process that is overseen by these viral constituents. By targeting host genes, these microRNAs can modulate the immune system and influence apoptosis, hence developing a permissive environment for neoplastic transformation. This highlights the need for more detailed research on the microRNA universes of oncogenic viruses, since an understanding of their dynamics would provide insight into effective therapeutic strategies against virus-induced cancers (Anderson et al., 2009) (Figure 4.2).

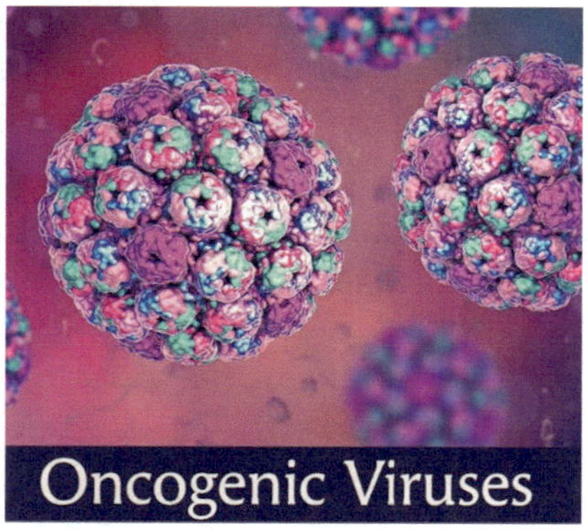

Figure 4.2. Oncogenic viruses.

Source: https://m.media-amazon.com/images/I/71c9U6gW72L._UF1000,1000_QL80_.jpg.

4.1. Classification of Herpesviruses

The taxonomy of herpesviruses is multifaceted, echoing the biological and genetic diversity of this family of viruses. Herpesviruses are primarily divided into three major subfamilies: Alpha, Beta, and Gammaherpesvirinae. Alpha-herpesviruses, such as notable pathogens herpes simplex virus (HSV) and varicella-zoster virus (VZV), possess the capacity to replicate rapidly and, in addition to that, also sustain latent infection within sensory nerve neurons. These viruses are most commonly associated with causing diseases ranging from oral and genital ulcers to chickenpox and shingles. Beta-herpesviruses, such as cytomegalovirus (CMV) and human herpesvirus 6 (HHV-6), tend to replicate slowly and have increased tissue tropism and are typically associated with more persistent disease. On the other hand, viruses like the EBV and *KSHV* belong to the Gammaherpesviruses and are normally linked with oncogenic processes due to their lymphotropic character and association with certain cancers. Marek's disease virus (MDV) is an intriguing case in the herpesvirus group that at one point was listed as a gammaherpesvirus. Recent phylogenetic research, however, proved that MDV is more closely related to the alpha-herpesviruses, specifically the neurotropic strains like HSV. MDV is an oncogenic avian herpesvirus responsible for widespread economic losses in poultry due to its capacity to induce lymphomas and neurologic disease. In-depth genomic analysis has identified some open reading frames (ORFs) in MDV's DNA with homology to those in alpha-herpesviruses, thus making it a complex virus as far as its past classification is concerned. These evolutionary observations also suggest that earlier categorizations based on disease characteristics and host tropism per se may have to be revisited as genomic data play an increasingly larger role in our understanding of viral lineage and pathology (Brunovskis & Velicer, 1995). Genetic information-based categorizations serve a much higher purpose than mere virology; they have huge implications for therapeutic interventions and disease control measures. The recent discovery of genome editing technologies, such as the CRISPR/Cas9 system, provides a revolutionary approach to the delivery of herpesvirus genomes within latent infections. The technology is capable of accurately modifying viral genes and has immense potential for eradicating latent infections if conventional antiviral treatments fail. Scientists suggest that the use of CRISPR/Cas9 technology could be a paradigm change for the treatment of herpesvirus-caused diseases, in particular those with oncogenesis (Chen et al., 2018). Understanding the classification of herpesviruses thus contributes not only to our biological knowledge but also guides the application of new therapeutic strategies to resist their disease-causing activity.

4.1.1. Major Types of Herpesviruses

Herpesviruses form a broad family of DNA viruses, classified into three general subfamilies: Alpha, Beta, and Gamma herpesviruses. They are characterized by specific attributes, e.g., the life cycles for replication, host range, and correlation with disease outcomes. Alpha herpesviruses, exemplified by Herpes Simplex Virus (HSV-1 and HSV-2) and Varicella-Zoster Virus (VZV), possess the ability to become latent in sensory neurons and then frequently recur. In contrast, Beta herpesviruses, like Cytomegalovirus (CMV) and Human Herpesvirus 6 (HHV-6), typically have a slower replication cycle and are more associated with immunocompromised individuals. Lastly, Gamma herpesviruses, which include EBV and Kaposi's Sarcoma-Associated Herpesvirus (KSHV), are notable for their associations with various malignancies, making them significant in the context of oncogenic viruses. The oncogenic potential of certain herpesviruses renders them critical to public health discussions and clinical research. Epstein-Barr Virus, well-known for its link to Burkitt's lymphoma and nasopharyngeal carcinoma, highlights the intersection of viral infection and cancer development. *Kaposi's Sarcoma*-Associated Herpesvirus contributes to the pathogenesis of Kaposi's sarcoma, particularly in immunocompromised populations, such as individuals with AIDS. The mechanisms by which such viruses facilitate oncogenesis are typically multifactorial interactions with host cellular machinery, so that they can facilitate uncontrolled growth and evade immune detection. Evidence indicates that viral manipulation of cellular metabolism of the host is central to these processes, implying a potential site of intervention in the therapy of malignancies induced by herpesviruses (Thaker et al., 2019) (Figure 4.3).

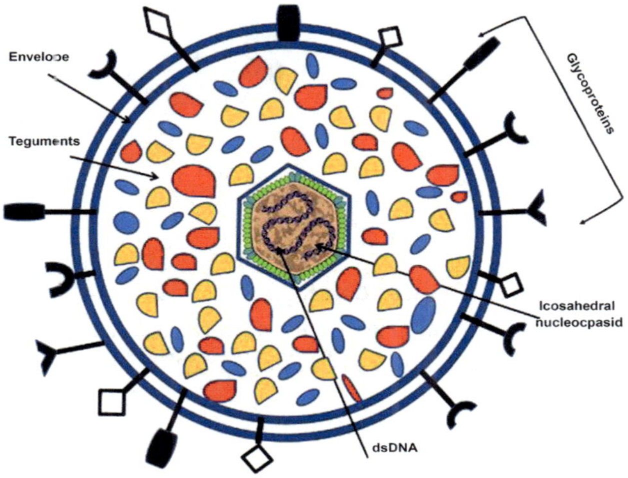

Figure 4.3. Structure of herpesviruses.

Source: https://glycopedia.eu/echapter/introduction-4/herpesviruses/.

Recent advances in genetic engineering, most notably in the CRISPR/Cas9 system, offer promising possibilities for overcoming herpesvirus challenges, especially latent infection. The technology has the potential to target and disrupt viral genomes selectively, and therefore represents a new avenue for possibly eradicating these infections from host cells. Of particular interest, its use has proved effective in engineering diverse herpesviruses like HSV, EBV, and CMV, indicative of a revolutionary method of treatment as opposed to conventional antiviral methods. Since most existing treatments fail in eliminating latent infections, continued research into the applications of CRISPR/Cas9 is crucial in creating novel antiviral approaches. With the use of this genetic tool, researchers aim to shed light on herpesvirus biology and also develop targeted therapy that would lessen the impact of this neoplastic disease induced by these oncogenic viruses (Chen et al., 2018).

4.1.2. Characteristics of Each Type

The herpesvirus family is heterogeneous, consisting of viruses with distinctive features but shared developmental and structural properties. One of their major categorizations is alpha, beta, and gamma herpesviruses, which are characterized by their growth patterns and host cell interactions. Alpha herpesviruses such as herpes simplex virus (HSV) and varicella-zoster virus (VZV) tend to establish latent infections in sensory nerve cells that periodically reactivate to produce symptomatic attacks. This cyclical regimen is challenging in therapy, particularly as the host's immune system is generally unable to clear the virus. Beta herpesviruses, like human cytomegalovirus (HCMV), primarily infect myeloid lineage cells and possess a more leisurely replication cycle. In contrast, gamma herpesviruses like EBV and *KSHV* are strongly known to be oncogenic, and their oncogenicity is facilitated by latent gene expression and various oncogenes (Thaker et al., 2019).

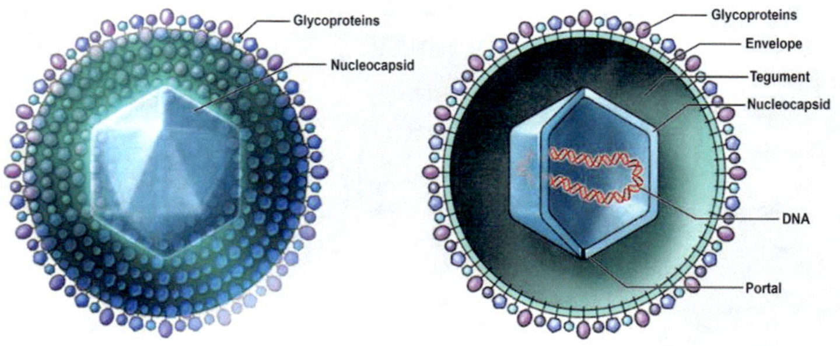

Figure 4.4. Herpes simplex virus structure.

Source: https://external-content.duckduckgo.com/iu/?u=https%3A%2F%2Fcdn.std.uw.edu%2Fdoc%2F361-1%2Fbasic-structure-herpes-simplex-virus.jpg&f=1&nofb=1&ipt=3bf711f8d4a0cd243f72e06ecbcb31724b9b62e92003a442dae61f3cc767bd27.

Oncogenic activities of some of the herpesviruses are based on their ability to hijack host cellular processes. Surprisingly, Epstein-Barr virus can cause growth and transformation of B cells, leading to lymphoma-type diseases. Similarly, *Kaposi sarcoma*-associated herpesvirus employs several mechanisms by which it manipulates the immune environment to promote tumorigenesis. Upregulation of pro-oncogenic signaling pathways and downregulation of host tumor suppressor mechanisms are the mechanisms involved in this manipulation, increasing the virus's pathogenic potential. The involvement of viral genes with host cellular pathways accounts for the oncogenic herpesviruses, highlighting the need for advanced therapeutic strategies. Knowledge of such traits is important for designing targeted antiviral treatments and enhancing existing treatment methods, especially in treating latent infections that are commonly recalcitrant to traditional treatments (Chen et al., 2018) (Figure 4.4).

In order to better understand the nature of herpesviruses, it is necessary to take into account new technologies applied in virology. Advances in CRISPR/Cas9 technology represent a milestone for accurate manipulation of viral genomes. Genome editing not only serves for in-depth studies of viral characteristics, but it is also important for creating new therapeutic approaches to managing herpesvirus-induced malignancies. When used correctly, CRISPR/Cas9 can stop dormant infections and target specifically those viral strains that enable oncogenesis, thereby possibly arresting the formation of herpesvirus-educated cancers. Integration of such methodology is a significant breakthrough in unraveling the complex dynamic between host cellular machinery and herpesviruses, thereby furthering our understanding of viral metabolism and its implications for cancer therapy (Thaker et al., 2019). By espousing our combined expertise in this arena, we can develop successful strategies for counteracting the continuing burden of herpesviruses and their oncogenic potential.

4.1.3. Transmission Methods

The transmission pathways of herpesviruses and oncogenic viruses are crucial to their epidemiology and public health significance. Herpesviruses are predominantly transmitted by direct contact with infected body fluid or lesions, and thus the most frequent route of transmission for most of them is by sex, such as for herpes simplex virus (HSV). In addition, they can also be transmitted vertically from mother to child during birth, and therefore screening in pregnant females is especially relevant.

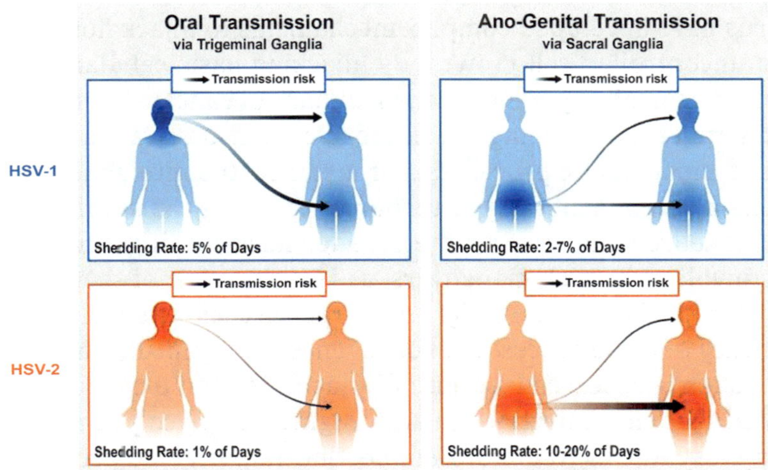

Figure 4.5. Transmission of HSV.

Source: https://cdn.std.uw.edu/doc/756-1/oral-ano-genital-transmission-hsv-1-hsv-2.jpg.

In contrast, oncogenic viruses, such as certain human papillomavirus (HPV) types, are sexually transmitted but may also be transmitted by skin abrasions or fomites. The heterogenic modes of transmission complicate public health interventions and need specific measures for reducing transmission and outbreak control. Zoonotic transmission of some herpetic and oncogenic viruses makes their epidemiology more complex. For instance, some viruses can cross the species barrier, which can potentially result in emergent infections in the human population. Surprisingly, macaques were extensively utilized as model animals to elucidate the pathways of transmission of various viral infections. Nonhuman primates are typically intermediaries in situations where zoonotic infections can be studied and therefore, knowledge regarding mechanisms of pathogenesis, as well as vaccine targets might be obtained. This supports the necessity for the identification and control of risks from zoonotic viruses, especially because these pathogens are able to carry oncogenic infections whose effects on human health are not known (Gardner & Luciw, 2008) (Figure 4.5).

Current prevention of transmission of herpesviruses and neoplastic viruses focuses more on advanced techniques of prevention and detection. For instance, xenotransplantation is a significant challenge with the transmission of pig viruses to human hosts, and there is a need for immediate screening of prospective donors from animals (Janich, 2018). The development of sensitive PCR-based assays and immunological tests has become critical in the identification of viral agents that are potentially risky. Enhanced detection processes are meant to provide assurance of the selection of virus-free donor animals for transplantation, a step that minimizes zoonotic transmission. Such strategies are of great significance not just to enhance public health controls to combat viral infection but also to enhance medical interventions safety whose faulty conduct may inadvertently transmit infectious disease.

4.2. Mechanisms of Oncogenesis

The oncogenic processes, particularly for herpesviruses, show a very complex interplay between viral infection and cellular dysfunction. Herpesviruses such as Epstein-Barr virus and *Kaposi sarcoma*-associated herpesvirus have developed complex mechanisms to hijack host cell signaling processes to ultimately lead to uncontrolled cell growth. By hijacking basic cellular processes, these viruses are able to cause genomic instability, which is the hallmark of cancer. The metabolic reprogramming due to these cancer viruses makes things even more complicated, as it plays with the host cells' energy production and biosynthetic processes. For instance, the interactions between viral protein and cellular metabolism reveal a shifting of resources favoring the survival and growth of cancer cells. This metabolic takeover underscores the broader need for ongoing research to reveal some of the viral proteins involved in such maneuvers, as identification of these interactions can reveal new therapeutic targets (Thaker et al., 2019). The herpesviruses' effect on the host cell metabolism underscores the intricacy of these processes of oncogenesis. By imposing a metabolic state favorable to their replication, such viruses can potentially facilitate tumorigenesis with high efficiency. Research has indicated that viral infection leads to augmented glycolytic flux and higher utilization of intermediates for biosynthesis, therefore supporting tumorigenic processes. Such a metabolic shift not only provides nutrients for virus growth but also sustains the malignancy of infected cells, driving them toward an aggressive cancer phenotype. The recent advances in viral metabolic research highlight the clinical significance of such interactions. These developments enable the identification and characterization of critical metabolic nodes that oncogenic viruses are attacking, giving rise to new therapeutic strategies that could potentially exploit these vulnerabilities (Modrow & Wolf, 1983). Furthermore, the revelation of lytic infection kinetics in herpesvirus-infected cells reveals certain temporal patterns of protein expression that contribute to oncogenesis. A case in point is provided by results demonstrating how the introduction of TPA in the course of the lytic cycle induces viral polypeptide production while simultaneously suppressing host protein synthesis. This dual action mechanism aids the viral life cycle as well as disrupts cellular function, lending a helping hand to malignancy. The identification of virus-induced protein, as illustrated in herpesvirus saimiri research, indicates the complexity of viral programming of host cells. Determining early and late protein synthesis following lytic infection allows researchers to best recognize the fine molecular interactions driving oncogenesis. This nature of information is a necessity for the development of specific therapies that will interfere with these oncogenic processes and restore normal cell function (Modrow & Wolf, 1983) (Figure 4.6).

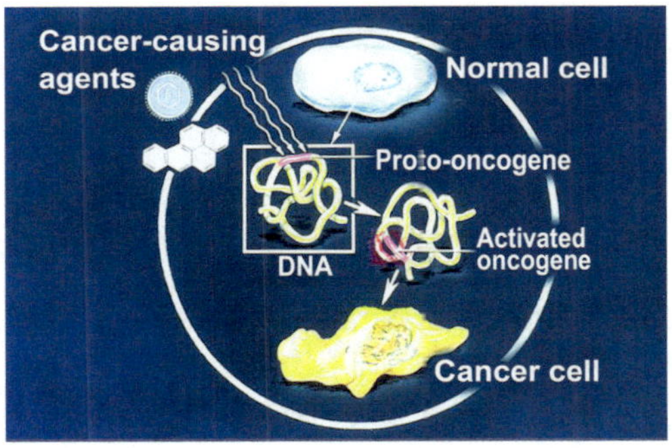

Figure 4.6. Normal cell is converted to a cancer cell when an oncogene becomes activated.

Source: https://en.wikipedia.org/wiki/Oncogene#/media/File:Oncogenes_illustration.jpg.

4.2.1. Viral Integration into Host DNA

The process through which herpesviruses integrate their genome into the host genome is one that determines the oncogenic potential of herpesviruses. Integration tends to modify the host cellular machinery for the virus to replicate and evade immune surveillance. For tumor viruses, such as EBV and *KSHV*, integration events generally coincide with the cellular transformation into cancerous cells. The virus may contain oncoproteins that take over tumor suppressor pathways to cause uncontrolled cell growth. Thus, the mechanisms of viral integration not only give way to means of viral persistence but also highlight the potential of such viruses in fostering oncogenesis in susceptible hosts, focusing on viral actions and host cell activities that will ultimately result in cancer. Improved genetic manipulation in recent years has opened up new approaches to understanding and potentially ameliorating the effects of viral integration. Technologies such as the CRISPR/Cas9 system have also emerged to be known to be very powerful tools with the potential to target and interfere with viral genomes, including herpesviruses. By the introduction of programmed mutations in the viral genome, scientists can analyze the contribution of individual viral genes to latent life and oncogenicity. The precision delivered by CRISPR/Cas9 not only facilitates thorough exploration of viral processes but also possesses therapeutic implications. Since current antitherapeutic approaches for herpesvirus infection are limited in eliminating the latent virus, utilization of CRISPR/Cas9 may bring forth novel treatments that will be able to eradicate viral DNA from the host genome at latent infection stages and thereby reduce oncogenic potential (Chen et al., 2018). Despite progress with genetic research, there remain significant gaps in understanding how viral integration reprograms host metabolism — particularly on the basis of oncogenesis. Metabolic rewiring induced by oncogenic virus-host cell interaction involves complex interactions which are either augmentative or inhibitory to host cell function. For instance, such viruses have been said to hijack metabolic pathways to enhance their own replication while simultaneously modulating the hosts metabolic profile for tumorigenesis support. It is crucial to investigate viral proteins implicated in such modifications because these proteins can serve as drug targets or biomarkers for viral-associated cancers. Future research that examines herpesvirus-induced changes to metabolism may yield valuable information and lead to novel methods of cancer therapy and antiviral medicines that act upon changes to metabolism resulting from viral infection (Thaker et al., 2019) (Figure 4.7).

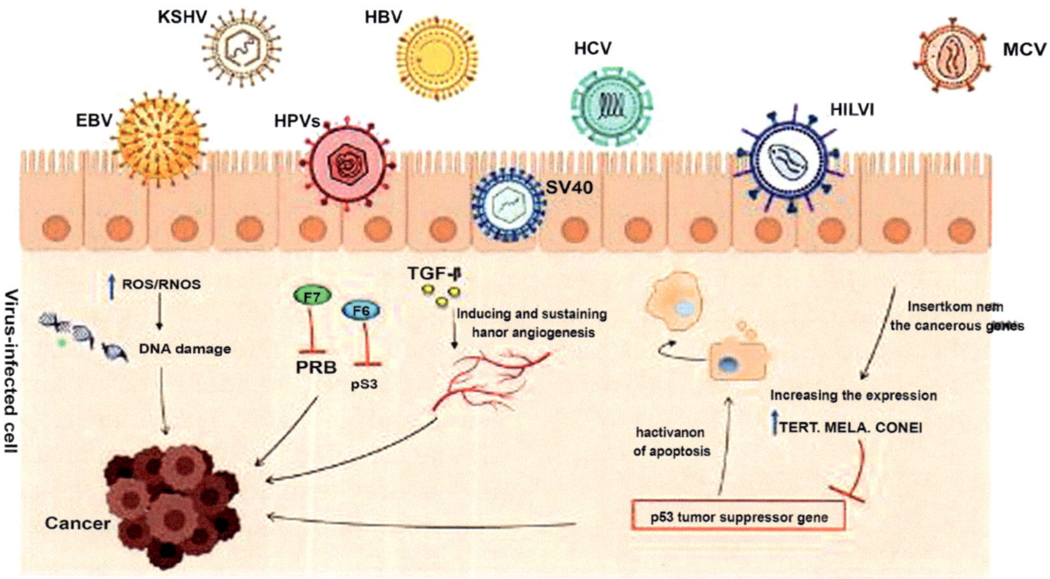

Figure 4.7. Oncogenesis mechanisms of viruses in cancer development.

Source: https://www.researchgate.net/figure/Oncogenesis-mechanisms-of-viruses-in-cancer-development-Viruses-induce-their-carcinogen_fig1_369061341.

4.2.2. Induction of Cellular Proliferation

The promotion of cell proliferation is a feature of some oncogenic viruses, including herpesviruses, which co-opt the machinery of the host cells to enhance their replication and survival. These viruses co-opt pathways of signaling that control cell division and, in the process, trigger uncontrolled cellular growth. Herpesviruses, for instance, can manipulate regulatory proteins such as p53 and Rb, which have an important function in cell cycle regulation. In doing so, they not only enable their own replication but also establish a cellular environment conducive to oncogenesis. The virus-host cell interaction demonstrates a multi-factorial relationship wherein the virus is capable in effect to usurp the hosts proliferative machinery for its own purposes, propagating its genomic presence while also establishing the foundation for forthcoming malignancies. In an increasingly competitive arena of oncogenic processes, identifying viral metabolism is most important. Herpesviruses, for instance, induce metabolic rewiring in the host cell in such a manner that the metabolic environment is optimized to favor their growth and development. This is amply observed in the manner in which herpesviruses interact with anabolic pathways, optimized cellular pathways, which, in effect, reprogram the host's metabolic state. Insertion of viral genes can trigger cascades of signals that commit resources to viral replication, creating an environment in which viral progeny and cancer-transformed cells thrive. Recent attention is given to the necessity of *in vivo* research to unravel the metabolic hijacking modes employed by such viruses, which remain central to rational therapy against virus-induced malignancy (Thaker et al., 2019). Further, herpesvirus impacts on cell growth exceed their replication since they have been shown to elicit immune responses that lead to disease conditions. Some recent studies have shown how pathogens, such as viruses, can initiate innate immune responses that, while initially protective, could inadvertently lead to chronic inflammation and dysregulation of cells. In particular, the relationship between herpesviruses and the innate immune system suggests that such viruses can become facilitators of immune dysregulation, providing a fertile ground for oncogenic transformation. Through the study of the relationship between viral infection and innate immune system activation, scientists can better envision how herpesviruses cause and sustain cancer-permissive conditions like systemic sclerosis (Farina & Farina, 2016). Explanation of these mechanisms will be useful for the development of new therapeutic interventions that aim to reverse the oncogenicity of such viral infections, and hence resolve the overall implications of viral infection-induced cell proliferation in cancer.

4.2.3. Evasion of Immune Responses

The ability of herpesviruses to evade immune responses lies in the genetic code for their survival and persistence in the host. Among the most significant mechanisms employed by the viruses is the modulation of the immune system's antigen-presentation machinery. Through disrupting major histocompatibility complex (MHC) pathways, herpesviruses scan decrease the host's capacity to identify and target infected cells. For example, EBV produces proteins that downregulate MHC class I molecules, the importance of which is in being recognized by CD8+ T cells. Not only does such an evasion mechanism shield the virus from immediate immune attack, but it also allows it to survive long term within the host, making individuals susceptible to oncogenic changes in the future. Therefore, understanding these immune evasion mechanisms is critical in determining the pathogenesis of these viruses and their link to the initiation of cancer. In addition to direct manipulation of MHC-associated processes, herpesviruses also employ microvesicle biogenesis to manipulate immune responses in the host. New findings indicate that extracellular vesicles of this type are able to carry viral components away from infected cells, thereby regulating local immune milieus and potentially skewing immune responses. Microvesicles contain a range of molecules that can induce immune suppression or immune enhancement. Some microvesicles, for example, can transfer viral antigens in a bid to disseminate the infection in the host, while others induce immune dysregulation. This bifunctional nature highlights the complexity of herpesvirus interactions with the immune response, as vesicles can drive both the efficiency of viral dissemination and hosts' capacity to enact effective immune responses to counteract infection, rendering therapeutic interventions targeted against efficient viral dissemination problematic (Wurdinger et al., 2012). Some viral proteins are also effective at countering immune surveillance through exploiting targeted mechanisms aimed against immune signaling pathways. Notably, EBV BILF1 protein demonstrates this strategy with physical interaction with MHC class I molecules, inducing them to be turned over quickly and hence reducing their cell surface expression. This interference blocks CD8+ T cell recognition of infected cells and therefore enables the virus to survive longer in the host without clearance by the immune system. Interestingly, the same mechanisms have been observed in other herpesviruses and exhibit a conserved evolutionary strategy to regulate host immune responses. By interfering in antigen presentation along with maintaining their replication and survival, these viruses not only maintain their existence but also contribute to the potential oncogenesis of their human hosts (Zuo et al.,

2009). Understanding the intricate interactions of herpesviruses with the immune system is crucial to creating new therapeutic approaches to combat viral infections and their associated cancers.

4.3. Herpes Simplex Virus (HSV) and Cancer

The relationship of Herpes Simplex Virus (HSV) with oncogenesis involves a specific area of interest within cancer research. HSV is best known for its causation of oral and genital herpes; however, its behavior in cancer has been of interest due to its ability to disrupt host cellular processes. Specifically, oncogenic viruses like some types of HSV have been observed to initiate metabolic reprogramming in cancer cells. This metabolic hijacking allows the replication of the virus but also seems to play a role in tumorigenesis by creating a permissive environment for cancer cell proliferation. Knowledge of how HSV manipulates cellular metabolism could shed light on pathways that are involved in cancer development and highlight the dual character of this virus as both pathogen and potential therapeutic target in oncology (Thaker et al., 2019). During the last decade, the application of CRISPR/Cas9 technology in virology has opened new avenues for studies on the interaction of HSV with cancer. The revolutionary genome-editing tool allows for the accurate manipulation of viral genomes and comprehension of the oncogenic capability of HSV with increased efficiency. By targeting CRISPR/Cas9 to induce breaks in viral genomes during latent infection, scientists can observe how interference with the viral life cycle can suppress the oncogenic processes of HSV. Moreover, the method also offers therapeutic potential to such an extent that CRISPR/Cas9 can be used to target and annihilate latent HSV infection, thereby reducing cancer risk presented by the virus." The precision and the speed provided by CRISPR/Cas9 point towards its potential as a novel method for not only understanding HSV-related oncogenesis but also antiviral therapy design (Chen et al., 2018) (Figure 4.8).

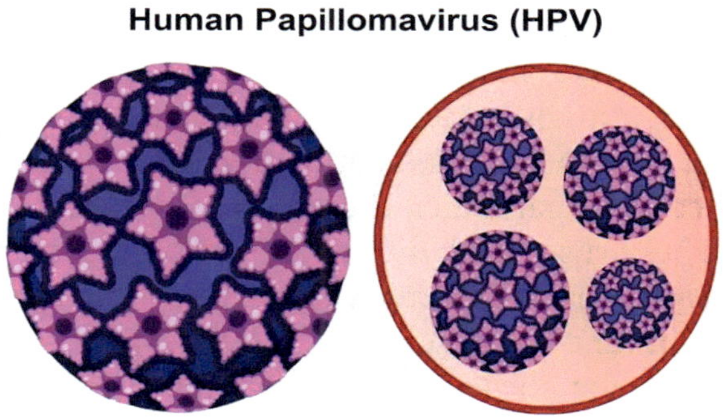

Figure 4.8. Human papillomavirus (HPV) infection.

Source: https://continentalhospitals.com/images/blogs/4ee9709c3d64e92a0420f4cf6576c63f.webp.

While the relationship between HSV and cancer is complex, evidence is accumulating that HSV can also be exploited as a vector for the treatment of cancer. Oncolytic virotherapy, or the use of genetically modified viruses to infect and kill cancer cells selectively, is being increasingly favored as a novel strategy for cancer treatment. Some HSV strains have been genetically engineered to enhance their oncolytic activity, infecting and lysing cancer cells with minimal cytotoxicity to normal tissues. Such a treatment modality leverages the inherent tropism of HSV for human cells with the potential of enhanced delivery of therapeutic agents to the tumor microenvironment. As research continues to shed light on mechanisms of HSV's activity in both cancer development and treatment, the therapeutic potential of the virus as a biotherapeutic agent may be fully exploited, connecting viral infection with oncologic therapy (Thaker et al., 2019).

4.3.1. Association with Cervical Cancer

The association between herpesviruses and cervical carcinoma has been of great interest in oncological research due to the role of human papillomavirus (HPV) as the most frequent etiological agent. While HPV is well established to be a sexually transmitted virus that causes nearly all cervical cancer cases, recent reports indicate other herpesviruses, like some members of the Gammaherpesvirus family, could also contribute to oncogenesis. Such viruses can alter normal cellular processes, including apoptosis — a critical pathway to avoid the development of potentially malignant cells. By evading the apoptotic machinery of the hosts, long-term herpesviral infection may create a favorable condition for the development and growth of cervical cancerous lesions, reflecting the complex interaction between viral infection and cancer development (Banerjee et al., 2016). Further, research utilizing next-generation sequencing has found herpesviruses, such as various forms of HPV, to occur in premalignant and malignant cervical lesions. In a study of cervical sample analysis, HPV was found to be detected in 95% of carcinomas and in all the CIN2/3 samples, showing a clear correlation between viral load and severity of cervical dysplasia (Mensaert et al., 2015) (Figure 4.9).

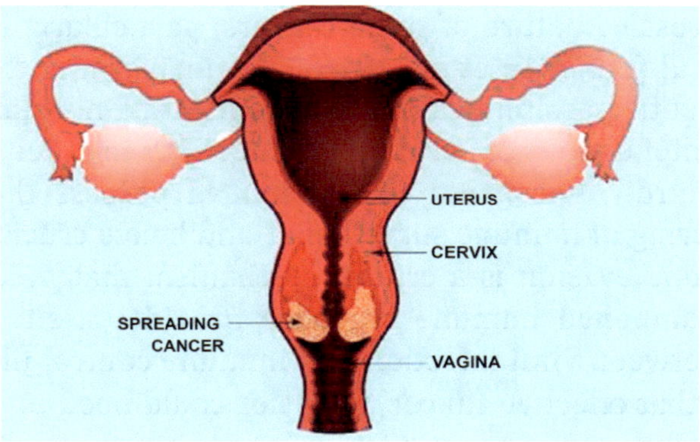

Figure 4.9. Cervical cancer.

Source: https://www.drshonanagbreastcancer.in/specialization/cervical-cancer.

The presence of these viral genomes alone indicates their role in the disease and the importance of viral interaction with host cell pathways. Viral load and epigenetic modification, such as DNA methylation, are some of the factors contributing to the differing rates of progression from benign lesions to malignant neoplasms. The interaction dynamics of viral presence and host cell response thus play a crucial role in understanding the cervical cancer's multifactorial etiology. Consequently, therapeutic methods that treat such viral infections are a foremost aspect of preventing and treating cervical cancer. Isolating and identifying the specific viral proteins blocking apoptotic processes will allow researchers to develop antiviral therapies that can restore apoptosis in infected cancer cells (Banerjee et al., 2016). Besides, the use of viral sequence information in cancer studies allows for a better understanding of the molecular role of herpesviruses in oncogenesis. This emphasis highlights the need for ongoing monitoring of viral disease in patients with cancer, particularly in cervical cancer screening programs, and that this may lead to earlier diagnosis and, in turn, improved patient outcomes. The intricate interaction between cervical cancer and herpesviruses creates opportunities and challenges to cancer biology and therapeutic advancement.

4.3.2. Role in Other Malignancies

Their sophisticated connection to tumors is more than just their proven association with specific cancers. Recent studies indicate a role for these viruses in creating a permissive environment for tumor growth in a wide range of malignancies. Through manipulation of host metabolic pathways, oncogenic herpesviruses can induce a metabolic reprogramming biased towards the growth and survival of cancer cells. For instance, the modulation of lipid and glycometabolism is used to supply the anabolic requirements of growing cancer cells, which are required for their growth and metastasis. Beyond that, this hijacking of metabolism reflects a two-way relationship between cancer and viral infection, suggesting that understanding these mechanisms could reveal new aspects of cancer biology and new targets for therapeutic intervention for various malignancies (Thaker et al., 2019). In addition to its metabolic functions, herpesvirus function in the regulation of apoptotic pathways is vital when thinking about tumors. The Gammaherpesvirus family, for instance, has evolved several mechanisms to disrupt the host cells' apoptotic processes such that infected cells can evade regular tumor suppressive mechanisms. By encoding viral proteins that interrupting both intrinsic and extrinsic apoptotic pathways, these viruses can guarantee the survival of infected cells, thus facilitating oncogenesis. This survival is not only beneficial to tumor cell survival but can also be responsible for the aggressive nature of some cancers, particularly if the balance of apoptosis is tilted towards cell survival (Banerjee et al., 2016). The insight into these viral mechanisms can provide insight into therapeutic possibilities aimed at reinstating normal processes of apoptosis in cancer cells. Secondly, the implications of herpesvirus infections in other cancers are their influence on the immune system. Thirdly, oncogenic viruses indeed possess the ability to alter immune reactions, leading to a lowering of immune surveillance and hence crucial in identifying and killing nascent tumors. This immune evasion is a critical mechanism that predisposes the pathogenesis of most cancers, as the dampened immune response provides a site for unrestrained cellular expansion. The interplay between viral infection and immune control illustrates the complexity of cancer onset and suggests that effective cancer therapies could need to incorporate measures that not only eliminate the virus but also enhance host immune capabilities. Through the understanding of these mechanisms, scientists will better understand the multifactorial etiology of cancer from herpesvirus infections (Banerjee et al., 2016; Thaker et al., 2019).

4.3.3. Mechanisms of TUMORigenesis

The processes of tumorigenesis linked with oncogenic herpesviruses are multifaceted and intricate and mainly consist of the reprogramming of cellular growth and survival pathways. The viruses make use of host cell mechanisms for their replication; however, at the same time, they indirectly modify the normal regulatory processes. Some of the characteristics of this metabolic remodeling include glycolytic pathway upregulation and promotion of anabolic metabolism, both being critical to the ability of the rapid growth characteristic of cancer cells. Such types of metabolic alteration are characteristic of viral pathogenesis and present fertile ground for oncogenic transformation. Investigation of the metabolic pathways of oncogenic viruses sheds light on therapeutic possibilities and emphasizes the interface between tumorigenesis and viral infection, thus providing a foundation for an enhanced understanding of tumorigenic mechanisms as a whole (Thaker et al., 2019). Among the diverse herpesvirus family, Marek's disease virus (MDV) offers a particularly good example of the action of distinct viral components in tumorigenesis. MDV causes lymphomas in chickens, and its pathogenicity is not just due to its ability to set up latency but also to its intricate interaction with host cellular components. Of particular interest, the involvement of some viral genes has been established in the oncogenic activity, mediating cell transformation by virtue of mechanisms that are still partially understood. Studies of MDV have indicated that some viral genes and their spliced products may influence tumor onset and development, which suggests a close interconnection of viral genetic components with cellular host processes. Understanding such intricate relationships is essential to appreciating how viral integration influences the growth of tumors, particularly through potential interference with cellular regulatory networks (You et al., 2022). Also, the integration of oncogenic viruses into host genomes is a primary tumorigenesis mechanism that causes permanent oncogenic signaling and cellular dysregulation. In MDV, viral integration usually occurs in telomere positions of the host genome, generating genomic instability and inappropriate gene expression profiles that predispose to malignancy. This mechanism not only highlights a process through which viruses may sustain their actions against host cells but is also representative of potential pathways for defining new therapeutic treatments. Additional studies on cellular components involved in viral integration will enhance our knowledge of herpesvirus tumorigenic processes, defining new avenues both for therapeutic targeting and the prevention of virus-induced malignancies (Thaker et al., 2019; You et al., 2022).

4.4. Epstein-Barr Virus (EBV) and Oncogenesis

The oncogenic mechanism of EBV is crucial to grasp in order to learn how certain viruses induce cancer. EBV is a herpesvirus and is linked with a variety of cancers, including Burkitt lymphoma and nasopharyngeal carcinoma. The virus creates a latent infection in which the virus produces several nuclear antigens and membrane proteins that interfere with normal cellular processes. By hijacking the host cell machinery, EBV promotes unchecked cell growth and inhibition of apoptosis, processes which are vital during oncogenesis. The complexity of the association of EBV with the host's immune system emphasizes the virus's adaptability and the challenge of being able to effectively target EBV-associated malignancies therapeutically. One of the most significant aspects of EBVs' oncogenic potential is the ability to manipulate host cell metabolism. Recent research is highlighting how viruses, including EBV, can induce metabolic reprogramming of infected cells to favor a tumorigenesis at ease.

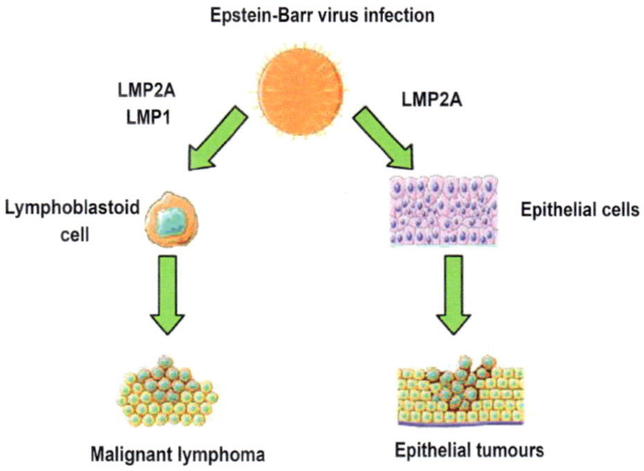

Figure 4.10. Pathogenetic mechanisms of Epstein-Barr virus on carcinogenesis.

Source: https://www.researchgate.net/figure/Pathogenetic-mechanisms-of-Epstein-Barr-virus-on-carcinogenesis-EBV-is-associated-with_fig1_353887422.

The metabolic shift that occurs here is not opportunistic but is strategic reprogramming to favor viral replication while boosting the anabolic processes beneficial for cancer cell growth and survival. EBV does this by coding and expressing viral proteins that modulate host metabolic pathways to induce dependency on certain metabolic substrates that favor the development of cancer. These findings are pivotal in understanding the overall implications of viral infection on metabolic pathways and how they contribute to oncogenesis, thus providing the scope for targeted intervention for the treatment of cancer (Thaker et al., 2019) (Figure 4.10).

EBV's influence is not confined to metabolism but also has a significant role in the control of apoptosis. The virus contains proteins that are capable of inhibiting both the extrinsic and intrinsic apoptotic pathways, which are necessary for removing infected or damaged cells. Through the inhibition of these pathways, EBV maintains its own life cycle but also assists the avoidance of immune mechanisms that would otherwise target tumorigenic cells. Current studies have identified the essential viral anti-apoptotic proteins involved in executing this process and have documented support for the potential of targeting these proteins as a new therapeutic approach. Based on understanding how EBV hijacks apoptosis through viral mechanisms, researchers can devise strategies toward the recovery of the process of apoptosis in EBV-associated cancers and improve treatment efficiency (Banerjee et al., 2016).

4.4.1. Link to Burkitt Lymphoma

The intricate relationship between herpesviruses, particularly EBV, and Burkitt lymphoma (BL) marks the multi-aspect interface between viral infection and oncogenesis. EBV, a member of herpesviruses, has been conclusively implicated in BL, particularly endemic forms that occur in regions of Africa. Such a connection highlights the pathogenic function of EBV as a key pathogen in the etiology of BL but whose mechanisms for precision remain in need of elaboration.

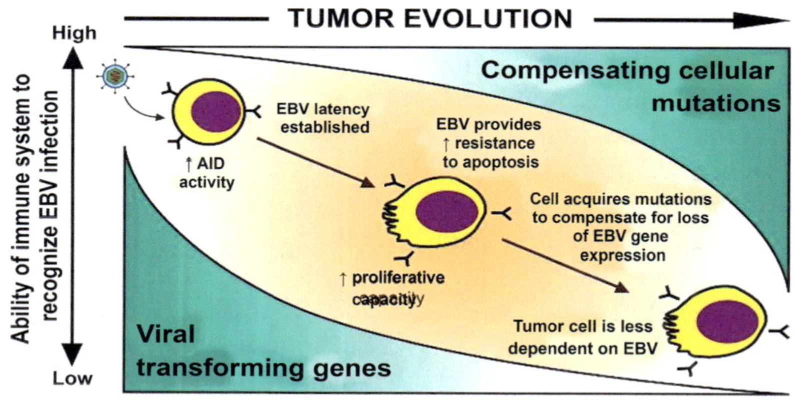

Figure 4.11. A model for EBV-positive Burkitt lymphomagenesis. Cells transformed with EBV are provided with oncogenic advantages, including the ability to proliferate and avoid apoptosis through the expression of viral transforming genes.

Source: https://www.frontiersin.org/files/Articles/606412/fcimb-10-606412-HTML/image_m/fcimb-10-606412-g001.jpg.

The understanding of such correlations is important, as it can provide information that not only explains the process of carcinogenesis but also prophylactic measures and therapeutic interventions. To firmly ground causality, it is imperative to expand on rudimentary criteria, keeping in mind the delicacy of asymptomatic long-term infections to significantly influence disease expression and prognosis (Gentile & Micozzi, 2016). Research indicates that although the presence of EBV is a strong predictor for BL, it is not a strict determinant; certain BL cases can shed the virus spontaneously, reflecting an intriguing complexity in the viral-disease front.

Experiments demonstrate that BL cells that have lost EBV are more apoptotic, reflecting the significant role of latent EBV genes in cell survival and tumorigenicity. In fact, EBV loss is associated with a phenotype that renders cells vulnerable to programmed cell death, which implies that EBV has a protective role by modulating pathways of apoptosis. This information brings to the limelight the need for further research into how the equilibrium between virus presence and absence impacts tumor severity and prognosis in BL patients, noting the role of EBV to sustain malignant transformations (Fitzsimmons et al., 2017) (Figure 4.11).

Additionally, the interactions between herpesviruses and the immune system complicate the situation in the context of Burkitt lymphoma. As emphasized in the majority of the studies, EBV immunity can regulate disease prognosis, and thus, the BL pathogenesis image is complicated. In seropositive asymptomatic infections, the virus may be suppressed by the immune system, but disruptions in this balance may induce malignant transformations.

The dual nature of EBV as both a disease-causing agent and a coactor in immune modulation speaks to the need for balanced thinking regarding host-virus interaction. Such interactions not only shed light on oncogenesis mechanisms but also define areas for therapeutic intervention. Current study of this interaction has potential for further interventions and a better understanding of how to neutralize the risks of EBV and its connection to Burkitt lymphoma (Gentile & Micozzi, 2016).

4.4.2. Role in Nasopharyngeal Carcinoma

The association of EBV with nasopharyngeal carcinoma (NPC) is emphasized by the pivotal role played by Epstein-Barr virus, a member of the herpesvirus family. NPC occurs quite frequently in certain geographic regions and among different ethnic populations, often in conjunction with EBV infection. Oncogenic potential of EBV is a result of its interference in host cell processes, particularly through the expression of latent membrane proteins (LMPs) that promote cellular proliferation and inhibit apoptosis. Such interaction between EBV and nasopharyngeal epithelial cells triggers a cascade of molecular events leading to tumorigenesis, highlighting the role of viral metabolism in tumorigenesis. A correct interpretation of these mechanisms is able to push forward the therapeutic interventions against NPC, thereby highlighting the relevance of herpesviruses in its etiopathogenesis (Thaker et al., 2019). Moreover, research into the metabolic reprogramming caused by EBV provides insightful information on the aggressiveness of nasopharyngeal carcinomas. Herpesviruses like EBV are also known to hijack the metabolism of host cells to develop a tumor-supportive environment and survival support. Studies have established that cells infected with EBV have been found to possess deranged glucose metabolism with enhanced glycolysis and production of metabolic end products that meet the biosynthetic demands of rapidly proliferating cancer cells. This metabolic rewiring not only facilitates the growth of malignant cells but also regulates their immunogenicity, influencing host immune response. Understanding of the metabolic alterations induced by EBV in NPC may unveil new therapeutic approaches, and thus most significantly the ones that particularly target the unique metabolic programs activated by oncogenic viral infections (Thaker et al., 2019) (Figure 4.12).

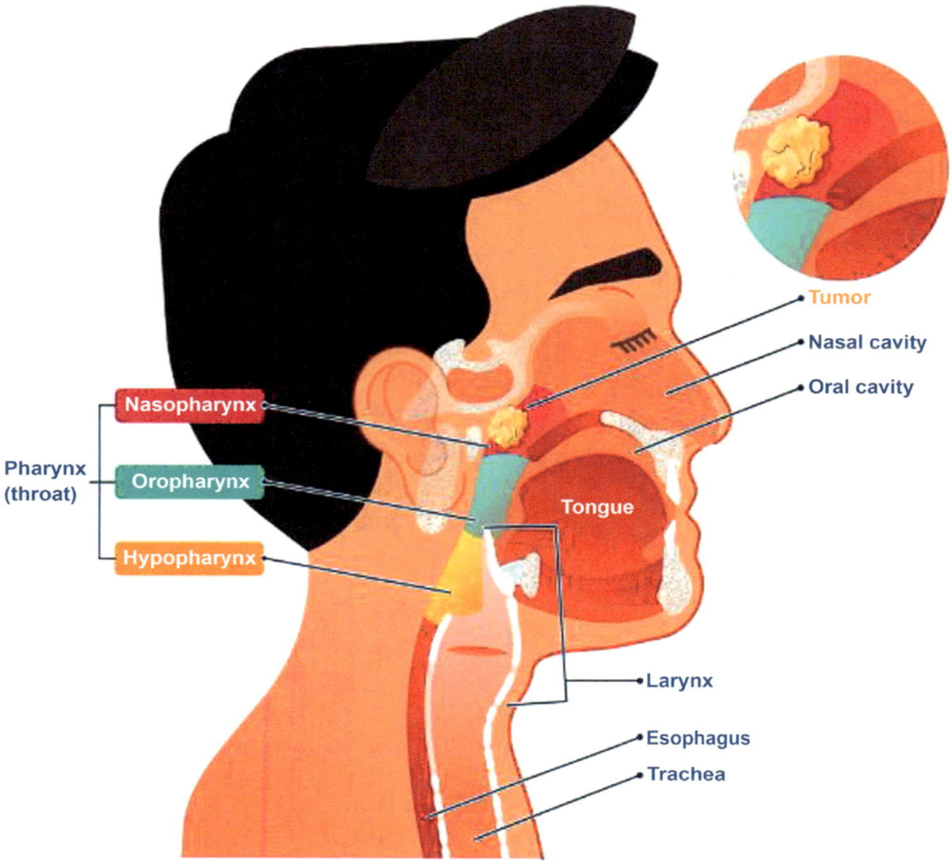

Figure 4.12. Nasopharyngeal carcinoma.

Source: https://www.cmuh.cmu.edu.tw//FileUploads/images/%E8%A1%9B%E6%95%99/84018-shutterstock_1667954575.jpg.

Apart from metabolic reprogramming, the development of advanced genomic editing technologies, such as CRISPR/Cas9, also provides a potential solution for treating herpesvirus-mediated oncogenesis of nasopharyngeal carcinoma. It facilitates specific manipulation of viral genomes that can result in disruption of EBVs latent infection, which is involved in NPC development. Fresh research shows that employing CRISPR/Cas9 to edit viral genes can not only reduce tumor development but also enhance existing antiviral treatments. As studies continue to advance with the complementarities between virology and cancer treatment, CRISPR/Cas9 is a groundbreaking tool, opening up new solutions to the management of latent herpesvirus infections and their oncogenic consequences in nasopharyngeal carcinoma.

4.4.3. Mechanisms of Immune Evasion

The mechanisms through which herpesviruses evade immune responses are a highly evolved process by which such pathogens can ensure survival in the host. One of the best examples of such an evasion mechanism is witnessed with EBV, which is a virus that actively inhibits major histocompatibility complex (MHC) class I antigen processing. The BILF1 gene for the lytic cycle has been identified as a major player in this response; it is a glycoprotein responsible for decreasing surface MHC class I molecules, thereby blocking CD8+ T cell recognition. Through direct interaction with MHC class I, BILF1 promotes its turnover from the cell surface and initiates lysosomal degradation. This interference is most vital during the lytic cycle of replication when the virus generates several potential targets for immune recognition, underlining the strategic function of immune evasion in perpetuating viral persistence and developing oncogenesis within susceptible hosts (Zuo et al., 2009). In addition to simple interference with antigen presentation, herpesviruses use extracellular vesicles as a tool of immune evasion. Microvesicles, including exosomes and shed microvesicles, carry a broad range of biological molecules to enable cell-to-cell communication and potentially modulate immune responses. In viral infection, viral components may be found within these vesicles and lead to a complex interaction between the virus and the host immune system. Herpesviruses co-opt the pathway of microvesicle biogenesis to enable their release or even produce noninfectious vesicles that can be employed to evade immune surveillance. Although some microvesicles possess the capacity to inhibit infection or trigger immune dysregulation, they also have the capacity to disseminate viral particles. This dual potential lends support to the need to examine more extensively how microvesicles function during viral infection because they may represent novel targets for therapeutic approaches to restore immune function (Wurdinger et al., 2012). The interaction between immune evasion and host immune responses highlights the dynamic nature of herpesvirus infections. Successful immune evasion not only allows viral persistence but also contributes to the malignant transformation potential of host cells. As such, viruses hijack the immune pathways; their control over the host immune landscape becomes increasingly complex. Elucidation of these mechanisms will be important for the development of successful prevention and therapy against herpesviruses and their oncogenic impacts. The deciphering of the immune modulation pathways and involvement of extracellular vesicles in the future will be relevant, as this might offer new therapeutic options to enhance host immunity while combating viral persistence. By fully characterizing the intricate relationships between herpesviruses and the immune system, researchers can lay the groundwork for new therapeutic approaches capable of mitigating the oncogenic risk of such viral infections.

4.5. Cytomegalovirus (CMV) and Cancer

The oncogenicity of Cytomegalovirus (CMV) has been a subject of intense scrutiny over the last several years, owing to its alleged oncogenicity. As a Herpesviridae virus, CMV has been known for many years to be capable of gaining latency within host cells and evading immunity, leading researchers to consider its association with malignancy. Surprisingly, research shows that CMV may play a key part in the pathogenesis of glioblastoma, an aggressive form of brain cancer with unfavorable prognosis and high recurrence rate. While some studies have shown measurable amounts of CMV within glioblastoma tissues, results have not been consistent and have been questioned by tissue sample size and method of diagnosis. Thus, ongoing research on CMV in cancer is essential within the context of appreciating the complex interactions of viral infections with tumorigenesis. Within the study of the interaction between CMV and other cancers, variable prevalence levels have been demonstrated, particularly in glioblastoma in comparison to other cancers. New studies that have utilized more advanced techniques, such as ddPCR, have attempted to quantify the amounts of CMV DNA within brain tissues. Although multiple studies indicated a potential correlation between the presence of CMV and glioblastoma, others could not detect the virus within tumor tissue, casting doubt on the virus's actual role in tumorigenesis. Additionally, although Cytomegalovirus is merely one of a number of viruses under investigation for its potential oncogenic capabilities, cancer virology as a field is multifaceted, involving interaction with host cell processes and cofactors such as immune modulation. Thus, further studies are required to clarify CMV's role because it is an area of contention within the general framework of herpesviruses and oncogenic viruses. Studies on CMV's mechanisms of action in cancer biology are required to determine its potential role in cancer progression. For example, CMV has been found to cause alterations in cellular pathways, e.g., regulation of apoptosis and stimulation of angiogenesis. These interactions have the potential to create a permissive environment for tumor progression and metastasis, particularly in highly proliferative tumors like glioblastoma. Further, CRISPR/Cas9 genome-editing research has been promising to correct latent CMV infections, and new therapeutic strategies are being offered. As current antiviral treatments are not entirely effective at eliminating latent herpesviruses, CRISPR/Cas9 use is a revolutionary strategy that not only can enhance fundamental virology but also has the potential to reveal insights into potential antiviral therapies that can be used to suppress cancer-related risk factors for CMV (Chen et al., 2018). Therefore, the search for CMV in cancer scenarios continues to be an essential part of cancer research worthy of investigation to further explore its particular role and contribution to tumor biology (Lin et al., 2016) (Figure 4.13).

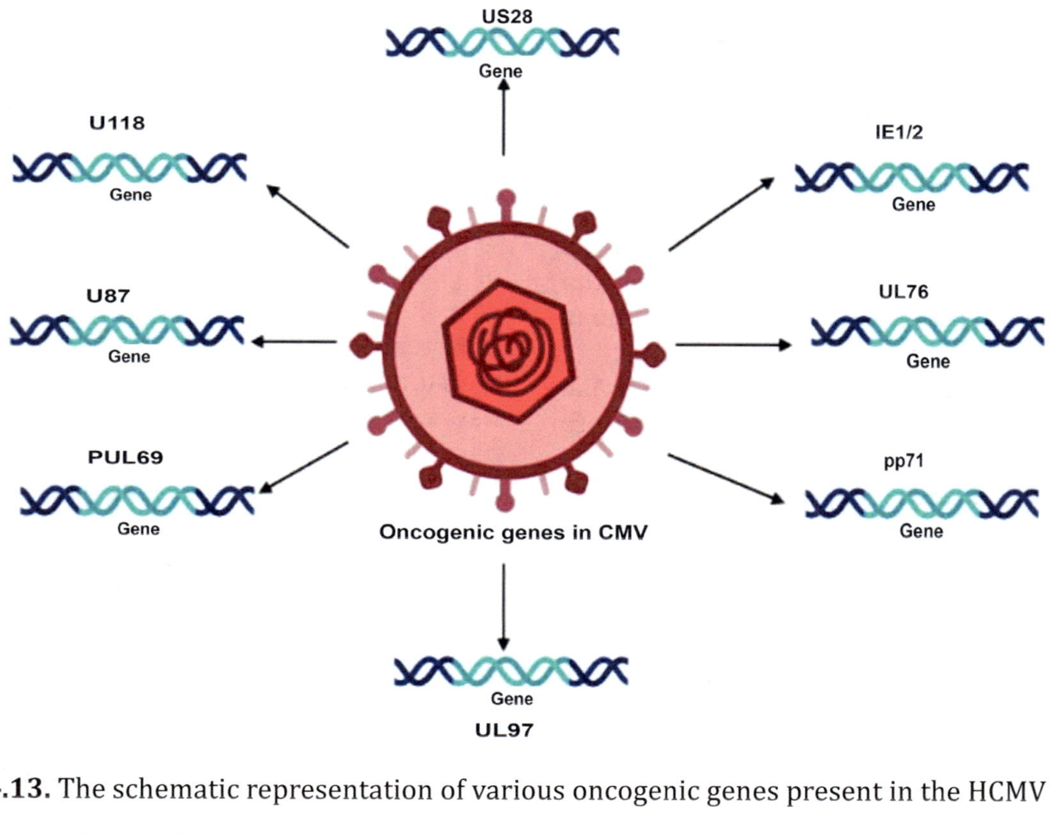

Figure 4.13. The schematic representation of various oncogenic genes present in the HCMV genome.

Source: https://www.frontiersin.org/files/Articles/1202138/fcimb-13-1202138-HTML/image_m/fcimb-13-1202138-g001.jpg.

4.5.1. Association with Glioblastoma

The relationship between glioblastoma, the most aggressive brain cancer, and the herpesviruses has drawn significant attention in the recent literature. Glioblastoma multiforme (GBM) accounts for a significant proportion of the primary central nervous system tumors, and it is an imposing foe with its unfavorable prognosis and high recurrence rate. A few recent reports have suggested potential associations between herpesviruses, namely cytomegalovirus (CMV), EBV, and human herpesvirus 6 (HHV-6), and glioblastoma etiology. However, the inconsistency in research findings casts doubt on the oncogenic nature of these viruses, with greater scrutiny required to ascertain an unequivocal cause-and-effect relationship in GBM formation and progression, especially since GBM patients typically exhibit only 12 to 18 months of survival when diagnosed (Lin et al., 2016). Experimental design has also been crucial in establishing the involvement of herpesviruses in glioblastoma. Sophisticated procedures such as droplet digital PCR (ddPCR) have been employed by scientists to explore the prevalence of viral DNA in GBM tissues with high efficacy. In one study comparing various samples from astrocytoma, EBV was observed to have a close association with GBM, indicating that the virus can exert an impact on tumor formation through processes such as immune modulation or direct transformation (Lin et al., 2016). Conversely, though, CMV was conspicuously absent in the glioblastoma population examined here, and its proposed role as an oncogenic stimulus in many earlier reports is brought into doubt (Figure 4.14).

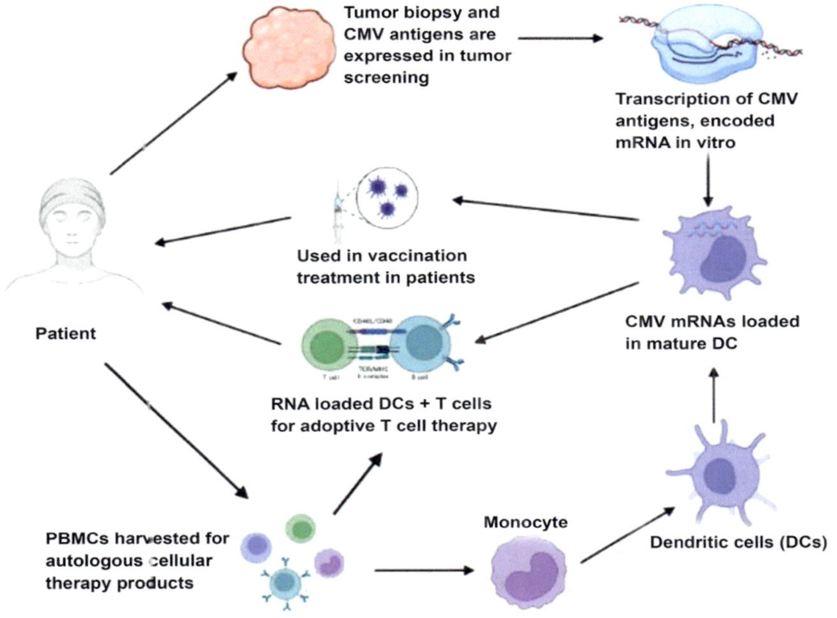

Figure 4.14. Clinical immunotherapy of glioblastoma multiforme (GBM) via dendritic cells (DCs) loaded with mRNA encoding CMV antigens.

Source: https://www.frontiersin.org/files/Articles/1202138/fcimb-13-1202138-HTML/image_m/fcimb-13-1202138-g002.jpg.

Variability in detection rates between studies is suited to a complicated picture around the relationship between herpesviruses and glioblastoma, and careful weighing of evidence before creating absolute conclusions. Moreover, research into the role viral infections play in glioblastoma extends the scope beyond mere association and raises questions regarding potential neuro-oncomodulatory mechanisms. It has been shown that some herpesviruses can create a microenvironment conducive to tumor growth, which is rich in inflammation and regulated immune responses. Neuro-oncomodulation is difficult and is an interesting hypothesis for future investigation, particularly in the clinical setting with limited direct evidence. With our increasing understanding of the molecular and epigenetic processes of glioblastoma comes the need for research into chronic infections and their ability to modify tumor biology. Further study is essential to the identification of new therapeutic targets and effective methods of treatment against a malignancy that continues to resist conventional therapies.

4.5.2. Role in Other Solid Tumors

The role of herpesviruses in solid tumor pathogenesis exceeds their documented association with lymphoproliferative neoplasms. For example, EBV has also been implicated in various cancers, particularly those originating from solid tissues. Apart from lymphomas, EBV's ability to influence immune responses is critical in solid tumors. EBV lytic replication serves a two-fold purpose; while initiating the replication of the virus, it also suppresses major histocompatibility complex (MHC) class I presentation on host cells via the BILF1 gene. Suppression avoids the recognition of infected cells by CD8+ T cells, something that is vital in controlling disease. Thus, as EBV-transformed immune surveillance and the altered tumor microenvironment interact, its role in solid tumors becomes increasingly obvious, supporting the assumption that herpesviruses participate in oncogenesis through immune evasion mechanisms (Zuo et al., 2009). Moreover, the link between other herpesviruses, such as *KSHV*, and solid tumors reveals an even broader scope of viral oncogenic potential. KSHV is most directly associated with *Kaposi's sarcoma* but seems to play a role in other malignancies, including primary effusion lymphoma and some types of multicentric Castleman disease. These cancers are serious problems within the world of solid neoplasms. The oncogenesis pathways employed by KSHV to induce disease most likely involve chronic infection and host regulatory pathway modulation, analogous to EBV. Furthermore, KSHV is also encoded with genes that can disrupt the functioning of cells, resulting in tumorigenesis. Based on the understanding of how herpesviruses disrupt tumor pathways and regulate the immune response, scientists can design targeted therapy and prevention against the cancers, giving vigor to the concept of the virus as a pivotal player in solid tumor biology (Saddawi-Konefka & Crawford, 2010).

The ongoing research in the participation of herpesviruses in solid cancers, particularly primary central nervous system (CNS) malignancies, is important due to the intricate biology of their viruses. Although there is controversy regarding the direct correlation between chronic viral infection and neuro-oncogenesis, the detection of herpesviruses in a variety of CNS tumor subtypes indicates an intriguing neuro-oncomodulatory potential. For instance, the presence of polyomavirus and herpesvirus in brain tumors suggests that the viruses can utilize the CNS environment to facilitate tumor growth or modulate pre-existing tumors. Current hypotheses concentrate on the need for further research to uncover the underlying molecular processes, including potential epigenetic alterations inherited via viral infections. As more evidence accumulates, an increasingly accurate image of the association between herpesviruses and solid tumors is required to clarify the multifaceted functions of these oncogenic viruses in human cancers (Saddawi-Konefka & Crawford, 2010).

4.5.3. Impact on Tumor Microenvironment

The communication between herpesviruses and the tumor microenvironment is central in understanding tumorigenesis and cancer progression. Oncogenic viruses, such as those in the herpesvirus family, exert a profound influence by reshaping the host's cellular microenvironment. They regulate several pathways that contribute towards sculpting the characteristics of the tumor microenvironment, including immune evasion and enhanced tumor cell survival. This manipulation is achieved through a variety of mechanisms, among them the regulation of type I interferons (IFNs), which play a pivotal role not only in antiviral immunity but also in orchestrating immune cell function and growth. By interfering with IFN signaling, herpesviruses create a permissive tumor microenvironment that favors tumor growth and support, emphasizing the bimodal role of IFNs as both tumorigenic sentinels and tumorigenic promoters (Iuliano et al., 2021). Herpesviruses influence cellular activities such as proliferation, apoptosis, and differentiation alongside immune modulation. For instance, the *Kaposi sarcoma*-associated herpesvirus (KSHV) is good at establishing a lifelong infection with both latent and lytic cycles. During latency, KSHV maintains its genome in a manner that produces viral genes sparingly, thereby evading immune surveillance while concurrently reprogramming host cell functions. Upon reactivation to the lytic cycle, KSHV dysregulation of cell signaling pathways is favoured by the expression of multiple viral proteins that lead to uncontrolled cell survival and proliferation. Such changes give rise to malignancies, including *Kaposi sarcoma* and primary effusion lymphoma, further substantiating the argument that herpesviruses significantly shape the tumor microenvironment (Damania et al., 2024). Moreover, the herpesvirus microenvironment is characterized by the release of soluble factors, extracellular vesicles, and alteration of cellular communication. It has been suggested that the viral infections promote the release of cytokines and chemokines that not only activate immune cells but also suppress their effective anti-cancer functions. These alterations allow cancer cells to settle in an unfavorable environment to enable metastatic capability. Through various viral mechanisms in shaping the tumor microenvironment, herpesviruses point to an evolutionary process that ensures their survival while simultaneously facilitating the development of oncogenic diseases at the same time. Such complex interaction is the multifunctional role played by oncogenic viruses within the tumor microenvironment, gaining important insight in future therapeutic interference against virus-induced tumorigenesis (Iuliano et al., 2021).

4.6. Prevention and Treatment Strategies

Prevention and therapy strategies for herpesviruses and cancer viruses are evolving rapidly, which points towards the need for comprehensive approaches addressing both viral persistence and active infection. Traditional antiviral drugs, such as acyclovir and valacyclovir, have been effective in suppressing symptomatic recurrent episodes, in addition to reducing viral shedding, but are deficient in completely eradicating the virus from the host. Also, these therapies do not target the herpesvirus-induced latent reservoirs that cause repeated infections. Therefore, there is a critical need for new strategies that, in addition to controlling active infection, target latent viral genomes to prevent recurrence and potential oncogenic modifications with these viruses. Realizing the limitations of existing therapies highlights the need to investigate new avenues that can address infection management and prevention in vulnerable groups comprehensively. Perhaps one of the most promising advances in the fight against herpesviruses is the use of the CRISPR/Cas9 genome-editing technology. The system allows targeted disruption and cutting of the viral DNA with great accuracy, providing a potential solution to eradicating latent infections that conventional therapies cannot. Through CRISPR/Cas9-mediated mutagenesis, researchers are able to edit the viral genome and add mutations, thus preventing the mode of reactivation and replication in the host. It is a milestone in fundamental virology as well as clinical therapeutics, as it can eradicate chronic infection, which is most often the etiological cause of oncogenic diseases. The ease of adaptation of CRISPR/Cas9 facilitates its being adapted for use across herpesvirus strains, testifying to its value as a general-purpose tool in the therapy and prevention of herpesvirus pathologies and their potential oncogenic implications (Chen et al., 2018). Moreover, the incorporation of a multi-dimensional understanding of herpesviruses' biological features is essential in designing interventions. A complete knowledge of the virus lifecycle, pathogenesis, and immune response of the host is critical to developing strategies that can prevent viral replication and persistence. Complete resources, such as updated texts that integrate scientific research and clinical applications, are used to inform healthcare professionals of the information necessary to institute effective prevention and treatment strategies. These resources not only enhance clinical herpesvirus infection control but also clarify the oncogenic potential of certain strains. Through summarizing extensive research findings and condensing them into comprehensible forms, clinicians can better understand the complexities of herpesviruses, which ultimately contributes to better patient outcomes and prevention strategies (Chen et al., 2018).

4.6.1. Vaccination Efforts Against Oncogenic Viruses

Protection against oncogenic viruses is a serious aspect of public health, especially in the context of preventing herpesvirus-causing diseases. Among these are infections caused by human papillomavirus (HPV) and EBV, which are causes of most cancers, including cervical and nasopharyngeal cancers. Furthermore, the presence of vaccines like Gardasil has rendered it progressively easier to fight malignancies caused by HPV. By immunizing individuals prior to becoming sexually active, these vaccines might eradicate cervical cancer almost entirely, showcasing the efficacy of preventive measures in oncogenic virus control. Furthermore, work continues towards the development of EBV vaccines and their potential to restrict incidence of related lymphomas, showcasing the potential inherent in vaccination as an approach to herpesvirus-mediated oncogenesis. There have also been remarkable advances in the superinfection dynamics of viral populations, particularly their significance in vaccine design. The phenomenon of inhibition of superinfection by research on Gallid herpesvirus 2 (GaHV-2) is an excellent indicator of the intricate behavior of the viruses when they are co-located within a host environment. This study emphasizes the vulnerability of homologous alphaherpesviruses that co-infect cells and the impact their interactions might have on the efficacy of vaccines (Figure 4.15).

While scientists capitalize on what is known about these mechanisms, they aim to design vaccines that not only target specific oncogenic strains but also limit the conditions for virulent recombination events that would be possible through superinfection. Knowledge of these interactions is therefore significant in optimizing vaccine preparations against oncogenic herpesviruses and informing public health policy. Application of animal models, particularly macaques, cannot be overemphasized in driving vaccination approaches against oncogenic viruses. These models have been critical to the duplication of human infectious diseases, enabling investigators to examine vaccine response and pathogenesis under controlled conditions. Macaques, for instance, have contributed to the understanding of a number of oncogenic viruses, including among them simian immunodeficiency virus (SIV) and its human counterpart, HIV. The insights gained through the study of macaques have influenced the creation of vaccines for the human condition, serving as a paradigm for strategies aimed at eradicating oncogenic herpesviruses. Through enabling the determination of new vaccines and treatment methods, the macaque model application demonstrates the vital interplay between clinical research and vaccination strategy in addressing the oncogenic virus-induced malignancy burden and hence determining future public health response.

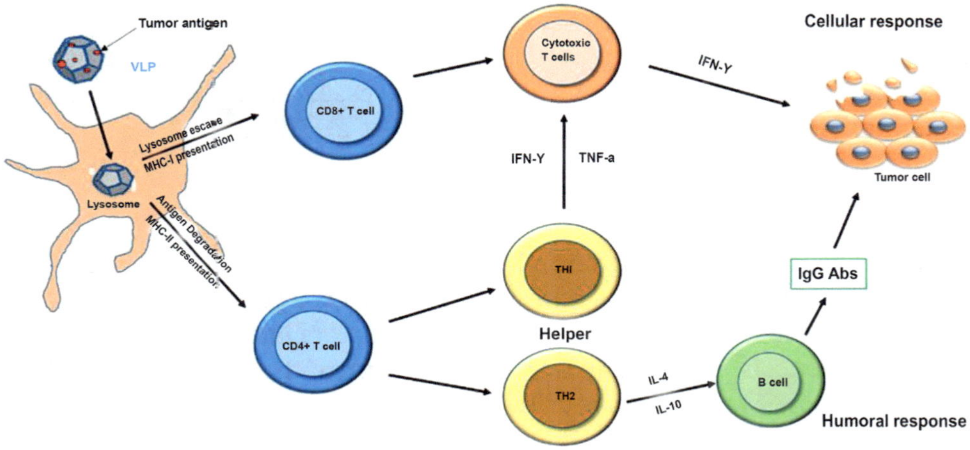

Figure 4.15. VLP-based vaccine: Mechanism of action against tumor cells.

Source: https://www.mdpi.com/vaccines/vaccines-10-00227/article_deploy/html/images/vaccines-10-00227-g001.png.

4.6.2. Antiviral Therapies and Their Effectiveness

Antiviral therapy plays an important role in the treatment of herpesvirus infections, which are known for their ability to establish latent infection and are associated with oncogenic processes. Traditional antiviral therapy primarily depends on inhibiting the virus replication by nucleotide analogs, such as acyclovir and valacyclovir, that are extremely effective in the treatment of HSV and VZV. While these therapies show remarkable efficiency in the reduction of symptoms and relapse prevention, they do not achieve complete eradication of the virus from the host. This is especially the case for latent infections, in which viral genomes remain present within the host's cell as a reservoir for onward infections and complicating treatment regimens. The long-term challenge has been to develop therapies that not only suppress symptoms but target the latent viral reservoirs of chronic herpesvirus infections. Recent advances in gene-editing technology, including the CRISPR/Cas9 system, offer an optimistic strategy to overcome the limitations of current antiviral treatments. This new method provides for targeted mutagenesis of viral genomes to successfully disrupt latent infections in herpesviruses like HSV, Epstein-Barr virus, and cytomegalovirus. With the precision of CRISPR/Cas9, researchers can potentially eliminate these viruses at their origin, providing a longer-lasting solution for repeated infections. As noted, CRISPR/Cas9 can insert mutations identical to those produced by standard recombination techniques, showing its viability not only for basic research but also as a treatment intervention. These advances represent a paradigm change in the fight against herpesviruses, with opportunities for improved patient outcomes through more effective removal strategies (Chen et al., 2018). A merging of a comprehensive understanding of herpesviruses' biology and oncogenic capacity will be required to formulate effective antiviral therapies. Current antiviral treatments cannot cure the full spectrum of clinical manifestations associated with herpesvirus infections, so emphasis is placed instead on ongoing research. Such close study of herpesviruses both scientifically and clinically directs the future development of therapeutic approaches, which could involve novel antiviral agents or adjuvant therapy such as immunotherapies. By combining data from the fragmented sciences and incorporating the latest breakthroughs, clinicians are better positioned to address the daunting issues posed by these viruses. The emphasis on a multi-disciplinary approach may unlock the door to new treatments that not only treat symptoms but also target the underlying processes of latency and viral oncogenesis, with the potential for more long-lasting solutions (Chen et al., 2018).

4.6.3. Future Research Directions

The study of herpesviruses and oncogenic viruses is at a crossroads, with the new evidence uncovering the sophisticated mechanisms by which these viruses co-opt host cellular function. The attention of future studies should be directed toward the complete understanding of viral metabolism and its impact on oncogenesis. Specifically, an understanding of the metabolic remodeling induced by these viruses will uncover the pathways critical for cancer initiation and growth. As emphasized in recent research, viral proteins involved in this metabolic takeover must be identified as a premise for correlation between virus presence and tumorigenesis (Thaker et al., 2019). Enhanced mechanistic studies that include newer methods will not only clarify herpesvirus participation in cancer biology but also provide valuable information on potential therapeutic modalities. Further, the application of innovative technologies such as CRISPR/Cas9 presents an exciting frontier in herpesvirus research, particularly in the context of latent infections. The ability to edit viral genomes with precision has opened new avenues for therapeutic intervention. Future studies could explore the effectiveness of this genome-editing technology in disrupting the latent reservoirs of oncogenic viruses like Epstein-Barr virus and Kaposi's sarcoma-associated herpesvirus. By analyzing CRISPR/Cas9's capacity to convert latent infections to productive lytic cycles, researchers can detect new directions towards eradication that have evaded current therapies (Chen et al., 2018). Such an exploration could rewrite treatment paradigms in virology to provide the scientific community with a solid foundation for combating these prevalent and often devastating viral infections. Furthermore, cross-disciplinary communication between virologists, oncologists, and metabolic scientists is crucial in facilitating new ways of looking into herpesviruses. The future research must focus on the integration of information from metabolic rewiring studies into viral pathogenesis to ensure that the full picture of how these interactions result in cancer generation can be attained. An in-depth understanding of the interplay dynamics between viral infection and host metabolism can potentially uncover novel therapeutic targets and biomarkers. An expansion of research methodologies to cover *in vivo* models will provide us with a better capacity to properly characterize such dynamics, as suggested in more recent work (Thaker et al., 2019). With the progress in the field, an alliance approach will definitely accelerate discovery that may transform our understanding of herpesviruses and their oncogenicity.

SUMMARY

Herpesvirus studies dealing with oncogenic processes are typified by a complex interplay between viral and host cellular processes. Herpesviruses, particularly gammaherpesviruses, employ highly subtle mechanisms to counter host protective mechanisms such as apoptosis, which is the most important aspect of cellular integrity and prevention of tumorigenesis. Through manipulation of apoptotic pathways, the viruses can enhance their survival within the infected cells and have also been implicated in the process of oncogenesis. The findings underscore the importance of deciphering such viral deceptions not just in virology but also in cancer biology, as they suggest potential sites for therapeutic intervention able to reconstitute normal apoptosis in infected cells. Elucidating the molecular cross-talks between herpesviruses and host cell pathways is thus pivotal for cancer therapy development and improved patient outcomes. Further exploration of the therapeutic utility of this information is highlighted by the exploration of such natural products as apigenin, which is cytotoxic to many cancers. For instance, the activity of apigenin against primary effusion lymphoma, KSHV-induced cancer, demonstrates how natural products can impact dominant oncogenic pathways. Apigenin stimulates p53, which in turn affects numerous downstream effects, including inhibition of STAT3, an essential pro-survival pathway in cancer cells. This suggests a highly important connection between food components and viral oncogenesis, perhaps opening new pathways for therapeutic strategies against herpesvirus-induced cancers. Having the ability to target pro-survival and pro-apoptotic pathways equally can potentially revolutionize the oncologic treatment of the future, particularly for fulminant cancers linked to viral etiology. In conclusion, the intersection of herpesvirus biology and oncogenic mechanisms is a critical frontier for both oncology and virology. Understanding how these viruses regulate cellular mechanisms, including apoptosis, could unlock new information that could lead to new treatment strategies. Furthermore, the use of chemicals like apigenin with the potential to modulate oncogenic signaling could be a double-edged approach in the treatment of malignancies induced by herpesviruses. Identification of viral anti-apoptotic proteins as therapeutic targets may be able to empower cancer therapy by triggering cell death among tumor cells without harming normal cells. As research progresses in this direction, it is crucial to stay focused on developing targeted therapies that can harness such viral mechanisms to effectively treat cancer, leading to better therapeutic outcomes for patients with herpesvirus-induced tumors in the future.

The intricate interaction of herpesviruses with oncogenic processes is reflective of the viral interference with host cellular processes with complexity. The area of manipulation of apoptosis, a highly regulated process important for cell integrity, is an important area of research. Oncogenic and latent members of the Gammaherpesvirus family have evolved intricate mechanisms to evade host apoptosis pathways. This evasion is achieved by the modification of both extrinsic and intrinsic apoptotic signals in a way that the viruses survive longer in infected cells than they would during normal infections. The existing findings indicate towards the mechanisms whereby such viruses can abrogate cellular signaling genes and introduce viral homologues that mimic cellular regulatory processes, ultimately contributing to tumorigenesis and ushering in new avenues towards therapeutic interventions targeting these viral proteins modulating apoptosis pathways (Banerjee et al., 2016). Vaccine technology is an important advancement in oncogenic viral disease prevention, namely, virus-induced cancer such as that caused by Marek's disease virus (MDV). Live-attenuated vaccine development, i.e., the CVI988/Rispens strain, has been very important in controlling this viral disease in poultry by preventing tumor formation. The adaptive nature of MDV is problematic because the virus continues to evolve despite vaccination efforts. Significantly, mutations in the viral oncogene, meq, have been identified as the main determinants for this pressure, and certain isoforms correlate with virulence levels. Such findings reveal a double narrative: tumor growth is prevented by vaccination but can at the same time induce the development of more virulent viruses capable of evading vaccination-generated immunity, illustrating the complexities surrounding viral evolution and vaccination programs (Conradie, 2021). The implications of herpesviruses and their oncogenic potential extend to the proximate clinical problems, disclosing broader epidemiological trends and therapeutic strategies. The development of viral strains between immunized and non-immunized groups calls for a grave reconsideration of current vaccination schedules and long-term efficacy. As is evident from the oncogene mutations of the meq oncogene, enhancing the virulence, continuous surveillance and genetic monitoring of the dominant viral strains becomes the norm of the day. Lastly, the information regarding the biochemical pathways through which herpesviruses usurp host cellular processes can be utilized to guide the design of antiviral therapy. As oncogenic processes and viral evolution are dependent upon one another, by realizing this dependency, researchers can better plan interventions that would disrupt these processes, ultimately resulting in more productive public health interventions against herpesvirus-linked cancers (Banerjee et al., 2016; Conradie, 2021).

CLOSER LOOK

VARICELLA-ZOSTER VIRUS (VZV)

Varicella-Zoster Virus (VZV) is a very contagious human herpesvirus and is a Human Herpesvirus 3 (HHV-3) of the family Herpesviridae. It is an enveloped double-stranded DNA virus that causes two diseases of clinical significance: varicella (chickenpox) in initial infection and herpes zoster (shingles) on reactivation. VZV is transmitted by respiratory droplets and contact with the lesions and has a global distribution, with a preponderance in children during primary infection.

During primary infection, the VZV enters the body through the respiratory mucosa or conjunctiva, replicates in local lymph nodes, and causes an early viremia that is short-lived. It is followed by viral replication in the liver and spleen and a second viremia during which the virus infects the skin and mucous membranes and causes the characteristic vesicular exanthem of chickenpox. The eruption typically starts on the trunk and face and progresses to the extremities, accompanied by fever and malaise. Lesions go through a sequence of — macules, papules, vesicles, and crusts — that may all occur simultaneously. Chickenpox is usually self-limited in healthy children but can be extremely severe in neonates, adults, and immunocompromised hosts, with complications of pneumonia, encephalitis, or secondary bacterial infection (Figure 4.16).

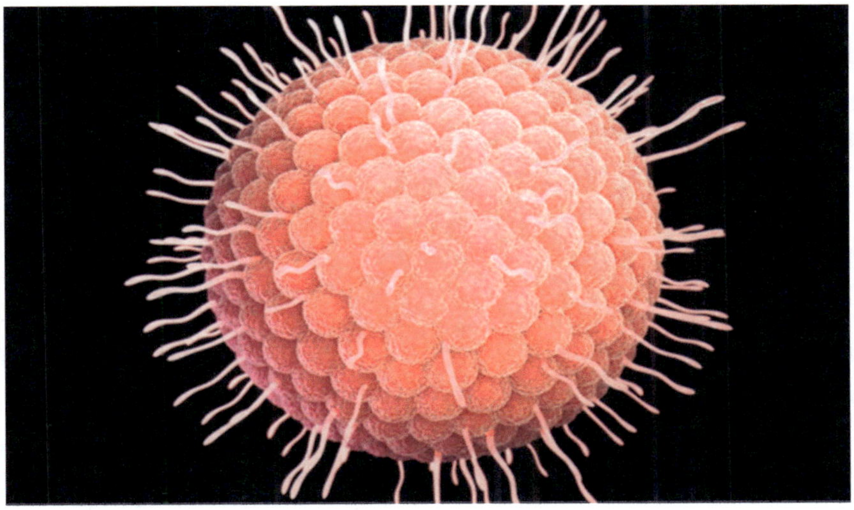

Figure 4.16. 3D rendering of the varicella-zoster virus (VZV), the causative agent of chickenpox and shingles, showing its icosahedral capsid and glycoprotein spikes.

Source: https://dimensionsofdentalhygiene.com/wp-content/uploads/2020/03/shingles-750x430.jpg.

After resolution of the primary infection, VZV is not eliminated from the host. Instead, it becomes latent within sensory nerve ganglia such as the dorsal root or cranial nerve ganglia. Latency is typical of herpesviruses and involves the persistent existence of the viral genome in a sleeping but nonreplicating state without clinical effects. Reactivation of a latent VZV causes herpes zoster (shingles), usually in older adults or immunocompromised patients. Shingles is a painful, vesicular rash that follows a dermatomal pattern, reflecting the reactivation of the virus within a single sensory nerve. Pain is severe and may precede the rash by days. A more serious shingles complication is postherpetic neuralgia (PHN), a pain condition that can persist for many months or years following the rash. VZV reactivation in unusual cases can also lead to herpes zoster ophthalmicus, encephalitis, or disseminated infection.

Diagnosis of VZV infection is usually clinical but can be confirmed by PCR, direct fluorescent antibody, or viral culture. Treatment of varicella is mainly symptomatic, though antiviral therapy (e.g., acyclovir) may be used in high-risk infections. Herpes zoster is treated with antivirals such as acyclovir, valacyclovir, or famciclovir, especially when used within 72 hours of the rash.

Preventive measures include the varicella vaccine in children and zoster vaccine (recombinant subunit vaccine, e.g., Shingrix) in adults. The vaccines have reduced the incidence of both shingles and varicella significantly.

REFERENCES

1. Gardner, M. B., & Luciw, P. A. (2008). Macaque models of human infectious disease. *ILAR journal, 49*(2), 220–255. https://doi.org/10.1093/ilar.49.2.220(accessed on 16th July 2025).
2. Lin, C. T., Leibovitch, E. C., Almira-Suarez, M. I., & Jacobson, S. (2016). Human herpesvirus multiplex ddPCR detection in brain tissue from low- and high-grade astrocytoma cases and controls. *Infectious agents and cancer, 11*, 32. https://doi.org/10.1186/s13027-016-0081-x(accessed on 16th July 2025).
3. Anderson, A. S., Bernberg, E. L., Burnside, J., Garcia, M., et al. (2009). *MicroRNAs of Gallid and Meleagrid herpesviruses show generally conserved genomic locations and are virus-specific.* https://core.ac.uk/download/pdf/82336562.pdf (accessed on 16th July 2025).
4. Wurdinger, T., Gatson, N. N., Balaj, L., Kaur, B., Breakefield, X. O., & Pegtel, D. M. (2012). Extracellular vesicles and their convergence with viral pathways. *Advances in virology, 2012*, 767694. https://doi.org/10.1155/2012/767694(accessed on 16th July 2025).
5. Baquero-Perez, B., Berndt, A., Hughes, D. J., Jackson, D., et al. (2014). *Utilizing proteomic approaches to understand oncogenic human herpesviruses.* https://core.ac.uk/download/29031635.pdf (accessed on 16th July 2025).
6. Bhella, D., McElwee, M., Rixon, F., Vijayakrishnan, S., et al. (2018). *Structure of the Herpes-Simplex Virus Portal-Vertex.* https://core.ac.uk/download/159994609.pdf (accessed on 16th July 2025).
7. Brunovskis, P., & Velicer, L. F. (1995). *The Marek's disease virus (MDV) unique short region: Alphaherpesvirus-homologous, fowlpox virus-homologous, and MDV-specific genes.* https://core.ac.uk/download/pdf/82126844.pdf (accessed on 16th July 2025).
8. Chen, Y. C., Liu, F., Sheng, J., Trang, T., et al. (2018). *Potential application of the CRISPR/Cas9 system against herpesvirus infections.* https://core.ac.uk/download/323080891.pdf (accessed on 16th July 2025).
9. Thaker, S. K., Ch'ng, J., & Christofk, H. R. (2019). Viral hijacking of cellular metabolism. *BMC biology, 17*(1), 59. https://doi.org/10.1186/s12915-019-0678-9(accessed on 16th July 2025).
10. Cirone, M., D'Orazi, G., Faggioni, A., Gilardini Montani, M. S., et al. (2017). *Apigenin, by activating p53 and inhibiting STAT3, modulates the balance between pro-apoptotic and pro-survival pathways to induce PEL cell death.* https://core.ac.uk/download/141695927.pdf (accessed on 16th July 2025).
11. Conradie, A. M. (2021). *Evolution of Marek's Disease virus Pathogenesis and Vaccine Resistance.* https://core.ac.uk/download/427638595.pdf (accessed on 16th July 2025).
12. Saddawi-Konefka, R., & Crawford, J. R. (2010). Chronic viral infection and primary central nervous system malignancy. *Journal of neuroimmune pharmacology : the official journal of the Society on NeuroImmune Pharmacology, 5*(3), 387–403. https://doi.org/10.1007/s11481-010-9204-0(accessed on 16th July 2025).
13. Banerjee, S., Uppal, T, Strahan, R., Dabral, P., & Verma, S. C. (2016). The Modulation of Apoptotic Pathways by Gammaherpesviruses. *Frontiers in microbiology, 7*, 585. https://doi.org/10.3389/fmicb.2016.00585(accessed on 16th July 2025).
14. Damania, B., & Yu, C. J. (2024). *Molecular mechanisms of Kaposi sarcoma-associated herpesvirus*

(HHV8)-related lymphomagenesis. https://core.ac.uk/download/624147501.pdf (accessed on 16th July 2025).

15. Fitzsimmons, L., Boyce, A. J., Wei, W., Chang, C., Croom-Carter, D., Tierney, R. J., Herold, M. J., Bell, A. I., Strasser, A., Kelly, G. L., & Rowe, M. (2018). Coordinated repression of BIM and PUMA by Epstein-Barr virus latent genes maintains the survival of Burkitt lymphoma cells. *Cell death and differentiation, 25*(2), 241–254. https://doi.org/10.1038/cdd.2017.150 (accessed on 16th July 2025).
16. Farina, A., & Farina, G. A. (2016). *Fresh insights into disease etiology and the role of microbial pathogens.* https://core.ac.uk/download/54530426.pdf (accessed on 16th July 2025).
17. Gentile, G., & Micozzi, A. (2016). *Speculations on the clinical significance of asymptomatic viral infections.* https://core.ac.uk/download/98344656.pdf (accessed on 16th July 2025).
18. Jarosinski K. W. (2012). Dual infection and superinfection inhibition of epithelial skin cells by two alphaherpesviruses co-occur in the natural host. *PloS one, 7*(5), e37428. https://doi.org/10.1371/journal.pone.0037428(accessed on 16th July 2025).
19. Iuliano, M., Mangino, G., Chiantore, M. V., Di Bonito, P., Rosa, P., Affabris, E., & Romeo, G. (2021). *Virus-induced tumorigenesis and IFN system.* https://core.ac.uk/download/534202570.pdf (accessed on 16th July 2025).
20. Janich, E. (2018). *Safety of xenotransplantation: Development of screening methods and testing for porcine viruses.* https://core.ac.uk/download/199423495.pdf (accessed on 16th July 2025).
21. Modrow, S., & Wolf, H. (1983). Herpesvirus saimiri-induced proteins in lytically infected cells. I. Time-ordered synthesis. *The Journal of general virology, 64 (Pt 1)*, 37–46. https://doi.org/10.1099/0022-1317-64-1-37(accessed on 16th July 2025).
22. Zuo, J., Currin, A., Griffin, B. D., Shannon-Lowe, C., Thomas, W. A., Ressing, M. E., Wiertz, E. J., & Rowe, M. (2009). The Epstein-Barr virus G-protein-coupled receptor contributes to immune evasion by targeting MHC class I molecules for degradation. *PLoS pathogens, 5*(1), e1000255. https://doi.org/10.1371/journal.ppat.1000255(accessed on 16th July 2025).
23. Mensaert, K., Van Criekinge, W., Thas, O., Schuuring, E., Steenbergen, R. D., Wisman, G. B., & De Meyer, T. (2015). Mining for viral fragments in methylation enriched sequencing data. *Frontiers in genetics, 6*, 16. https://doi.org/10.3389/fgene.2015.00016 (accessed on 16th July 2025).
24. You, Y. (2022). *Novel genetic factors in Marek's disease virus pathogenesis and establishment of a cell culture-based viral integration system.* https://core.ac.uk/download/541748738.pdf (accessed on 16th July 2025).

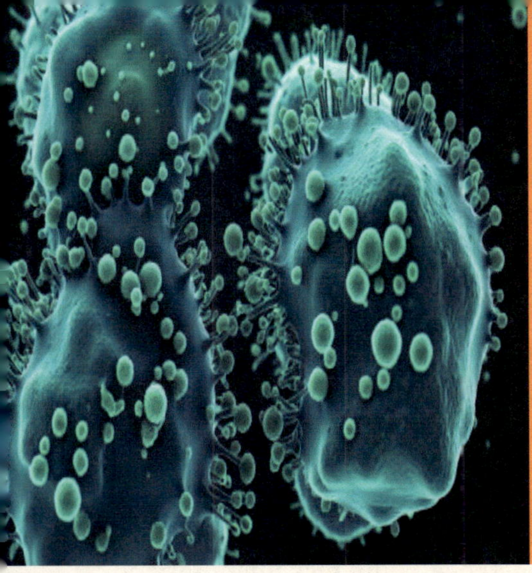

Chapter 5

EMERGING AND RE-EMERGING VIRAL INFECTIONS

Contents

Introduction

The epidemiology of infectious diseases is dynamic, and it poses a significant threat to public health systems globally. As populations grow and become urbanized, the interface between humans and animals becomes greater, with the potential for new viral pathogens to emerge. Emerging viral infections, as commonly defined, are referred to as pathogens from non-human reservoirs, i.e., animals, and spill over to the human reservoir. These infections possess complex dynamics that rely on environmental, ecological, and sociopolitical factors. For instance, the rising zoonotic diseases, driven by ecological and behavioral changes, accentuate the need for public health examination and investigation to forecast and avert likely outbreaks (Ludlam et al., 2006). An understanding of the processes underlying these transmissions is critical to the development of effective preventive and control measures against viral emergence. Viral re-emerging diseases introduce yet another layer of public health worry, since previously known pathogens have the capacity to re-emerge or develop methods of evading previously implemented control measures.

Viral diseases such as tuberculosis and measles are harsh reminders of this fact, erupting anew in environments where vaccination has decreased or where public health budgets have been reduced. The resurgences of these diseases not only indicate shortcomings in healthcare delivery but also highlights the capacity of viruses to undergo adaptation due to human activities, including land use and climatic changes. Like in recent disease outbreaks of diseases such as hepatitis or HIV, effective management is largely dependent on synthesizing scientific research, public health policy, and global collaborations. New strategies will need to take into consideration the evolving nature of these viruses and build rigorous surveillance systems to enable timely and suitable reactions to outbreaks (Ludlam et al., 2006). The intricacies of new and re-emerging viral diseases require an interdisciplinary approach that combines several disciplines such as virology, epidemiology, ecology, and social sciences. While the globe wrestled with pandemics, it is certain that traditional methods of managing infectious diseases are no longer sufficient. New technology and strategies, including advanced mathematical modeling and better diagnostic tools, hold out the prospect of reshaping our capabilities in predicting viral infections and controlling them. These new advances also hold out the promise of unleashing targeted surveillance, whereby dangerous pathogens are identified ahead of time before they cause widespread harm. By promoting joint research work globally, the scientific community can strive to reverse the paradigm of strategies from reactive to proactive prevention, ultimately leading to our preparedness against the ever-changing threat of viral infections (Morse et al., 2012).

Definition of Emerging and Re-Emerging Viral Infections

The concept of re-emerging and emerging viral infections is core in understanding the public health problems worldwide. Emerging viral infections are those that have newly emerged in a population or were known whose incidence or geographic distribution is increasing at a very rapid rate. These infections typically embody an innovative human-zoonotic reservoir interface, which could be with various animal reservoirs, thus reflecting the dynamic interrelationship in ecosystems. The rapid evolution of viral genotypes further contributes to the complexity, underlining the constant adaptation of viruses that have the potential to cause outbreaks. Influenza viruses that spill over from animal reservoirs, for instance, could pick up mutations that enable them to infect humans more effectively and present a pandemic risk that is ever-present and needs to be monitored carefully and responded to quickly. On the other hand, re-emerging infections are those that had already declined before but are now reviving, often due to environmental change, human action, or public health response. Such infections can be due to antimicrobial resistance, population movement, and disruption of vaccine coverage. Notably, epidemics of infectious illnesses like measles and tuberculosis demonstrate the manner in which altered social conditions and public health measures can renew the threat of infection that had been deemed under control. Moreover, populations whose immune systems are compromised, as with people who have HIV, are at greater risk of these re-emergent perils. The increase in cases among high-risk populations further calls for continuous education and healthcare to mitigate the public health burden of such infections (Harris et al., 2016). The distinction between emerging and re-emerging infections is critical when preparing for and responding to pandemics. Emerging threats can prompt preemptive action based on genetic and biological research, such as in flu virus research that emphasizes the identification of those strains with the highest potential for infecting humans (Barclay et al., 2016). With knowledge of the parameters behind viral adaptation, such as receptor binding affinity and polymerase activity, health agencies can focus surveillance and control. Through the complex interactions between hosts, pathogens, and the environment, stakeholders can develop combined systems of surveillance and control of these viral diseases. This is a multi-disciplinary approach essential to addressing the dynamic pattern of viral pathogens and safeguarding public health against new and re-emerging threats (Figure 5.1).

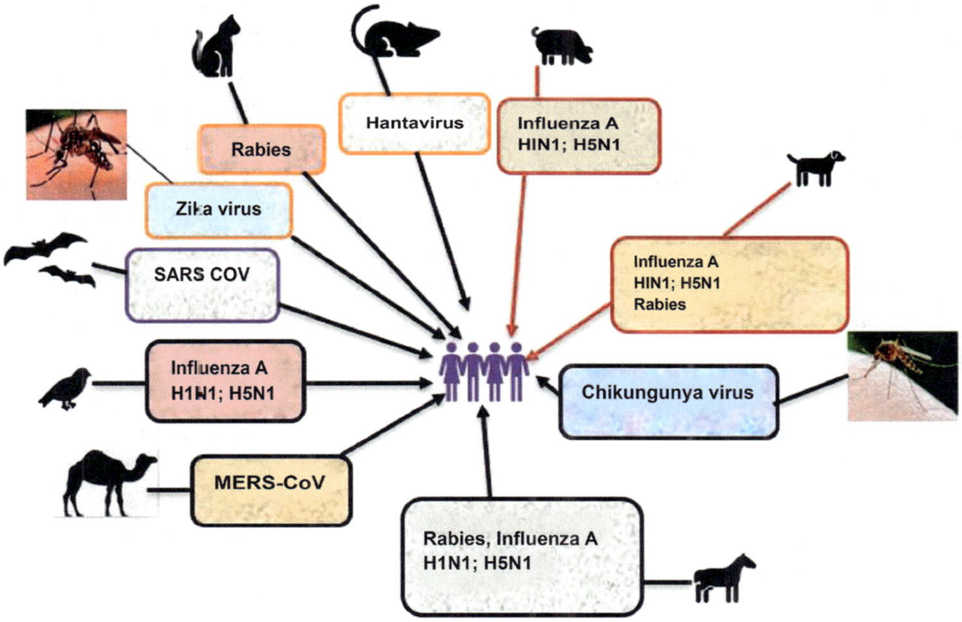

Figure 5.1. (Re)-emerging viral diseases: Vectors, reservoirs, and routes of transmission.

Source: https://clinmedjournals.org/articles/ijva/international-journal-of-virology-and-aids-ijva-7-067.php?jid=ijva.

Importance of Studying Viral Infections

It is significant to know viral infections since, through their continuous and rapid mutagenesis and adaptation to the host, they pose daunting public health issues in terms of emergence or re-emergence of viral infections. For instance, ranaviruses, which affect mostly amphibians, reptiles, and fish, are being perceived more and more as risks to biodiversity throughout the globe, leading to massive die-offs in affected groups. These viruses' capacity to evolve and spread reiterates the need for ongoing monitoring and research. Investigation into such viral diseases is important not only for protecting wildlife but also to gain insight into potential spillover events that can have an impact on human populations. With these viruses replicating in new environments, the stakes for ecological balance and human health cannot be overstated, which is why scientific work in this area is important for science and society (Brunner et al., 2014). Moreover, interaction between wildlife and human society complicates the epidemiology of viral disease. Wild birds, especially migrant birds, can act as carriers of numerous microorganisms, some of which are several viruses that are associated with human disease. Although direct transmission from wild birds to human beings is rather rare, their role as reservoirs for pathogens like the influenza A virus and West Nile virus cannot be overlooked. An appreciation of the pathways for these pathogens to propagate in wildlife is of the utmost importance for public health interventions to succeed. Continual follow-ups on migratory patterns, altering habitats, and human impacts will define a more comprehensive epidemiological picture, creating the capacity to predict and minimize the danger of impending outbreaks. Thus, a vision for studying viral infections, particularly of free-roaming animals, is imperative to help in guaranteeing public health actions (Tsiodras et al., 2008). Moreover, the scientific significance of viral infection research extends beyond ecological concerns to public policy and global health security. From recent pandemics across the globe, the ability of viral infections to cross species can lead to widespread health crises and economic instability. The public health workforce and policymakers must be advised by good epidemiological research in putting in place robust monitoring and response systems. Improved understanding of viral transmission dynamics provides a foundation for the development of efficient vaccines and treatment regimes and thereby reduces the threats from emerging and re-emerging infections. Preparation for future epidemic is based on a robust scientific foundation addressing both the biological essence of viruses and the socio-economic factors impacting disease transmission. Briefly, viral infections research is not only scholarly work but a vital part of humankind protection from the ever-present threat of epidemic diseases (Figure 5.2).

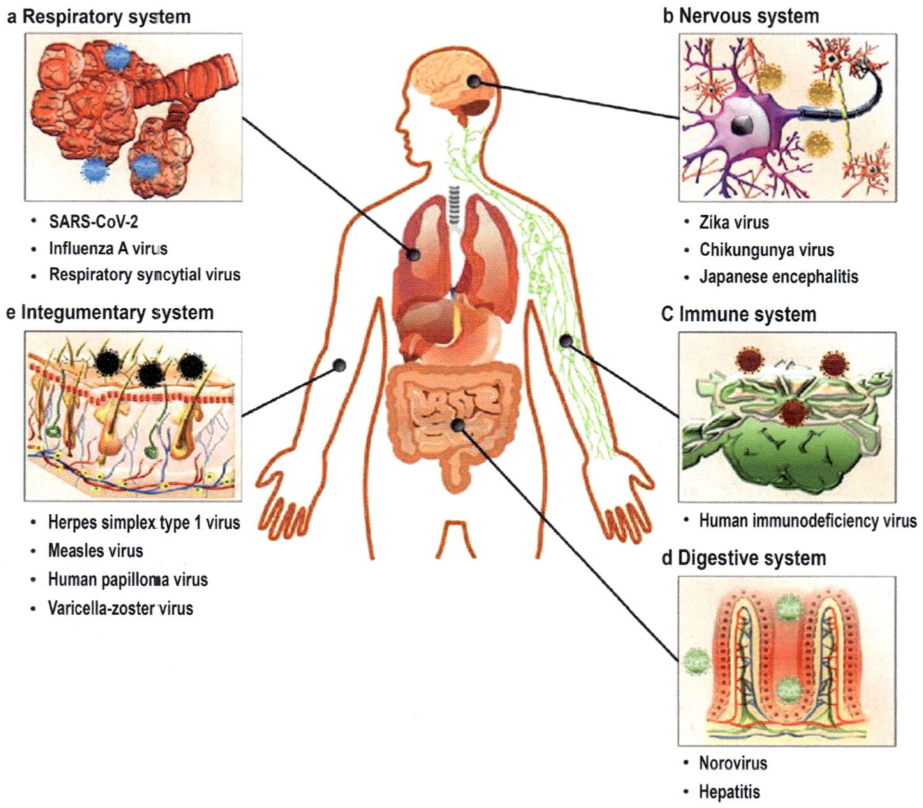

Figure 5.2. Schematic illustration of viral infection in organ systems.

Source: https://www.researchgate.net/publication/363775332/figure/fig1/AS:11431281088705685@1665246151709/Schematic-illustration-of-viral-infection-in-organ-systems-Viral-infection-in-human.png.

5.1. Historical Context of Emerging and Re-Emerging Viral Infections

In tracing the historical context of re-emerging and emerging viral infections, it is crucial to realize that how the conditions of society and public health intervention influence disease dynamics determines its trajectory. The HIV pandemic, which started to develop in the early 1980s, is the best example of the entwining of social processes with virology. Originally perceived in a myopic mode, pointing at high-risk groups, the HIV response was weak and often became a helper in spreading the virus instead of limiting its growth. Health disparities and social stigmatization of the disease were indicative of inequalities embedded in the healthcare system and society at large. This provides the background against which to reflect on how public health programs evolve and are shaped by new diseases, typically reflecting more general societal concerns and historical injustices. As awareness of HIV increased, the development of initiatives like the Getting to Zero campaign in San Francisco represented a significant shift in public health policy. From a city that was once thought to be the epicenter of the HIV epidemic, this campaign not only aims for zero cases but also addresses the primary social determinants of health, such as housing, which have significant influences on public health outcomes. Even though it was innovative in its methodology, the campaign highlights shortcomings in managing intersections of socio-economic determinants with health. Leaving housing problems out of regular interventions indicates a general failure to take into account the management of health emergencies and how a comprehensive plan is essential in realizing public health interventions in preventing increasing viral infections (Zaragoza, 2019). The past history of viral illnesses also provides useful lessons for current global health crises. The patterns of zoonotic spillover, such as with viruses Ebola and SARS, demonstrate the effects of climate change and globalization on infectious disease patterns. Historical events, like the 1918 flu pandemic, have shaped current epidemiological understanding and responses, but similar trends occur with present diseases. Emerging viral diseases are likely to take advantage of the weaknesses in societies, magnified by processes including urbanization and climate change. While societies try to respond to such complex challenges, the examination of the past historical paths of viral threats imposes the imperative need for an integrated response that not only sees the pathogens but also considers the socio-economic and political systems where they succeed (Zaragoza, 2019).

5.1.1. Notable Past Viral Outbreaks

The etiological evolution of viral epidemics provides us with essential data regarding the balance of emerging and re-emerging infectious diseases. A case in point is the 2014–2016 Ebola Virus Disease (EVD) epidemic in West Africa, which directly reminded us of the enormous public health dangers of new pathogens. Characterized by a high fatality rate of over 40% in certain regions, the outbreak underscored the imperative for united global public health responses. The rapid spread was facilitated by a wide range of factors, ranging from cultural burial practices, poor health infrastructure, and medical intervention resistance at the level of culture. Consequently, this outbreak not only revealed the vulnerabilities of local health care systems but also prompted reevaluation of global surveillance and response strategies with particular focus on the importance of preparedness in the face of such new threats from zoonotic diseases. A greater example is the Zika virus outbreak, first reported in Africa's central and eastern regions in the 1940s but brought into infamy in the Americas in 2015. What began as a solitary infection quickly became a global public health crisis, responsible for severe birth defects such as microcephaly in newborns. The outbreak was particularly alarming due to the virus's vector-borne nature of transmission, which spread its transmission at lightning speed across continents by vector.

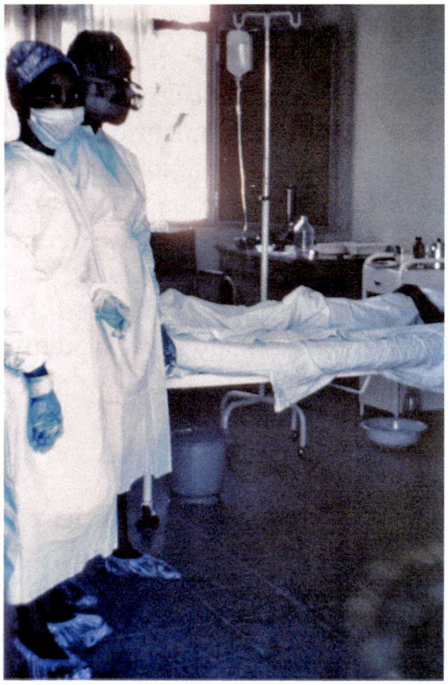

Figure 5.3. Two nurses standing near Mayinga N'Seka, a nurse with Ebola virus disease during the 1976 outbreak in Zaire.

Source: https://upload.wikimedia.org/wikipedia/commons/thumb/a/ab/7042_lores-Ebola-Zaire-CDC_Photo.jpg/800px-7042_lores-Ebola-Zaire-CDC_Photo.jpg.

The occurrence prompted an investigation of the epidemiology of the Zika virus as well as its broader consequences for maternal and child health. After the eruption, it was evident that there was a requirement for robust global collaboration and viral genomics and pathogen dynamics research, more evidence of the need for a One Health response to prevent future viral outbreaks (Lewnard & Reingold, 2019). The historical lessons of viral epidemics documented in the books have transformed the field of infectious disease epidemiology, heralding the constant dynamic face of pathogens and the necessity of being flexible with public health interventions. The ongoing pandemic of COVID-19 highlights the lessons from past epidemics, wherein it has been exhibited that the interplay between human behavior, ecological alteration, and viral biology presents multifaceted challenges. With the developing of contemporary epidemiology embracing breakthroughs in data collection and analysis, the value of multi-disciplinary response is increasingly being appreciated. Through such combined understanding involving veterinary science, ecology, and epidemiology, public health networks can better respond to new infections, applying the experience gained through past outbreaks to inform future responses and preparedness (Lewnard & Reingold, 2019) (Figure 5.3).

5.1.2. Factors Contributing to the Emergence of Viruses

The appearance of viruses presents major global public health concerns, and it is necessary to determine the drivers of this phenomenon for the formulation of efficient preventive measures. Among the main determinants is the relationship between humans and animals, or the human-animal interface. As the globe becomes more integrated, the rate of contact between humans and wildlife increases, hence increasing the potential for zoonotic transmission. This interface is a central point for the spillover of pathogens from animals to people, a spillover that is facilitated by ecological drivers such as habitat loss and climate change. Also, as urbanization extends to rural and natural environments, the uprooting of animal populations may lead to unanticipated viral epidemics, thus the need for a more profound understanding and monitoring of these interfaces to contain risks of emergent infections (Pike et al., 2010). Anthropogenic forces significantly contribute to the occurrence of new viral infections, with the highest effects via activities such as deforestation, agriculture, and wildlife trade. As human activities bleed into the natural environments, they undermine ecosystems and open up space for viruses to make jumps from animal hosts to human populations. The interactions are also influenced by changing climate patterns, which can potentially redirect animal migration routes and behaviors. This further amplifies the danger of disease transmission. Industrial farming methods also create ideal conditions for viruses to replicate and mutate effortlessly, especially in dense livestock corridors. International trade in goods and human travel have the potential to facilitate the rapid exchange of both viral pathogens and infected individuals, facilitating the swift emergence and re-emergence of disease. Addressing these environmental and industry factors is thus pivotal in disease prevention and control (Al-Tawfiq et al., 2018). Social behavior and public health interventions also play a key role in the viral emergence dynamics. Social mobilization, health education, and behavior change interventions are required to reduce the risk of epidemic occurrence, particularly in highly affected regions. Weak global surveillance mechanisms for zoonotic diseases hinder response and preparedness, allowing viruses to spread unrestricted. Recommended changes include intensifying communication efforts to sensitize populations to emerging health and community-based interventions that engage local populations in the monitoring and response effort. Moreover, understanding the socio-economic milieus within which these viruses circulate can facilitate targeted prevention interventions, highlighting the requirement for a multi-disciplinary approach that balances scientific inquiry, public policy, and community participation. Therefore, addressing these socio-environmental determinants is the way to deal with the impacts of emerging and re-emerging viral diseases (Pike et al., 2010).

5.1.3. Lessons Learned from Historical Pandemics

Learning from historical pandemics provides valuable lessons about interventions that are effective in stemming the impact of emerging and perennial viral infections. The historical experiences of pandemics such as the 1918 flu and the recent COVID-19 pandemic emphasize the critical roles of early warning and timely response actions in preventing the spread of viruses. For instance, rapid implementation of public health measures, including social distancing, face mask covering, and immunization campaigns, was essential in curbing COVID-19 cases. From the history, it was observed that countries that acted promptly, like Taiwan and South Korea, were able to contain their infection rates compared to those countries that arrived late." Besides, the importance of international collaboration has also been underscored, as pooled data and resources come in handy in monitoring and predicting potential outbreaks. Such measures, as the case of the Mpox outbreak reveals, are not mere recommendations but are inevitable methods of ensuring global health security in the future (Enitan et al., 2024). Public health interventions based on evidence and epidemiological surveillance have become integral parts of the fight against viral infections. Past pandemics have shown us that monitoring and surveillance systems play a fundamental role in reacting to outbreaks. During the Ebola outbreak in West Africa, inaccurate data collection led to slow response and limited containment measures. Efficient surveillance systems, with the help of technology and bioinformatics advancements, can now process data in real-time and present key findings on viral evolution and transmission. This was seen in the COVID-19 pandemic when genomic sequencing played a core role in tracking mutations of variants. This makes financing robust surveillance systems, as well as healthcare facilities' improvement, critical in managing potential pandemics. The need for access equality to the systems also brings to the fore the lessons that have been learned, with gaps that must be bridged in future public health approaches (Enitan et al., 2024). Finally, previous pandemics reveal the fundamental relationship between public health measures' effectiveness and societies' behaviors. Disparities in medical care distribution and vaccine distribution, highlighted by the COVID-19 pandemic, highlight the structural disparities that can increase infectious disease spread. No less significant is the fact that the social culture plays a crucial role in dictating populations' reactions to public health crises; widespread disinformation can erode public confidence in health authorities. Educating communities, open communication, and culturally appropriate health promotion interventions are essential in building compliance with health mandates. Health interventions, based on the lessons learned from experience, should involve participation from the communities and meet localized needs in order to build public trust and public effectiveness. Lastly, the experience gained from previous pandemics reiterates a multi-dimensional approach that combines scientific interaction, organizational organization, and global coordination in tackling novel viral infections and re-emerging viral infections effectively (Enitan et al., 2024) (Figure 5.4).

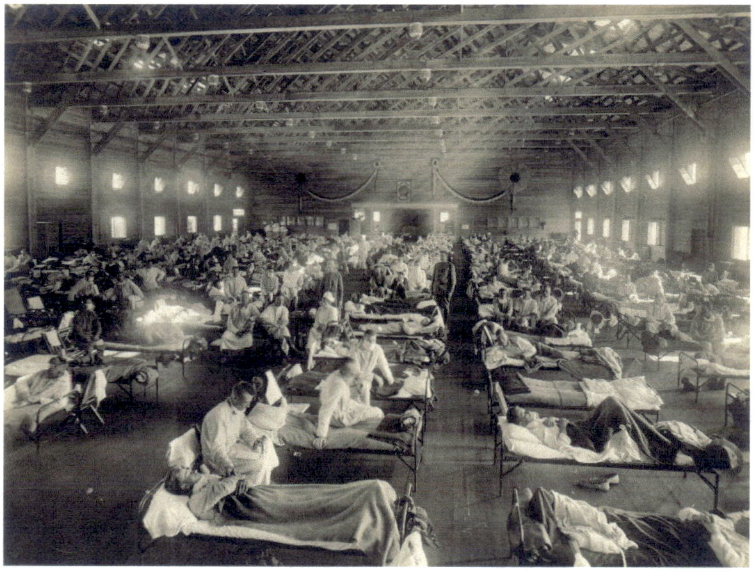

Figure 5.4. Influenza pandemic of 1918–1919: A temporary hospital in Camp Funston, Kansas, during the 1918–1919 influenza pandemic.

Source: https://upload.wikimedia.org/wikipedia/commons/2/20/Emergency_hospital_during_Influenza_epidemic%2C_Camp_Funston%2C_Kansas_-_NCP_1603.jpg.

5.2. Mechanisms of Viral Emergence

The emergence of viruses is a multifaceted phenomenon that occurs due to countless factors, most of which stem from zoonotic transmission — how viruses jump from animals to humans. This process is of great importance in studying pandemics, as the majority of recent pandemics, such as HIV/AIDS and SARS, have shown that animal reservoirs are very important for new human viruses. Ecological modifications like habitat disturbance and land use change play a major role in this process by augmenting human contact with animals. Moreover, behavioral and socioeconomic factors such as urbanization and poverty can amplify these contacts to enable the transmission of viruses to human hosts. The challenge of predicting such outbreaks is in the confines of our understanding of the intricacy of such zoonotic linkages, and this requires a concerted approach to be in a position to comprehend the mechanisms of viral emergence and how it influences global public health (Morse et al., 2012). The pursuit of predictive surveillance of potential viral outbreaks is now considered to be critical in averting human infection. Studies have shown that the merging of genetic and ecological data can potentially provide valuable insights into the prediction of high-risk viruses before they attain the ability to infect humans. Researchers in the fields of virology, ecology, and computational biology have conducted workshops that have sought to establish the feasibility of making such predictions. By looking into the species that act as reservoirs or vectors, scientists have hoped to better understand the biological determinants of virus transmission. This not only involves the detection of endemic viruses but also the establishment of systems that can effectively predict imminent species jumps. The value of this predictive capability cannot be emphasized enough because it represents a proactive approach to addressing incipient zoonotic disease risks and could significantly enhance public health preparedness (Flanagan et al., 2012). Moreover, existing surveillance strategies are more likely to react after the emergence of disease and not to prevent it, indicating a significant lack in public health interventions being carried out. Solving this problem involves upscaling actions for screening wild animals and domesticated animals for potential zoonotic viruses. Research has proven that wild animals, particularly rodents and bats, have a high amount of viruses with the potential to spill over to human beings. This calls for the convergence of science and government agencies to establish an integrated and robust surveillance system. By embracing the new technologies and strategies that address high-risk interfaces of humans and animals, we can develop predictive models. These methods would not only improve our response to new viral threats but also aid in making a shift from reactive to proactive prevention, ultimately to minimize the likelihood of future pandemics (Flanagan et al., 2012; Morse et al., 2012).

5.2.1. Genetic Mutations and Recombination

The genetic complexity of viral genomes is an emergent functional characteristic of viral emergence and re-emergence, primarily through mechanisms of genetic mutation and recombination. Through viral replication, genetic errors in the nucleotide sequence may occur, resulting in mutations that can alter viral features, including transmission and pathogenicity. Genetic diversity can be the origin of quasispecies, a diverse population of similar viral variants. A perfect example is HIV, which has shown tremendous genetic diversity as a consequence of mutations accumulated during replication in the infected hosts. The dynamic nature of such quasispecies enables the virus to adapt to neutralize immune pressures, facilitating its survival and persistence in populations even more. Lastly, the interplay of genetic mutations and the selective forces of the host immune environment is the foundation on which the genetic fluidity observed in initial viral pathogens (Eberle & Gürtler, 2012) is established. Mutations are complemented by recombination as a means for the formation of viral diversity. Recombination occurs when two different viral strains infect the same host cell, leading to the exchange of genetic information and the creation of novel viral genotypes. Recombination can greatly enhance pathogenicity and virulence, as evidenced by many emergent viruses with altered host ranges or increased virulence through recombination events. Re-emerging and emerging viruses, such as those belonging to the HIV family, provide significant insight into how recombination contributes to viral adaptation, in this case, with respect to co-infection situations. A relevant finding with plant viruses also illustrates how genetic recombination allows viruses to switch hosts or overcome resistance factors, a reflection of the increased evolutionary significance of this mechanism (Acosta-Leal et al., 1995). The importance of recombination of viruses and genetic mutation extends beyond the evolution of viruses; they also influence public health policy and treatment plans of emergent diseases. An understanding of the viral genetic processes is crucial for designing effective vaccines and antiviral medicines. For instance, the identification of conserved areas within highly variable viruses can inform vaccine development that induces broad immunity. In the same way, tracking viral mutations can give clues on drug resistance to antiviral therapies so that timely adjustments can be made in the treatment regimen. With new and re-emerging virus populations threatening global health, a thorough understanding of genetic mutations as well as recombination will be crucial for anticipatory actions in disease prevention and outbreak control (Acosta-Leal et al., 1995; Eberle & Gürtler, 2012) (Figure 5.5).

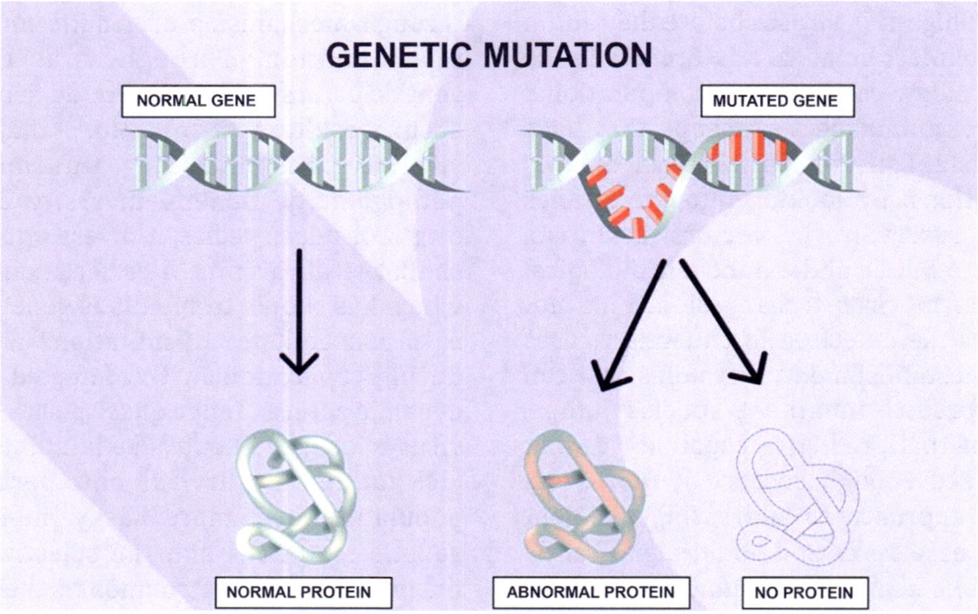

Figure 5.5. Genetic mutation.

Source: https://www.health.com/thmb/7UPmUcOC32y23eEXnKKjbbDzOjk=/1500x0/filters:no_upscale():max_bytes(150000):strip_icc()/Health-Genetic-Mutation-background-light-purple-a6ad7969c03e4780ae174b4c9f705c0c.jpg.

5.2.2. Zoonotic Transmission and Animal Reservoirs

Zoonotic transmission, by which pathogens are transferred from animals to humans, is a key force behind viral infection emergence. Observations have demonstrated that zoonoses account for a remarkable 60% of emergent new human infections, with over 71% of these emergent pathogens coming from wildlife reservoirs. This direct linkage emphasizes the relevance of studying animal reservoirs as potential incubators for emergent infectious dangers. As zoonotic diseases change, they may gain new genetic characteristics, thus improving their pathogenic potential. In addition, several ecological, behavioral, and socio-economic changes may affect the transmission of the pathogens, making it difficult for us to predict their emergence. Thus, it becomes critical to comprehend the intricate interactions between wildlife, domestic animals, and human populations so that preemptive public health measures may help avert future pandemics, for the previous patterns of viral infections have diversified into extensive outbreaks (Morse et al., 2012). Animal reservoirs are point sources in the chain of transmission of emergent viruses. The host behavior and habitat, along with the changing environmental conditions, have a great impact on the dynamics of infectious diseases. For instance, climate change and habitat loss can result in increased human-animal contact, providing new chances for spillover events where the pathogens are transmitted from wildlife to humans. Additionally, species adaptation in response to these changes can present new infections affecting human health. This is an interdisciplinary approach to bringing ecological data together with public health theory. Improved surveillance systems and mathematical modeling can expand our ability to estimate and predict the emergence of zoonotic pathogens, ultimately informing strategic ways to avoid epidemics from occurring (Cutler et al., 2010). From these intricacies, it is evident that mitigation of zoonotic transmission involves an extensive understanding of animal reservoirs and their role in viral infection. The interaction between pathogens and their animal hosts is governed by countless variables like ecological disruptions and altered host behavior. To govern effectively, scientists have to put a lot of emphasis on identifying the ecological niches where the zoonotic pathogens will be found. This involves not only monitoring wildlife populations but also addressing the broader socio-economic forces that facilitate zoonotic spillover. Through the development of strategies incorporating predictive analytics and real-time animal health surveillance, we can substantially reduce the risk posed by new infectious diseases. These efforts will transform our public health policy from a response to a viral invasion into a proactive, preventive measure that can save thousands of lives when there are viral invasions (Cutler et al., 2010; Morse et al., 2012) (Figure 5.6).

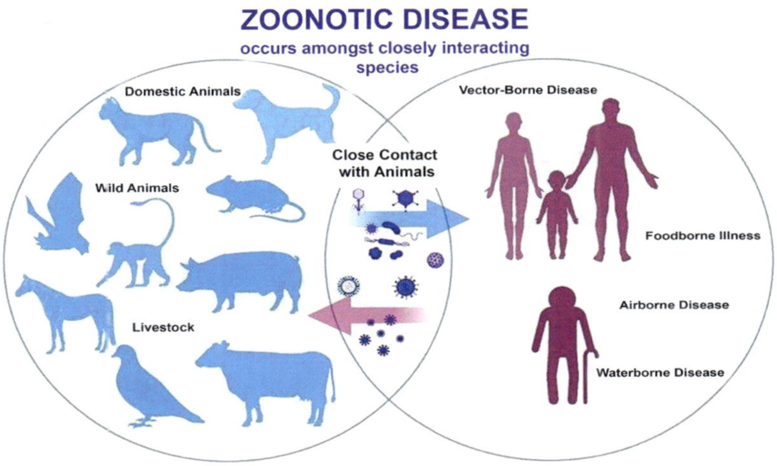

Figure 5.6. Zoonotic transfer of pathogens occurs when close contact encourages species-jumping transmission between animals — such as domestics, wildlife, or livestock — and humans.

Source: https://www.researchgate.net/profile/Abdullah-Channo/publication/377089354/figure/fig1/AS:11431281215539863@1704285706071/Zoonotic-transfer-of-pathogens-occurs-when-close-contact-encourages-species-jumping.jpg.

5.2.3. Environmental Changes and Their Impact on Viral Spread

The intricate dynamics of environmental change and virus spread are quickly being unraveled with ecosystems experiencing unprecedented alteration due to climate change, deforestation, and urbanization. Environmental modification directly impacts the habitats of animals in the wild, which serve as reservoirs for most emerging and re-emerging viral diseases. As species migrate or lose their habitats, they unavoidably come into contact with new ecological processes that alter the routes of virus transmission. For instance, human population expansion into wildlife reserves can enhance the possibility of zoonotic spillover of viral infections such as HIV/AIDS and SARS that have significantly impacted human health. Understanding the ecological forces behind these viral transmissions is key to developing measures to slow their transmission and inform educated antiviral interventions and policies to minimize human-animal contact (Morse et al., 2012). In addition to habitat alteration, human activities such as agricultural extension and land use dynamics contribute to the determination of viral emergence patterns. All of these enhance viral emergence factors that facilitate close contact between domestic, wild, and human species, thus increasing the likelihood of spillover events. Agricultural intensification, for example, creates a conducive environment for viral transmission by nurturing viral spread through agricultural practices that ignore natural ecosystems. Besides that, climate change is also modifying vector-borne diseases by redistributing vector and pathogen geographic ranges and behaviors. This points to the necessity of integrating ecological alongside virological research in order to unravel the complexities of emergent infections and therefore facilitate proactive surveillance and intervention strategies in endemic regions (Flanagan et al., 2012). The demand for sophisticated surveillance and predictive models stems from the awareness that most future viral outbreak incidents can be prevented with proactive efforts. Cross-disciplinary efforts involving virology, ecology, and public health are essential to determine high-risk locations for likely viral spillover before their occurrence. For example, genetic and ecological data can be used to identify species and environments where zoonotic transmission risk is higher. All of this anticipation can, in fact, move pandemic preparedness from response to pre-emptive. By building on our understanding of environmental drivers of viral spread, we can design integral frameworks that enhance our abilities to forecast and avert emerging and re-emerging viral threats, thereby protecting global health in the context of changing ecosystems (Flanagan et al., 2012; Morse et al., 2012) (Figure 5.7).

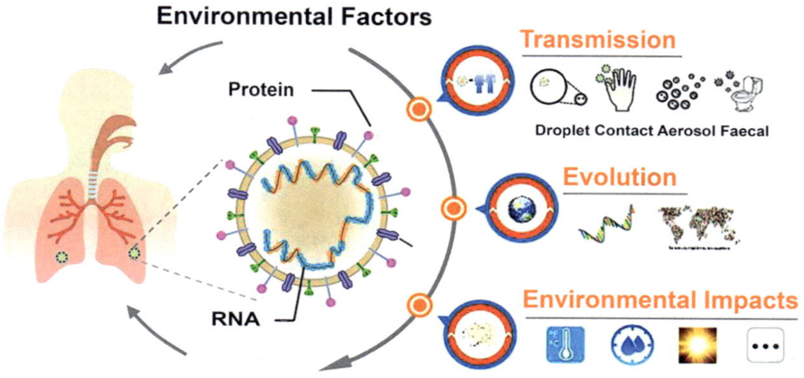

Figure 5.7. Environmental factors.

Source: https://ars.els-cdn.com/content/image/1-s2.0-S0269749120363090-fx1_lrg.jpg.

5.3. Case Studies of Emerging Viral Infections

In the last ten years, the incidence of viral disease has been one of the most formidable challenges to public health, reflecting on the complex interplay of pathogen biology, environmental determinants, and human behavior. For instance, the re-emergence of the Zika virus, originally discovered in the 1940s but emerging to the forefront in the 2010s, showed how urbanization and globalization may augment the spread of viruses long thought to be geographically fixed. Causes like intensified travel and the widening of the habitat of mosquitoes because of climate change were the key factors in the virus's quick spread. Understanding these dynamics is crucial as it highlights the need to have new surveillance and response systems in place to pre-empt and contain subsequent outbreaks, supporting the need to have comprehensive studies on pathogen and vector emergence, as echoed in the findings under emerging viral diseases (Morse et al., 2012). Another pertinent case study is the West African Ebola virus epidemic of 2014–2016, which brought to the foreground the ghastly effects of zoonotic transmissions. Having appeared primarily from fruit bats and causing widespread human infections, this outbreak emphasized the critical connection between environmental change and human well-being. The social health determinants, including poverty and inferior healthcare infrastructure, aggravated the crisis, and the interventions must address broad socioeconomic determinants in order to be effective. Flanagan et al. (2012) also support this by providing predictive surveillance to detect risk viruses before infecting humans. Through the implementation of proactive measures that consider ecological data and animal behavioral characteristics, health systems can better predict zoonotic spillovers in the future, in the long term, focusing on the prevention of emerging infection incidence and impact. In the end, awareness of the surveillance role as a forward-looking measure paves the way to improving global health security against emerging viral infections. With advances in the analysis of ecologic and genetic information, researchers can identify potential viral threats in wildlife reservoirs and vectors and thereby allow for early intervention. The Nipah virus case is a poignant reminder of the interconnectivity of health outcomes with environmental alteration and agricultural practice. As Flanagan et al. (2012) point out, workshops on predictive surveillance illustrate collaboration between virologists, ecologists, and computational biologists. This interdisciplinary approach can significantly enhance our capacity to anticipate potential outbreaks, indicating the necessity of an integrated health framework considering animal and human health. By embracing such comprehensive surveillance policies, the global community can effectively address the complexities of emerging viral infections.

5.3.1. Ebola Virus Outbreak in West Africa

The 2014 West African Ebola virus outbreak is a strong indicator of how quickly a spreading disease becomes a global public health threat. Spurred by the zoonotic transmission of the Ebola virus from animal reservoirs to humans, the outbreak highlighted the large gaps in the healthcare facilities and response in affected areas. Initially, the outbreak was contained within Guinea, but before long broke into Sierra Leone and Liberia, with thousands of infections and deaths. The quick geographical expansion showed how vulnerable public health infrastructures are to magnifying the effects of emerging viral infections. The incident also showed that countries that had long been considered to be free of such debilitating diseases were not, pinpointing the interconnected nature of global health security in order to respond to viral outbreaks effectively.

Enhanced vigilance and international cooperation were the order of the day to avoid another such future crisis, with a focus on systemic improvement in the health preparedness space. The key to the back-to-the-future counterattack against Ebola was an appreciation of the need for the world health community to operate under cooperative frameworks. Active engagement of the World Health Organization and non-governmental organizations provided invaluable resources, but the response indicated gross failures in preparedness and execution. Countries inexperienced in dealing with such infection outbreaks struggled to implement proper quarantine measures and medical interventions. This was exemplified most clearly by the relationship between local medical professionals and international aid agencies, tending to create communication breakdowns and a lack of trust. The need for effective training and deployment of health workers is evident, as was stated while deliberating on the establishment of the upgraded screening and detection systems in airports and borderposts to facilitate early detection of probable cases and prevent further spread (Adu-Gyamfi, 2019). In addressing the Ebola outbreak, it should be noted that adopting a One Health approach based on the interconnectedness of human, animal, and environmental health is necessary. The existence of zoonotic pathogens like Ebola demonstrates how human activities that encroach upon wildlife habitats can create viral spillover events. This multi-level feedback involves coordination across various stakeholders, including public health organizations, veterinary departments, and environmental scientists, to facilitate an integrated understanding of zoonotic transmission trends (Abdulaziz et al., 2016). Through formation of multidisciplinary coalitions, affected regions can enhance more effective surveillance and intervention approaches, ultimately bridging the gap between emerging viral threats and public health responses. As illustrated by West Africa's Ebola outbreak, cooperative efforts are most essential to improving the security of health and preparedness for possible viral pandemics (Figure 5.8).

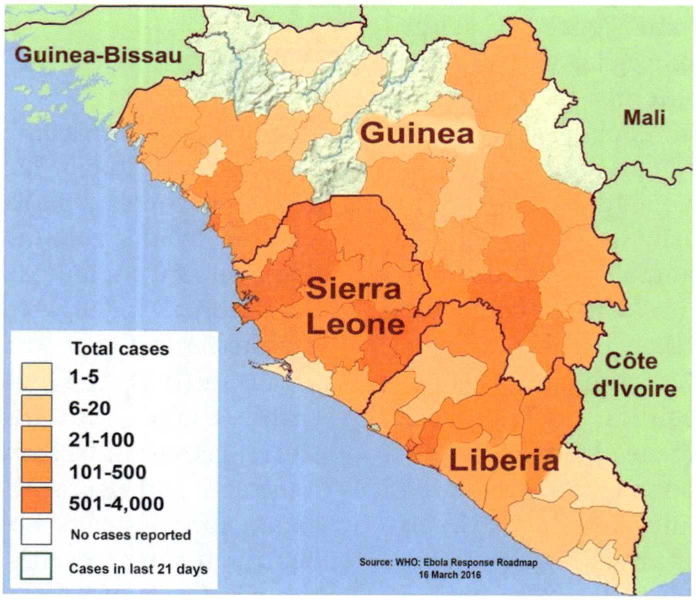

Figure 5.8. Ebola virus outbreak distribution map affected part of Western Africa.

Source: https://upload.wikimedia.org/wikipedia/commons/thumb/f/f3/2014_West_Africa_Ebola_virus_outbreak_situation_map.jpg/1024px-2014_West_Africa_Ebola_virus_outbreak_situation_map.jpg.

5.3.2. Zika Virus and Its Global Implications

The Zika virus outbreak is a global public health emergency due to its capacity to spread rapidly, where the pathogen was previously unknown. Originally reported in Africa, the virus gained notoriety through outbreaks in the Pacific and later in Latin America, the concern being its potential to cause neurological diseases such as microcephaly in newborns. The Zika virus is primarily spread by the Aedes mosquito, making it possible for its rapid distribution in susceptible groups. Hence, concerted global health efforts must be implemented to understand the entire spectrum of Zika's implications, including the need for effective surveillance systems to monitor its transmission and the establishment of preventive interventions to interrupt transmission in high-risk areas where vector control still remains a challenge (Marano et al., 2016) (Figure 5.9).

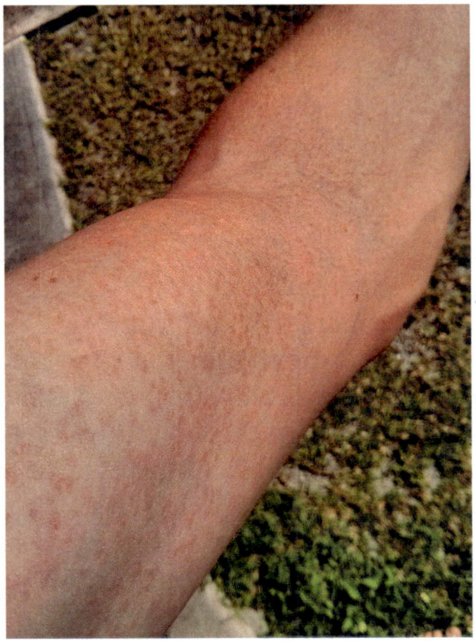

Figure 5.9. Rash on an arm due to Zika.

Source: https://upload.wikimedia.org/wikipedia/commons/thumb/b/b8/Zika.Virus.Rash.Arm.2014.jpg/800px-Zika.Virus.Rash.Arm.2014.jpg.

The global implications of the Zika virus extend beyond immediate health concerns, affecting socio-economic stability and public health infrastructure. The countries with severe outbreaks experienced disruptions in healthcare systems, increased expenditure on maternal and child health programs. Moreover, Zika-infected groups have been stigmatized, making it challenging to provide them with important treatment, raising anxiety and fear among the public.

As recurrent similar viral outbreaks are a risk factor, nations must execute wide-ranging strategies encompassing vector control, education, and preparedness in healthcare. Learning from the Zika epidemic can boost global responses to looming viral threats, focusing resource allocation and research priority on novel infectious diseases (Lewnard & Reingold, 2019). Further, the Zika virus outbreak has underscored the imperative for interdisciplinarity to combat emerging viral infections. The combination of epidemiology and new technologies can enhance the monitoring of diseases and facilitate the real-time exchange of data by public health practitioners. Further, understanding social determinants of health that predispose populations to disease transmission is essential in order to implement effective interventions.

Global health agencies must focus on building robust infrastructures that promote interdisciplinary research, local community engagement, and capacity development at the local level. Ongoing vigilance and responsive actions are necessary to counteract future outbreaks of the Zika virus and other emerging pathogens, which will eventually result in proactive and effective global health programs to address health threats worldwide (Marano et al., 2016) (Figure 5.10).

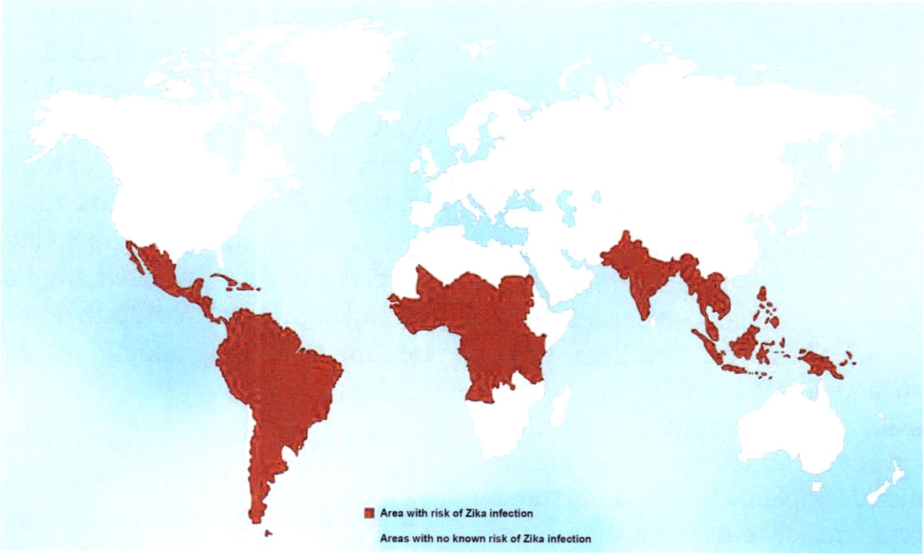

Figure 5.10. Global map of Zika virus infection.

Source: https://www.researchgate.net/profile/Morteza-Zaim/publication/330422906/figure/fig7/AS:716724374605824@1547891815243/Global-map-of-Zika-virus-infection-Content-source-Centers-for-Disease-Control-and.png.

5.3.3. COVID-19 Pandemic and Its Effects on Society

The COVID-19 pandemic has drastically changed social norms, resulting in changes in public health policy and individual practices. The unexpected emergence of SARS-CoV-2 generated the creation of fast responses by all aspects, like the healthcare, education, and economic sectors. Lockdowns and social distancing were implemented by governments in an attempt to contain the spread of the virus, hence altering community interaction. Moreover, these interventions placed in the spotlight technology disparities and healthcare access, in that those at-risk populations were less able to adhere to public health measures. As social institutions learned to contend with this new environment, companies everywhere embraced remote work, a phenomenon that could persist long after the pandemic. Health facilities and other public services altered operational procedures to restrict the risk of transmission, thereby actualizing the essence of community responsibility in public health. Long-term implications of these changes reveal a society that is more susceptible to virus threats and necessitate preparedness in the occurrence of new infectious diseases. Faced with the pandemic caused by COVID-19, researchers and policymakers have increased efforts to understand the virus-borne connections with built environments. As detailed in current research, the epidemic put the importance of minimizing transmission in indoor environments into focus, followed by attempts to investigate environmental drivers of viral or microbial transmission. With greater emphasis on ventilation, finish surfaces, and sanitizing procedures, an understanding of the microbiology of the built environment now informs corporate and public administrators' choices. This new information base supports the development of strategies that attempt to reduce transmission risks, resulting in ongoing environmental assessment along with modifications to building design and operation (Figure 5.11).

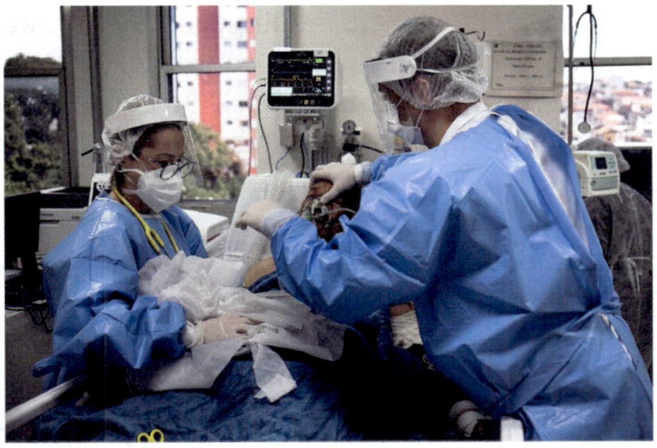

Figure 5.11. Medical professionals treating a COVID-19 patient in critical condition in an intensive care unit.

Source: https://upload.wikimedia.org/wikipedia/commons/thumb/f/f6/Covid-19_SP_-_UTI_V._Nova_Cachoeirinha.jpg/1280px-Covid-19_SP_-_UTI_V._Nova_Cachoeirinha.jpg.

By combining knowledge of microbial interactions within indoor spaces, stakeholders can initiate practical measures to enhance defense against outbreaks of viruses, and through the exercise, they gain valuable lessons from the ongoing pandemic (Dietz et al., 2020). The aftermath of the COVID-19 pandemic provides valuable lessons in preparedness against and response to new and re-emerging viral diseases. As revealed in the vulnerabilities of the pandemic, there's an urgent awareness of the deficiencies in the current healthcare infrastructure and the need for integrated surveillance systems. The need to enhance the safety of blood-derived products and medical practice has been brought out by stakeholders from various industries, highlighted by new recombinant technologies aimed at minimizing the reliance on human plasma and thus safety against potential viral risk (Ludlam et al., 2006). The unpredictable dynamics of viral infection and lessons from the COVID-19 pandemic have generated global debate regarding the merits of pre-emptive responses, rapid response strategies, and comparative studies. Future reaction must prioritize a multisectoral response, synthesizing virology, public health, and environmental science to build resilience to inevitable future pandemics (Figure 5.12).

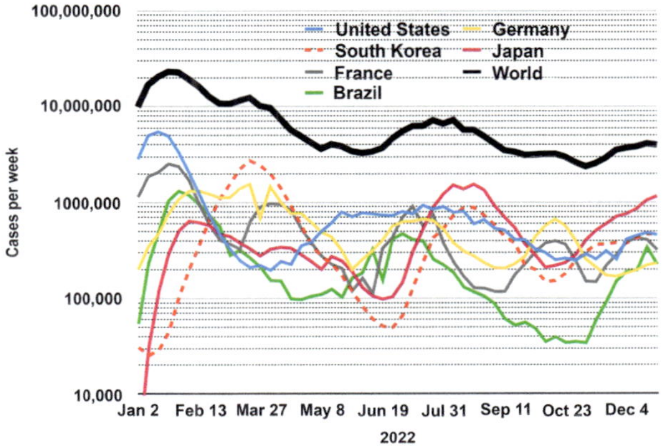

Figure 5.12. Semi-log plot of weekly new cases of COVID-19 in the world and the top six countries in 2022.

Source: https://upload.wikimedia.org/wikipedia/commons/4/4e/Covid-19_new_cases_in_top_5_countries_and_the_world.png.

5.4. Global Health Implications

In global health, the consequences of re-emerging and emerging viral diseases are extensive and complex. The coming together of globalization, urbanization, and climate change has led to an environment that nurtures infectious disease transmission. As populations migrate and people interact more than ever before, viruses find new channels of transmission. The Hajj pilgrimage, one of the largest mass gatherings on the globe, is the prime example of this phenomenon, in which millions of pilgrims from various countries gather, necessitating stringent health precautions to avoid endangering them by causing a risk of disease spread. This is the optimal scenario for requiring vaccination, such as the quadrivalent meningococcal vaccine, which is essential for protecting pilgrims and preventing outbreaks that would have international implications, such as outbreaks of diseases such as cholera or MERS-CoV. Lack of continuous monitoring and increased vaccination, the threat of imminent mass health crises remains high (Al-Tawfiq & Memish, 2019). Spillover of zoonotic diseases is yet another global health challenge. About 60% of emerging human pathogens are zoonotic, and wildlife is the main reservoir for these pathogens. Their passage into the human species is mediated by various routes, commonly triggered by environmental changes, wildlife trade, and human intrusion into the wild. These zoonoses often undergo extreme genetic changes, enhancing their infection rate in novel hosts or demonstrating enhanced pathogenicity. It is thus of critical need to know how zoonotic disease emergence occurs to inform effective prevention and response interventions. The interconnection of the health of animals, humans, and the environment emphasizes the necessity to address these complex interlinks in a One Health approach, which includes cooperation between many sectors to address these several complex interlinks (Cutler et al., 2010). Moreover, the control of re-emerging and emerging viral diseases must integrate global public health policies into local healthcare systems. There should be a robust health infrastructure with effective surveillance, early reporting, and collaborative research. As worldwide travel and trade increase connectivity, rapid identification and containment of outbreaks are critical to preventing the widespread transmission of infection. Initiatives such as the Global Health Security Agenda aim to enhance countries' ability to detect and respond to infectious disease threats. Hearteningly, there is a growing perception of the need for equitable access to vaccines and treatments in low-resource settings so that the world's efforts against viral dangers do not expand current health disparities. Ultimately, global cooperation and support for local capacities are most important in safeguarding international health in the context of emerging viral diseases (Figure 5.13).

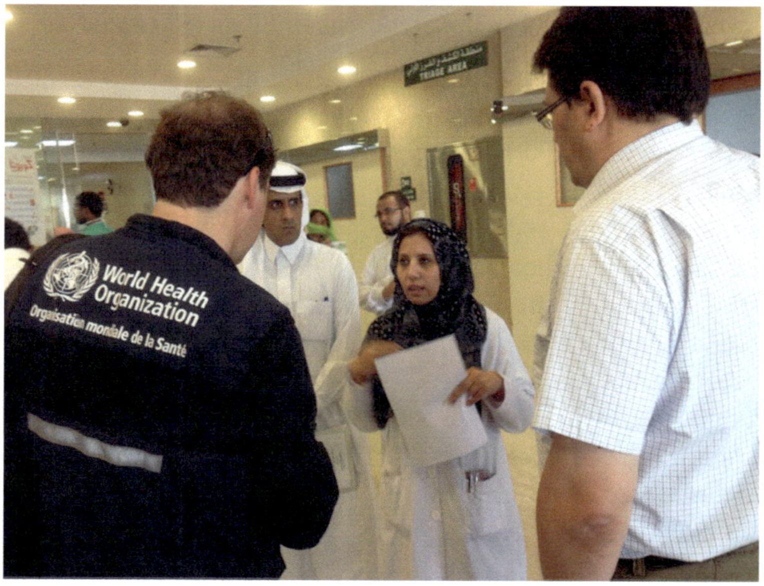

Figure 5.13. Training workers in health facilities can help to reduce health care-associated outbreaks of MERS-CoV.

Source: https://www.emro.who.int/images/stories/csr/mers_copy_copy.jpg.

5.4.1. Impact on Healthcare Systems

Viral infection re-emergence and emergence have a significant influence on the health care systems of the world, requiring integrated responses that tend to stretch available resources. With new pathogens being formed, health care infrastructures have to mobilize fast to deal not only with the short-term implications on health but also with the long-term repercussions on public health policy and resource distribution. The uncertainty surrounding new viral infections may lead to significant economic costs, with direct costs experienced through increased hospitalization, medication, and labor shortages. Apart from that, the cost burden of healthcare does not merely end at treatment but also includes prevention, as justification for robust surveillance mechanisms to ensure early detection and response. This strain highlights the imperative value of a One Health approach, which integrates human, animal, and environmental health in an effort to increase overall resilience against future outbreaks (Dar et al., 2015). Apart from treatment and management expenses due to emergent viral infections, healthcare systems worldwide have been strained by antimicrobial resistance (AMR). The cross-talk between viral infections and AMR not only complicates the treatment regimen but also compromises the effectiveness of existing antimicrobial agents vital for the control of secondary bacterial infections. With healthcare professionals scrambling to navigate these complexities, consequences could ripple throughout the system, pushing hospital stays longer and death greater. The heterogeneity of treatment regimens and infection control practices adds to exacerbating these problems, further highlighting the necessity of region-focused interventions grounded in local health realities. International collective action aimed at strengthening policy frameworks serves to enhance understanding regarding AMR dynamics, thereby enabling enhanced practice (Cookson et al., 2002). It demands new models re-examining screening and treatment processes. For instance, hospitals can implement cost-effective laboratory screening interventions aimed at high-risk wards and thereby improve the patient outcome for individuals with compounded bacterial and viral infections. Such interventions involve scrutiny — identifying the sensitivity and specificity of tests has a finalizing impact on infection control. Secondly, costing various clinical interventions can empower healthcare systems to deliver optimal resource allocation along with focused responses to emerging threats. Lastly, encouragement of flexibility within healthcare frameworks will be critical in order to improve resilience against future viral outbreaks and minimize their systemic impact (Cookson et al., 2002).

5.4.2. Economic Consequences of Viral Outbreaks

The economic impact of viral epidemics extends well beyond the expense of healthcare in the immediate moment, as it impacts several sectors and causes long-term financial instability. An outbreak puts enormous strain on healthcare networks, calling for greater utilization of funds for treatment, research, and prevention. The expense of increased healthcare can lead to resource issues in public health systems. Additionally, viral outbreaks tend to cause disruptions in the workforce through sickness and resulting quarantines that can reduce productivity. For example, those industries that depend on maintaining a steady workforce, such as manufacturing and agricultural production, can have serious operational losses, thus contributing to the overall economic decline that follows an outbreak. The interconnectedness of global economies means that outbreaks of viruses locally can have spillover impacts, affecting trade and travel on a larger scale and thus doubling the economic implications. Apart from this, viral outbreaks also result in tremendous indirect costs that amplify their cost implications. Panic of infection can lead to a drop in consumer confidence, resulting in smaller expenditure and investment. For example, businesses in tourism and hospitality are likely to suffer significant losses as safety concerns and travel restrictions deter clients. In addition, agricultural sectors face possible financial loss due to disease of livestock or infestation of crops, with costly avoidance measures or eradication programs being undertaken. The financial impact is further compounded when businesses must add new safety measures, further straining their budgets. Studies have identified that the collective effect of these indirect costs can be staggering, creating a total assessment of economic loss encompassing direct healthcare costs and the broader economic climate generated by consumerism and market forces. In the control of the economic effects of viral outbreaks, effective surveillance and control measures must exist. The Bovine Viral Diarrhea Virus (BVDV) case illustrates the complexity involved in managing a widespread viral disease in agriculture. In spite of its far-reaching impact on cattle well-being and economic efficiency, a significant percentage of farms are even oblivious to their BVDV status, which indicates the most urgent need for enhanced surveillance programs. Implementation of effective monitoring protocols not only aids in real-time management of disease but also serves as a preventive measure to protect economic interests. By incorporating preventive interventions, such as vaccination and overall testing, the long-term economic viability of affected industries can be ensured. Therefore, such symbiosis between economic paradigms and health policies can effectively combat the challenges presented by viral epidemics, strengthening both economic and public health resilience (Figure 5.14).

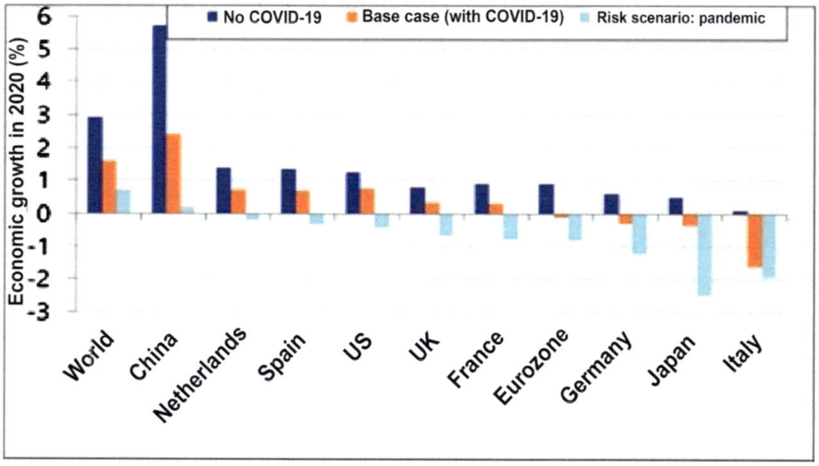

Figure 5.14. The economic impact on world and different countries due to COVID-19 outbreak.

Source: https://www.researchgate.net/publication/348106175/figure/fig1/AS:976152336293890@1609744261285/The-economic-impact-on-world-and-different-countries-due-to-COVID-19-outbreak-Source.png.

5.4.3. Importance of Global Surveillance and Response

The increasing trend of re-emerging and emerging viral infections necessitates strict international surveillance and response mechanisms. The mechanisms are important in monitoring viral epidemics and identifying pathogens before establishing a foothold in human populations. Records of the past reveal that most pandemics, including HIV/AIDS and severe acute respiratory syndrome, are created by zoonotic pathogens, which are typically driven by ecological, behavioral, or socioeconomic change. These developments highlight the necessity of understanding the interface among animal, human, and environmental health. Enhanced surveillance mechanisms, therefore, not only help recognize potential dangers but also provide insights for timely intervention, which can effectively halt the effect on public health. Mathematical modeling, diagnostic methods, and emerging communication technology can augment the ability to forecast and respond to viral threats more effectively, thereby enabling the transition from reactive to proactive global health management (Morse et al., 2012). Early identification of high-risk viruses able to spill over from animals to humans is one critical aspect of global surveillance. Current strategies are likely to act after the virus has already crossed over to humans, and this showcases a vital deficit in our capacity. Appraise the need for predictive surveillance, and this has driven workshops where virologists, ecologists, and computational biologists come together to exchange frameworks that are meant to anticipate viral species jumps. By combining genetic and ecological data, scientists are able to determine possible viral threats prior to infecting humans. This forecasting method has the capability of reducing the occurrence of outbreaks by allowing health authorities to take preventive measures in high-risk areas, thereby safeguarding global health (Flanagan et al., 2012). Moreover, the dangers of emerging viral illnesses require international coordination in the form of surveillance efforts. Interconnectedness of our world today means that an outbreak in one region can be a global pandemic within a few days. Cooperative structures based on shared scientific understanding and capability are vital as they enable countries to respond promptly and efficiently. The development of common guidelines for surveillance measures, exchange of information, and response to outbreaks will improve the preparedness of the world. These collaborative efforts not only enhance local responses but also give the world a complete overview of virus ecology and transmission patterns. By investing in such global programs, we equip ourselves with the arsenal with which to combat future viral threats and thereby reduce the public health burden of emerging and re-emerging infections (Morse et al., 2012).

5.5. Prevention and Control Strategies

Viral infection re-emergence and emergence call for wide-scale prevention and control to counter their impacts on global public health. The framework for such control should involve robust surveillance mechanisms that can identify and follow up viral transmission patterns. This is the foundation for the identification of outbreaks at the earliest stage possible, enabling rapid public health response. As was experienced in the case of tuberculosis (TB) during the COVID-19 pandemic, there can be widespread disruption to regular healthcare services, including disease management as well as control measures. Disruptions of TB care during lockdowns have been shown to result in increases in prevalence and mortality. It is therefore essential to restore regular services and realign healthcare delivery to ensure continuity, even during pandemics (Chaturvedi et al., 2023). Another crucial aspect of effective prevention is the development and deployment of vaccines. Immunization programs have the ability to reduce the incidence of new viruses significantly, thereby reducing the burden on the healthcare system. History has shown that in the past, vaccines have been utilized to control diseases such as influenza and Ebola, but new and novel methods need to evolve to meet emerging threats. Researchers emphasize the necessity of attacking viral reservoirs through cross-species surveillance and investigation of ecological drivers of zoonotic transmissions. By integration of mathematical modeling and informatics tools, health authorities would be able to better predict potential outbreaks and employ preemptive vaccination policies for the safeguarding of risk populations (Morse et al., 2012). Lastly, education and awareness programs are part and parcel of efficient prevention and control programs. Active community engagement to adopt health protocols — hand hygiene, mask wearing, and vaccination — is key to limiting viral infection transmission. Communication frameworks need to be structured for translation into diverse communities, with the target of reaching vulnerable populations with critical health information. Additionally, learning from the COVID-19 pandemic reveals that communicators should ensure clarity and transparency in messages to minimize public anxiety and ensure compliance with health measures. For emerging and re-emerging viral diseases, strengthening an informed society can strengthen resilience and foster a united response to future health challenges (Chaturvedi et al., 2023).

5.5.1. Vaccination and Its Role in Prevention

The role of vaccination in the prevention of re-emerging and emerging viral diseases grows more important with changing global health challenges. The last few decades have witnessed a resurgence of some of the viral pathogens whose incidence was previously considered under control and now pose serious threats to public health. The need for an effective vaccination strategy has grown larger to combat the outbreaks of such pathogens in areas with no immunity. Vaccination offers a crucial line of defense by triggering protective immunity, thereby decreasing the incidence of disease and curbing outbreaks. Infectious disease epidemiology indicates that herd immunity by mass vaccination can actually protect immunologically naive groups of people, thereby curtail transmission and reduce the likelihood of rebound, as emphasized in recent public health assessments (Noorulhuda, 2022). Vaccine development against such novel viruses is particularly tricky due to the rapid mutation rate and adaptive capabilities of such viruses. Traditional approaches may fall short, and the identification of new vaccine technologies is thus of the utmost urgency. The progress in molecular biology has also given rise to new vaccine development strategies such as mRNA vaccines and viral vector platforms. These emerging technologies allow for quicker response to emerging dangers and assist in creating vaccines that are effective and scalable. They also provide opportunities to tackle not just new viruses but also advance existing vaccines for re-emerging diseases. With a variety of platforms and an increased understanding of viral biology, public health can better prepare for future pandemics and epidemics. Thus, the merging of new technologies with conventional approaches is necessary to support our immunization strategies (Noorulhuda, 2022). Additionally, the growing awareness of the intricacies in viral epidemiology requires a targeted approach to vaccine assessment and deployment. Contemporary epidemiology has developed to close gaps between conventional chronic disease practices and infectious disease dynamics, recognizing the distinct challenges presented by new or re-emerging pathogens. This change demands robust data-driven approaches to measure vaccine efficacy, pathogen transmission patterns, and the overall impact of public health interventions. Integration of molecular and digital data sources allows for enhanced surveillance and understanding of vaccination efficacy across populations. Furthermore, novel causal inference techniques are the future of vaccine science, allowing for the assessment of the impact of vaccines on public health outcomes. As the field continues to grow, the position of vaccines as a pillar in the control of emerging and re-emerging viral infections continues to be promising and central to health care strategies globally (Figure 5.15).

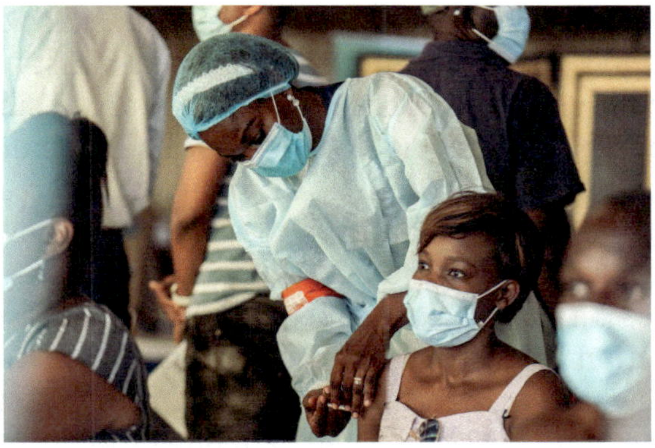

Figure 5.15. Vaccination for viral infection prevention.

Source: https://www.afro.who.int/sites/default/files/2022-05/vaccination_efficacy.jpg.

5.5.2. Public Health Policies and Education

Public health policy plays a significant role in controlling and limiting emerging and re-emerging viral diseases. Policy must be evidence-based and consider the particular socio-economic and cultural environments of different nations, particularly in low- and middle-income countries. A good policy-making approach includes an assessment of existing measures in the areas of infection prevention and control, judicious use of resources, and surveillance. As Dar et al. (2015) state, the complexities in translating effective public health interventions across sectors necessitate localized approaches that understand the distinct needs and conditions of every locality. Policy makers must invest in the development of standardized frameworks for evaluating the cost-effectiveness and generalizability of health interventions, such that policies have the capacity to adapt over time to fit the evolving landscape of infectious diseases. Education is a critical foundation of public health policy, particularly in the context of emerging viral infections. Establishing firm educational programs in populations has the potential to sensitize people to hygiene behaviors, vaccine value, and epidemiological dynamics of new pathogens. Such programs must have the general goal of equipping local populations with the information and skills necessary to immunize and guard themselves and their populations against health hazards. The collaborative effort between international research agencies and local institutions, as in Molia et al. (2012), identifies the possibility of training modules being set to develop a highly informed workforce that is able to address issues of health. By making use of already established networks in disease control and training, public health programs are able to develop a culture of readiness and responsiveness, improving the resilience of society against future pandemics. Moreover, the promotion of a One Health approach emphasizes the interconnectedness of human, animal, and environmental health in tackling viral infections. The integration of the veterinary and public health disciplines is required to obtain comprehensive disease surveillance and risk evaluation of zoonotic pathogens. For example, intensive training and research on zoonotic diseases like rabies might yield critical insight into pathogen transmission patterns and potential control measures, as suggested by Molia et al. (2012). Such a model of collaboration not only offers a venue for the sharing of information between disciplines but also enables the development of sensitive policies that consider the complex interdependencies between ecosystems and public health. Finally, a coordinated effort in health policy and education can have a profound impact in making responses to re-emerging and emerging viral infections more effective, ensuring global health security in a more interlinked world.

5.5.3. Research and Development of Antiviral Treatments

The area of antiviral treatment drug development and research remains dynamic, especially in the face of novel and re-emerging viral infections. The most interesting area is how viruses can escape host immune responses. Understanding this allows researchers to design antiviral therapies that can target viral replication and transmission effectively. New advances in molecular biology techniques have opened the door for scientists to identify viral genes and pathways that are critical for survival and replication in host organisms. For instance, mechanisms by which the feline infectious peritonitis virus (FIPV) escapes immune detection indicate the way forward for potential therapeutic intervention. Despite the progress, finding curative therapy remains a monumental challenge, pointing towards the need for a novel approach in antiviral drug research (Pedersen, 2014). In addition to the traditional antiviral drugs, work on the application of RNA interference (RNAi) as an antiviral therapeutic has also been of importance. RNAi possesses a natural mechanism of action against viral infections with the ability to target and kill viral RNA. Dramatic research has indicated that certain viruses are able to both take advantage of and suppress the RNAi system, constituting a complicated challenge to creating successful therapies. Antiviral defense research in animals such as bumblebees has indicated surprising findings, whereby infection through the IAPV virus actually enhances the RNAi system, contrary to traditional expectations of viral suppression. This finding accentuates the importance of understanding the molecular host-virus interactions and suggests that manipulation of the RNAi mechanism can create new therapeutic strategies against viral infections (Cappelle et al., 2016). The complexity of viral infections and their correlation with host systems necessitates an interdisciplinary approach towards developing antiviral therapies. Direct antiviral drugs combined with immunomodulators are also promising methods against viral infections. Furthermore, the application of high-throughput screening technology and bioinformatics helped to identify new antiviral compounds at faster rates. Since new viruses tend to mutate in order to adapt to ongoing treatments, the research efforts should be kept constant in responding to the dynamic character of these pathogens. Ongoing investment in research and development will be vital to creating a robust portfolio of antiviral drugs that can treat both current and future viral threats, thereby safeguarding public health in an increasingly interdependent world.

SUMMARY

As the research into emerging and re-emerging viral diseases progresses, it increasingly becomes apparent that the global terrain is deeply conditioned by intricate interactions among pathogens, hosts, and their environment. The historical record places emphasis on the fact that a majority of pandemics are the result of zoonotic viruses, transmitted mainly from animals to humans, and this serves to underscore the importance of a sensitive appreciation of the ecological and behavioral forces conditioning viral emergence. Although a lot has been done in the detection and response to outbreaks, no pandemic has been forecast before its human infection, which translates into major gaps in surveillance and preparedness. Closing these gaps is important to improving public health outcomes and requires a multidisciplinary approach involving cutting-edge technology and science (Morse et al., 2012). Efforts to strengthen viral surveillance have come into prominence, particularly for application in predictive modelling, which implies discovering future outbreaks ahead of time before they turn into large-scale ones. Proactiveness on this aspect brings into perspective the necessity of early warning methods and the application of genetic and ecological information to identify risky viruses. By identifying where and how these zoonotic transmissions occur — particularly in wildlife populations such as bats and rodents — scientists can develop risk assessment plans that precisely predict upcoming species jumps. The workshop discussions of virologists, ecologists, and computational biologists provide an elemental source for building a virus surveillance system that is capable of predicting future infections (Flanagan et al., 2012). Such inter-disciplinary cooperation will be necessary since it integrates scientific research into harmony with realistic public health policy. In short, community concern about emerging and re-emerging viral diseases necessitates a coordinated approach that involves research, community policy, and international partnership. With the integration of advanced surveillance systems, genetic information usage, and interdisciplinary partnerships, the scientific community can significantly enhance its ability to anticipate and deter viral dangers. The need for swift innovation and robust preparedness plans is highlighted by the growing number of pandemics that are caused in a globally interconnected world. Continuing on the path to the future while emphasizing prevention and building a predictive model will not only limit existing threats but may well prevent future outbreaks from arising, in turn, protecting public health globally (Flanagan et al., 2012; Morse et al., 2012).

In the context of emerging and re-emerging viral diseases, the requirement for better surveillance systems has been at the forefront. Existing workshops have highlighted the necessity to develop predictive models that can identify high-risk viruses prior to their jumping from animal reservoirs to humans. This prevention strategy is based on learning about zoonotic disease dynamics, with the debate revolving around the convergence of genetic and ecological information to predict impending species leaps. What comes out of these workshops is that the involvement of multidisciplinary teams, such as virologists, ecologists, and computational biologists, is necessary in order to develop effective surveillance systems. Such proactive strategies would significantly limit the instances of zoonotic spillovers and steer public health interventions to stem infectious diseases before they spread into large-scale outbreaks (Flanagan et al., 2012). In addition, the interaction between the physiology of animals and viral transmission dynamics has grown to hold significant importance for the prediction of zoonotic infection. Bat studies, specifically those related to henipavirus dynamics, draw attention to the complexity of these interactions. Antibody titer analysis of captive groups has demonstrated not just maternal antibody persistence but also how maternal parameters influence rates of viral transmission, especially during critical life events such as pregnancy and lactation. These findings add to our knowledge of reservoir host infection persistence and illuminate how seasonal ecological events may propel infection dissemination. Equipped with such information, public health officials and researchers can enhance forecasting of when and where spillover events would occur, resulting in enhanced outreach activities and preparedness strategies imperative in the case of emergent viral outbreaks (Baker et al., 2014). Finally, elucidation of ecological and behavioral drivers of viral infection cannot be exaggerated. The linkage between human encroachment and wildlife habitat tends to increase the potential for infectious diseases to transfer from animals to humans. Care must therefore be taken in the monitoring of reservoir habitats for newly emerging viruses. This entails consideration of the conditions favoring the survival of such viruses and the environmental forces underpinning their dynamics — information that is central to effective surveillance programs. By uniting ecological data and virological studies, researchers are able to formulate a clearer picture of minimizing the risks generated by impending zoonotic diseases. A unified approach embracing these elements will fortify efforts against both known and unknown viral risks, paving the way for an even safer public health landscape (Flanagan et al., 2012; Baker et al., 2014).

CLOSER LOOK

INFLUENZA PANDEMICS

Pandemics of influenza are global epidemics of a novel strain of influenza virus that infect large numbers of individuals in two or more nations or continents. Seasonal influenza, which results from anticipated mutations of already circulating human influenza viruses, differs from pandemics that appear when a new strain for which most of the population lacks immunity appears. These new strains typically arise by antigenic shift, a process where the influenza A viruses undergo major genetic change, typically viral RNA segment reassortment between species, for example, birds, pigs, and humans (Figure 5.16).

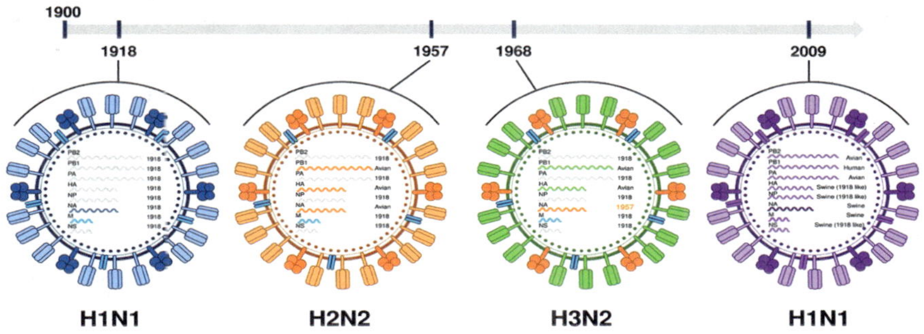

Figure 5.16. Timeline and structural comparison of major influenza A virus subtypes (H1N1, H2N2, H3N2) responsible for past pandemics, highlighting changes in hemagglutinin and neuraminidase surface proteins and genome segment composition.

Source: https://www.nature.com/articles/s12276-021-00603-0/figures/1.

Historically, influenza pandemics have inflicted terrible damage on world health and economies. The 1918 H1N1 "Spanish flu" pandemic was the most lethal, infecting an estimated one-third of the earth's population and killing an estimated 50 million people around the globe. The pandemic was characteristic because it had an unusually high death rate in young, healthy adults, possibly because of an overactive immune response called a "cytokine storm.

The 1957 H2N2 "Asian flu" and the 1968 H3N2 "Hong Kong flu" pandemics were less severe but still caused significant illness and death, particularly in the elderly and those with underlying conditions. The 2009 H1N1 "swine flu" pandemic was the first pandemic in the 21st century of influenza. It had started as a triple reassortment of swine, avian, and human influenza viruses and most notably struck among younger age groups. Although its mortality rate amongst seniors was lower than that of regular flu, its rapid transmission pointed to the challenge involved in identifying and controlling early pandemics.

Influenza A virus is the principal cause of pandemics due to its ability to infect a diverse range of animal species and become engaged in widespread genetic reassortment. Wild birds, particularly waterfowl, are natural reservoirs of all subtypes of influenza A. Avian influenza viruses that infect intermediate hosts, including pigs that may harbor human strains, can lead to mixing of the genes and produce new strains that are communicable among humans.

Pandemic preparedness necessitates global surveillance, accelerated virus identification, vaccine production, and coordination of global public health response. Organizations such as the World Health Organization (WHO) and the Centers for Disease Control and Prevention (CDC) are essential in keeping influenza virus activity surveillance, issuing alerts, and guiding policy during pandemic events.

Control measures against pandemics include vaccination, antiviral medications (such as oseltamivir and zanamivir), social distancing, quarantine, travel restrictions, and information campaigns. Their effectiveness depends on the speed and accuracy of the detection of the new strain and the capacity to produce and deliver vaccines within a short timeframe.

Influenza pandemics still remain a threat since the virus mutates frequently and is infectious between species. Emerging zoonotic viruses like H5N1 and H7N9 avian influenza viruses are still under constant surveillance since they have the potential to start future pandemics.

REFERENCES

1. Dar, O. A., Hasan, R., Schlundt, J., Harbarth, S., Caleo, G., Dar, F. K., Littmann, J., Rweyemamu, M., Buckley, E. J., Shahid, M., Kock, R., Li, H. L., Giha, H., Khan, M., So, A. D., Bindayna, K. M., Kessel, A., Pedersen, H. B., Permanand, G., Zumla, A., ... Heymann, D. L. (2016). Exploring the evidence base for national and regional policy interventions to combat resistance. *Lancet (London, England)*, *387*(10015), 285–295. https://doi.org/10.1016/S0140-6736(15)00520-6(accessed on 16th July 2025).
2. Acosta-Leal, R., Duffy, S., Xiong, Z., Hammond, R. W., et al. (1995). *Advances in plant virus evolution: Translating evolutionary insights into better disease management.* https://core.ac.uk/download/pdf/36058493.pdf (accessed on 16th July 2025).
3. Enitan SS, Akele RY, Cmoare AA, Dogonyaro BB, Iduh MU, Digban KA, et al. Mpox resurgence: preventing a potential pandemic through lessons learned from COVID-19 experience and future research directions. Avicenna J Clin Microbiol Infect. 2024; 11(4):191-203. doi:10.34172/ajcmi.3564 (accessed on 16th July 2025).
4. Adu-Gyamfi, S. (2019). *Ebola Hemorrhagic Fever in Africa: A Necessary Highlight.* https://core.ac.uk/download/480549437.pdf (accessed on 16th July 2025).
5. Alagaili, A. N., Zumla, A., Arabi, Y., Azhar, E. I., Briese, T., et al. (2016). *Taking forward a 'One Health' approach for turning the tide against the Middle East respiratory syndrome coronavirus and other zoonotic pathogens with epidemic potential.* https://core.ac.uk/download/45467901.pdf (accessed on 16th July 2025).
6. Al-Tawfiq, J. A., & Memish, Z. A. (2014). *Emerging respiratory viral infections: MERS-CoV and influenza.* https://core.ac.uk/download/322846911.pdf (accessed on 16th July 2025).
7. Al-Tawfiq, J. A., & Memish, Z. A. (2019). The Hajj 2019 Vaccine Requirements and Possible New Challenges. *Journal of epidemiology and global health*, *9*(3), 147–152. https://doi.org/10.2991/jegh.k.190705.001(accessed on 16th July 2025).
8. Al-Tawfiq, J. A., Benkouiten, S., & Memish, Z. A. (2018). *A systematic review of emerging respiratory viruses at the Hajj and possible coinfection with Streptococcus pneumoniae.* https://core.ac.uk/download/322846904.pdf (accessed on 16th July 2025).
9. Eberle, J., & Gürtler, L. (2012). HIV types, groups, subtypes and recombinant forms: errors in replication, selection pressure and quasispecies. *Intervirology*, *55*(2), 79–83. https://doi.org/10.1159/000331993(accessed on 16th July 2025).
10. Ansari, A., Chang, C., Gershwin, M. E., Ortiz, L., et al. (2016). *The Zika Outbreak of the 21st Century.* https://core.ac.uk/download/323068480.pdf (accessed on 16th July 2025).
11. Calderon, Guzman, Salazar-Bravo, Figueiredo, Mattar, and Arrieta (2016). *Viral zoonoses that fly with bats: A review.* MANTER: Journal of Parasite Biodiversity (September 30, 2016) number 6doi: 10.13014/K2BG2KWF(accessed on 16th July 2025).
12. Baggaley, R. F., Ferguson, N. M., & Garnett, G. P. (2005). *The epidemiological impact of antiretroviral use predicted by mathematical models: A review.* https://core.ac.uk/download/pdf/3765667.pdf (accessed on 16th July 2025).
13. Baker, K. S., Barr, J., Boots, M., Broder, C. C., et al. (2014). *Viral Antibody Dynamics in a Chiropteran Host.* https://core.ac.uk/download/9357743.pdf (accessed on 16th July 2025).

14. Barclay, W., Beauchemin, C. A. A., Bedford, T., Belser, J. A., et al. (2016). *Viral factors in influenza pandemic risk assessment.* https://core.ac.uk/download/74230057.pdf (accessed on 16th July 2025).

15. Tsiodras, S., Kelesidis, T., Kelesidis, I., Bauchinger, U., & Falagas, M. E. (2008). Human infections associated with wild birds. *The Journal of infection*, *56*(2), 83–98. https://doi.org/10.1016/j.jinf.2007.11.001(accessed on 16th July 2025).

16. Booth, R., De Vliegher, S., Deprez, P., Dewulf, J., et al. (2013). *Assessment of two essential elements of BVDV control on selected Flemish dairy and beef farms.* https://core.ac.uk/download/55761867.pdf (accessed on 16th July 2025).

17. Molia, S et al. (2012). *Mission to Indonesia to participate to the 1st Indonesia-France Seminar in Medicine & Public Health and investigate potential collaborations on animal health: 2nd–9th of November 2012.* http://agritrop.cirad.fr/567354/1/document_567354.pdf (accessed on 16th July 2025).

18. Ludlam, C. A., Powderly, W. G., Bozzette, S., Diamond, M., Koerper, M. A., Kulkarni, R., Ritchie, B., Siegel, J., Simmonds, P., Stanley, S., Tapper, M. L., & von Depka, M. (2006). Clinical perspectives of emerging pathogens in bleeding disorders. *Lancet (London, England)*, *367*(9506), 252–261. https://doi.org/10.1016/S0140-6736(06)68036-7(accessed on 16th July 2025).

19. Brunner, J. L., Duffus, A. L. J., Gray, M. J., Miller, D., et al. (2014). *Second International Symposium on Ranaviruses: A North American herpetological perspective.* https://core.ac.uk/download/289166243.pdf (accessed on 16th July 2025).

20. Flanagan, M. L., Parrish, C. R., Cobey, S., Glass, G. E., Bush, R. M., & Leighton, T. J. (2012). Anticipating the species jump: surveillance for emerging viral threats. *Zoonoses and public health*, *59*(3), 155–163. https://doi.org/10.1111/j.1863-2378.2011.01439.x(accessed on 16th July 2025).

21. Cappelle, K., Dhaenens, M., Meeus, I., Smagghe, G., et al. (2016). *Israeli acute paralysis virus infection leads to an enhanced RNA interference response and not its suppression in the bumblebee Bombus terrestris.* https://core.ac.uk/download/84042020.pdf (accessed on 16th July 2025).

22. Morse, S. S., Mazet, J. A., Woolhouse, M., Parrish, C. R., Carroll, D., Karesh, W. B., Zambrana-Torrelio, C., Lipkin, W. I., & Daszak, P. (2012). Prediction and prevention of the next pandemic zoonosis. *Lancet (London, England)*, *380*(9857), 1956–1965. https://doi.org/10.1016/S0140-6736(12)61684-5(accessed on 16th July 2025).

23. Ch'ng, J., Christofk, H. R., & Thaker, S. K. (2019). *Viral Hijacking of Cellular Metabolism.* https://core.ac.uk/download/323078193.pdf (accessed on 16th July 2025).

24. Chaturvedi, T., Gupta, S., & Rajput, S. (2023). *Impact of the COVID-19 pandemic on tuberculosis management in India: A brief overview.* https://core.ac.uk/download/579951024.pdf (accessed on 16th July 2025).

25. Chrisafis, G. C. (2017). *Historical patterns of arboviral seroprevalence across Africa and Asia.* https://core.ac.uk/download/84397690.pdf (accessed on 16th July 2025).

26. Harris, C. M., Wu, H. M., Li, J., Hall, H. I., Lee, A., Zell, E., Harrison, L. H., Petit, S., Farley, M. M., Lynfield, R., Miller, L., Nichols, M., Reingold, A., Schaffner, W., Thomas, A., MacNeil, J. R., Clark, T. A., & Cohn, A. C. (2016). Meningococcal Disease in Patients With Human Immunodeficiency Virus Infection: A Review of Cases Reported Through Active Surveillance in the United

States, 2000-2008. *Open forum infectious diseases, 3*(4), ofw226. https://doi.org/10.1093/ofid/ofw226(accessed on 16th July 2025).

27. Dietz, L., Horve, P. F., Coil, D. A., Fretz, M., Eisen, J. A., & Van Den Wymelenberg, K. (2020). 2019 Novel Coronavirus (COVID-19) Pandemic: Built Environment Considerations To Reduce Transmission. *mSystems, 5*(2), e00245-20. https://doi.org/10.1128/mSystems.00245-20(accessed on 16th July 2025).
28. Cookson, B., Kibbler, C., Kunori, T., Roberts, J., et al. (2002). *Cost-effectiveness of different MRSA screening methods.* [No DOI provided].
29. Cowden, J., Forbes, K. J., MacRae, M., Maiden, M. C. J., et al. (2013). *Operationalizing factors that explain the emergence of infectious diseases: A case study of the human campylobacteriosis epidemic.* https://core.ac.uk/download/18601300.pdf (accessed on 16th July 2025).
30. Cutler, S. J., Fooks, A. R., & van der Poel, W. H. M. (2010). *Public health threat of new, reemerging, and neglected zoonoses in the industrialized world.* https://core.ac.uk/download/pdf/29238214.pdf (accessed on 16th July 2025).
31. Pike, B. L., Saylors, K. E., Fair, J. N., Lebreton, M., Tamoufe, U., Djoko, C. F., Rimoin, A. W., & Wolfe, N. D. (2010). The origin and prevention of pandemics. *Clinical infectious diseases : an official publication of the Infectious Diseases Society of America, 50*(12), 1636–1640. https://doi.org/10.1086/652860(accessed on 16th July 2025).
32. Marano, G., Pupella, S., Vaglio, S., Liumbruno, G. M., & Grazzini, G. (2016). Zika virus and the never-ending story of emerging pathogens and transfusion medicine. *Blood transfusion = Trasfusione del sangue, 14*(2), 95–100. https://doi.org/10.2450/2015.0066-15(accessed on 16th July 2025).
33. Khalaf, N. F. (2022). *Viral Vaccine Strategies.* https://core.ac.uk/download/629276972.pdf (accessed on 16th July 2025).
34. Lewnard, J. A., & Reingold, A. L. (2019). Emerging Challenges and Opportunities in Infectious Disease Epidemiology. *American journal of epidemiology, 188*(5), 873–882. https://doi.org/10.1093/aje/kwy264(accessed on 16th July 2025).
35. Pedersen, N. C. (2014). *An update on feline infectious peritonitis: Diagnostics and therapeutics.* https://core.ac.uk/download/323070220.pdf (accessed on 16th July 2025).
36. Wiethoelter, A. K., Bengis, R. G., Chardonnet, P., Beltrán-Alcrudo, D., Dehove, A., Kock, R., et al. (2015). *Global trends in infectious diseases at the wildlife–livestock interface.* https://core.ac.uk/download/36778662.pdf (accessed on 16th July 2025).
37. Zaragoza, G. (2019). *Getting to zero HIV cases in San Francisco: Reconceptualizing housing as public health infrastructure in the framework of HIV prevention and treatment.* https://core.ac.uk/download/287522090.pdf (accessed on 16th July 2025).

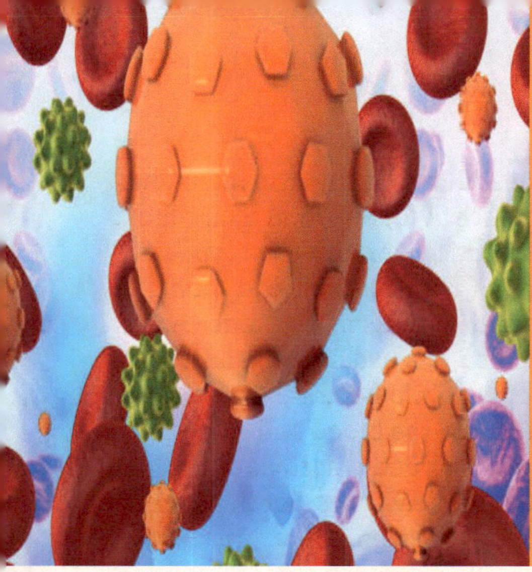

Chapter 6

HEPATITIS AND BLOODBORNE VIRUSES

Contents

Introduction

The beginning of the new era of hepatitis and bloodborne viral diseases has uncovered key public health problems that must be taken seriously. Being diseases that can lead to serious morbidity and mortality, hepatitis B and C are at the center of this complicated picture. They infect millions of individuals all over the globe with liver disease and hepatocellular carcinoma. Their spread is predominantly by blood, sexual contact, and mother-to-child transmission, thereby necessitating the need for extensive education and effective intervention strategies. The significance of the epidemiology knowledge of hepatitis and bloodborne viruses towards this end cannot be overestimated, as it is the foundation for formulating targeted public health policy for prevention, early detection, and control. The role of vulnerable populations in the spread of hepatitis and bloodborne viruses is of particular concern, and this is particularly true among marginalized populations. To mention one example, Indigenous Australians experience far higher rates of hepatitis B and C than their non-Indigenous counterparts. The gap is more than numerical; it is a manifestation of a complex of historical disadvantages and socioeconomic determinants that undermine access and equity in health. The social context of mistrust of conventional health care, fostered by the distrust, further complicates the situation, and health inequalities continue to persist. It is hence imperative to address both the social and public health dimensions of bloodborne viruses and hepatitis. New strategies, including culturally sensitive health education and outreach in the community, might promote awareness and encourage testing and treatment among these populations, ultimately leading to the reduction in transmission rates. Medical science and technology have also brought more understanding to the issue and potential remedies in the case of hepatitis and bloodborne diseases. Hepatitis C has been a top global health concern, and the demand for better detection methods and specialized treatment has followed suit. Serological testing and epidemiological studies have proven effective in making the disease less complex and more manageable within populations. With hepatitis C, an active treatment approach is capable of achieving significant patient and healthcare system cost reductions. Falzon et al. (1997) stress the importance of treating this serious, potentially progressive, infectious disease early in young individuals. By looking to preventive interventions and patient management, public health programs aim to reduce the long-term costs of these viral illnesses, and thus, the door is opened to healthier populations and improved health outcomes.

Definition of Hepatitis

The term hepatitis is applied to an inflammation of the liver, whose cause could be a variety of factors, including viral infections, autoimmune disease, and toxic substances like alcohol. The disease is not only useful in itself due to its direct impact on liver function, but also when applied to more sophisticated complications. Out of the many causes of hepatitis, viral infections, particularly hepatitis A, B, C, D, and E, are most prevalent. All hepatitis viruses of each type have a different mode of transmission and a unique symptomology and long-term outcome. As an illustration, hepatitis A is usually transmitted by the fecal-oral route, while hepatitis B and C are usually transmitted by the blood and secretions, hence being most directly associated when dealing with bloodborne viruses. For hepatitis, it is equally necessary to recognize the threat posed by injection drug use because this population is disproportionately affected by bloodborne illnesses, such as hepatitis B and C. A study found that among injecting drug users (IDUs), infection incidence at the injection site was highly correlated with such drug-using activities as needle sharing, which directly increases the risk of infection with hepatitis B and C (Hope et al., 2008). This suggests an interdependent mutual relationship between drug use, health care access, and public health. Knowledge of these factors is important in addressing the hepatitis epidemic, as it is both biological and socio-economic. Actions against stemming the spread of hepatitis should therefore involve targeted interventions towards the education of high-risk groups in safe injecting practices.

The effectiveness of preventive measures also lies in the understanding of universal precautions (UP) by health workers and emergency responders. Research on fire department EMS personnel has shown that non-compliance with UP has been a significant factor in escalated risk of exposure to bloodborne pathogens, such as hepatitis viruses (Wrentz-Hudson, 2015). This is an open call for comprehensive training and compliance with safety protocols in high-risk care environments. Better knowledge of universal precautions and their deep meaning can lead to better compliance and, in the end, a reduction in the transmission of contagious diseases. Therefore, hepatitis needs to be addressed through both public health and enhanced occupational safety procedures in order to secure a reduction in its impact on bloodborne virus-involved communities (Figure 6.1).

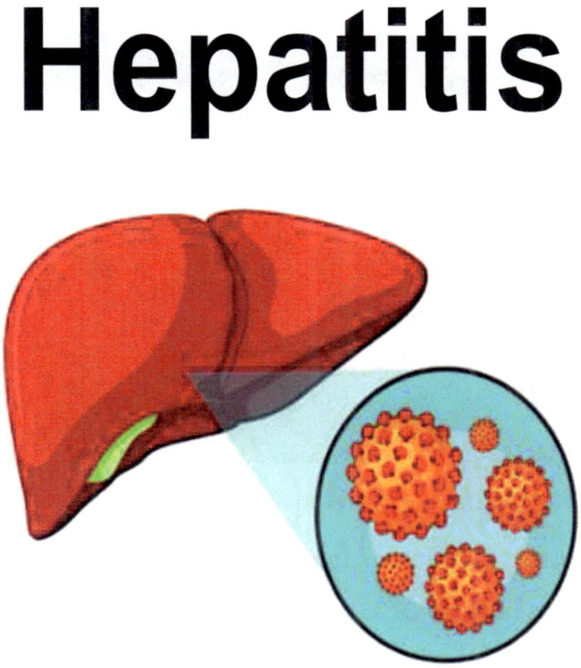

Figure 6.1. Hepatitis virus.

Source: https://continentalhospitals.com/uploads/mceu_16317320111724051300712.jpg.

Overview of Bloodborne Viruses

Bloodborne viruses, including hepatitis B (HBV) and hepatitis C (HCV), present a significant public health issue globally. These viruses are spread primarily through exposure to infected blood, and their transmission patterns are thus central for prevention. With millions of individuals having chronic infections of hepatitis, health systems in most countries find it difficult to manage the socio-economic impacts of these diseases. Highlighting the gravity of this issue, recent studies have brought to attention the increasing prevalence of hepatitis C in adolescent populations, pointing towards an alarming pattern that is bound to translate into greater healthcare costs and ill health among patients as well as society (Falzon et al., 1997). An examination of the transmission patterns helps to form targeted interventions and educate at-risk groups to check the prevalence of these frequently debilitating diseases. In addition to HBV and HCV, human immunodeficiency virus (HIV) is also a significant bloodborne pathogen that affects the health of the world significantly. All three viruses share the same modes of transmission and the same problems with public education and prevention. Despite the advancements in the treatment of HIV, HBV, and HCV, many individuals remain uninformed about their risk for infection or even testing. This lack of awareness is the primary cause of the ongoing spread of these viruses. Preventive care programs for the general and high-risk populations are crucial to developing a prevention culture. Greater awareness about bloodborne pathogens ensures that individuals make safe decisions and get tested and treated when necessary (Hunter, 2017) (Figure 6.2).

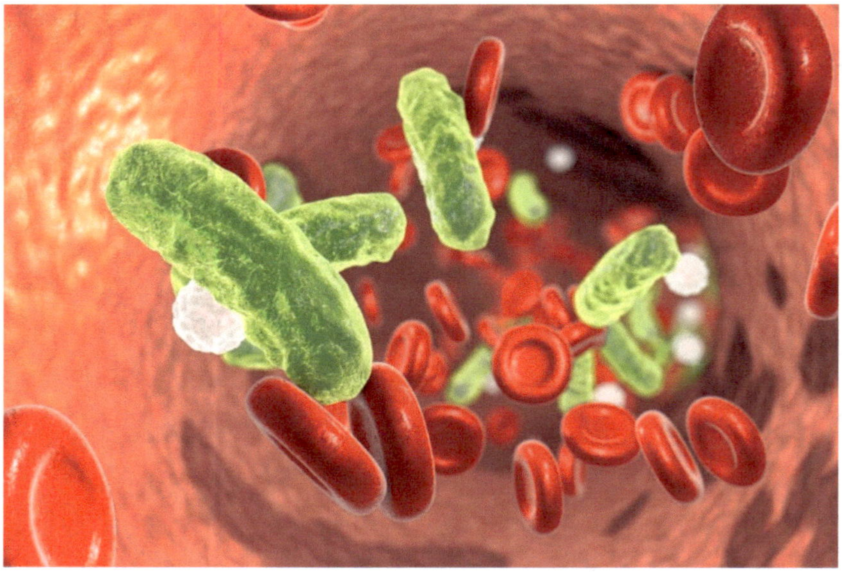

Figure 6.2. Bloodborne pathogens.

Source: https://cprcare.com/wp-content/uploads/2018/07/Bloodborne-Pathogens.jpg.

Furthermore, the socioeconomic effects of bloodborne viruses are not only confined to individual health but also affect families and communities. Stigma and discrimination affect individuals with chronic infection, leading to further marginalization and rendering it more difficult for them to access care. The healthcare cost of treating, managing, and maintaining ongoing medical care for hepatitis and other bloodborne diseases encompasses treatment, ongoing medical care, and prevention. Policymakers should take note of these intricate factors concerning bloodborne viruses. Strategies involving educational outreach, early detection, and comprehensive care are able to significantly reduce the incidence of these viruses. Prevention and care management effectively mitigate the broader public health effect of hepatitis and other bloodborne diseases on public health systems and enhance public health outcomes (Falzon et al., 1997).

Importance of Understanding Hepatitis and Bloodborne Viruses

In-depth understanding of hepatitis and bloodborne viruses is pertinent to public safety and health, particularly in light of their prevalence and factors contributing to risks. The said viruses – Hepatitis B (HBV), Hepatitis C (HCV), and the Human Immunodeficiency Virus (HIV) – are severe health threats to the global community. They primarily transmit through contact with infected blood and body fluids, thereby making education and sensitization key to intervention. By learning about the fundamental characteristics of these infections, including how they are spread and their potential impact on health, individuals can better protect themselves and others. Learning about these viruses can also lead to informed discussion on the use of vaccines, infection control within healthcare settings, and the stigmatization implications of these illnesses. As put, "learning the who, what, when, where, and why of bloodborne pathogens allows us to better understand the world we live in" (Hunter, 2017). Occupational exposure to bloodborne pathogens in healthcare environments is high-risk, and strict adherence to safety standards is required. The importance of valuing such risks cannot be overstressed, particularly for health care workers who are at risk of exposure to bloodborne pathogen exposures (BBPE) in the course of their daily practice. Safe management and prevention measures are absolutely essential components of health care systems to ensure patient and health worker safety. Implementing rigorous reporting and post-exposure follow-up mechanisms is critical to reducing exposure-related hazards. Despite these regulations, findings indicate that there is a high percentage of healthcare professionals who fail to comply with follow-up monitoring, generating compliance and best practice training issues. The findings identify a clear demographic pattern affecting medical centers and emphasize the necessity of improved training and awareness initiatives in raising levels of compliance (Chongswatdi et al., 2022). Secondly, increased understanding of hepatitis and bloodborne viruses results in increased sympathy in public discourse about individuals who carry these diseases. Stigma often stems from ignorance and misconceptions about the spread and treatment of viruses. An educated population can fight against societal stigma and promote supportive environments for individuals who have hepatitis and other associated infections. Such consciousness highlights the value of education for prevention but also for advocacy and empathy in healthcare settings and society as a whole. Having an awareness of the human sides of such diseases has a tendency to galvanize inclusive policy and practice that benefits the victims. Lastly, a good understanding of hepatitis and bloodborne viruses is required in order to develop a health-respecting community, a community that values safety and the welfare of persons at risk or infected with such.

6.1. Types of Hepatitis

Hepatitis is associated with various forms, each induced by different viruses that have in common the fact that they target the liver. Among these, the best known are Hepatitis A, B, C, D, and E.

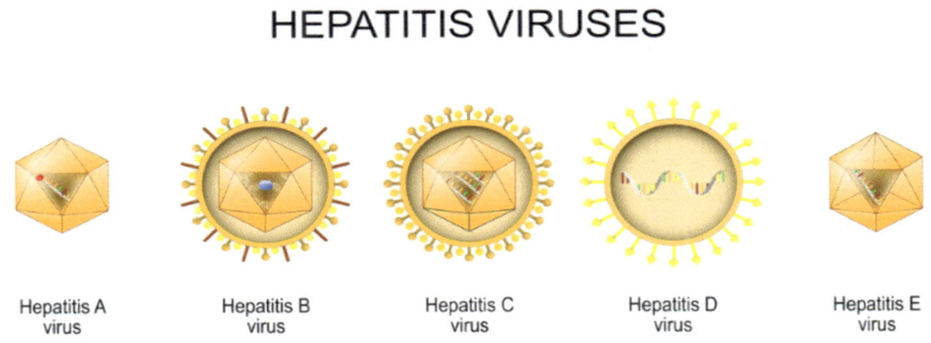

Figure 6.3. Types of hepatitis virus.

Source: https://cdn3.vectorstock.com/i/1000x1000/56/17/hepatitis-virus-structure-a-b-c-d-e-vector-49795617.jpg.

Hepatitis A virus (HAV) is commonly spread through the fecal-oral route, frequently associated with food or water contamination, causing acute but not usually chronic disease. Conversely, Hepatitis B virus (HBV) is mainly spread through blood and body fluids and causes both acute and chronic liver disease. Chronic HBV infection is a serious global health concern as it is linked to advanced liver disease, such as cirrhosis and hepatocellular carcinoma. Both forms of hepatitis have distinctive epidemiologic features that require specific public health responses. Hepatitis C virus (HCV) is also a major problem, mainly spread by blood exposure, most commonly among injecting drug users. Research shows that awareness of HCV status can affect injecting drug users' risk behavior, and therefore, it might result in decreased rates of transmission (Palmateer et al., 2008). In contrast to HAV and HBV, which are vaccine-preventable, no vaccine exists for HCV, so prevention becomes difficult. Chronic HCV tends to be asymptomatic until extensive liver injury develops, which makes timely diagnosis and treatment challenging. One of the major breakthroughs in the management of HCV is the introduction of direct-acting antiviral agents that have transformed the treatment paradigm and dramatically improved cure rates (Figure 6.3).

An understanding of the epidemiology of the transmission of HCV is important in the establishment of successful harm reduction measures among high-risk groups. Hepatitis D (HDV) and E (HEV) are other types of the virus that lead to public health issues, but in more limited environments. HDV is unique in the sense that it only affects those who are already infected with HBV, leading to more severe liver injury. The co-infection increases the risk of fulminant hepatitis, and therefore, treating HBV as a preventive measure against HDV infection is important. HEV, on the other hand, is primarily transmitted by the fecal-oral route and is predominantly a third-world problem with poor sanitation. Although generally self-limiting, HEV poses extremely hazardous risks in pregnant females. Current research shows that exposure to bloodborne viruses is also experienced by healthcare professionals, and thus, education on occupational exposure (Mashoto et al., 2013) needs to be emphasized. Thus, the knowledge of all forms of hepatitis is crucial in successful public health interventions.

6.1.1. Hepatitis A

Of the hepatitis and bloodborne viruses, hepatitis A stands out as a viral hepatitis that is spread primarily by the fecal-oral route, usually through ingestion of contaminated water or food. Unlike its bloodborne siblings, hepatitis B and C, hepatitis A is not a chronic infection and is most often an outbreak-causing cause in unclean environments. The virus is particularly difficult in vulnerable groups, including Indigenous Australians, who may be more at risk and have worse outcomes due to social determinants of health. It is because of this discrepancy in health status that public health interventions, particularly aimed at improving sanitation and hepatitis A education, are crucial in preventing outbreaks in high-risk populations. Despite the general weak pathogenicity of hepatitis A, its epidemiologic importance cannot be overstated, particularly in settings where clean water is not available. As other studies have shown, Indigenous Australians carry a twofold burden of heightened infectious disease and mainstream health service distrust (Strobel & Ward, 2012) (Figure 6.4).

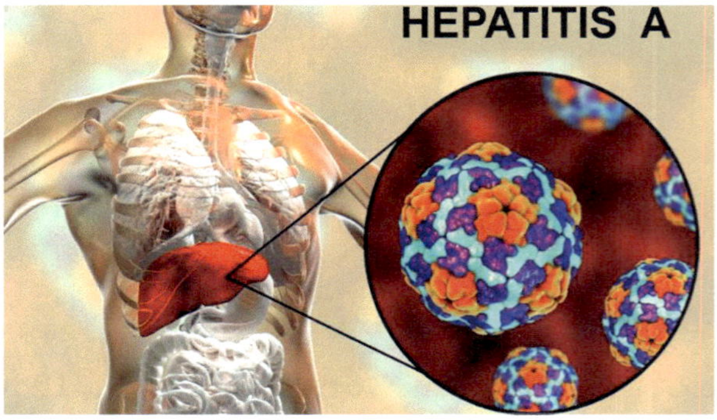

Figure 6.4. Hepatitis A.

Source: https://newsnetwork.mayoclinic.org/n7-mcnn/7bcc9724adf7b803/uploads/2019/05/shutterstock_1122823709_Fotor-16x9-1024x576.jpg.

This background contributes to the challenges of preventing the transmission of hepatitis A since individuals with such backgrounds will be less likely to seek medical care for treatment or a vaccine, thus contributing to increased prevalence in such communities. In addition, the relationship between socio-economic determinants and health further suggests the necessity of overall health strategies that focus not only on vaccination strategies but also on efforts to reduce the broader inequalities. Prevention of hepatitis A involves a multifaceted approach that includes health education and vaccination campaigns. Vaccination has significantly reduced the spread of hepatitis A, yet public health interventions need to continue to include populations with intermittent access to health care services (Palmateer et al., 2008). Public education programs that sensitize individuals to safe handling of food and the importance of vaccine use can also reduce the risk of spread. This combined approach is crucial not only for the prevention of hepatitis A epidemics but also for building community resilience among disproportionately affected liver disease populations. Ultimately, addressing hepatitis A in bloodborne viruses requires commitment to equal access to care and universal education towards protecting vulnerable populations.

6.1.2. Hepatitis B

Hepatitis B is a bloodborne and extremely endemic viral disease with significant global public health implications. Hepatitis B virus (HBV) infection due to this disease primarily affects the liver and can lead to both acute and chronic conditions. HBV infection is caused by contact with bodily fluids, including semen, blood, and vaginal discharge. Besides, certain risk groups are unevenly vulnerable to infection, for instance, injecting drug users and individuals who have multiple sexual partners. Due to the transmission mode, Hepatitis B is often associated with other bloodborne viruses and consequently leads to a complex interaction calling for unique public health intervention. In Aboriginal Australians, for instance, the prevalence of Hepatitis B infection is typically high compared to socioeconomic conditions, reflecting systemic healthcare barriers and cultural determinants that aggravate health inequities between them (Strobel & Ward, 2012). The increasing burden of Hepatitis B underscores the need for effective prevention and treatment interventions.

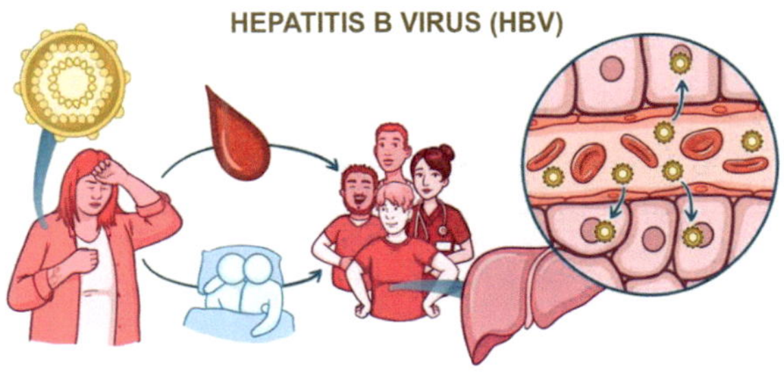

Figure 6.5. Hepatitis B virus.

Source: https://www.osmosis.org/_next/image?url=https%3A%2F%2Fd16qt3wv6xm098.cloudfront.net%2FG4Qb2kpsQxSKNI7UfNlZdC1iS1mEKhyM%2F_.jpg&w=3840&q=75.

Vaccination has emerged as the key tool against HBV transmission because it provides robust immunity and can even reduce transmission rates by a great deal. Hepatitis B vaccine has been recommended by the World Health Organization for all children, with the target of curbing the number of cases of the disease at the earliest possible point. Knowledge about the risk factors of Hepatitis B also plays a significant role in preventing it. Literature indicates that certain populations, such as injecting drug users, have high prevalence rates of Hepatitis B as well as other viral infections like Hepatitis C and HIV. The literature indicates that the risk of Hepatitis B increases according to certain drug use behaviors and history, and thus the relevance of focused interventions in such high-risk groups (Keenan et al., 1998) (Figure 6.5). Education and accessibility of healthcare services, apart from immunization, play a key role in successfully managing Hepatitis B infection. Chronic Hepatitis B patients require regular medical checkup and can be treated with antiviral drugs to suppress the virus and avoid complications due to the liver. Cultural bias against Hepatitis B prevents some individuals from visiting medical facilities, particularly vulnerable groups. It calls for an intermultiplied approach that includes community outreach and culturally modified delivery of healthcare to empower the affected to seek treatment and engage in prevention. This integrated understanding of Hepatitis B, coupled with the intersection of the social determinants of health, renders it necessary for multi-stakeholder interventions that address both the medical and environmental roots of the virus persistence (Strobel & Ward, 2012).

6.1.3. Hepatitis C

Hepatitis C, a viral disease spread through blood, is a serious public health problem everywhere. A study by the Centers for Disease Control and Prevention estimates that approximately 3.2 million people in the United States are chronically infected with this virus. IDUs are the most exposed among the risk group, as needle sharing raises the risk of exposure by far. Prevalence of hepatitis C and other bloodborne illnesses was evaluated among IDUs who attended a rehabilitation center in a 2004 study.

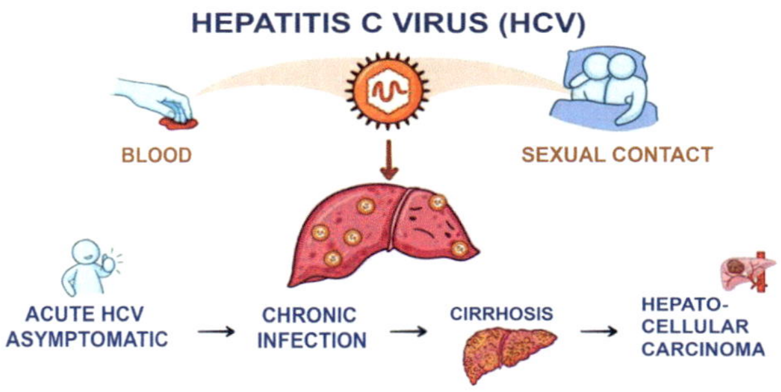

Figure 6.6. Hepatitis C virus.

Source: https://www.osmosis.org/_next/image?url=https%3A%2F%2Fd16qt3wv6xm098.cloudfront.net%2FBc46jFC9TB6PwkPnX9mNgAR6T4SWSggm%2F_.jpg&w=3840&q=75.

The findings indicated that a significant 11.2% of the participants were HCV positive, which supports the direct association between syringe sharing and risk of acquisition of not only HCV but also other bloodborne viruses such as HIV and HBV (Imani et al., 2008). These statistics underscore the pressing need for targeted interventions aimed at reducing transmission in this group. Education and awareness among the public regarding Hepatitis C constitute critical components in its prevention of transmission. Many individuals are unaware that they are infected due to the typically asymptomatic nature of the presentation of the disease. When symptoms do manifest, they may only appear after several years of concealed infection, which complicates early diagnosis and treatment. Therefore, effective health policy development and outreach campaigns are important to recognize at-risk populations and connect people to testing and treatment. The latest discussions among health and social care professionals highlighted the necessity to establish an all-round regional policy to respond to Hepatitis C infection. Such initiatives would not only focus on treatment but prevention and education, hence enhancing an informed populace that can actively participate in actions to curb the spread (Strobel & Ward, 2012) (Figure 6.6).

Besides, treatment progress has transformed Hepatitis C from a slow, lethal disease to a controllable one, greatly improving the prognosis of the victims. The revolution in the use of direct-acting antivirals (DAAs) has transformed the face of treatment, with cure rates now standing at more than 95% in the majority of cases. Not only does this empower patients but also presents an opportunity for public health officials to eliminate the virus entirely in targeted populations. However, access to such treatments is variable, usually based on socioeconomic status and access to healthcare. As a result, multidisciplinary measures — focusing on education, policy formulation, and treatment availability — are needed to combat the intricate challenges presented by Hepatitis C. Cooperative efforts from healthcare professionals, policymakers, and community groups need to be accomplished for implementing effective control of the epidemic of this bloodborne pathogen.

6.2. Transmission of Bloodborne Viruses

Transmission of bloodborne illnesses such as hepatitis C and B occurs primarily through direct contact with infected blood, and therefore, certain groups, particularly injecting drug users (IDUs), are particularly vulnerable. Sharing equipment such as needles, syringes, and other drug paraphernalia offers a suitable route for the spread of these viruses. Transmission of hepatitis B and C is possible through tiny quantities of blood, and these remain on the surface or equipment for weeks after the act. The prevalence of IDUs reflects a serious public health problem since unsafe injecting practices directly relate to an elevated rate of transmission. The population also doesn't usually have complete access to prevention education and health care, which creates a vicious cycle of infection and disease progression. Social settings in which drug injecting is engaged in exacerbate bloodborne virus transmission rates. An in-depth study revealed that the majority of IDUs, who are usually isolated from the general health services, possess a distrust that is based on historical injustices within healthcare systems. This distrust can deter individuals from acquiring necessary screenings and treatments, thereby further perpetuating the spread of hepatitis as well as other bloodborne diseases. Besides, the taboo associated with drug consumption can lead to feelings of shame, thereby preventing individuals from seeking health services that will provide countermeasures for risk behaviors. Latent social issues need to be addressed to engage with efficient public health interventions against the transmission of bloodborne viruses, particularly among vulnerable populations. When examining IDUs' behavior towards hepatitis C testing and their subsequent injecting behavior, research has identified complex dynamics that inform transmission patterns. Those participants who were aware of their hepatitis C status had defined injecting risk behaviors distinct from those who were unaware of their status. Especially, among the hepatitis C-negative ones, the likelihood of sharing needles and other paraphernalia was reduced, a sign that an individual's health status awareness can lead to safer conduct. The cross-sectional analysis in this case points towards a need for longitudinal studies to definitively prove causality since correlation is not necessarily causation and does not necessarily reflect direct behavioral change. Inclusion of education regarding hepatitis C and targeted interventions has the potential to play a significant role in reducing transmission rates and ultimately contribute to better health outcomes for at-risk populations.

6.2.1. Routes of Transmission

The routes of transmission of hepatitis and other bloodborne viruses are significant to the epidemiology of the infections. Hepatitis B, C, and D viruses are primarily spread through contact with infected blood, either by percutaneous exposure, such as sharing needles among intravenous drug users or mucous membranes, especially during sexual intercourse.

Hepatitis Transmission Methods

Viral Hepatitis Type	Fecal-oral transmission and food contamination	Blood and body fluid contact	Close personal contact	Saliva and infected droplets, such as from coughing
A	✓	✓	✓	✗
B	✗	✓	✓	✗
C	✗	✓	✗	✗
D	✗	✓	✗	✗
E	✓	rarely	rarely	✗

Figure 6.7. Hepatitis transmission methods.

Source: https://dims.healthgrades.com/dims3/MMH/d1138cf/2147483647/strip/true/crop/1024x759+0+0/resize/800x593!/quality/75/?url=https%3A%2F%2Fucmscdn.healthgrades.com%2Fdc%2Ff2%2F37e2cc283691fcc1168c9455898a%2F303398-is-hepatitis-contagious-types-and-transmission-explained-1296x961-body-1024x759.jpg.

In addition, the virus is vertically transmitted from mother to infant during birth. Such consciousness favors the effectiveness of preventive strategies, including needle exchange programs and safe sex, which have helped to decelerate the rate of transmission among groups at high risk. The multifaceted mode of transmission channels demands continuous public health intervention to educate high-risk groups on the routes of transmission as well as strategies for reducing exposure. In the clinical setting, the risk of transmission of hepatitis remains a problem, particularly in nosocomial infections. The presence of bloodborne viruses is a risk to the patient as well as to the healthcare staff, which demands strict adherence to infection control practices, such as the application of personal protective equipment and disinfection protocols. Despite robust surveillance systems, the identification of hospital-acquired infections continues to be troublesome because of factors such as long incubation periods and microbiological diagnostic issues. For instance, occult infections may remain undetected for extensive intervals of time, and hence, the management of infected patients becomes problematic. Therefore, hospitals must prioritize introducing such focused surveillance programs that can counter these issues and limit the risk of nosocomial infections of hepatitis to provide a secure environment for both patients and professionals. The understanding of the various modes of transmission of hepatitis and bloodborne viruses directs the overall public health strategy aimed at containment and prevention. Occupational exposure remains a primary concern for health care workers, who risk possible infection by needlestick injuries or contact with contaminated surfaces. Transmission through non-sexual horizontal transmission, such as sharing personal items such as razors or toothbrushes, defines the need for mass education on habits of hygiene. Public health initiatives that promote mandatory hepatitis immunizations, particularly among risk groups, can significantly reduce the rate of transmission. By enhancing the significance of medical as well as individual preventive measures, the population can assist in decreasing the prevalence and incidence of hepatitis infection, thereby improving public health outcomes (Petignat et al., 1998; Shorten & Wilson-Davies, 2017) (Figure 6.7).

6.2.2. Risk Factors for Infection

Risk factors for infection in the case of bloodborne viruses and hepatitis are also complex and strongly interwoven with determinants of a sociocultural nature. Disadvantaged populations, such as Indigenous Australians, have exceptionally high infection rates of hepatitis due to systemic access barriers to healthcare and previous injustices predominant in their societies. The unequal healthcare system often results in engendering suspicion, which raises these groups' susceptibility to infection. Individuals may be afraid to seek preventive care or treatment of sexually transmitted infections (STIs) because they fear being stigmatized or having had bad experiences with the healthcare system, deterring an effective public health approach. This complex interdependence of cultural background and availability of care to foster greater emphasis on specialized health programs that take into account the unique circumstances of Indigenous people and seek to build trust within those groups (Strobel & Ward, 2012). In addition to sociocultural factors, risk-taking behaviors also has a significant contribution to the transmission risk for hepatitis and bloodborne viruses. Injecting drug use and unprotected sex are among the high-transmission modes. Intravenous drug users also tend to share needles, which not only facilitates the spread of hepatitis C but also increases the risks of other bloodborne infections. Likewise, individuals practicing unsafe sex might inadvertently expose themselves to the risk of hepatitis B and other STIs. The normalization of these dangerous behaviors in certain populations is therefore proof that there has been a gap in education on safer practices as well as effective harm reduction methods. By bridging such behavior-related gaps, public health interventions are better positioned to tackle the spread of hepatitis and general community health (Shorten & Wilson-Davies, 2017). Systemic health inequalities and structural hazards then further amplify the likelihood of hepatitis and bloodborne disease within and between populations. Economic disadvantage, limited access to good-quality care, and the lack of health education all contribute to central roles in susceptibility to disease. Individuals from lower socioeconomic groups are more likely to be subject to barriers interfering with their ability to access proper health care, thereby leading to delayed diagnosis or untreated infection. Moreover, geographic differences make rural populations underserved, and this is another reason why infection rates are higher. Solution to such issues demands inter-disciplinary solutions that include policy changes for strengthening healthcare funding, enhancing equitable access to healthcare, and spending on community-based health education programs. Such interventions are essential in curbing the prevalence of hepatitis as well as enabling vulnerable groups to take proactive measures for their protection against disease (Strobel & Ward, 2012) (Figure 6.8).

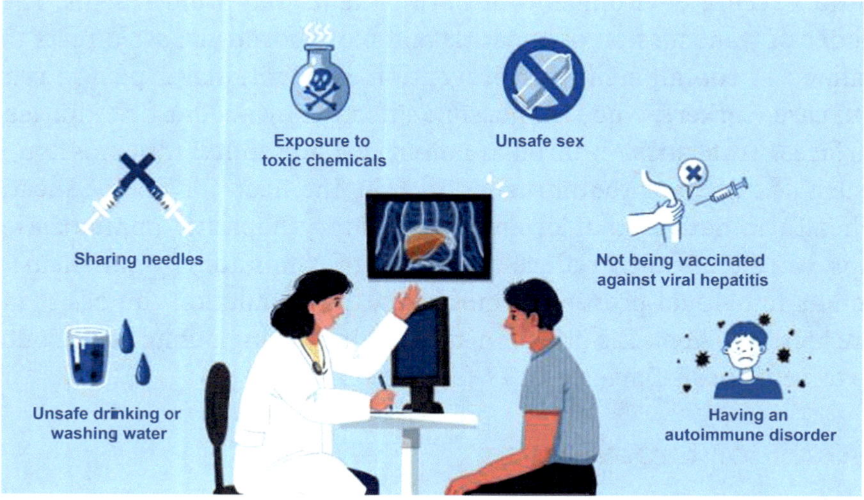

Figure 6.8. Hepatitis risk factors.

Source: https://www.verywellhealth.com/thmb/eB_WOXJnLlmUhxloyI_bbcrroXQ=/1500x0/filters:no_upscale():max_bytes(150000):strip_icc()/hepatitis-causes-and-risk-factors-4689127_color-1c8b56f0bbf04615826acd3e581716ab.gif.

6.2.3. Global Prevalence

The hepatitis and bloodborne virus burden is a complex case decided by various social, economic, and healthcare determinants. The hepatitis B and C viruses are the most notable globally, with the World Health Organization estimating that around 296 million are infected with hepatitis B and around 58 million with hepatitis C. Disparities in prevalence can be attributed to differences in access to healthcare services, the quality of screening programs, and heterogeneity in public health programs aimed at prevention and education. They are also determined by local variations in injection drug use, which is central in determining the transmission dynamics of these viral infections. In addition, social stigmatization of both hepatitis and bloodborne viruses often leads to the affected individuals being deprived of proper treatment, but another factor that perpetuates the epidemic. Social determinants play a large role in hepatitis and bloodborne virus incidence and prevalence, particularly among vulnerable populations. For instance, Aboriginal and Torres Strait Islander Australians have disproportionately higher rates of such infections as reflected in their high rates of bloodborne viruses and STIs, such as hepatitis B and C. This tragic situation reflects systemic access inequalities in health and cultural mistrust of mainstream health care, mainly based on historical injustices. The prevalence rates in Indigenous Australians demonstrate an intersection of healthcare, social, and historical determinants that are strongly influencing their health outcomes. Intervention strategies to close these disparities must recognize and work to satisfy cultural considerations to enhance uptake and efficacy of services among these groups, bringing an end to the burden of hepatitis and related healthcare needs. The influence of risk behaviors on global prevalence rates cannot be overstated. Studies indicate that injecting drug users (IDUs) exhibit varying levels of risk based on their knowledge of hepatitis status and the uptake of test schemes. Studies have observed that HCV-negative individuals were significantly less likely to engage in risk injection than untested subjects, suggesting an apparent motivational effect of knowing one's status. However, the cross-sectional study design of such research limits the potential to definitively determine causal relationships. Importantly, interventions and harm reduction strategies of a specific type are needed in response to the risk factors of injection behavior, especially where the prevalence of hepatitis and bloodborne viruses is high within targeted populations. The utilization of large-scale educational programs and available testing sites can make significant contributions to prevalence decline in these populations, enabling a broader public health impact.

6.3. Symptoms and Diagnosis

Symptoms of hepatitis can also be very diverse, depending on the specific virus — Hepatitis A, B, C, D, or E — and the course of the disease. Acute hepatitis is often accompanied by non-specific symptoms such as weakness, malaise, and loss of appetite, which can escalate to jaundice, dark urine, and pain in the abdomen. While others remain asymptomatic, others develop acute illness that could go on to become chronic infection, particularly in the case of Hepatitis B and C. Chronic hepatitis can be in the form of gradual liver damage over a long duration, typically quietly until there is severe liver dysfunction. Early detection of symptoms is thus crucial for public health interventions since untreated cases would make significant contributions to the overall transmission of such bloodborne viruses in populations. The need for systemic screening is self-evident, especially with the potential for severe health implications if not addressed. Hepatitis diagnosis typically starts with a full medical history and physical exam, often followed by serologic tests that detect specific antibodies or antigens of each of the hepatitis viruses. Laboratory testing, such as the hepatitis panel, can provide valuable information regarding the nature of the hepatitis, the infection stage, and liver function markers. For instance, Hepatitis C antibody evidence with polymerase chain reaction (PCR) testing confirms current infection, serving as the basis for further treatment. Furthermore, in some populations — namely Indigenous Australians, who are overrepresented in their burden of hepatitis and bloodborne viruses — a targeted screening program will reveal early infection, eventually leading to better treatment and reduced transmission rates. Culturally appropriate healthcare is central to breaking down barriers to diagnosis and treatment in these populations (Strobel & Ward, 2012). Improved technology in diagnostic procedures has enhanced the identification of hepatitis C, whose status as a global public health concern is increasingly being realized. Improved serological test methods not only increase the reliability of diagnosis but also enable broad epidemiological studies that are central to the understanding of the spread and effect of the virus (Falzon et al., 1997). In a majority of cases, hepatitis C is diagnosed by screening instead of by symptomatic presentation, and mass testing, particularly in risk groups, is therefore indicated. Active screening measures are important to counterbalance the healthcare cost of undiagnosed infection and avert liver disease in young individuals at risk for chronic liver disease. Therefore, finding a balance between early diagnosis, public health awareness, and particular interventions is key in reducing the prevalence of hepatitis and improving health outcomes in affected communities.

6.3.1. Common Symptoms of Hepatitis

Hepatitis, a viral infection that is most often of the liver, has a range of signs and symptoms that can vary greatly in severity. The majority of individuals experience common onset symptoms such as exhaustion, nausea, and stomach discomfort, particularly in the upper right quadrant, where the liver is located. This exhaustion can be especially crippling to day-to-day activities, leading to reduced productivity and overall health. With infection, other usual characteristics like jaundice may ensue, which involves yellowing of the skin and eyes with the rise in bilirubin levels as a result of compromised liver function. This initial stage points to the importance of early diagnosis and treatment as inadequate treatment will lead to severe complications of the liver in the long run (Figure 6.9).

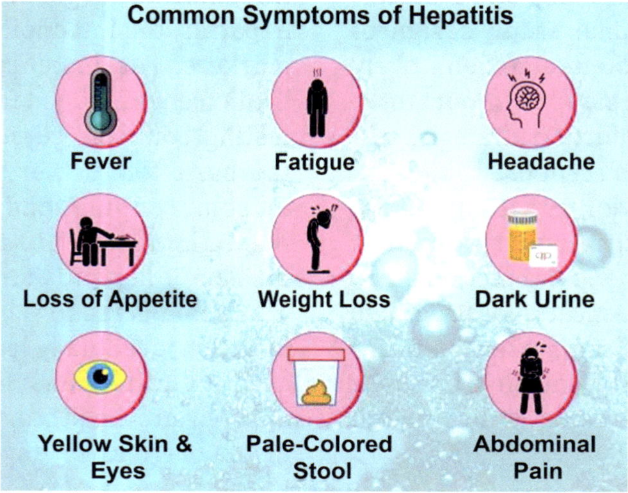

Figure 6.9. Common symptoms of hepatitis.

Source: https://www.facebook.com/HealthyIndiaPage/photos/its-worldhepatitisday%EF%B8%8Fworld-hepatitis-day-is-observed-on-july-28-every-year-it-a/620137988631097/.

As hepatitis progresses, patients will experience a shift in their symptomatology that will help differentiate between the different types of the virus. For instance, acute hepatitis will usually present as a flu-like illness with fever and muscle aches, which is misleading and usually leads to delayed diagnosis. Chronic infection with hepatitis B and C, on the other hand, will be symptom-free for many years, which will hinder public health programs from controlling these diseases. Later on, there might be symptoms like dark-colored urine, light-colored stools, and severe weakness that reflect the ongoing liver damage. The wide range of symptoms proves that hepatitis infections vary in nature and need frequent screening, especially in high-risk populations, to avoid the risk of serious liver diseases and complications in the long term. The presentation of hepatitis symptoms might be most challenging in particular groups, such as Indigenous Australians, in that they have disproportionately higher infection rates with hepatitis compared to the general population. This is in part related to ineffective access to culturally appropriate health service delivery and an extensive lack of trust within mainstream health care systems.

As highlighted, Indigenous Australians also carry high rates of hepatitis B and C, and other sexually transmitted diseases, which call for public health programs targeted towards them alone. These programs must attend to the social and historical determinants that create these health disparities, looking to establish accessible screening and treatment programs sensitive to the particular needs of Indigenous groups in order to most effectively combat the spread of hepatitis and generally improve health outcomes (Strobel & Ward, 2012).

6.3.2. Diagnostic Tests for Hepatitis

The diagnostic testing setting of hepatitis, that is, hepatitis B and C, is of prime value in disease control as well as public health planning. Hepatitis serologic testing plays a vital role in detecting antibodies or antigens in the blood, providing information regarding current as well as past infection.

For hepatitis B, testing generally assesses the presence of Hepatitis B surface antigen (HBsAg) to determine an active infection and antibody tests, such as Anti-HBs and Anti-HBc, that help determine immunity and history of exposure. Similarly, hepatitis C diagnosis typically employs serological tests for detecting antibodies against the virus. Early and accurate diagnosis of the infections enables prompt medical care since untreated hepatitis can progress to chronic liver disease and increased healthcare costs, particularly in the younger age group, who may be disproportionately affected by this illness (Falzon et al., 1997) (Figure 6.10).

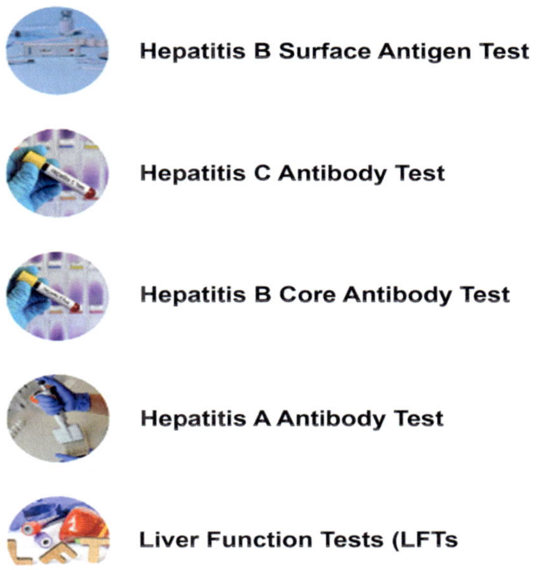

Figure 6.10. Hepatitis diagnostic tests.

Source: https://images.drlogy.com/assets/uploads/img/admin/health_blog/editor-img/hepatitis_diagnosis_-_drlogy.webp.

In addition to serological tests, molecular testing has emerged as an important diagnostic tool for hepatitis, especially for hepatitis C. The HCV RNA test is a significant test in the detection of active infection and measurement of the viral load, which is very important in determining how severe the disease is and whether or not treatment is effective. These molecular diagnostic technologies enable medical professionals to tailor antivirals to the individual genotype of the virus and the personal response of the patient. As has been highlighted in more recent articles, advances in diagnostics have enabled increased detection of cases so that most at risk can receive the necessary attention. This technological advancement in testing is a fundamental aspect of a broad-ranging public health initiative aimed at curbing the spread of hepatitis and optimizing patient outcomes (Shorten & Wilson-Davies, 2017). Furthermore, integration of RDTs in screening for hepatitis is transforming the approach by clinicians and public health professionals to address the disease. RDTs offer an instantaneous and straightforward method of detecting hepatitis infections, and as such, it is incredibly useful in resource-scarce environments. These tests are simple to administer with little training and will normally yield results immediately, enabling immediate counseling and referral for care. This accessibility is also very essential when one is thinking about the barriers that marginalized populations face that would deter them from utilizing standard healthcare services. With RDTs used in combination with standard laboratory methods, health systems are able to increase screening rates, thus enhancing the detection and control of hepatitis cases efficiently (Falzon et al., 1997).

6.3.3. Importance of Early Detection

Early detection of hepatitis and other bloodborne viruses is crucial for effective treatment and control. Detection of infection in early stages enables clinicians to apply interventions in due time that not only stop disease progression but also lead to improved patient outcomes. Because asymptomatic phases are characteristic of viral infections, the majority of individuals do not know the fact, increasing the opportunity for transmission to others. Enhanced surveillance schemes, specifically intended to detect such infections at the time of inception, can effectively reduce the incidence of complications due to hepatitis, i.e., liver cancer and cirrhosis. Also, implementing routine screenings, especially among high-risk populations, can facilitate early medical care and enhanced resource allocation, and ultimately assist in public health programs against bloodborne pathogens (Petignat et al., 1998). The implications of early diagnosis extend beyond individual health to impact broader epidemiological trends associated with hepatitis and bloodborne viruses generally. With the sine qua non of diagnosis and surveillance, patterns of infection and outbreaks can be tracked and identified by health authorities before their spread. Forensic control of the transmission of viruses such as hepatitis B and C, which take years to become active but present imminent threats to health, is best exercised in averting their spread. Through the application of advanced diagnostic techniques, health systems can ensure equity and evidence for interventions, leading to an informed approach to controlling such viral infections. Ultimately, the integration of early detection mechanisms into health policies encourages a prevention and education culture, core to reducing cumulative disease burden among populations (Hunter, 2017) (Figure 6.11).

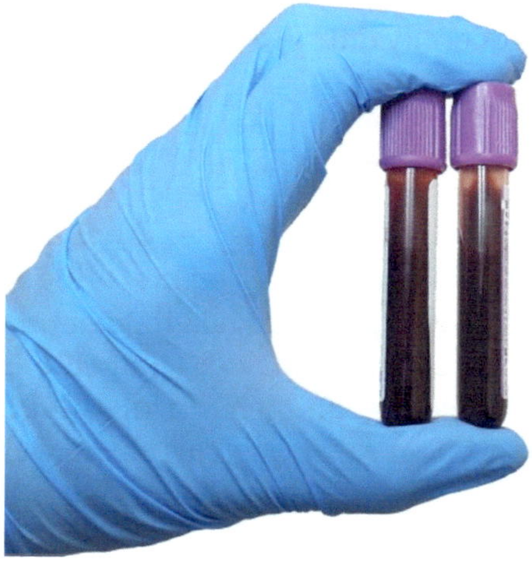

Figure 6.11. Hepatitis early detection.

Source: https://www.stitest.london/cdn/shop/products/hiv-hepatitis-test.jpg?v=1719068194.

Apart from improving health results and reducing transmission rates, early diagnosis of hepatitis and bloodborne illnesses can also improve the overall well-being of afflicted individuals. Those diagnosed at an early stage of the disease tend to be provided with better care, which can reduce the long-term effects of the illness. Early detection also eliminates the psychological trauma caused by living in ignorance of one's health status. Community education initiatives focusing on the necessity of regular testing and awareness about bloodborne viruses can empower individuals to become active managers of their own health. Together with holistic health programs, this empowerment can lead to an enhanced public health environment where individuals are better positioned to manage risks and advocate for their health (Petignat et al., 1998).

6.4. Treatment Options

Treatment options for bloodborne viruses and hepatitis have also changed dramatically over the past few decades and offer numerous choices of both pathogen and patient. As an illustration, the direct-acting antiviral (DAA) medications have revolutionized hepatitis C treatment. The DAAs target a precise point in the viral life cycle and yield over a 95% cure rate.

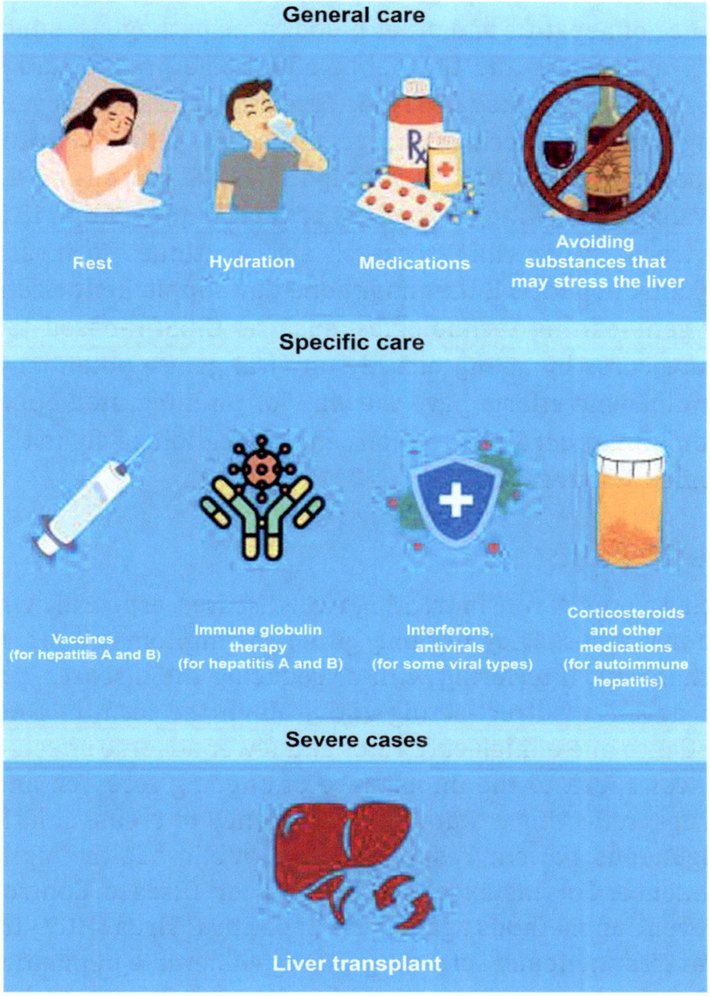

Figure 6.12. Hepatitis treatment options.

Source: https://liverdiseasenews.com/wp-content/uploads/2024/02/HEPATITIS-TREATMENT-OPTIONS.png.

Likewise, with hepatitis B, while a cure is not easily achieved, the use of antiviral medications like tenofovir and entecavir can successfully down-regulate viral replication and thereby avoid liver damage and other consequences. With a greater understanding of these viruses, treatment protocols become increasingly targeted and individualized, addressing the specific needs of the patient based on their viral load and the condition of the liver. In the control of bloodborne viruses, treatment strategies surpass antiviral medication to include preventive interventions that aim to reduce the risk of transmission.

Harm reduction techniques, for example, emphasize safe disposal of medical waste, which forms a crucial part in the prevention of infection transmission. As indicated in current research, public awareness and policy interventions, such as the Medical Waste Treatment Act (MWTA), underscore the importance of appropriate treatment and disposal practices to abate problems stemming from medical waste exposure (Battle, 1994). Such interventions underscore the interactive function between treatment interventions and public health policies since both of them work toward minimizing the prevalence of hepatitis and other bloodborne pathogens. Educational programs that teach both healthcare practitioners and the public about safe practice are vital to compounding the effectiveness of these treatment modalities. As research continues, novel treatments are under consideration, including potential vaccines and gene therapy. The effectiveness of preventing the transmission of the hepatitis A and B viruses through effective prevention using hepatitis A and B vaccines is currently available, showing the success of vaccine prevention in avoiding transmission of hepatitis A and B viruses. Meanwhile, research also continues to investigate the promise of therapeutic vaccines against hepatitis C that might one day supplement existing antiviral regimens (Hunter, 2017). Other gene-editing technologies, such as CRISPR-based technologies, also have promise to deliver future cures by acting directly on viral genes, potentially making a functional cure possible. These trailblazing efforts pave the way for an integrated approach to hepatitis and bloodborne viruses, combining cure, prevention, and education to fight the complex challenges wrought by these illnesses (Figure 6.12).

6.4.1. Antiviral Medications

Antiviral medications play a crucial role in treating viral diseases, especially when involving hepatitis and other blood-borne infections. They not only provide symptomatic control but also target the viral reproductive mechanisms, interfering with or reducing the diseases' propagation, such as in hepatitis B and C. The advent of direct-acting antivirals in the form of DAAs has revolutionized treatment for hepatitis C into one of high cure rates and fewer adverse effects compared to previous treatments. Such advances speak to the importance of ongoing research and advancement in the creation of antiviral drugs, reflecting a state of high urgency to create solutions that combat viral resistance and heterogeneous patient responses. The public health implications of successful antiviral drugs are immense. For instance, the Centers for Disease Control and Prevention has created widespread prevention methods against the hepatitis C virus (HCV) transmission, including easier access to antiviral treatment and screening among vulnerable populations. By using stringent guidelines that not only cure but also educate and avert such infections, health workers attempt to reduce their incidence (Figure 6.13).

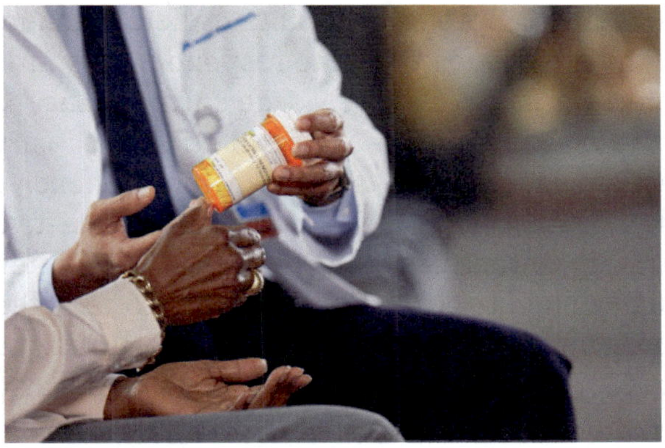

Figure 6.13. Antiviral medications used to treat hepatitis C.

Source: https://external-content.duckduckgo.com/iu/?u=https%3A%2F%2Fdoctorsatkaisertpmg.com%2Fwp-content%2Fuploads%2F2024%2F06%2Fhepc-19DEC_34388-1.webp&f=1&nofb=1&ipt=8242e89d8d05bf535d86db8ddb1aec1281949b7af7dee305bcc239785851dc86.

Furthermore, antiviral drugs must be incorporated into regular healthcare to alleviate the burden of complications from hepatitis, reinforcing the need for cooperation between public health professionals, healthcare providers, and policymakers in formulating sustainable healthcare systems (N/A). Apart from clinical efficacy, the availability of antiviral drugs also offers opportunities and challenges within the healthcare system. Despite greater advances, cost, insurance, and patient education continue to serve as obstacles to access. This inequality puts focus on resolutions for the social determinants of health and addressing the necessity for equal policies that address susceptible populations. Awareness and screening programs can significantly contribute to early detection and compliance with treatment, which is especially important in the situation of chronic viral infections. By facilitating an integrative approach that incorporates both medical and socioeconomic factors, we can better enhance the overall effectiveness of antiviral medications in combating hepatitis and bloodborne viruses within multicultural populations (Hunter, 2017).

6.4.2. Supportive Care

Supportive care is imperative in managing patients who have a diagnosis of hepatitis and other bloodborne infections, in that it is meant to palliate symptoms and enhance quality of life. Curative treatment directed toward the pathogen is in comparison to supportive care, which comprises a range of interventions focused on alleviating complications as well as rendering the patient more comfortable. This strategy regularly incorporates pain relief, nutritional therapy, and psychological therapy, which are very important in managing the complex challenges experienced by those with chronic infection. Under comprehensive care approaches, health professionals can reduce the disease burden considerably and enhance compliance with therapy regimens, which is of high importance for those suffering from chronic hepatitis infection, which could have severe long-term consequences. In addition, the incorporation of education and awareness programs is important in hepatitis and bloodborne virus supportive care. Education programs for healthcare providers as well as patients enhance awareness about modes of transmission, prevention, early detection and treatment. Evidence has shown that utilization of formal training programs can bring about a significant decrease in the incidence of events related to needle-stick injuries among health workers, who are normally the first line of defense against these infections. Such training improves the overall climate of safety, hence protecting health workers and, subsequently, patients through quality improvement in care and minimizing the risk of outbreaks (Zafar et al., 2009). Lastly, facilitating both the patients and the provider by using information leads to a more effective supportive care system. Apart from education, the significance of permanent surveillance and monitoring cannot be overstated in supportive care for bloodborne viruses and hepatitis. Permanent monitoring of practice in healthcare and patient outcome enables the identification of which practices need to be changed and allows quality improvement projects to be set up. For instance, after data analysis showing inordinate needle-stick injuries, interventions aimed at risk reduction can be implemented within specific healthcare settings (Zafar et al., 2009). Creating a safe environment that is aware of hazards leads to a robust, supportive care model and ultimately to better patient outcomes. This ongoing cycle of training, learning, and surveillance is the basis of hepatitis and bloodborne virus management, where the needs of affected people are met holistically and respectfully.

6.4.3. Emerging Therapies

New drugs for hepatitis and bloodborne diseases are evidence of a seismic shift in treatment models that take into account the complexity of these illnesses. One of the most thrilling developments is the development of direct-acting antiviral agents (DAAs), which specifically inhibit one or more processes in the virus life cycle. DAAs have achieved unparalleled cure rates for hepatitis C virus (HCV) infection, evidence of their status as patient-care revolutionaries. Interestingly, the mechanism of action by which these treatments operate minimizes the likelihood of resistance, and clinicians can use several DAAs together for better efficacy. Further, apart from reducing hepatitis morbidity, these drugs have also been of potential benefit in lowering the more universal public health impacts of bloodborne disease, often complicated by zoonotic elements aggravating pathogen dynamics, as attested to by the development of new zoonotic strains in contemporary settings (Cutler et al., 2010). With pharmaceutical advancements, public health interventions are significant in affecting these new treatments effectively. Formulation of policies that address a whole region, through qualitative approaches, facilitates field planners in the area of healthcare to respond to hepatitis infection most effectively. One such instance is from a recent forum of health and social care leaders focusing on creating a comprehensive plan against hepatitis C, evidencing a positive strategy towards handling the epidemic (Hunter, 2017). Such conversations can lead to targeted screening programs and education campaigns that promote informed decisions and early treatment. This integrated approach is capable of bringing therapeutic progress to high-risk populations, thereby reducing the rates of transmission and ultimately resulting in disease incidence of viral hepatitis and its complications. Moreover, the application of technology in delivering developed therapies creates new opportunities for enhancing patient care. Telemedicine and mobile health applications have also become key tools in the battle against bloodborne viruses and hepatitis. It is through such applications that better patient monitoring, follow-up, and compliance support become possible, especially for vulnerable communities with limited access to healthcare. With these advances in technology, the treatment method of healthcare providers can be improved by increasing patient empowerment and participation. As emerging treatments take hold, alignment between new treatment modalities and policy health environments will be crucial in the battle against hepatitis and enhancing patient outcomes in all groups.

6.5. Prevention Strategies

Effective prevention strategies go a long way in reducing hepatitis and other BBVs transmission. Foremost among these prevention strategies is the facilitation of safe practices, particularly among those at high risk, such as injectors of drugs. Needle exchange programs and injecting facilities have been found to be highly effective in reducing BBV transmission. These programs, in addition to providing clean needles, also act as a point of contact for health education and care services. These programs are aimed at creating an environment that will encourage the reduction of harm that is associated with injecting drug use and lower the frequency of hepatitis B and C infections among vulnerable individuals. Highlighting harm reduction indicates an important step towards addressing public health problems involving the transmission of hepatitis and is in line with overall public health objectives.

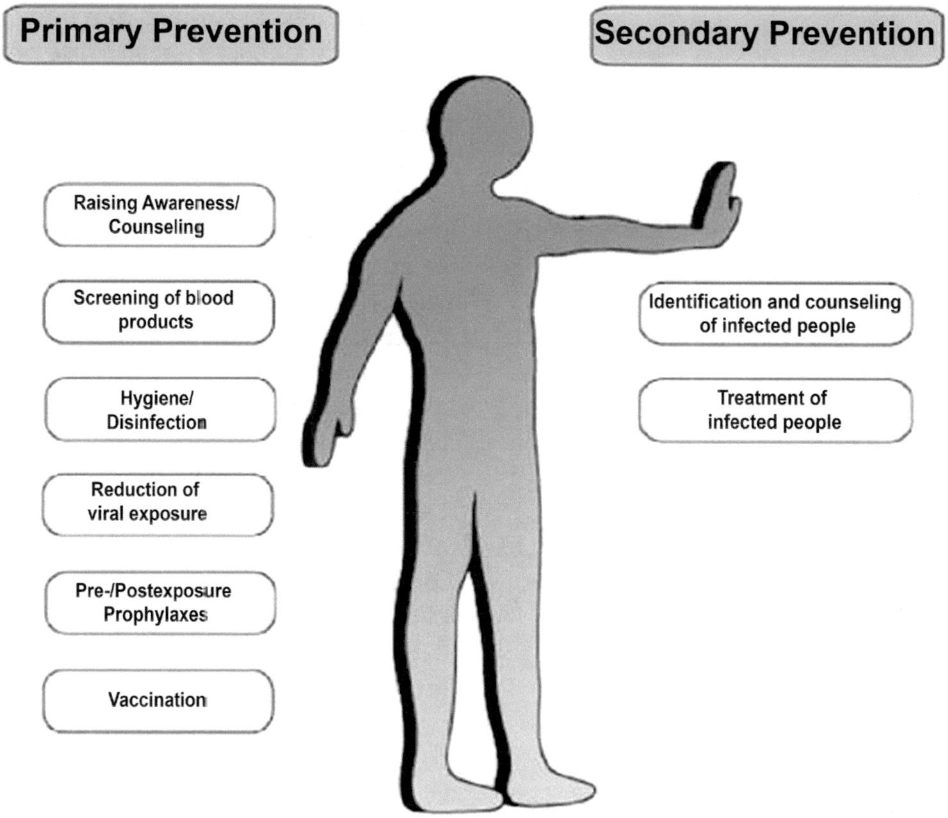

Figure 6.14. Primary and secondary prevention strategies for blood-borne viral infections. These strategies help reduce the transmission of blood-borne viral infections.

Source: https://www.researchgate.net/figure/Primary-and-secondary-prevention-strategies-for-blood-borne-viral-infections-Prevention_fig1_303317132.

Thorough education campaigns are central to fostering awareness of hepatitis and BBVs, particularly in marginalized groups. Interventions based on cultural sensitivity that are individualized can facilitate more interaction with vulnerable groups. For instance, Indigenous Australians have their own unique health concerns that are linked with past grievances toward their relationship with mainstream healthcare. The higher incidence of hepatitis and other STIs among Indigenous Australians necessitates focused efforts that not only consist of education on prevention and treatment but also building trust within the communities. Such programs must react to the history of medical care in addressing how to encourage participation in immunization and screening campaigns, and hence eliminate stigma concerning BBV care seeking (Strobel & Ward, 2012). Effective community outreach develops an enabling environment through which individuals are able to obtain prevention interventions. Routine testing and vaccination remain important components of hepatitis prevention policy. Widespread application of hepatitis B immunization has worked to prevent transmission of the virus, and awareness-raising on the issue of hepatitis C testing can lead to early diagnosis and treatment and subsequently lowered infectivity. Research indicates that individuals aware of their hepatitis status can use safer injecting and hence reduce harm to themselves and others effectively (Palmateer et al., 2008). However, gaps persist in the utilization and availability of these measures among at-risk groups. Barriers such as socioeconomic determinants and mistrust in the health system need to be addressed to enhance screening activity. Incorporating testing and vaccination into combined prevention programs can significantly lower overall hepatitis and bloodborne virus burden in the community (Figure 6.14).

6.5.1. Vaccination for Hepatitis A and B

The global health scenario demands an overall strategy towards both Hepatitis A and Hepatitis B vaccination, bearing in mind their significance in the public health sector and their association with bloodborne viruses. Hepatitis A, which is transmitted mostly through the fecal-oral route, can be avoided through vaccination, especially in communities of populations in areas that have poor sanitation facilities. Vaccination not only guards the individual but is also useful in generating herd immunity, which significantly reduces the transmission of the virus in populations. Through studies, it is noted that widespread vaccination campaigns are capable of curtailing Hepatitis A outbreaks to a great extent, thus safeguarding individuals who cannot receive the vaccine because of certain medical conditions. Therefore, it is important to enhance vaccination centers, particularly in risk areas, in order to combat this avoidable disease as part of the overall plan to manage and control bloodborne pathogens effectively. Hepatitis B, however, is a more difficult problem due to its modes of transmission, which are perinatal, sexual contact, and body fluid contact. High-risk groups, i.e., healthcare providers, must be accorded priority vaccination to prevent occupational contact with bloodborne pathogens. As is evident from evidence that individuals with a history of Hepatitis B infection (with evidence of past exposure) have increased risks of poor outcomes to the liver when coinfected with Hepatitis C, not only does immunization protect individuals against diseases, but also prevents risks of chronic liver disease (Allen et al., 2018). Proper immunization reduces viral load within the overall population and fortifies healthcare systems by lowering Hepatitis B-related diseases. Guaranteeing universal access to vaccination for all groups is thus vital to reducing the burden of Hepatitis B. From an education-in-health perspective, for instance, dental education, vaccination processes help lower the risks of bloodborne exposure to future practitioners. Studies have also demonstrated that dental students experience high exposure to blood and body fluids during their training, and the majority of them lack proper knowledge of their Hepatitis B immunity status (Dantas et al., 2017). This calls for institutions to make mandatory Hepatitis B vaccination and screening at the start of their programs to equip students with complete protection before they can carry out clinical practice. In addition, enhancing education in occupational safety and infection control can also reduce exposure risks, thereby making the environment safer for the patients and students. Hence, the inclusion of vaccination strategies in healthcare education can have a significant impact on the control of Hepatitis and the related bloodborne viruses (Figure 6.15).

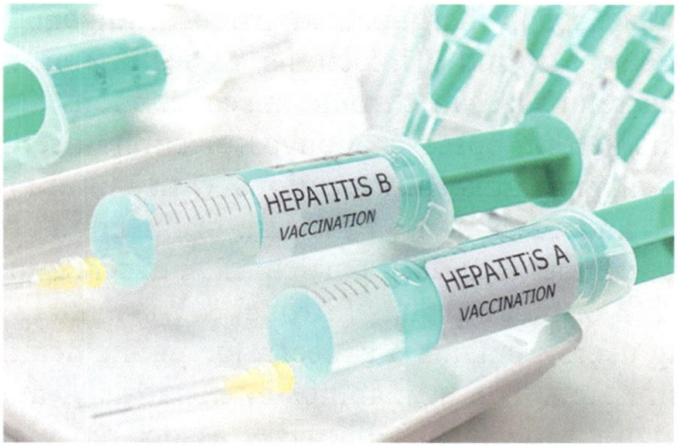

Figure 6.15. Vaccination for hepatitis A and B.

Source: https://samitivej-prod-new-website.s3.ap-southeast-1.amazonaws.com/public/uploads/contents/ab708034dceed83138aef1344d0cac65.jpg.

6.5.2. Safe Practices to Avoid Transmission

In answering the safe practices for averting the spread of hepatitis and other bloodborne infections, standard precautions in clinical practice must be underscored. Medical practitioners always need to wear proper personal protective equipment (PPE), such as gloves, masks, and gowns, to present a barrier against blood and bodily fluids that may harbor infectious agents. Furthermore, regular training sessions in infection control procedures may allow healthcare personnel to remain vigilant and, in the loop, as far as the latest safety protocols are concerned. According to the most recent studies, appropriate adherence to such preventive measures continues to reduce occupational exposure risk among healthcare providers, which ultimately translates to a secure working environment for healthcare workers as well as patients. It is important that health centers accord these practices high priority in their overall program to combat the transmission of hepatitis effectively (Falzon et al., 1997). Used needles and sharp objects also pose a serious risk of hepatitis transmission and need to be handled with extreme caution. The application of a tightly controlled regimen for disposing of sharps and encouraging the use of needleless systems can significantly lower the risk. Training on the dangers of unsafe injection practice is important because it informs the patients and the health workers of the danger of injury and harm in case of carelessness. Additionally, promotion of harm reduction strategies, such as needle exchange, has also been effective in lowering the rates of infection with hepatitis in certain populations. By giving people access to clean needles and guaranteeing safe disposal is accessible, these schemes not only work to safeguard public health but also promote a sense of responsibility among users. Overall, the combination of proper methods of disposal with education awareness is essential in the fight against bloodborne viruses (Strobel & Ward, 2012). Lastly, public involvement is essential in disseminating information on the prevention of hepatitis and bloodborne viruses through safe practices. Public health education campaigns aimed at boosting awareness of the transmission modes and regular screening can greatly influence community engagement in prevention. Special care must be exercised for vulnerable groups, who may be at higher risk of infection based on social determinants of health. Actions taken to build trust among healthcare workers and these groups are crucial, particularly for Indigenous Australians, who experience multiple health services use barriers. By developing positive rapport, healthcare workers are able to provide culturally appropriate education and information targeted at the specific requirements of these groups. An informed and engaged public is important in establishing a healthier society as well as effective control of hepatitis and other transmissions of bloodborne viruses (Strobel & Ward, 2012).

6.5.3. Public Health Campaigns

Public health action against hepatitis and bloodborne viruses (BBVs) is crucial in addressing the disproportionate prevalence of these diseases in marginalized groups. Indigenous Australians, for instance, have very high levels of hepatitis B and C infections, as well as other sexually transmitted infections, with the underlying factor based on chronic misconceptions and institutional prejudice within healthcare systems. This setting poses challenges to public health practitioners tasked with creating responsive outreach programs. Interventions with culturally appropriate messages, outreach work in communities, and education on the risk of infection are required. Such interventions can regain confidence and facilitate increased participation in screening and immunization, and consequently enhance the health of these groups (Strobel & Ward, 2012). Furthermore, targeting high-risk groups, such as drug users, remains a concern for public health campaigns with the aim of reducing hepatitis transmission. The availability of hepatitis A and B vaccines under license has provided the key opportunity to decline the risks associated with drug use. There is evidence that successful vaccination programs can be implemented among drug users, which demonstrates the effectiveness and practicability of health education among drug users. By employing strategies such as needle exchange programs and focused vaccination drives, public health programs can efficiently limit the transmission of hepatitis infections, again highlighting the need for ongoing funds and funding for such initiatives (Lugoboni et al., 2009). Evaluation of the effectiveness of public health campaigns is essential to strategy improvement and longer-term health goals. Data collection and analysis regarding campaign coverage, participant demographics, and outcomes such as vaccination rates and reduced infection rates are pertinent. Community engagement not only leads to policy support but also the possibility of a collective response in understanding how barriers and facilitators of accessing health services could vary. Through the utilization of this knowledge, public health campaigns can adjust and refine their messages and delivery mechanisms, making interventions more effective in combating hepatitis and BBVs. Ultimately, these campaigns will play an important role in reducing health inequalities and improving population health in the long term.

SUMMARY

The public health emergency that is posed by hepatitis and bloodborne viruses to vulnerable populations must be answered by swift, multifaceted interventions. It is not only a health responsibility but a profound social responsibility — especially in the aftermath of the disparities facing Indigenous Australians, whereby they experience far greater infection rates compared to their non-Indigenous peers. The systemic and historical mechanisms of distrust and the resulting health inequities must be addressed; health care alone is insufficient without an acknowledgment of and a reaction to the social setting that these groups are a part of. In this manner, bridging the gap between Indigenous peoples and health services is necessary in order to promote health literacy and culturally competent care. Such efforts need to extend beyond clinical interventions to involve community engagement and advocacy that acknowledges the historical injustices that frame health behavior and access to services, thus opening the door to improved health outcomes. Changes in the treatment of hepatitis C also underscore the necessity of balancing innovative medical practice with inclusive public health policies. The recent developments in the serological detectability and treatment protocols have thrown new light on methods of controlling this infection, but the innovations must be accompanied by the education program aimed at eradicating stigma. As noted, the outcomes of neglected hepatitis C can cause serious financial costs not only to the patient but also to the healthcare system and society at large (Falzon et al., 1997). Considering this, prevention, early detection, and proper management in a concerted effort becomes the urgent call. Patient education and ensuring equal access to treatment are important components of an expansive strategy with the aim of not only stopping the hepatitis C epidemic but also contributing towards a healthier and better-educated populace. Lastly, the conclusion from the ongoing discussion regarding hepatitis and bloodborne infections is that collaboration and community-based approaches are essential to bringing about change. Since the prevalence of these infections continues to burden healthcare systems, stakeholders must shift toward complementary approaches that encompass prevention, treatment, and education at the community level. This is particularly essential for Indigenous populations, where systemic inequalities have placed barriers to care (Strobel & Ward, 2012). By connecting healthcare practices with the cultural habits and experiences of these groups, there is a capacity for trust-building and facilitation of engagement with healthcare. In doing so, public health initiatives can become more effective, connecting with the larger goal of reducing rates of hepatitis and bloodborne viruses while also endeavoring to address the social determinants that drive health inequities. This holistic approach is not just to address the current crisis but also to open up paths for a healthier future.

Understanding the complexities of hepatitis and bloodborne viruses entails embracing a series of main points that guide public health policy and policymaking. The detail on hepatitis C, for instance, highlights the significance of particular health programs. These programs aim to address the mind-boggling infection rates and identify successful prevention strategies. A key component of this situation is the necessity for health planners to acknowledge and address issues relevant to the regional impact of hepatitis C. As seen in the dialogue between health authorities, the determination of these key factors assists in developing a concerted response to the disease and increasing awareness among infected communities (Hunter, 2017). This targeted strategy not only raises the level of treatment measures quality but also facilitates educational outreach, particularly among the more vulnerable groups. Additionally, demographic determinants of health behaviors, particularly among young men, provide important information in understanding the broader picture of hepatitis and other infections. It is revealed that males aged 0–24 years possess significant health disparities, particularly in behaviors that could render them more vulnerable to infections like hepatitis. For instance, aggressive behavior, such as use of drugs or unsafe sex, accounts for the prevalence of bloodborne viruses in this group. Therefore, measures for better health have to focus on how to reverse such behavior and offer young men both prevention tools and information on the risks of hepatitis and other similar diseases. Identifying this connection between age-related health behavior and susceptibility to infection is important for developing successful health policy. Lastly, it is important to understand the larger public health implications of hepatitis and bloodborne viruses beyond personal health consequences. The social costs of untreated infections can be high, including healthcare costs, loss of productivity, and the possibility of transmitting infection in community settings. Thus, formulating comprehensive policies that address prevention as well as treatment of hepatitis is not only a health necessity but also an economic. By making use of the results of research that clearly indicate the sexual and injury-related health disparities in young men, public health programs can target more effectively the most vulnerable areas (Hunter, 2017). In the attempt to reduce the incidence of hepatitis and bloodborne viruses, concerted efforts must be made in terms of education, early treatment, and commencement of supportive health services across communities.

CLOSER LOOK

HIV PATHOGENESIS

Human immunodeficiency virus (HIV) is a retrovirus causing acquired immunodeficiency syndrome (AIDS) by increasingly debilitating the immune system. HIV preferentially infects CD4+ T lymphocytes, which are critical for immune modulation and mounting immunity. Pathogenesis of HIV arises from complex interactions between the host immune system and the virus, ultimately leading to immune suppression, opportunistic infection, and, unless treated, mortality.

HIV enters the body through mucosal surfaces, blood, or perinatal exposure. The virus primarily infects CD4+ T cells, macrophages, and dendritic cells. Host cell entry occurs through interaction between the viral envelope glycoproteins (gp120 and gp41) and the host CD4 receptor and a co-receptor — CCR5 (most importantly during primary infection) or CXCR4 (most importantly during late infection). Upon entering the host cell, HIV uses its enzyme reverse transcriptase to convert its single-stranded RNA genome into double-stranded DNA, which is then integrated into the host genome by the enzyme integrase. The integrated viral DNA, also known as a provirus, can be latent or transcriptionally active to form new virions (Figure 6.16).

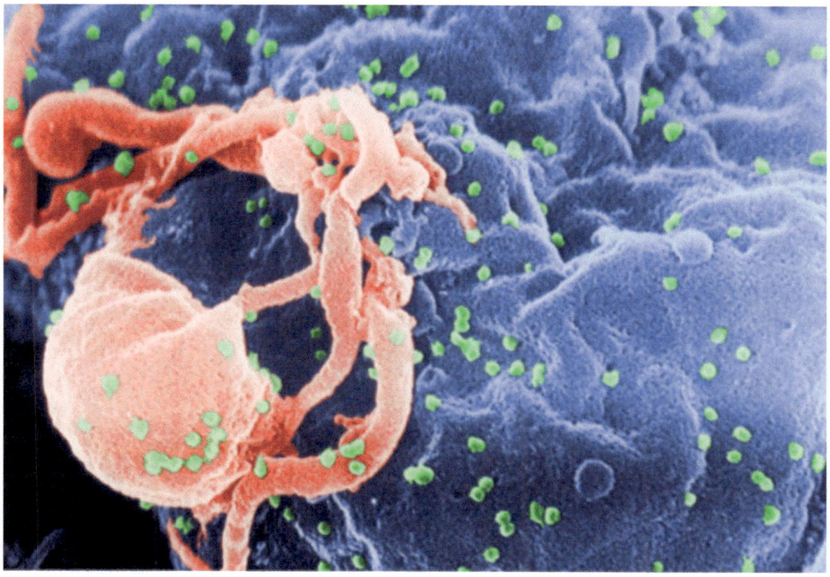

Figure 6.16. Colorized scanning electron micrograph showing HIV (green) budding from the surface of a cultured human immune cell (blue), with cellular filopodia (red) aiding in viral spread.

Source: https://upload.wikimedia.org/wikipedia/commons/1/1a/HIV-budding-Color.jpg.

In the acute infection phase, which arises in weeks following exposure, the virus replicates extensively to induce high viral load and aggressive CD4+ T cell depletion. The syndrome can be preceded by influenza-like illness, but is otherwise not diagnosed. The body responds by initiating cytotoxic T lymphocytes (CTLs) and neutralizing antibodies that retard the viral load. However, HIV is highly mutable and quickly develops resistance to the immune system.

Following the acute phase is the clinical latency phase, which could be several years. During this phase, the virus is still active at low levels and CD4+ T cells slowly diminish. Although the patient could be asymptomatic, the immune system still deteriorates progressively. The ability of HIV to create latent reservoirs in resting memory CD4+ T cells and other tissues is primarily responsible for its persistence and renders eradication challenging.

As the CD4+ T cell count continues to fall, the individual enters the AIDS phase, defined by a CD4+ count below 200 cells/mm^3 or the presence of specific AIDS-defining illnesses such as Pneumocystis pneumonia, Kaposi's sarcoma, cytomegalovirus retinitis, or tuberculosis. The immune system is severely compromised, leaving the individual vulnerable to opportunistic infections and malignancies.

HIV pathogenesis is also marked by chronic inflammation and activation of the immune system that results in the gradual loss of CD4+ T cells. Mechanisms involve direct killing of the infected cells by the virus, immune-mediated lysis of the infected and uninfected bystander cells, and destruction of the gut-associated lymphoid tissue (GALT), causing microbial translocation and systemic immune activation.

Antiretroviral therapy (ART) treatment can suppress viral replication, reconstitute CD4+ counts, and slow progression to AIDS. ART is not a cure and should be taken lifelong due to ongoing existence of reservoirs.

REFERENCES

1. Lugoboni, F., Quaglio, G., Civitelli, P., & Mezzelani, P. (2009). Bloodborne viral hepatitis infections among drug users: the role of vaccination. *International journal of environmental research and public health*, *6*(1), 400–413. https://doi.org/10.3390/ijerph6010400 (accessed on 16th July 2025).
2. Ali, N., Gilbert, R., & Pervaiz, M. (2018). *The prevalence and under-reporting of needle-stick injuries among dental healthcare workers in Pakistan: A systematic review*. https://core.ac.uk/download/159074647.pdf (accessed on 16th July 2025).
3. Allen, S., Barclay, S. T. Bhattacharyya, D., Dillon, J., et al. (2018). *Impact of previous hepatitis B infection on the clinical outcomes from chronic hepatitis C? A population-level analysis*. https://core.ac.uk/download/293863732.pdf (accessed on 16th July 2025).
4. Palmateer, N., Anderson, N., Wadd, S., Hutchinson, S., Taylor, A., & Goldberg, D. (2008). Exploring associations between perceived HCV status and injecting risk behaviors among recent initiates to injecting drug use in Glasgow. *Substance use & misuse*, *43*(3-4), 375–388. https://doi.org/10.1080/10826080701202908(accessed on 16th July 2025).
5. Aung Thein, O., Crawford, G., Davis, K., Hallett, J., et al. (2024). *Review of epidemiology, prevention and management of blood-borne viruses experienced by Aboriginal and Torres Strait Islander peoples*. https://core.ac.uk/download/638727696.pdf (accessed on 16th July 2025).
6. Battle, L. C. (1994). *Regulation of Medical Waste in the United States*. https://core.ac.uk/download/46711429.pdf (accessed on 16th July 2025).
7. Petignat C, Blanc DS, Francioli P. Occult Nosocomial Infections. *Infection Control & Hospital Epidemiology*. 1998;19(8):593-596. doi:10.1086/647880(accessed on 16th July 2025).
8. Brown, N. J. (2019). *Communicable Diseases and the Workplace*. https://core.ac.uk/download/219377207.pdf (accessed on 16th July 2025).
9. Fábio Fernandes Dantas Filho, Eunice Beatriz Martins Chaves, Maria Carlota Borba Brum , Francisco Jorge Arsego Quadros de Oliveira (2017). *Risk factors affecting occupational exposure to blood and body fluids among dental students: A cross-sectional study in a Brazilian federal university*. Clin Biomed Res 2017;37(1) https://core.ac.uk/download/303956346.pdf (accessed on 16th July 2025).
10. Chongswatdi, N. N., Franks, A. M., Harman, M. J., et al. (2022). *Analysis of blood borne pathogen exposure monitoring protocol adherence in an academic medical center: A seven-year analysis and literature review*. https://core.ac.uk/download/519836119.pdf (accessed on 16th July 2025).
11. Cox, A. L., Orkin, C., Centers for Disease Control and Prevention (CDC), Cohen, D. M., Conway, D. P., Lamoury, F. M. J., et al. (2018). *Point-of-care screening for a current hepatitis C virus infection: Influence on uptake of a concomitant offer of HIV screening*. https://core.ac.uk/download/286027388.pdf (accessed on 16th July 2025).
12. Cutler, S. J., Fooks, A. R., & van der Poel, W. H. M. (2010). *Public health threat of new, reemerging, and neglected zoonoses in the industrialized world*. https://core.ac.uk/download/pdf/29238214.pdf (accessed on 16th July 2025).
13. Zafar, A., Habib, F., Hadwani, R., Ejaz, M., Khowaja, K., Khowaja, R., & Irfan, S. (2009). Impact of infection control activities on the rate of needle stick injuries at a tertiary care hospital

of Pakistan over a period of six years: an observational study. *BMC infectious diseases*, *9*, 78. https://doi.org/10.1186/1471-2334-9-78(accessed on 16th July 2025).

14. Falzon, D., Gauci, C., Mallia Azzopardi, C., Portelli, A., et al. (1997). *Hepatitis C: An Emerging Concern*. https://core.ac.uk/download/46601989.pdf (accessed on 16th July 2025).
15. Hope, V., Kimber, J., Vickerman, P., Hickman, M., & Ncube, F. (2008). Frequency, factors and costs associated with injection site infections: findings from a national multi-site survey of injecting drug users in England. *BMC infectious diseases*, *8*, 120. https://doi.org/10.1186/1471-2334-8-120(accessed on 16th July 2025).
16. Hunter, S. (2017). *The five W's of bloodborne pathogens: Who, what, when, where, and why*. https://core.ac.uk/download/143838338.pdf (accessed on 16th July 2025).
17. Imani, R., Karimi, A., & Rouzbahani, A. (2008). *Seroprevalence of HBV, HCV and HIV infection among intravenous drug users in Shahr-e-Kord, Islamic Republic of Iran*. https://core.ac.uk/download/143842202.pdf (accessed on 16th July 2025).
18. Mashoto, K. O., Mubyazi, G. M., Mohamed, H., & Malebo, H. M. (2013). Self-reported occupational exposure to HIV and factors influencing its management practice: a study of healthcare workers in Tumbi and Dodoma Hospitals, Tanzania. *BMC health services research*, *13*, 276. https://doi.org/10.1186/1472-6963-13-276(accessed on 16th July 2025).
19. Keenan, E., O'Connor, J. J., & Smyth, B. P. (1998). *Bloodborne viral infection in Irish injecting drug users*. https://core.ac.uk/download/34711516.pdf (accessed on 16th July 2025).
20. Shorten RJ, Wilson-Davies E (2017) The risk of transmission of a viral haemorrhagic fever infection in a United Kingdom laboratory. PLoS Negl Trop Dis 11(5): e0005358. https://doi.org/10.1371/journal.pntd.0005358(accessed on 16th July 2025).
21. Strobel, N. & Ward, J. (2012). *Education programs for Indigenous Australians about sexually transmitted infections and bloodborne viruses*. **ISBN:** 978-1-74249-300-8 https://core.ac.uk/download/pdf/30678470.pdf (accessed on 16th July 2025).
22. Wrentz-Hudson, D. A. (2015). *Emergency medical service worker knowledge of and compliance with occupational exposures to infectious diseases*. https://core.ac.uk/download/147834489.pdf (accessed on 16th July 2025).

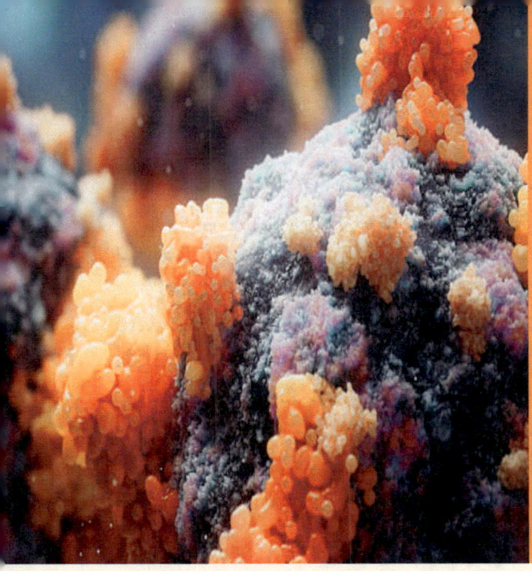

Chapter 7

FUNGAL PATHOGENS AND MYCOSES

Contents

Introduction

The research on fungal infections and mycoses is increasingly significant in modern medical practice because these organisms pose hazardous risks to human health. Fungi are present everywhere and are highly flexible, with crucial roles in the environment, but certain species possess severe infection potential, particularly among immunocompromised individuals. Mycoses, or fungal infections, can take numerous forms, ranging from cutaneous superficial infections to systemic invasive infections. Understanding the mechanisms of fungal infection and growth within the human host is central to the development of effective therapy. The alarming rate of invasive fungal infections requires enhanced awareness and the diagnostic capabilities to manage such infections appropriately. Immunological responses elicited by fungal infection are exemplified in studies of host-pathogen interactions that are complex in nature. Elevated cytokine levels of interleukin (IL)-6 and IL-8 following mold infections illustrate the state of immune activation and response of the body to combat fungal attackers. For instance, one study highlighted the prognostic value of IL-6 and IL-8 among patients with underlying hematological malignancies and suspected mold infection, suggesting that these biomarkers may be predictors of mortality among patient cohorts (Rawlings et al., 2019). A sound understanding of these immune reactions is not only useful in the diagnosis of mycoses but also in treatment regimen planning, particularly when antifungal therapy should be initiated. In addition, the design and management of antifungal therapy, such as itraconazole, are important considerations in fungal infection management. It has been proven by research that therapeutic drug monitoring can significantly enhance treatment outcomes by ensuring that patients are maintained at optimal drug levels (Vogeser et al., 2003). It is important to focus on pharmacokinetics and individualized treatment strategies, particularly in tertiary care institutions where infection is prevalent among immunocompromised patients. Conquering the limitations of fungal pathogens requires repeated innovations in diagnostic protocols as well as treatment monitoring, which will allow practitioners to effectively treat these complex infections and improve patient prognoses. Through steady inquiry and interdisciplinary exchange, the field can work to vanquish the severe challenges presented by fungal pathogens and mycoses.

Definition of Fungal Pathogens

Fungal pathogens are organisms belonging to the kingdom Fungi and possess the capability to infect plants, animals, and humans. Fungi are not like bacteria or viruses as they are eukaryotic organisms, i.e., they possess complex cell structures such as membranes and organelles. Fungal pathogens can broadly be categorized into yeasts, molds, and dimorphic fungi, each possessing its own characteristics and mechanisms of pathogenicity. Yeasts, such as *Candida* species, are mostly unicellular and often opportunistic pathogens, especially in immunocompromised hosts. Molds, on the other hand, are multicellular and can grow as extensive networks of hyphae, which are indeed for their ability to invade tissues and generate biofilms. These characteristics highlight the importance of proper classification of fungal pathogens, as such information is very crucial to the effective diagnosis and treatment of mycoses, the diseases caused by them.

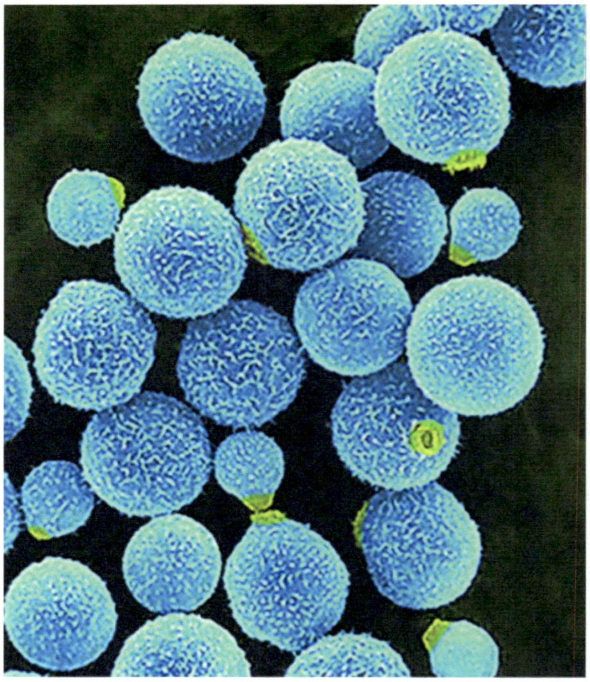

Figure 7.1. Fungal pathogens of humans, animals, and plants.

Source: https://www.ncbi.nlm.nih.gov/books/NBK549988/bin/AAMCol.18Oct.2017.fig09.jpg.

One of the most striking characteristics of fungal pathogens is their biofilm production, which enhances their virulence and makes them more resistant to treatment. Biofilms are complex communities of attached microorganisms embedded in a self-produced extracellular matrix, and they are highly resistant to antifungal therapy. *Candida albicans* is usually the best studied organism regarding biofilm formation, but non-*Candida albicans* species are also becoming increasingly targeted due to their clinical relevance. The heterogeneity and structural complexity of biofilms contribute to differential patient reactions during infection, as various strains may show variations in pathogenic potential. The clinical observation emphasizes the relevance of considering the genetic diversity of fungal pathogens while formulating treatment in view of the fact that, in the case of widespread antifungal resistance and increased incidence of opportunistic infections, taking this factor into consideration becomes relevant (Kean et al., 2018) (Figure 7.1).

Knowledge of the definition and medical implications of fungal pathogens is crucial for the control of mycoses' large-scale public health problems. The latest approaches to the study of these organisms highlight the multifaceted nature of the research, including both environmental and clinical isolates, in order to document their diversity and accommodation. Key findings in molecular biology approaches have unveiled the means through which such pathogens thrive and interact with host systems, thus making it possible to achieve better diagnosis and targeted therapy. Furthermore, the association between fungal pathogens and their human hosts is more and more framed in relation to immunology and host-pathogen interactions. This perspective is not only significant in the development of antifungal drugs but also in understanding the immune response in combating fungal infections, which remain underappreciated in the broader infectious diseases arena (King et al., 2017).

Importance of Studying Mycoses

It is of critical relevance to appreciate the significance of knowledge regarding mycoses in addressing public health concerns, especially considering the growing number of fungal infections. Mycoses, those infections caused by pathogenic fungi, pose a significant threat, especially in immunocompromised individuals and patients with chronic illnesses. The rapid emergence of some fungi, including *Candida auris*, raises the need for intense inquiries into their pathogenicity mechanisms, epidemiology, and drug resistance. Current studies have shown that the clades of *Candida auris* have special traits that render it virulent and versatile, hence its treatment is challenging and demands ongoing monitoring and research (Kean et al., 2020). Knowledge gained through studies of such fungi will enable medical practitioners to implement improved diagnostic, therapeutic, and preventive strategies and, in the long run, bring about improved health outcomes and reduced healthcare costs. In addition, the environmental aspects of mycoses reveal how conditions outside impact the dissemination of fungal pathogens. Studies monitoring fungal loads in various environments, such as healthcare facilities, have come to the forefront of how hygiene protocols contribute to the inhibition of fungal growth. For example, a study at the University of Johannesburg found high microbial levels on chiropractic tables, demonstrating poor disinfection processes and the presence of bacteria and fungi (Kingham, 2019). The finding emphasizes the necessity of strict hygiene protocols in the clinical environment. Through investigating routes of transmission and extrinsic determinants influencing fungal infection, researchers can come up with improved public health interventions that raise awareness and even hinder the prevalence of disease-causing fungi within various populations. Finally, increasing resistance among fungal pathogens to conventional therapy necessitates further investigation into mycoses' biology and genetics. The emergence of resistant strains, such as *Candida auris*, highlights a significant knowledge gap in understanding fungal adaptive mechanisms and the implementation of effective antifungal therapies. Investigations into the genetic causes of resistance and virulence will provide researchers with the knowledge to fashion targeted therapies and novel antifungals. Furthermore, the multidisciplinary nature of mycology requires collaboration between clinical practitioners, microbiologists, and public health professionals. These efforts combined will make us more resilient in the battle against fungal infections, protecting vulnerable groups, and informing research agendas to follow, solidifying the importance of continued research into mycoses and their repercussions (Kean et al., 2020) (Figure 7.2).

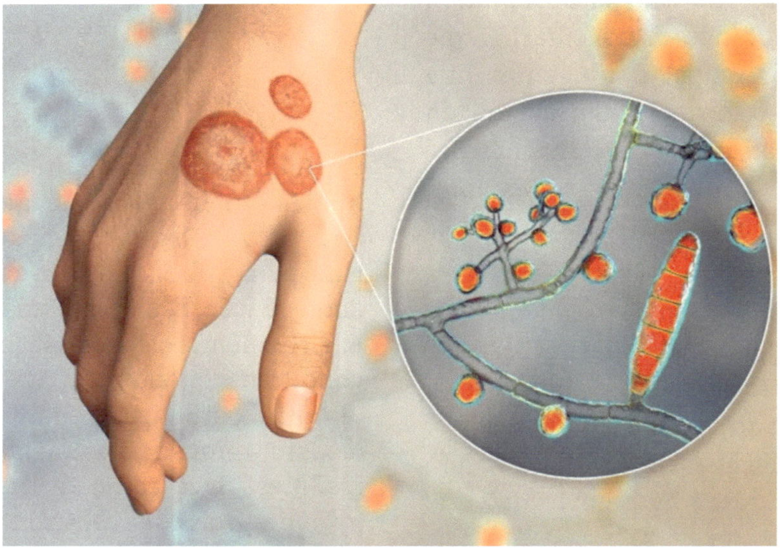

Figure 7.2. Skin mycoses.

Source: https://medissmedical.pl/wp-content/uploads/2024/06/grzybica-skory-mediss-medical-gdansk.webp.

7.1. Types of Fungal Pathogens

Fungal path diversity is diverse, and every species shows specific pathogenicity mechanisms as well as environmental niches. One of the prominent classes of such pathogens is yeast fungi that include species such as *Candida* and *Cryptococcus*, typically involved in opportunistic infections in human hosts. Yeasts are opportunistic pathogens that are found within various types of environments, both in nature and in the clinical environment. *Candida*, particularly *Candida albicans*, is the causative agent of mucosal infections and can cause systemic infection, especially in immunocompromised individuals. Rising cases of multidrug-resistant yeasts have emphasized the need for new diagnostic and therapeutic approaches. New technologies such as high-throughput sequencing are being researched to further detect these pathogens and reveal their resistance mechanisms in a bid to improve patient outcomes (Consortium OPATHY, & Gabaldón, 2019). In contrast to yeast fungi, filamentous fungi play a significant part in human disease as well, and *Aspergillus* and Mucor are the most significant genera. These molds tend to produce invasive infections, particularly in immunocompromised hosts, wherein they have the capacity to rapidly become invasive and pose serious clinical problems. *Aspergillus* species, for example, can be the cause of invasive aspergillosis, which is a highly morbid and lethal disease. Filamentous fungi are primarily entered through inhalation of conidia, resulting in lung infections that may progress to other organs. The identification of the pathogen could be complicated by its unique growth needs and the hardness of the environment. As a result of the unique pathogenic mechanisms, such as production of toxic secondary metabolites, understanding of the behavior and virulence of filamentous fungi is essential for successful clinical management (Nasr et al., 2010). Fungal pathogens are also differentiated on the basis of their mode of pathogenicity: primary pathogens and opportunistic pathogens. Primary fungal pathogens, including Histoplasma and Coccidioides, infect immunocompetent hosts in general and can produce serious disease, especially in areas where they are endemic. They are most commonly acquired by inhalation of spores and can resist host defense mechanisms by several tactics, such as modulation of the immune response. Opportunistic pathogens, on the other hand, generally infect individuals with compromised immune systems or underlying health conditions. Grasping this difference is central to the epidemiology and therapy of fungal infection. As the science of mycology continues to progress, ongoing research into mechanisms of pathogenicity, virulence factors, and host-pathogen interaction remains integral to the evolving development of targeted therapies and improved clinical outcomes in infected patients.

7.1.1. Yeasts

The contribution of yeasts to mycoses and fungal pathogens cannot be overemphasized, as they form a heterogeneous group of opportunistic fungi that can produce severe infections, particularly among immunocompromised patients. Among the numerous species, *Candida* spp. merits special mention for its ability to thrive in diverse environments within the human body. As a matter of fact, *Candida albicans* is a normal inhabitant of the human microbiota, but in certain conditions, it can proliferate unchecked and cause candidiasis, which has a broad range of clinical presentations from superficial infection to life-threatening systemic disease. Also, the increasing incidence of yeast infections is alarming, more so with these pathogens becoming increasingly resistant to antifungal agents, complicating treatment options and requiring new diagnostic tools and therapeutic interventions (Consortium OPATHY, & Gabaldón, 2019) (Figure 7.3).

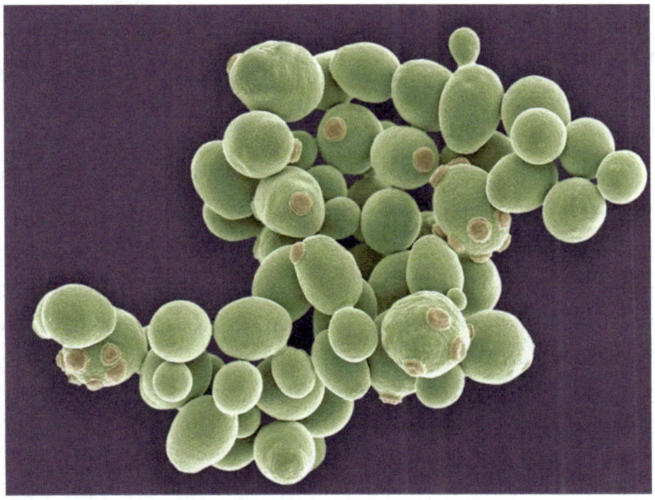

Figure 7.3. Yeast: Budding yeast cells.

Source: https://www.britannica.com/science/yeast-fungus.

The issues raised by yeasts like *Candida* spp. are not just their pathogenicity, but also their potential to evade the host immune system and produce recurrent infections. The production of proteolytic enzymes in these yeasts is of special significance in their potential to colonize host tissues and degrade the host's protective proteins. Specifically, research has shown that secreted aspartyl proteinases of *Candida* species can effectively break down precursors of kininogen, thereby disrupting the inflammatory processes of the hosts and favoring the establishment of infection (Nasr et al., 2010). Enzymatic activity during the process not only favors tissue invasion but also regulates the host's immune response, thereby allowing the pathogen to develop and survive in different niches of the human body. Hence, understanding the pathogenesis mechanisms used by yeasts is important in planning effective treatment and prophylactic strategies for fungal infections. The advent of new diagnostic technologies within the recent past has offered new methods for the detection of yeast pathogens and their detection for drug resistance. Traditional culture methodologies are often time-consuming and tend to lead to delayed diagnosis, which is particularly deleterious in the treatment of severe cases of yeast infection. On the other hand, novel high-throughput technologies such as next-generation sequencing and proteomics hold the promise to provide sensitive, quick, and precise detection of yeast pathogens. These groundbreaking techniques enable clinicians to achieve a greater understanding of the causative organisms and the resistance mechanisms, which is crucial for the development of proper antifungal treatment (Consortium OPATHY, & Gabaldón, 2019). However, translation of these technologies into the clinic is not without challenges, such as the need for standardized protocols and testing across different healthcare facilities. As research continues, one would expect these new modalities to enhance clinical outcomes and improve treatment regimens for infection by these virulent fungal pathogens (Figure 7.4).

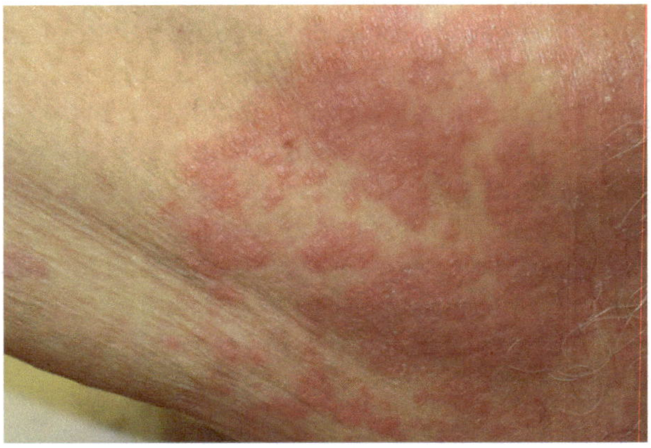

Figure 7.4. Yeast infection on the skin.

Source: https://www.verywellhealth.com/thmb/BIdTrVY7T7jCB5b3xHQwgf8jexs=/1496x1000/filters:no_upscale():max_bytes(150000):strip_icc()/VWH_DermNet_Intertrigo-Candida_011-438df9c065c24f82a0a37f4bedda98bd.JPG.

7.1.2. Molds

Molds, as one of the most common classes of fungal pathogens, are infamous for their ability to cause a range of mycoses, particularly in immunocompromised subjects. Mold growths are highly adapted to diverse environments and express themselves in diverse forms, ranging from filamentous structures known as hyphae. Molds' pathogenicity is most commonly related to their tendency to grow into host tissues, forming deadly diseases such as aspergillosis and mucormycosis. These infections are most prevalent among the population with underlying illnesses, such as hematological malignancies or diabetes mellitus, in whom they exhibit compromised immunity. Understanding mold biology and pathogenic mechanisms is important in developing effective treatments and preventive interventions, and this makes it critical that research is ongoing in mycology and the management of infectious diseases (King et al., 2017). The immune reaction to mold infection is a delicate dance of cytokines, and this can directly influence the clinical course of infected individuals. Among these signaling molecules, IL-6 and IL-8 have been identified as important biomarkers in the context of exposure to and infection by mold. Elevated levels of these cytokines have been associated with increased morbidity and mortality among infected patients. Specifically, IL-6 and IL-8 levels in blood and bronchoalveolar lavage fluid (BAL) have been demonstrated to be capable of predicting 30-day all-cause mortality in patients with assumed mold infections (Rawlings et al., 2019). Hence, timely analysis and interpretation of cytokines may provide valuable prognostic hints, underlining the importance of cytokine kinetics in mold pathologies. Apart from cytokine reactions, identification of mold-specific biomarkers is important for accurate and timely diagnosis of fungal infections. Biomarkers such as galactomannan (GM) and β-D-glucan (BDG) are at the forefront of the early detection of invasive mold infections. These substances, which occur in body fluids, correlate with the occurrence of fungal cell wall components and have been established to be in good correlation with the severity of infection and patient outcomes. The integration of biomarker testing into clinical practice can potentially enhance the diagnostic accuracy for practitioners and provide the opportunity for early intervention. It is most important in high-risk populations, including patients with hematological malignancies, where detection and treatment of mold infection can make a profound impact on survival rates, underlining the importance of expanding our knowledge of mold pathogenesis and diagnostics in the clinical environment (King et al., 2017).

7.1.3. Dimorphic Fungi

Dimorphic fungi studies depict how they possess a unique characteristic of existing in two disparate morphological states, directly associated with their pathogenicity in humans. Dimorphic fungi are capable of undergoing transition between the yeast form, most frequently encountered during the parasitic state, and the filamentous or mycelial form, most frequently encountered under environmental conditions. It is a key aspect of their virulence and host survival, allowing them to become accommodated in various habitats within hosts as well as evade immune assault. Their pathogenicity relies heavily upon this morphological shift, since it is that which allows the fungi to infect tissues and cause disease, leading to severe clinical complications in immunocompromised hosts or those with underlying disease. Explanation of the mechanisms governing this transition is a relevant area of study for fungal pathogens since it holds promise for new therapeutic approaches to the treatment of mycoses due to these pathogens. Of the principal dimorphic fungi, those belonging to the Onygenales order, such as *Histoplasma capsulatum* and *Blastomyces dermatitidis*, are of great clinical importance since they produce severe conditions such as histoplasmosis and blastomycosis. These fungi normally inhabit specific geographic regions, typically with environmental niches like soil enriched with bird or bat dung. Once inhaled, the spores can become their yeast form in the host, yielding a range of respiratory and systemic manifestations. Pathogenic mechanisms employed by these fungi are complex, most often involving manipulations of host cell milieus to maximize fungal survival and dissemination. Recent genomics have hopefully enriched our understanding of the special adaptations of these fungi, underscoring the importance of gene family expansions and contractions of each species that are fundamental to understanding their evolutionary success and pathogenicity in human life (Whiston & Taylor, 2015). Reactive research is interested in the evolutionary developments that occur in the dimorphic fungi with a view to how these fungi have evolved with strategies of surviving harsh host conditions. Phylogenomic studies reveal that the capacity of these fungi to increase their gene family while concomitantly decreasing others is a hallmark of their adaptability in various ecological situations. For instance, studies have elucidated Coccidioides spp.'s particular genes responsible for their particular parasitic phase, including the formation of spherules. Such evidence determines that gene family dynamics are not only important in the evolutionary adaptation of the fungi but also in infecting and causing illness. By crossing genomic data with clinical data, researchers are able to find specific targets for antifungal therapy that may shatter these pathogenic cycles, thereby enhancing treatment prospects for severe mycoses caused by dimorphic fungi (Chakrabarti et al., 2018) (Figure 7.5).

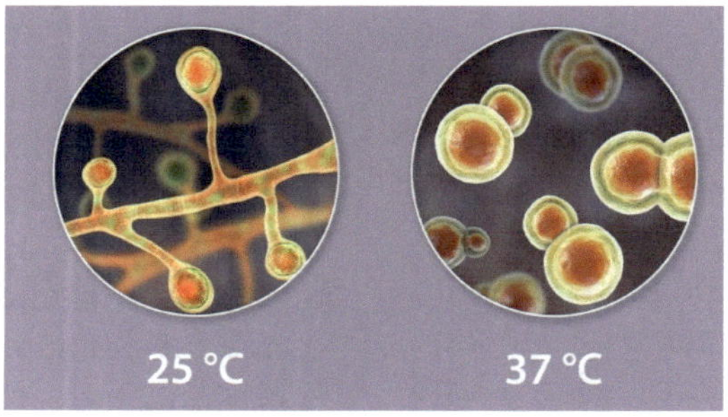

Figure 7.5. Dimorphic fungus.

Source: https://microbialnotes.com/wp-content/uploads/2023/03/dimorhpic-fungi.webp.

7.2. Mechanisms of Pathogenicity

The pathogenicity mechanisms utilized by fungal pathogens are multifarious and varied, allowing these pathogens to cause infections in their hosts. A major mechanism is the secretion of virulence factors such as enzymes and toxins that are used to invade and damage tissues. For example, some fungi secrete proteases and phospholipases that can digest host tissue, thereby promoting the dissemination and colonization of fungi. Furthermore, the ability to adhere to host cells by specific surface proteins enhances their potential to occupy niches within the host environment. The application of host immune evasion mechanisms is also vital; most fungal pathogens have developed the sophisticated mechanisms that allow them to evade or manipulate the innate immune response, enabling them to survive and proliferate in seemingly inhospitable environments. *Candida auris* exemplifies the complexity of fungal pathogenicity. This yeast also possesses a remarkable ability to adapt between various environments, which increases its virulence and survival in clinical settings. The existence of emergent distinct clades suggests the dynamic nature of the organism's epidemiology and potential to become resistant to antifungal treatment, rendering treatment difficult. The mechanisms can either be via changes in membrane composition or the increased efflux of the antifungal drugs, thereby impairing the effectiveness of treatment. With these adaptations, *C. auris* not only occurs but thrives, proving that being familiar with some of the genetic and phenotypic features that enhance its pathogenicity is of significance, as shown in the extensive library of literature elucidating its unique pathogenic features and clinical significance (Kean et al., 2020). Another feature of fungal pathogenicity is the ability of some fungi to form biofilms, a type of growth that complicates treatment and eradicability. Biofilms are composed of densely packed aggregates of fungal cells embedded in a self-produced extracellular matrix and offer more resistance to host immunity and antifungal agents. Biofilm formation is of paramount significance in the context of device-associated infection, in which fungi can infect device surfaces such as catheters and prostheses. The pathogenesis mechanism of biofilm resistance involves the extrusion of polysaccharides and proteins that protect the fungal cells from environmental stresses. Such biofilm dynamics reveal new insights into the development of strategies to combat fungal infections efficiently, and constant research on cellular and molecular mechanisms of fungal pathogenesis is warranted (Mayer et al., 2013).

7.2.1. Adherence and Invasion

The initial stages of fungal infections involve two processes that are crucial: invasion and adherence. Fungal pathogens' capacity to adhere to tissue is the gateway to effective colonization by them. Adherence is typically brought about by many surface structures, for instance, adhesins and biofilms, through which fungi become established in their separate niches within the host. For instance, *Candida albicans*, an opportunistic pathogen, uses a range of adhesion molecules to adhere to epithelial surfaces and result in infection. Its ability to form biofilms is vital to its virulence since such multicellular populations protect the fungal cells from host immune assaults as well as antifungal therapy. Also, adherence is not always a passive process but is rather a dynamic process that involves the host-pathogen interaction and can affect the resulting inflammatory response and allow further invasion into the deeper layers of tissue. Solidly adherent fungal pathogens can set the stage for the invasion process and lead to tissue damage and systemic infection. The modes of invasion vary among the different species of fungi, but usually involve degradation of the host's extracellular matrix substances and immune evasion. For example, *C. albicans* is able to secrete proteolytic enzymes that can hydrolyze the host tissues, enabling its invasion across mucosal barriers. This invasive capacity becomes crucial in immunocompromised hosts, where the host's defense mechanisms fail to destroy the expanding population of the fungus. The mortality and morbidity associated with invasive fungal infections underscore the importance of understanding the processes involved, for it offers the possibility of creating more effective therapeutic and preventive strategies. Innovation in research employing animal models has significantly advanced our understanding of the dynamics of adherence and invasion in fungal pathogenesis. The interaction between host immune responses and fungal adherence and invasion is complex and multifaceted. In particular, the immune response is essential to prevent or allow fungal colonization. The innate immunity detects fungal pathogens through pattern recognition receptors that recognize conserved fungal structures. Successful pathogens, such as *C. albicans*, developed the mechanism to manipulate host immune response in order to facilitate their adhesion and invasion. Greater insight into these interactions is of importance when building new immunotherapeutic strategies to manage fungal infection. Through the utilization of data from omics technologies and potential biomarkers, scientists are delineating how *C. albicans* develops in host environments, further elucidating host-pathogen interaction mechanisms. This research is highly significant, particularly in light of the fact that mortality due to *Candida* infection rises with numerous factors, including drug resistance and the growing numbers of immunocompromised hosts (Mayer et al., 2013; Basir et al., 2016).

7.2.2. Immune Evasion Strategies

Immune evasion strategies employed by fungal pathogens play a crucial role in their pathogenicity and survival within host organisms. *Candida* and *Aspergillus* are fungal pathogens that have developed many strategies to avoid the host immune response. Modulated cell wall constituents represent one of the primary strategies by which the pathogenic fungi become hidden from the immune system. Modulation of surface antigens allows such fungi to escape immune cell recognition, thereby permitting their invasions and proliferation. The alteration not only prevents attachment by antibodies but also phagocytosis, which permits such organisms to proliferate under unfavorable conditions. It has been found that changes in the polysaccharides present in the cell wall can significantly alter the immune response, and the sophistication with which fungi play upon host immunity has been firmly established. The other important immune evasion strategy observed during fungal infections is the secretion of immunomodulatory factors. These directly affect the function of immune cells, regulating the host's inflammatory response to the benefit of fungal survival. For instance, certain fungi release proteases that degrade cytokines and chemokines, stopping signal transduction pathways important for immune responses. This interference not only inhibits the activation of the immune cells but can also skew the immune response towards a tolerant or inefficient one. This stealthy approach allows such pathogens as *Candida auris* to survive within the host despite the presence of a normal immune system. As highlighted in recent studies, conservation of the pathogenic features across different clades of fungi poses significant concerns, suggesting wider applicability in the understanding of fungal pathogenesis and the development of effective treatments (Kean et al., 2020). Understanding these immunoevasive mechanisms is of paramount importance for designing therapeutic measures against fungal infection and mycoses. Targeting fungal pathways will enhance the immune response of the host, and this will result in better outcomes in infection treatment. Targeted research has focused on creating drugs that can inhibit the synthesis or action of immunomodulatory molecules produced by fungi, enabling the hosts to neutralize the infection. Furthermore, enhancing vaccine efficacy by presenting antigens that provoke robust immune responses can also prove beneficial against these smart pathogens. The constantly evolving and adapting character of fungal pathogens necessitates continuous efforts towards research and innovation, as seen with the funding drive towards medical mycology (Bain et al., 2015). Lastly, a better comprehension of immune evasion mechanisms will provide opportunities for developing more effective and targeted therapies for fungal infection.

7.2.3. Toxin Production

Toxin production is a key element in the pathogenicity exhibited by most of the fungal genera, and it is significant in the pathogenicity of human mycoses. Mycotoxins, being secondary metabolites of the fungi, possess the capability to alter host physiological processes, compromise immune reactions, and support disease. The synthesis of aflatoxins, for instance, by *Aspergillus flavus* strains, is widely known to be highly dangerous, leading to acute and chronic diseases in individuals affected. The toxins also pose food safety and consumption concerns for farm produce. Moreover, the ability of fungi to produce various mycotoxins aids their survival and fitness across most ecological niches and attests to their opportunistic pathogenicity in both immunocompetent and healthy hosts. The biosynthetic mechanisms of these toxins guide the design of treatment and prevention strategies against fungal infection. Antifungal properties of certain natural compounds, such as *Zataria multiflora* extracts, have opened up new avenues for the regulation of fungal toxin production. The report indicates that the essential oil constituent separated from this plant exerts an inhibitory effect on aflatoxin production at a transcriptional level, which has the potential to be used therapeutically for the regulation of the condition of mycotoxin diseases. The antifungal activities of carvacrol and thymol, the active compounds, are accompanied by induced morphological changes in fungi, which further inhibit toxin synthesis. Naturally, then, their inclusion in treatment regimens may endow a double action of inhibiting fungal growth while concurrently repressing toxin synthesis. This is a promising approach to limiting the health hazard of mycotoxins, thus enhancing patient outcomes of mycotic disease and generating a healthier environment. Additionally, the association between the growth of biofilms and the production of toxins among fungal pathogens like *Candida albicans* renders them challenging to treat. Biofilms, due to their structurally heterogeneous composition of numerous different cellular morphologies, provide a protective niche for fungi, as well as the secretion of toxins. Biofilms are extremely resistant to conventional antifungal therapy, enhancing the persistence of mycotoxin production within clinical settings. It is hence vitally important for the design of interventions to comprehend biofilm dynamics and their involvement in toxin expression. Analysis of clinical isolates also determines the genetic and phenotypic variation that influences toxin production and biofilm growth. This multi-disciplinary approach emphasizes the necessity for tailored treatment strategies that consider both the pathogenic action of the fungus and the resulting mycotoxin risks with an eye toward successful fungal infection control and resultant effects on health.

7.3. Common Human Mycoses

The prevalence of usual human mycoses has risen dramatically over the past several decades and is a public health issue worth attention from scientists and medical professionals alike. Of all fungal pathogens, *Candida* species are most notable in their capacity for acclimation to the human condition and the rising infection rates reported among immunocompromised individuals. Infections with *Candida* can occur in numerous forms, ranging from superficial mucosal infections such as oral thrush and vaginal candidiasis to more serious invasive candidiasis, which can lead to bloodstream infections. The spectrum in severity reflects the opportunistic nature of *Candida* spp., a feature again evidenced by their natural ability to produce biofilms on medical devices, thereby becoming progressively resistant to standard treatments. The continuous emergence of resistant *Candida* strains continues to justify vigilant monitoring and innovative therapeutic modalities to address such infections (King et al., 2017). As parallel with *Candida*, another crucial fungal pathogen is *Aspergillus* species, and more particularly *Aspergillus fumigatus*, with a range of respiratory infections, including allergic bronchopulmonary aspergillosis and invasive aspergillosis. These conditions affect most those with compromised immune status or underlying lung disease, producing a high morbidity and mortality. The airborne dispersion of *Aspergillus* spores leads to ubiquitous environmental exposure, but it is the host's immunity that ultimately decides whether the infection succeeds or fails. Recent studies indicate enhanced susceptibility to *Aspergillus* infection by co-morbid states such as cystic fibrosis and chemotherapy-induced neutropenia. Because of the rising global occurrence of such infections, it is critical to research their pathophysiology in a bid to design efficient prevention and treatment measures, given that the treatments could be limited for infected patients with resistant organisms (Wissing et al., 2013). Dermatophytes such as Trichophyton, Epidermophyton, and Microsporum are also among the most common fungal pathogens that infest human beings, leading to superficial infection to develop dermatophytosis. These infections can occur as ringworm, athlete's foot, and onychomycosis, compromising the quality of life of the infected individuals. Dermatophytes thrive best in warm and moist conditions and can easily be transmitted through direct contact with infected humans or contaminated surfaces, and their transmission hard to prevent. Treatment in most cases involves topical or oral antifungal drugs; however, resistant infections can necessitate long-term treatment and follow-up. The socio-economic burden of dermatophytosis need not be overemphasized since, in this case, work or school absenteeism occurs due to the infections. The attractiveness of effective public health interventions aimed at prevention as well as education would be the outcome. Discovering the complex mechanisms of resistance of the dermatophytes will equip health workers with the knowledge through which they will be able to combat the ubiquitous fungal infections (King et al., 2017).

7.3.1. Superficial Mycoses

Superficial mycoses are a category of fungal infections that primarily affect the outermost layers of skin, hair, and nails. They are usually caused by dermatophytes, yeasts, and non-dermatophyte molds and are characterized by their superficiality of invasion. Some common examples include tinea (ringworm), candidiasis, and pityriasis versicolor. Superficial as they are, they can cause a lot of distress, both to appearance and psychological well-being. The global spread of superficial mycoses is owing to environmental factors such as favorable weather, hot and humid climate, and greater exposure to potential fungal sources, typically within public facilities including swimming pools and locker rooms. Control of the public health problem entails awareness of the modes of transmission and the importance of correct diagnosis and treatment for the healing of the disease and prevention of complications. Treatment of superficial mycoses is usually with topical antifungals, which are adequate for infections in a localized form, and systemic in the more disseminated form. Azoles, allylamines, and polyenes are drugs that target the fungal cell membrane or block the cell wall biosynthesis and result in the destruction of the fungus cells. Cure of these infections depends frequently on timely diagnosis and adherence to regimens. Though not usually life-threatening, superficial mycoses are quite uncomfortable and can cause secondary bacterial infections if left untreated. Chronic superficial mycoses can even occasionally cause psychological distress due to the visible nature of the infection. Understanding the clinical relevance of these diseases, as well as pharmacologic options, is critical to healthcare providers in order to give the best patient care possible (Figure 7.6).

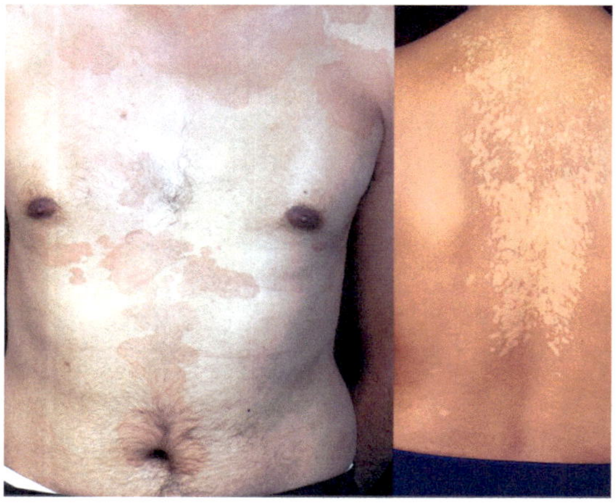

Figure 7.6. Superficial mycoses.

Source: https://www.adelaide.edu.au/mycology/sites/default/files/styles/ua_image_landscape/public/media/images/2021-09/pity-clin1.jpg?h=c4dd2c7b&itok=L0Ma0AIj.

Public education and awareness of superficial mycoses are basic components of prevention programs. Promotion of hygiene practices, such as drying the skin and not sharing personal items, can moderately but effectively reduce the risk of contagion. Moreover, individuals living or working in high-risk environments, such as athletes or individuals in tropical countries, should be more cautious. Enhanced public health programs aimed at encouraging awareness of these infections can encourage an approach to disease prevention. Moreover, as new research continues to reveal new fungal pathogens that may be capable of causing similar superficial infections, continued surveillance and further studies are needed. Lastly, an awareness, education-based solution with satisfactory treatment will better manage the incidence of superficial mycoses within different populations (Green et al., 1991; Schäfer et al., 2014).

7.3.2. Systemic Mycoses

The establishment of systemic mycoses as significant health problems emphasizes the complex interplay of fungal pathogens and immune mechanisms of the host. Systemic mycoses, typically caused by fungi such as *Histoplasma capsulatum*, *Coccidioides immitis*, and *Aspergillus* species, have the potential to be life-threatening, severe infections in immunocompromised hosts.

The pathogenesis of such an infection is usually environmental exposure and inhalation of spores, which become disseminated in other organs following initial lung colonization. Presentation is from acute respiratory distress syndrome to chronic debilitating disease and therefore highlights the need for early diagnosis and intervention. Identification of such pathogens requires cutting-edge laboratory techniques, encompassing sophisticated molecular diagnostics, which are crucial in guiding effective treatment strategies against such devious fungal foes (Liu & Paterson, 2011) (Figure 7.7).

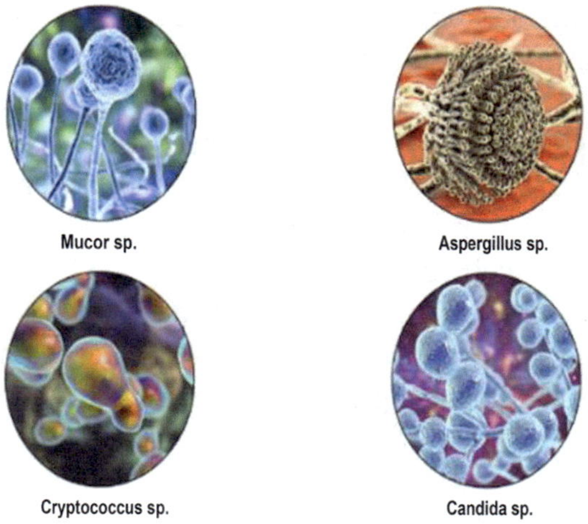

Figure 7.7. Systemic mycoses.

Source: https://microbialnotes.com/wp-content/uploads/2023/03/systemic-mycoses.webp.

Therapeutic interventions for systemic mycoses are dictated by the specific fungal pathogen and the clinical context of infection. Traditional therapy is primarily with systemic antifungal agents such as amphotericin B and its liposomal formulations. Advances in antifungal pharmacotherapy have introduced new drugs such as voriconazole, which is noted for its excellent oral bioavailability and broad-spectrum activity. It also offers both intravenous and oral modes of administration, facilitating half of the issue of logistics involved in long-term courses of treatment and enhancing patient adherence. Because infection typically requires therapy for several months, successful management hinges on both modalities being present in an effort to surmount complications arising from venous access (Abrahamse-Berkeveld et al., 2004). Furthermore, chronic challenges in the treatment of systemic mycoses are the need for long-term therapy and potential antifungal resistance. The character of the cell wall of fungi, inherently different from bacterial cells, necessitates certain antifungal modes of action that can have extremely dissimilar differences within pathogens. The costly realities of long-term therapies and the emergence of resistant organisms only add to the complexity of treating these diseases. Therefore, constant monitoring and study of the biology and treatment of systemic mycoses are essential. Constant research into the epidemiology, virulence determinants, and resistance mechanisms will ensure clinical practices and the creation of new antifungal strategies to manage the infection effectively (Liu & Paterson, 2011).

7.3.3. Opportunistic Mycoses

Opportunistic mycoses are of specific interest in the broad sense of the larger category of fungal pathogens and mycoses, and they nearly always develop among immunocompromised hosts. The pathogens are usually fungi that, in normal situations, are not particularly problematic for healthy hosts but become extremely pathogenic among hosts with compromised immune mechanisms, causing severe disease in the instance of patients undergoing chemotherapy, HIV/AIDS patients, or recipients of organ transplants. As the incidence of such predisposed states is rising globally, opportunistic mycoses too are bound to make a corresponding rise. This shift poses huge challenges to healthcare systems, as observed in recent studies, which point toward a notable rise in fungal infection rates within hospital settings, with an eerie emergence of antifungal resistance, necessitating heightened monitoring and new treatment strategies to combat such infections effectively (Schäfer et al., 2014). Critical to the pathogenesis of opportunistic mycoses is the virulence of certain fungal species, particularly those of the genera *Aspergillus*, *Candida*, and *Cryptococcus*. *Aspergillus fumigatus*, a well-characterized pathogen, is known to cause invasive aspergillosis, especially in patients who have impaired lung function or other clinical risk factors. *Candida* species, such as *Candida albicans*, also may lead to candidemia, which is revealed by infections within the blood and dissemination in the body. The challenge of diagnosing these infections is further aggravated by their broad clinical presentation, which has a tendency to imitate other diseases. Physicians are therefore required to adopt a high index of suspicion and employ advanced diagnostic techniques to differentiate fungal mycoses from other disease processes, thereby enabling early and relevant therapeutic interventions (Paterson & Lima, 2017).

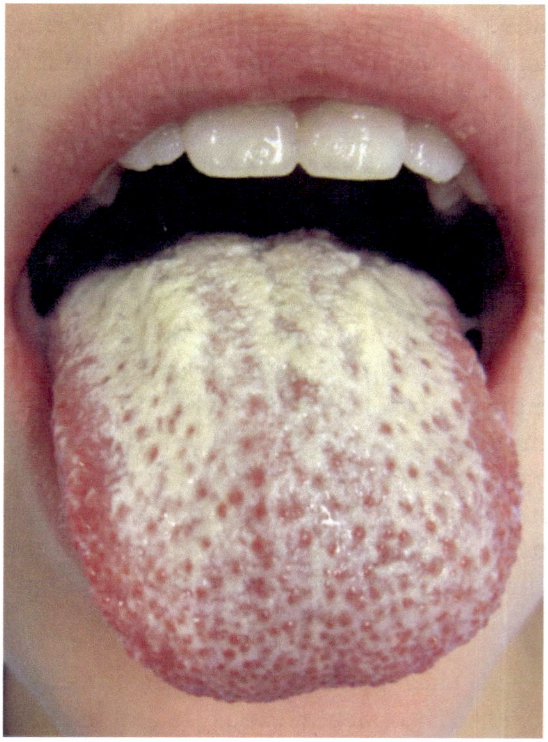

Figure 7.8. Opportunistic mycoses.

Source: https://upload.medbullets.com/topic/104077/images/human_tongue_infected_with_oral_candidiasis.jpg.

The interconnection of food reservoirs and opportunistic mycoses has been increasingly recognized by scientists and healthcare professionals in general. Research has indicated that certain fungal pathogens can be isolated from foods, a situation that is a cause of concern regarding their potential reservoir role for the infections of humans. Public health implications are of high priority, particularly among vulnerable groups. As a result, it is now necessary to have knowledge of the epidemiology of foodborne and human-infective filamentous fungi. It brings to the foreground the need for interdisciplinarity when food safety, medical mycology, and public health programs have to work together. By comprehensively navigating these areas of overlap, the scientific community is able to generate much increased awareness and reduce the occurrence of opportunistic mycoses and, consequently, alleviate a growing health issue (Paterson & Lima, 2017) (Figure 7.8).

7.4. Risk Factors for Fungal Infections

Risk determinants of fungal infections are multifactorial and typically entail the combination of intrinsic and extrinsic factors to create an appropriate environment for the pathogenic fungi. Intrinsic factors like diabetes, cancer, and immunosuppressive diseases are some of the conditions that compromise the body's defense mechanisms. For instance, patients undergoing chemotherapy have impaired immune responses, making them susceptible to opportunistic fungi. The diabetic contribution is particularly significant because elevated blood glucose promotes increased fungal growth. In addition, patient age contributes heavily, with the young and elderly being most vulnerable due to an underdeveloped or failing immune system. Knowledge of these intrinsic risk factors is valuable for clinicians in identifying populations at risk and implementing prevention measures. Extrinsic variables also occupy a primary role in fungal infection epidemiology. Environmental exposure is a significant determinant since certain ecological niches carry high densities of fungal spores. For example, individuals with occupational mold exposure, i.e., farmers or builders, are at increased risk. In addition, broad-spectrum antibiotic treatment disrupts normal microbiota such that opportunistic fungi, e.g., *Candida* species, have a niche to colonize. Hospital settings merely increase such risks, particularly intensive care units in which invasive procedures penetrate mucosal and skin barriers. An intensive care unit patient study, for instance, names the incidence of *Candida* infection as being large-scale, with many patients undergoing intravenous fluconazole administration but with a high rate of resulting concern regarding resistance, indicating the difficulty of delivering effective treatment to such infections (Wissing et al., 2013). Furthermore, clinical behavior significantly influences the risk of fungal infections. Growing numbers of immunocompromised subjects, due to improvements in medicine in therapy and treatment, need close monitoring for fungal pathogens in clinical settings. With more organ transplant recipients and HIV-infected subjects being treated, so also is increased the demand for individualized antifungal prophylaxis to guard against risks. Use of antifungal stewardship programs within hospitals has been effective in managing and limiting fungal infection cases among susceptible populations. These programs emphasize the importance of appropriate prescribing and even limit the growth of resistant fungal isolates, as shown by evidence demonstrating that a high percentage of *Candida*-infected patients were likely to be resistant to antifungal agents (Wissing et al., 2013). Collectively, in managing the risk factors, public health interventions to reduce the burden of fungal infections among various patient populations are crucial to be enhanced (Figure 7.9).

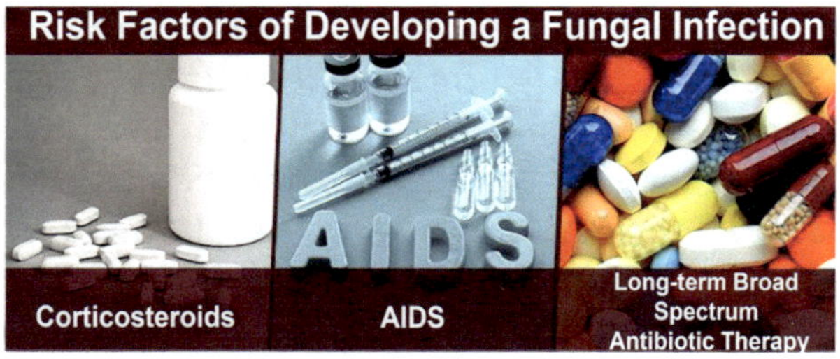

Figure 7.9. Risk factors of fungal infections.

Source: https://external-content.duckduckgo.com/iu/?u=https%3A%2F%2Fimages.medindia.net%2Fpatientinfo%2F950_400%2Frisk-factors-of-fungal-infections.jpg&f=1&nofb=1&ipt=e4b3fdd123dbdab96064f55747e397a239737cff6889374c706e3f2e3a246074.

7.4.1. Immunocompromised Individuals

The susceptibility of immunocompromised individuals to fungal infections is a critical problem in the domain of mycoses. These individuals experience compromised immunity due to diseases such as HIV/AIDS, cancer, or autoimmune diseases and are thus at risk of various fungal infections. *Aspergillus* and *Candida* species are the most prevalent fungal pathogens that infect these individuals and are known to cause severe systemic infections. The deficient ability to mount an effective immune response not only makes one susceptible to initial infection but also complicates treatment, leading to greater morbidity and mortality (Schäfer et al., 2014). Hence, understanding the mechanisms of the increased susceptibility of immunocompromised patients is extremely crucial in planning effective prevention and treatment strategies. Further, the clinical management of fungal infection in immunocompromised patients has to be handled with care, often involving the use of antifungal drugs that have to be properly selected based on the patient's own vulnerabilities. To illustrate, intravenous fluconazole is often applied in intensive care units to treat invasive candidiasis in patients with compromised immunity. A study revealed that approximately 32% of patients with evidence of *Candida* infection harbored potentially fluconazole-resistant strains, thereby reinforcing the importance of susceptibility testing in the treatment of antifungal therapy (Wissing et al., 2013). The multifactorial nature of drug resistance reinforces the need for ongoing investigations into potential alternative therapies such as novel antifungal drugs and combination regimens, which may enhance the treatment efficacy among this vulnerable group. In addition, the intrinsic heterogeneity of immune function among immunocompromised individuals necessitates a personalized approach to treatment. Factors such as the type of underlying condition, the level of immunosuppression, and the occurrence of concomitant infections significantly influence the susceptibility of a patient to fungal infections as well as the response to therapy. Such heterogeneity necessitates vigilance in monitoring and multidisciplinary management regimens that optimize both prophylactic and therapeutic regimens. With every new advance in the knowledge of the fungal pathogens and their interaction with the immune system, healthcare providers must remain vigilant and responsive in their management to reverse the imminent dangers these patients are exposed to (Schäfer et al., 2014). Effective control not only prevents deaths but is also essential in coping with the growing case load of fungal disease among this vulnerable population.

7.4.2. Environmental Exposures

Environmental exposures play an essential role in the presence and diversity of fungal pathogens, conditioning mycoses' epidemiology. A variety of natural and anthropogenic factors, such as climate change, land use changes, and urbanization, predispose the emergence of pathogenic fungi. For instance, temperature and humidity variations could facilitate the growth of certain fungi, particularly in subtropical and tropical areas. In addition, environmental disturbance by types of deforestation and industrial pollution can suppress natural ecological balance, promoting more contact among human beings and fungal spores and infection rates. All these serve to emphasize the need for persistent environmental monitoring, since environmental change can rather quickly be implicated in emerging fungal disease outbreaks, thereby requiring public health interventions that incorporate knowledge of determinants in the environment to curtail risk (Carver et al., 2009). In addition, urban environments present certain exposures that result in mycotic infections. Built-up areas tend to have a condensation of moisture and organic filth, which can support the development of opportunistic pathogens like *Aspergillus* spp. and *Cryptococcus neoformans*. The opportunistic pathogens thrive in organic-containing habitats, like the ones found in built-up areas with tendencies towards moisture and rot. The interaction of human populations with such urban microenvironments increases the susceptibility to infection, particularly among immunocompromised hosts. Furthermore, based on the Mycoses Study Group Education and Research Consortium research, it is suggested that knowledge of these environmental determinants and their implications for public health is critical for effective intervention measures. With growing urbanization, awareness of such urban-related exposures to fungal pathogens will only continue to play a significant role in preventing related mycoses (Little et al., 2024). Occupational exposure also plays a critical role in the risk of acquiring fungal infections, particularly in those occupations that involve the processing of organic material, such as agriculture, construction, and waste handling. Occupational employees are typically exposed to larger amounts of fungal spores, leading to increased opportunities for respiratory and systemic mycoses. For instance, farm laborers may inhale spores of soil-borne pathogens like *Histoplasma capsulatum*, especially where the environment is contaminated. The issue is even worse by climate uncertainty that may alter the location of these pathogens in the future. With more awareness of such occupational hazards, care should be taken to safeguard them and educate them on how to recognize symptoms of fungal infection. Finally, controlling these environmental and occupational exposures is critical to establishing overall strategies focused on managing fungal pathogens and decreasing mycoses' burden among affected groups (Carver et al., 2009).

7.4.3. Antimicrobial Therapy

Antimicrobial therapy remains the cornerstone of therapy for infections caused by fungal pathogens, particularly in the recent increase in nosocomial infections caused by pathogens such as *Candida*. The multiplicity of fungal infections necessitates a thorough understanding of mechanisms of microbial resistance. Intravenous fluconazole is one such commonly used first-line drug in intensive care. Research shows that despite the wide application of fluconazole, nearly 32% of patients with a confirmed *Candida* infection can harbor strains that may be resistant to the antifungal agent (Wissing et al., 2013). This statistic underlines the pressing need to follow antifungal susceptibility cautiously in a clinical setting and tailor treatment to the patient's microbial condition. An intimate understanding of the habitat in which fungal pathogens persist is crucial for effective antimicrobial design. Habitats in soil, termed heterogeneous microbial reservoirs, are difficult to treat with antifungal therapy due to the potential for resistance. Studies have shown that certain soil fungi possess resistance against conventional antifungal drugs, e.g., fluconazole, indicating potential mechanisms of resistance established under natural conditions (Nandkumar et al., 2010). This resistance may be due to selective pressures associated with antifungal usage, highlighting the cyclic nature of antimicrobial therapy problems. Thus, as these antifungal-resistant isolates are defined, they may potentially assume primary human pathogen status and need ongoing research and modification of therapy approaches. Antifungal resistance not only complicates treatment regimens but necessitates more emphasis on innovation in antifungal drug development. With the changing landscape of fungal infections, resistance surveillance becomes critical. Isolation of novel strains with the capacity to be resistant to several antifungal drugs can inform the discovery of new areas of therapy and treatment protocols. This becomes particularly critical in immunocompromised populations or where fungal infection has a high endemic rate. By recognizing the limitations and advances of antimicrobial treatments, medical professionals are able to enhance patient outcomes and prevent the devastating impact of pathogenic fungal disease.

7.5. Diagnosis of Fungal Infections

Diagnosis of fungal disease is a sophisticated process that involves extensive expertise in clinical presentation, patient history, and various laboratory methods. The clinician first evaluates the patient's symptoms, which may include chronic cough, fever, and lethargy, along with risk factors such as immunosuppression or ongoing antibiotic treatment. This clinical assessment culminates in laboratory confirmation, which often employs direct microscopy, culture, and serology to identify specific fungal pathogens. Notably, culture methods, while being gold standards, can take days to yield results, hence the need for rapid diagnostic tools. New molecular techniques, such as polymerase chain reaction (PCR), hold the potential for quicker diagnosis by direct detection of fungal DNA and enhancing the speed and accuracy of diagnostic processes in the clinical setting. New biomarkers have revolutionized the diagnosis of some fungal infections, particularly in immunocompromised individuals. For instance, biomarker quantification, such as galactomannan and β-D-glucan, has proven invaluable to diagnose invasive aspergillosis and candidiasis, respectively. These biomarkers are often detectable earlier during the disease process than traditional culturing methods, and they have been found to be of prognostic value. For instance, higher levels of cytokines interleukin-6 (IL-6) and interleukin-8 (IL-8) have been linked with poor clinical outcomes in infected individuals with fungal infections, particularly those who have hematologic malignancies (Rawlings et al., 2019). Hence, inclusion of these biomarkers in routine diagnostic procedures not only facilitates early diagnosis but also facilitates tracking of disease progression and the response to therapy, thus guiding patient management decisions. It is mandatory that attending physicians and clinical microbiologists collaborate closely to optimize the diagnosis of fungal infections. This interdisciplinarity also enhances the interpretative power of diagnostic tests and enables antifungal treatments to be tailored based on the specific fungal pathogens and resistance patterns. To mention just an example, as noted by Wellcome Trust-supported research (King et al., 2017), antifungal susceptibility testing via standardized protocols, for example, can significantly influence treatment decisions and patient outcomes. In addition, continuous education on new fungal pathogens and their resistance mechanisms must take place in both laboratory and clinical settings. A well-educated health care workforce will be able to better identify unusual presentations of fungal infections and, as a result, earlier and more accurate diagnoses, thus reducing morbidity for these infections.

7.5.1. Clinical Symptoms

The clinical manifestation of fungal infections is highly variable and generally dependent on the specific pathogen, infection site, and host immune status. Fungal pathogens such as

Candida spp., *Aspergillus* spp., and *Cryptococcus neoformans* are known to produce characteristic clinical features that can make their diagnosis and management challenging. Early symptoms can be in the form of nonspecific symptoms such as fever and malaise, which are often mistaken for other infectious or inflammatory diseases. Symptoms may also present locally depending on the location of infections; for example, pulmonary fungal infections would manifest symptoms such as cough, chest pain, and dyspnea, while cutaneous infections cause rashes or skin lesions. This diversity emphasizes the value of appreciating the clinical presentation of symptoms associated with mycoses to facilitate early intervention and enhance patient outcomes. In critically ill individuals, especially those in intensive care units, the presentation of invasive fungal infections may be indistinguishable from other more frequent entities, thus emphasizing the necessity of early diagnosis. For instance, the development of candidemia, an infection of the blood with *Candida* spp., typically develops nonspecifically and can lead to early detection and treatment difficulty. A study that examined intravenous use of fluconazole in the event of such instances noted that 32% of patients carried potentially resistant *Candida* strains, again highlighting the clinical importance of caution when managing such patients (Wissing et al., 2013).

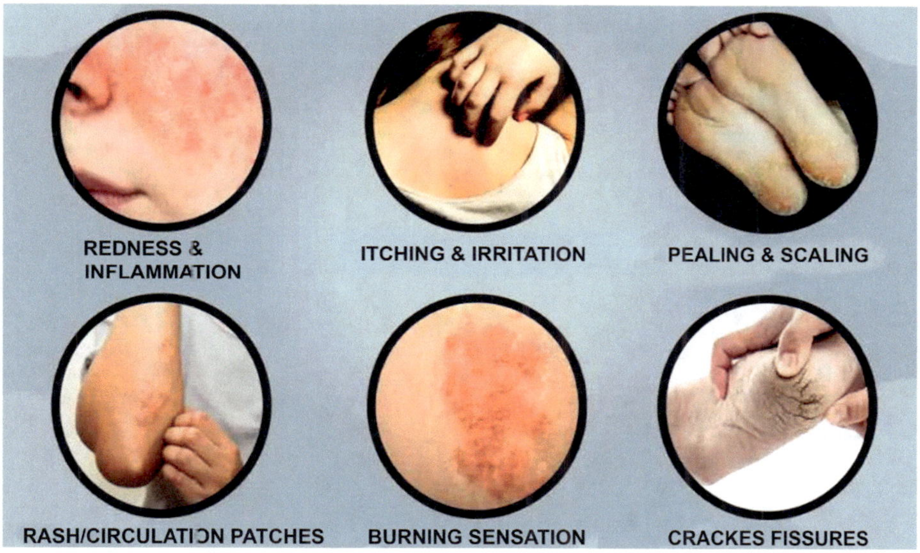

Figure 7.10. Symptoms of fungal infections.

Source: https://www.awishclinic.com/wp-content/uploads/2024/11/SYM-FUNGAL-1024x683.webp.

Symptoms may progress rapidly, especially given the patient's underlying health conditions, emphasizing the importance of standardized diagnostic protocols and surveillance approaches in the intensive care unit so as to promptly and accurately diagnose fungal infections. The consequences of neglected or misdiagnosed fungal infections may be severe, even involving high rates of morbidity and mortality. Patients with impaired immune systems, i.e., those on immunosuppressive treatment or those with chronic diseases, are particularly susceptible to the aggressive progression of mycoses. In fact, the general mortality rate among such patients suffering from such infections is usually very high, as evident in the numerous clinical reports on invasive fungal infections (King et al., 2017). This group puts significant importance on clinicians having a heightened index of suspicion for fungal infections, especially when presented with an atypical clinical presentation.

Proper knowledge of the diverse presentations of fungal pathogens and careful look-out for such infections are imperative steps that healthcare providers should take in order to avoid the potential high risks of fungal disease (Figure 7.10).

7.5.2. Laboratory Techniques

In clinical mycology, laboratory techniques are crucial to the quick and specific identification of fungal infections and their associated mycoses. Classical culture methods, while in the preparatory stage, are insensitive and nonspecific enough to successfully recognize opportunistic fungal infections. The importance of rapid and precise diagnosis has come into the spotlight due to increasing instances of antifungal drug resistance in species, emphasizing the identification of the pathogen as well as the susceptibility pattern. Recent advances have introduced new diagnostic technologies such as next-generation sequencing and proteomics, which are of great potential in enhancing detection efficiency.

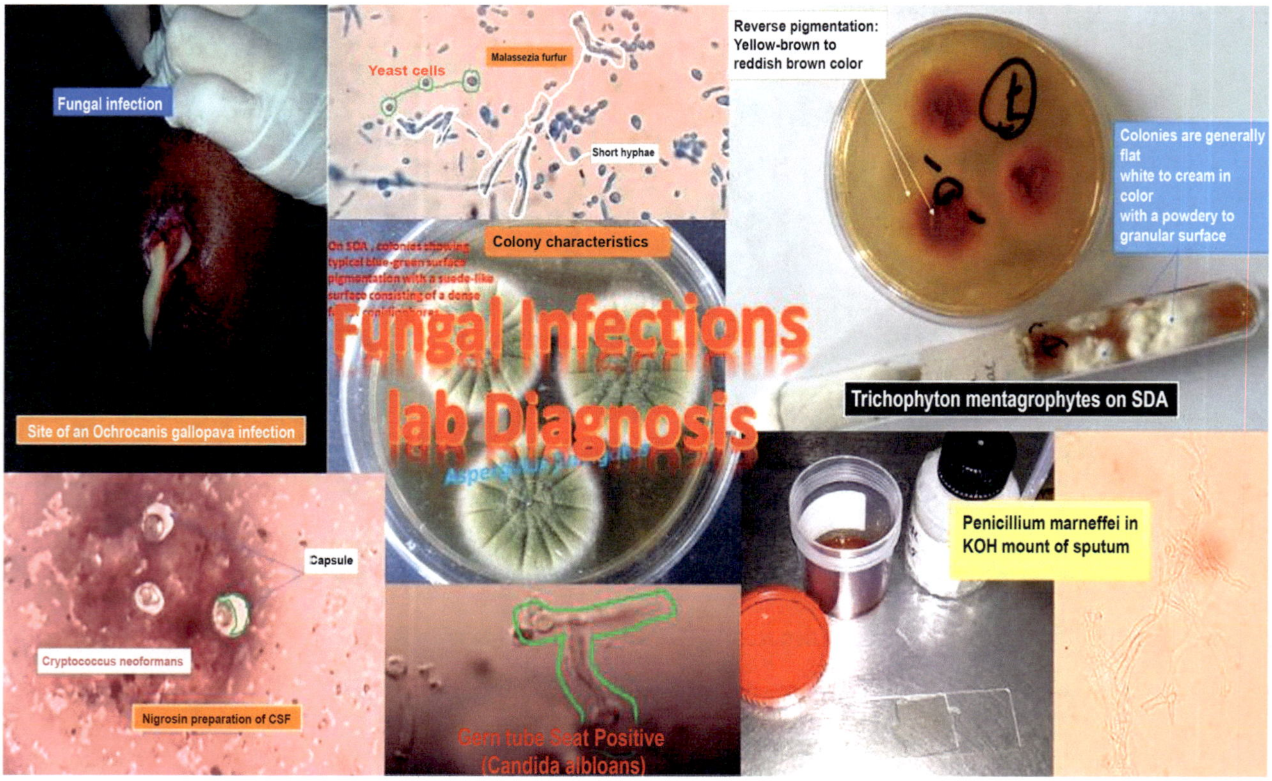

Figure 7.11. Fungal infections laboratory diagnosis.

Source: https://universe84a.com/wp-content/uploads/2020/04/Fungal-infection-Laboratory-diagnosisIntroduction-sample-collections-and-procedure.jpg.

These approaches not only curtail diagnostic time but also provide a comprehensive understanding of the phenotypic and genetic characteristics of causative fungi, hence making personalized therapeutic interventions possible (Consortium OPATHY, & Gabaldón, 2019). In addition, laboratory techniques utilized for the quantification of antifungal drugs provide an important interface of mycology and pharmacology. Therapeutic drug monitoring (TDM) has acquired growing significance, particularly in the case of drugs like itraconazole, which are virtually indispensable in the treatment of invasive fungal infections. The concomitant analysis of itraconazole and active metabolite hydroxyitraconazole by advanced methods such as liquid chromatography tandem-mass spectrometry and automated solid-phase extraction reflects the sophistication of current laboratory methodologies. Not only are they specific and precise, but they also yield rapid turnaround times essential for clinical decision-making. With changing resistance profiles of fungi, the incorporation of such advanced quantification methods into routine laboratory practice is inevitable for the optimization of patient outcome and ensuring successful prophylaxis and therapy regimens (Vogeser et al., 2003). Further, the adaptation of new laboratory technologies in clinical settings also points toward the potential of overcoming problem-solving due to the dynamic character of fungal pathogens. With hope generated by high-throughput approaches, eventual clinical application is fraught with difficulties in terms of standardization and validation of new techniques. Laboratories are placed on a tightrope of training on traditional methods while embracing innovations that have the potential to significantly enhance diagnostic capability. With continued research unveiling cutting-edge pathogen detection and surveillance techniques against fungi, lab personnel must see to it that operational procedures and quality control also keep abreast with the new developments. Combined, they will not only increase the accuracy of diagnostics, but they will also enable timely initiation of treatment that is effective, thus resulting in better clinical outcomes against evolving mycological threats (Consortium OPATHY, & Gabaldón, 2019) (Figure 7.11).

7.5.3. Imaging Studies

Imaging studies have emerged as a pillar in the diagnostic armory of mycoses and fungal infections, particularly for invasive fungal infection. Traditional methods such as culture and microscopy are necessary but are often plagued, for example, by difficult collection of sufficient clinical specimens and by prolonged turnaround time for cultures. As a result, imaging techniques such as computed tomography (CT) and magnetic resonance imaging (MRI) have become more pertinent to enhance the early detection and assessment of fungal infections. Current imaging technology can visualize lesions in organs, allowing for assessing disease burden and disease progression. These developments are critical in intervention timing since the effectiveness of treatment heavily depends on the rapid detection of the causative fungal etiology, as emphasized in the literature on management of invasive fungal infections (Dornbusch et al., 2010). The imaging tests not only aid in detection but also determine clinical decision-making for antifungal treatments. For instance, within immunocompromised patients, in whom invasive mold disease risk is elevated, precise imaging features can guide clinicians as to how to maximize antifungal prophylaxis and initiate appropriate treatment regimens. Such controversies on existing treatment paradigms highlight the controversy over the optimal time to institute mold-active antifungals, particularly during the early treatment stages. These imaging tests allow for the early diagnosis of fungal infection, thereby enabling pre-emptive treatment, which can significantly enhance oncology and hematology patient outcomes (Maertens et al., 2017). By facilitating a better-informed management plan for treating fungal infection, imaging technologies aid in attaining a more advanced level of management strategy, eventually leading to best-in-class patient care. Imaging technologies have also been programmed with new modalities that complement traditional diagnosis processes. These developments include the combination of imaging with molecular approaches to diagnosis, enabling the detection of circulating fungal components, i.e., cell wall structures and DNA, in corresponding body fluid or tissues. By bringing imaging-derived structural data together with molecular data, clinicians can get a more comprehensive view of the infection's status and extent. This association not only enhances the diagnostic sensitivity for invasive mycoses but also paves the way for individualized treatment regimens according to the particular demands of the patient. Thus, imaging tests represent an essential cornerstone in the care of fungal infections, particularly in high-risk patient populations, to achieve significant gains in early diagnosis and therapy (Dornbusch et al., 2010).

7.6. Treatment and Management

Effective treatment and control of fungal infections are crucial in alleviating the impact of mycoses on the health of patients. The approach is likely to be dependent on the form of the fungal pathogen, infection site, and the patient clinical status. Antifungal agents are the cornerstone of therapy, differentiated primarily based on their mode of action. Azoles, for instance, inhibit the production of the cell membrane of fungi, whereas echinocandins have an effect on cell wall synthesis. Therapy choice can then be influenced by patient tolerance, concurrent medical illness, and potential drug interactions. Clinical practice guidelines updates also strive to reflect prevailing research, acknowledging the necessity to adjust management protocols appropriately to keep pace with evolving evidence and resistance trends. Balancing these variables is essential to optimizing curative outcomes and avoiding treatment failures in mycoses-affected patients. With dermatophyte infection, such as tinea pedis, cure has improved with the introduction of specific antifungal therapy.

Terbinafine, a semisynthetic allylamine, is an excellent example of advancement in this direction, as it has fungicidal activity against dermatophytes only. Short-course treatment of terbinafine has been proven in clinical trials to be as effective as long-course treatment with topical azole antifungals, with reduced rates of relapse. Importantly, there has been the option of a single-application terbinafine 1% formulation suitable for long-term exposure of the skin and improved drug penetration. Such a novel strategy gives a reservoir of the drug in the epidermal layers — systematically where dermatophytes are localized — hence resulting in more effective eradication of the pathogens without the need for lengthy therapy. Hence, terbinafine's distinctive attributes facilitate effective and prompt control of tinea pedis. Prevention activities also play a significant role in managing and treating mycoses. Public health measures that encourage the population to be aware of hygiene and environmental factors play a vital role in preventing mycoses. For instance, encouraging proper foot care and the use of air-permeable shoes can contribute immensely to preventing tinea pedis. Besides, understanding the epidemiology of fungal infections enables clinicians to identify those at risk and offer tailored interventions. Knowledge of the evidence of fungal infection by the communities makes early detection and timely treatment possible. All these preventive measures put together are vital in reducing the incidence of fungal infections and promoting good health. In this interdisciplinary approach, integrating education, treatment, and ongoing research forms part of a cohesive framework for delivering effective management of the fungal pathogens and ensuing mycoses (Figure 7.12).

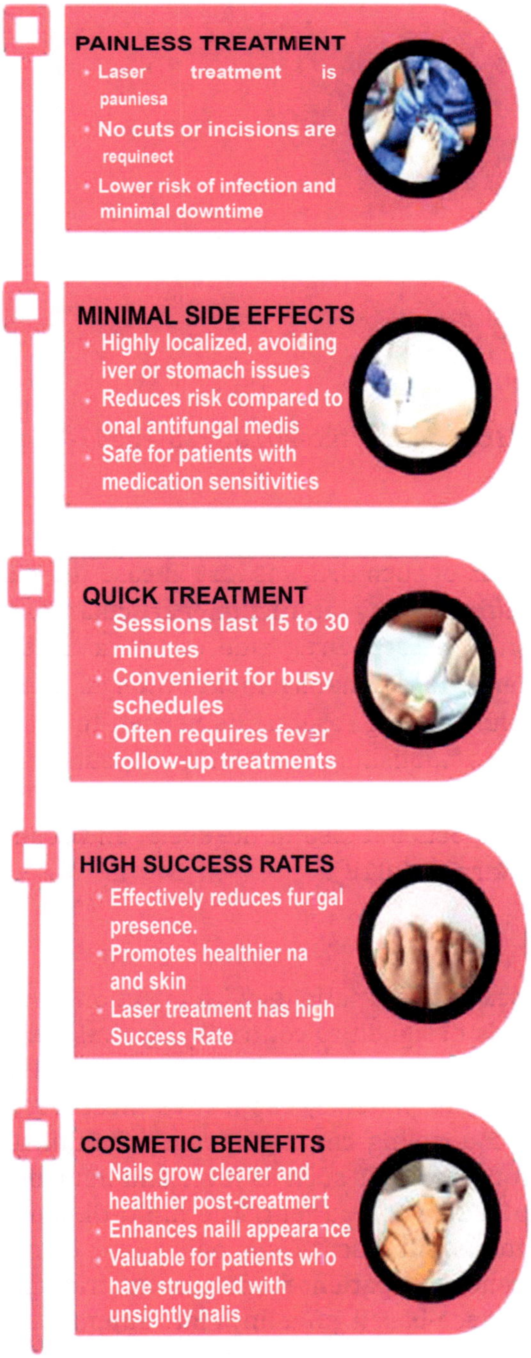

Figure 7.12. Benefits of laser treatment of fungal infections.

Source: https://athenaskinclinic.com/wp-content/uploads/2024/11/benefits-of-laser-treatment-for-fungaal-infections.png.

7.6.1. Antifungal Medications

Antifungal therapy plays a significant part in the management of fungal infections, particularly those involving opportunistic pathogens such as *Candida* species. The infections commonly occur in immunocompromised individuals, and effective antifungal therapy is thus essential. One of the most employed agents, intravenous fluconazole, is also frequently employed in intensive care. A recent survey demonstrated that around 98.4% of patients infected with *Candida* received first-line treatment with fluconazole, indicating the significance of the drug in clinical practice. However, the survey also recorded important resistance issues, with 32% of patients exhibiting infections caused by potentially fluconazole-resistant *Candida*. This underscores the importance of vigilance in monitoring antifungal efficacy and resistance patterns as a component of effective infection control, particularly in high-risk populations (Wissing et al., 2013). Beyond fluconazole, other agents such as posaconazole have been investigated for prophylactic use in high-risk patients, particularly those undergoing treatment for hematologic malignancy. The use of posaconazole has been extensively examined in terms of its pharmacoeconomic utility, especially in facilities like the National Center for Cancer Care in Qatar. Evidence indicates that although posaconazole may provide a marginally improved outcome in terms of prevention of invasive fungal infection, it is considerably more costly than fluconazole. This cost invites clinical decision-makers to weigh clinical benefit against cost, requiring tailored antifungal prophylaxis optimized for maximum cost-effectiveness. Findings of cost-analysis partitioned therapy failure as a major outcome of invasive fungal infections, depicting the complex interplay among treatment selection, result, and cost (Al-Marridi, 2018) (Figure 7.13).

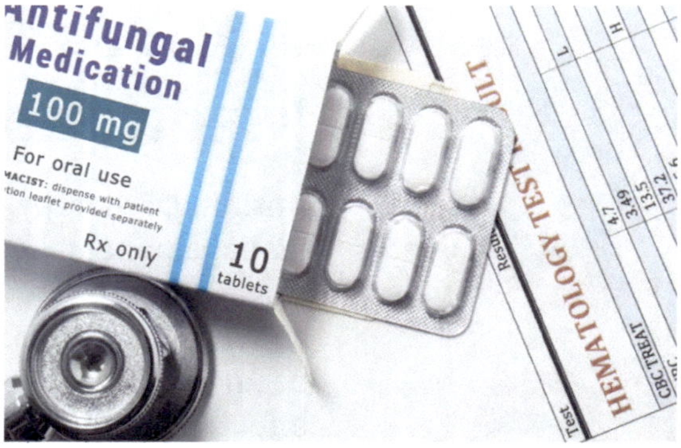

Figure 7.13. Antifungal medications.

Source: https://images.theconversation.com/files/238436/original/file-20180928-48647-12ud27s.jpg?ixlib=rb-4.1.0&q=45&auto=format&w=926&fit=clip.

Understanding antifungals extends from their clinical application to patient compliance, drug interaction, and side effects. The therapeutic effectiveness of such drugs is lost in case the patient does not complete the drug regimen or encounters significant drug interaction, particularly among patients who are on a cocktail of drugs for comorbid illnesses. Drug side effects also lead to therapy disruption, which presents an additional challenge to the management of fungal infection. As new antifungal products and drugs become available, ongoing research is needed to establish full treatment protocols that ensure patient safety while establishing the best therapeutic results. Knowledge of these complex factors is important for health practitioners in establishing effective antifungal programs that not only cater to the medical aspects but also to the social and economic factors of patient treatment (Wissing et al., 2013; Al-Marridi, 2018).

7.6.2. Supportive Care

Supportive treatment is an integral component of the treatment of patients with infection by fungal pathogens and associated mycoses. Supportive therapy is designed to control symptoms, enhance quality of life, and optimize overall outcomes, particularly in immunocompromised individuals at higher risk for fulminant fungal infections. Among these patients, supportive measures such as adequate pain relief, nutrition, and psychological counseling can significantly minimize the disease severity. In the event of fungal infection with complications such as fever and neutropenia, intensive supportive treatment becomes critical in stabilizing the patient. The multi-dimensional supportive care intervenes not just on physical symptoms but also psychological and emotional needs, highlighting the role of supportive care in comprehensive patient management strategies for fungal disease (Agyeman et al., 2014). Integration of evidence-based guidelines into supportive care is crucial for improving outcomes in fungal infections. For instance, strict compliance with defined guidelines has been shown to be useful in enhancing the effectiveness of empiric antibiotic treatment in febrile neutropenia episodes of microbiologically defined infection. In these episodes, early recognition of fungal pathogens, combined with appropriate supportive care maneuvers, has been shown to be followed by reduced hospital stay and improved recovery rates. Particularly in children with cancer, for whom the burden of fungal infections can be tremendous, effective utilization of supportive care practices heavily dictates clinical management (Boogaerts et al., 2007). Prioritizing these recommendations by healthcare workers can not only address present-day complications but also prevent future complications, making it all the more essential to adopt a proactive approach in settings where fungal pathogens are highly risky. Lastly, the psychosocial component of supportive care cannot be ignored, particularly for patients with the burden of mycoses due to compromised immune status. Emotional distress can secondarily worsen physical symptoms and impede treatment compliance, thus causing a deleterious effect on recovery. Thus, supportive care should encompass counseling and mental health support services to provide psychological handling of anxiety, depression, or fear that often accompanies severe fungal infections. Open communication regarding treatments, side effects, and outcomes between the healthcare professionals and the patients encourages a conducive atmosphere that is supportive of healing. Additionally, studies have indicated that inadequate management of emotional and psychological demands has been associated with greater hospitalization and unnecessary morbidity in patients with severe infections, again pointing out the multidimensional nature of supportive care in the management of fungal pathogens and mycoses (Agyeman et al., 2014).

7.6.3. Preventive Measures

Preventive measures against fungal infections and mycoses are needed to decrease incidence levels and enhance the quality of patients, particularly among immunocompromised patients. Awareness in the healthcare setting is crucial as fungal infections, including those due to *Candida* spp., have a tendency to arise among intensive medically managed patients. Prophylaxis measures have been developed, including the use of antifungal medication like intravenous fluconazole, which has been found to reduce the incidence of infection in high-risk subjects. In one research study, it was observed that while fluconazole as initial treatment was used successfully, slightly more than 32% of the patients presented with *Candida* species infection that was possibly resistant to the drug, highlighting the need for proper monitoring and early intervention strategies (Wissing et al., 2013). This underlines the importance of tailoring preventive interventions to patients' own risk profiles to ensure optimal efficacy of antifungal therapy. Apart from pharmaceutical interventions, infection and environmental control measures are also a critical component of fungal infection prevention. Compliant adherence to rigorous hygiene protocols within healthcare institutions can go far in reducing the risk of nosocomial infection. These include daily cleaning and disinfection of the environment, full hand hygiene, and adequate ventilation within patient-care areas. Application of these practices is particularly vital in intensive care units, where patients are at greater risk of infection due to invasive interventions and underlying disease states. Novel strategies, such as vaccination and modulation of the innate immune response, are also under investigation to supplement existing preventive structures. These new technologies can provide additional protection in environments with a high risk, where the fungal pathogens are a formidable enemy (Carvalho et al., 2012). Education of patients is yet another critical component of a multiple-pronged strategy against the prevention of mycoses. Patients must be taught about the risks of mycoses, especially those who have comorbidities or are on immunosuppressive therapy. Education that empowers patients can make them recognize the signs of early infection and enhance the importance of following prevention, for example, frequent follow-ups and monitoring of symptoms. Public health programs' awareness campaigns can also enhance knowledge and compliance with prevention procedures. By developing an active prevention culture of fungal infections, doctors have the potential to make widespread contributions to relieving the mycoses burden and improving the health status among high-risk groups, and thus it remains a fundamental aspect of modern clinical practice.

SUMMARY

While examining the intricate relationship of the fungal pathogens and mycoses, it is evident that a multidisciplinary framework has to be applied to reflect the intricacy of issues they exhibit. Their extensive spread reflects vast knowledge gaps that restrict our apprehension of their ecological roles and meaning in ecosystems worldwide. Despite advances in microbiological methodology, an understanding of the environmental and ecological conditions under which these pathogens thrive continues to evade us. As is seen from this essay, insufficient knowledge of the ecological role of fungal organisms not only impacts our knowledge of aquatic conservation but also food safety in general, particularly for populations reliant on fish as a primary source. Shared knowledge is significant, serving as a point of reference for future research and intervention strategies for inhibiting the menaces posed by fungal infections among wildlife and human health. Also, the emergence of fungal pathogens as primary agents of decline in animal and plant populations illustrates a compelling need for additional monitoring and study. Of more than local concern, the threat these pathogens present extends into ecosystem dynamics and biodiversity itself. Existing studies indicate that fungal diseases have increased in frequency in agricultural and aquaculture settings, where practices such as the international movement of fish can unknowingly disperse them. Such dispersion emphasizes the need for enhanced ecological consciousness and surveillance measures, which can yield useful information on the development, transmission, and ecological influence of such pathogens on fish populations. Through encouraging an interdisciplinary response, marrying ecological science with agricultural practice, we can develop rational overall strategies that safeguard ecosystem well-being and conserve biodiversity. In addressing the crisis involving fungal pathogens and mycoses, scientific collaboration among scientists, policymakers, and stakeholders is critical. Sharing knowledge and resources may give rise to innovative solutions that are both scientifically justifiable and socially responsible. Institutions and funders play a vital role in funding research that bridges such knowledge gaps, as shown through the many grants aimed at researching fungal and fungus-like pathogens. Overall effort must go into bridging the gap between research outcomes and prospective uses so that information is accessible and used for the greater good. Because emerging infectious diseases continue to threaten different organisms, our commitment to understanding and minimizing the impact of fungal pathogens will eventually determine an appropriate response towards reviving and safeguarding our ecosystems' delicate balance, thereby opening the door towards sustainable man-nature relationships.

Fungal pathogens have attracted significant interest in recent years owing to the increasing incidence and the challenge of mycoses diagnosis and treatment. Specifically, opportunistic yeast infections are also increasing, particularly among the immunocompromised population. The sheer variety of species causing the infections creates a problem for prompt and correct diagnosis since the traditional approach involves the need for preliminary culturing. Correspondingly, efforts have been on to develop diagnostic methods that have the potential to give more rapid and accurate identification of the causal agents. The new technologies, such as next-generation sequencing and proteomics, hold potential in enhancing the detection sensitivity, but the major challenges still remain in their clinical applications. This diagnostic advancement is not just crucial for effective treatment but also to minimize the load of antifungal resistance, which is rapidly emerging as a major challenge in fungal infection management (Consortium OPATHY, & Gabaldón, 2019). Among the many fungal pathogens, *Aspergillus fumigatus* has emerged as a cause of concern due to its association with increased mortality among immunocompromised individuals. The innate immune response also plays a crucial role in combating this as well as other fungal infections, as is indicated by the function of H-Ficolin in enhancing the host's defense against *A. fumigatus*. H-Ficolin functions through binding to some of the residues present in fungi, triggering the lectin complement pathway, and boosting the immune response by enhancing greater production of interleukin-8 from lung epithelial cells. This dialogue identifies a critical feature of the immune system's capacity to recognize and respond to fungal pathogens and places on the forefront probable diagnostic biomarkers, such as H-Ficolin in bronchoalveolar lavage fluid. Further research is required to account for the implications of this knowledge for therapeutic treatments and diagnostic development in fungal infection (Dagenais & Keller, 2015). In summary, the overall scenario of fungal pathogens and mycoses is a balance between pathogen biology, host immune response, and the ever-evolving diagnostic tools. The continued rise in opportunistic fungal infections highlights the importance of creating novel approaches towards diagnosing as well as treating the infections efficiently. Continued research observations continue to elucidate the immuno-dynamics, such as the role of H-Ficolin in boosting immunity against *A. fumigatus*, and the potential for new therapeutic and diagnostic strategies grows. Ultimately, these concerns will be addressed in a synergy of numerous disciplines with the goal not only to improve survival rates among such groups but also to implement cut-and-dried protocols for the prevention and treatment of fungal disease in an increasingly dynamic medical landscape.

CLOSER LOOK

ATHLETE'S FOOT

Athlete's foot is a fungal infection of the skin on the feet, particularly between the toes. It is brought about by dermatophyte fungi, predominantly Trichophyton rubrum, T. mentagrophytes, and Epidermophyton floccosum. The infection thrives in warm, moist environments such as locker rooms, public showers, and around swimming pools, thus its name, and therefore athletes and people wearing tight, closed shoes for prolonged periods are more at risk.

The symptoms of athlete's foot include itching, burning, and stinging between the toes or on the soles of the feet. The infected tissue will be red, scaly, cracked, or blistered. In some cases, the infection can spread to the toenails (onychomycosis) or the hands (Tinea manuum), particularly if the person scratches or touches the affected area frequently (Figure 7.14).

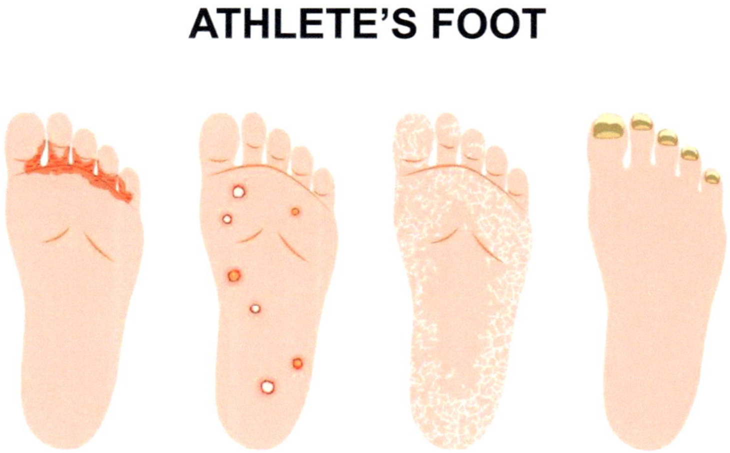

Figure 7.14. Illustration of various clinical manifestations of athlete's foot, a common fungal infection, including cracked skin, blisters, scaling, and discolored toenails.

Source: https://www.aurorahealthcare.org/-/media/Project/Health-System-Enterprise/AuroraHealthCareOrg/aurorahealthcare/images/services/dermatology/athletes-foot-symptoms.webp?h=800&iar=0&w=1200&rev=674b6e6eeb144084bc8b0bd9b913a092&hash=D9DE79C02D40674396A6D4B5D405EF42.

Transmission occurs by direct contact with the fungi or indirectly through dirty towels, socks, shoes, or surfaces. Walking barefoot in public areas or sharing personal items increases the chances of getting the infection. Good foot hygiene, dry skin, and frequent change of socks are preventive needs.

Treatment is typically with topical antifungals such as clotrimazole, miconazole, or terbinafine. Oral antifungals can be employed in advanced or chronic infections. Treatment must be completed as advised, even after the early disappearance of the symptoms, to prevent recurrence.

Athlete's foot, although not generally dangerous, can lead to complications if neglected and not treated, including secondary bacterial infections and spread to other body areas. Early identification and successful treatment are therefore crucial. Foot hygiene and drying, avoidance of going barefoot in public places, and disinfection of shoes can help to prevent future attacks and minimize risk of transmission to others.

REFERENCES

1. Paterson, R. R. M., & Lima, N. (2017). Filamentous Fungal Human Pathogens from Food Emphasising Aspergillus, Fusarium and Mucor. *Microorganisms, 5*(3), 44. https://doi.org/10.3390/microorganisms5030044(accessed on 16th July 2025).
2. Abrahamse-Berkeveld, M., Kegler, D., Oosting, A., Ringler, R., et al. (2004). *Oral versus intravenous therapy in the treatment of systemic mycosis.* https://core.ac.uk/download/pdf/82397595.pdf (accessed on 16th July 2025).
3. Agyeman, P., Ammann, R. A., Beck-Popovic, M., Bodmer, N., et al. (2014). *A prospective multicenter SPOG 2003 FN study of microbiologically defined infections in pediatric cancer patients with fever and neutropenia.* https://core.ac.uk/download/77166207.pdf (accessed on 16th July 2025).
4. Dagenais, T. R., & Keller, N. P. (2009). Pathogenesis of Aspergillus fumigatus in Invasive Aspergillosis. *Clinical microbiology reviews, 22*(3), 447–465. https://doi.org/10.1128/CMR.00055-08(accessed on 16th July 2025).
5. Alcazar-Fuoli, L., Armstrong-James, D., Bertuzzi, M., Bignell, E., et al. (2014). *The pH-responsive PacC transcription factor of Aspergillus fumigatus governs epithelial entry and tissue invasion during pulmonary aspergillosis.* https://core.ac.uk/download/30435716.pdf (accessed on 16th July 2025).
6. Al-Marridi, W. Z. (2018). *Pharmacoeconomics evaluation of the systemic antifungal posaconazole for prophylaxis against invasive fungal infections among immunocompromised cancer patients in Qatar.* https://core.ac.uk/download/161995723.pdf (accessed on 16th July 2025).
7. Mayer, F. L., Wilson, D., & Hube, B. (2013). Candida albicans pathogenicity mechanisms. *Virulence, 4*(2), 119–128. https://doi.org/10.4161/viru.22913(accessed on 16th July 2025).
8. Consortium OPATHY, & Gabaldón, T. (2019). Recent trends in molecular diagnostics of yeast infections: from PCR to NGS. *FEMS microbiology reviews, 43*(5), 517–547. https://doi.org/10.1093/femsre/fuz015(accessed on 16th July 2025).
9. Wissing, H., Ballus, J., Bingold, T. M., Nocea, G., Krobot, K. J., Kaskel, P., Kumar, R. N., & Mavros, P. (2013). Intensive care unit-related fluconazole use in Spain and Germany: patient characteristics and outcomes of a prospective multicenter longitudinal observational study. *Infection and drug resistance, 6*, 15–25. https://doi.org/10.2147/IDR.S38945 (accessed on 16th July 2025).
10. Basir, R., Chin, V. K., Chong, P. P., Tze, W. Y., et al. (2016). *Dissecting Candida albicans infection from the perspective of C. albicans virulence and omics approaches on host–pathogen interaction: A review.* https://core.ac.uk/download/153830058.pdf (accessed on 16th July 2025).
11. Ben Nasr, A., Bergmann, S., Boskey, E. R., Colman, R. W., De Bernardis, F., Frick, I. M., et al. (2010). *Degradation of human kininogens with the release of kinin peptides by extracellular proteinases of Candida spp.* https://core.ac.uk/download/19418372.pdf (accessed on 16th July 2025).
12. Carvalho, A., Cunha, C., Bistoni, F., & Romani, L. (2012). Immunotherapy of aspergillosis. *Clinical microbiology and infection : the official publication of the European Society of Clinical Microbiology and Infectious Diseases, 18*(2), 120–125. https://doi.org/10.1111/j.1469-0691.2011.03681.x(accessed on 16th July 2025).

13. Boogaerts, M., Cagnoni, P. J., Collins, C. D., DePestel, D. D., Donowitz, G. R., Mackler, E. R., et al. (2007). *Institutional experience with voriconazole compared with liposomal amphotericin B as empiric therapy for febrile neutropenia.* https://deepblue.lib.umich.edu/bitstream/2027.42/90034/1/phco.27.7.970.pdf (accessed on 16th July 2025).

14. Kean, R., Brown, J., Gulmez, D., Ware, A., & Ramage, G. (2020). *Candida auris*: A Decade of Understanding of an Enigmatic Pathogenic Yeast. *Journal of fungi (Basel, Switzerland)*, *6*(1), 30. https://doi.org/10.3390/jof6010030(accessed on 16th July 2025).

15. Carver, P. L., DePestel, D. D., & McCoy, D. (2009). *Primary antifungal prophylaxis in adult hematopoietic stem cell transplant recipients: Current therapeutic concepts.* https://deepblue.lib.umich.edu/bitstream/2027.42/90237/1/phco.29.11.1306.pdf (accessed on 16th July 2025).

16. Bain, J., Gow, N. A., & Erwig, L. P. (2015). Novel insights into host-fungal pathogen interactions derived from live-cell imaging. *Seminars in immunopathology*, *37*(2), 131–139. https://doi.org/10.1007/s00281-014-0463-3(accessed on 16th July 2025).

17. Chakrabarti, A., Synytsya, A., Rodrigues, A. M., Deng, B., et al. (2018). *Cell walls of the dimorphic fungal pathogens Sporothrix schenckii and Sporothrix brasiliensis exhibit bilaminate structures and sloughing of extensive and intact layers.* https://core.ac.uk/download/156963567.pdf (accessed on 16th July 2025).

18. Conrado, P. C. V. (2019). *Effect of photodynamic therapy with hypericin nanoencapsulated in P123 on Fusarium spp.* https://core.ac.uk/download/655371505.pdf (accessed on 16th July 2025).

19. Maertens, J., Groll, A. H., Cordonnier, C., de la Cámara, R., Roilides, E., & Marchetti, O. (2011). Treatment and timing in invasive mould disease. *The Journal of antimicrobial chemotherapy*, *66 Suppl 1*, i37–i43. https://doi.org/10.1093/jac/dkq440(accessed on 16th July 2025).

20. Kean, R., Delaney, C., Rajendran, R., Sherry, L., Metcalfe, R., Thomas, R., McLean, W., Williams, C., & Ramage, G. (2018). Gaining Insights from Candida Biofilm Heterogeneity: One Size Does Not Fit All. *Journal of fungi (Basel, Switzerland)*, *4*(1), 12. https://doi.org/10.3390/jof4010012(accessed on 16th July 2025).

21. Schäfer, K., Di Pietro, A., Gow, N. A., & MacCallum, D. (2014). Murine model for Fusarium oxysporum invasive fusariosis reveals organ-specific structures for dissemination and long-term persistence. *PloS one*, *9*(2), e89920. https://doi.org/10.1371/journal.pone.0089920 (accessed on 16th July 2025).

22. Dornbusch, H. J., Groll, A., & Walsh, T. J. (2010). *Diagnosis of invasive fungal infections in immunocompromised children.* https://core.ac.uk/download/pdf/81151526.pdf (accessed on 16th July 2025).

23. Rawlings, S. A., Heldt, S., Prattes, J., Eigl, S., Jenks, J. D., Flick, H., Rabensteiner, J., Prüller, F., Wölfler, A., Neumeister, P., Strohmaier, H., Krause, R., & Hoenigl, M. (2019). Using Interleukin 6 and 8 in Blood and Bronchoalveolar Lavage Fluid to Predict Survival in Hematological Malignancy Patients With Suspected Pulmonary Mold Infection. *Frontiers in immunology*, *10*, 1798. https://doi.org/10.3389/fimmu.2019.01798(accessed on 16th July 2025).

24. Green, M., Starzl, T. E., Todo, S., Tzakis, A., et al. (1991). *Aspergillosis of the CNS in a pediatric liver transplant recipient: Case report and review.* https://core.ac.uk/download/12204611.pdf (accessed on 16th July 2025).

25. Gozlan, R. E., Marshall, W. L., Lilje, O., Jessop, C. N., Gleason, F. H., & Andreou, D. (2014). Current ecological understanding of fungal-like pathogens of fish: what lies beneath?. *Frontiers in microbiology, 5*, 62. https://doi.org/10.3389/fmicb.2014.00062(accessed on 16th July 2025).

26. Kamat, N. M., & Velho-Pereira, S. (2010). *Exploring hidden dimensions of soil fungal biodiversity: A simple technique to detect soil fungi resistant to antifungal compounds.* https://core.ac.uk/download/pdf/289013.pdf (accessed on 16th July 2025).

27. King, J., Lehrnbecher, T., Pana, Z. D., Steinbach, W. J., et al. (2017). *Recognition and clinical presentation of invasive fungal disease in neonates and children.* https://core.ac.uk/download/131024549.pdf (accessed on 16th July 2025).

28. Kingham, M. C. (2019). *Monitoring treatment table hygiene in a chiropractic training clinic.* https://core.ac.uk/download/323341146.pdf (accessed on 16th July 2025).

29. Schäfer-Korting, M., Schoellmann, C., & Korting, H. C. (2008). Fungicidal activity plus reservoir effect allow short treatment courses with terbinafine in tinea pedis. *Skin pharmacology and physiology, 21*(4), 203–210. https://doi.org/10.1159/000135636(accessed on 16th July 2025).

30. Little, J., McCarthy, T., Pappas, P., Perfect, J. R., et al. (2024). *Clinical mycology today: Emerging challenges and opportunities.* https://core.ac.uk/download/619402138.pdf (accessed on 16th July 2025).

31. Liu, D.; Paterson, R. R. M., Phialophora. In Dongyou Liu, Molecular Detection of Human Fungal Pathogens, Boca Raton: CRC Press, 2011. ISBN: 9781439812402, 345-350(accessed on 16th July 2025).

32. Vogeser, M., Spöhrer, U., & Schiel, X. (2003). Determination of itraconazole and hydroxyitraconazole in plasma by use of liquid chromatography-tandem mass spectrometry with on-line solid-phase extraction. *Clinical chemistry and laboratory medicine, 41*(7), 915–920. https://doi.org/10.1515/CCLM.2003.139(accessed on 16th July 2025).

33. Molly Smith & Sara Selby (2017). *Microbiology for Allied Health Students.* https://core.ac.uk/download/217306147.pdf (accessed on 16th July 2025).

34. Sharifzadeh, A., & Shokri, H. (2015). *Zataria multiflora* Boiss.: A review study on chemical composition, antifungal and anti-mycotoxin activities, and ultrastructural changes. https://core.ac.uk/download/143844707.pdf (accessed on 16th July 2025).

35. Whiston, E., & Taylor, J. W. (2015). Comparative Phylogenomics of Pathogenic and Nonpathogenic Species. *G3 (Bethesda, Md.), 6*(2), 235–244. https://doi.org/10.1534/g3.115.022806(accessed on 16th July 2025).

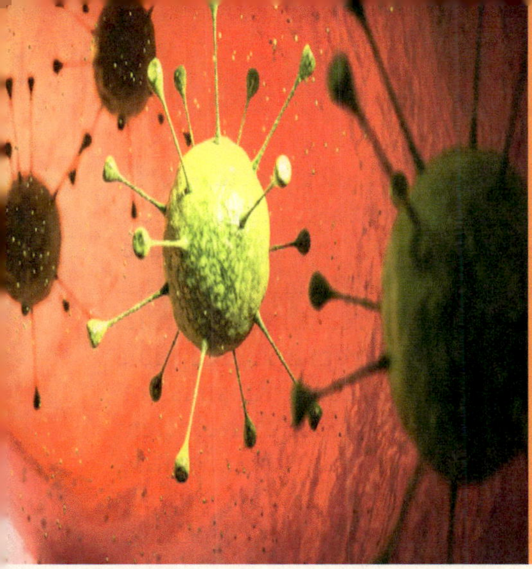

Chapter 8

PROTOZOAN INFECTIONS

Contents

Introduction

Protozoan infections represent a considerable international health problem, infecting millions of individuals, particularly in tropical and subtropical regions. The infections are caused by single-celled protozoan parasites, most notably those of the genera *Trypanosoma*, *Plasmodium*, and Leishmania, among others. The World Health Organization has classified certain protozoan diseases, such as malaria and Chagas disease, as neglected tropical diseases due to the fact that not much research and funding have been allocated to their prevention and treatment. The complexity of such infections — from the difference in their life cycle to modes of transmission — combined with the socio-economic status present in affected zones, aggravates their effect. The aim of this chapter is to examine the complex nature of protozoan infections, describe vectors for transmission, and indicate complications within their epidemiology and control, to bring to the forefront the important need for further research and public health measures. The results of recent studies point to the important interaction between socio-environmental conditions and protozoan disease transmission. For instance, vector-borne illnesses caused by protozoan parasites commonly take place in areas of ecological transformation, in which human contact with infected vectors becomes greater. A prime example is Chagas disease, in which the *Trypanosoma cruzi* parasite is transmitted primarily through triatomine bug feces and infects millions of individuals within Latin America. Contrary to major breakthroughs in its epidemiological knowledge, treatment guidelines remain behind, and millions remain susceptible to serious health complications. Ongoing endeavors in demarcating the disease transmission dynamics provide useful information utilized in the design of targeted interventions and efficient management of outbreaks, emphasizing the necessity of interdisciplinary approaches in confronting protozoan infections (Sherman, 2019). The use of new diagnostic tools and techniques has the potential to revolutionize the way protozoan infection is understood and managed. For instance, the use of high-throughput microfluidic real-time PCR technology has proved useful in defining the tick-borne pathogens of areas like the Caribbean. This advancement is making it possible to conduct large-scale epidemiological studies, generating data quickly and accurately that are essential for assessing the threat of disease emergence and designing public health interventions. Particularly, the ability to identify not only known pathogens, but even those then-unrecognized microorganisms, can significantly aid in understanding the dynamic shifts in protozoan threats and their vectors. By integrating such advanced methods into surveillance interventions, researchers can enhance the predictability of patterns of infection and develop responsive actions against the impact of protozoan infections (Gondard et al., 2020).

Definition of Protozoan Infections

Protozoan infections are caused by single-celled eukaryotic organisms known as protozoa, which live in different environments, including soil, water, and living hosts. The pathogens can be categorized into various groups depending on the modes of locomotion, for example, amoebae, flagellates, ciliates, and sporozoans. Protozoan infections primarily occur due to fecal contamination of food and drinking water sources or vectors like mosquitoes and ticks. These pathogenic agents can exploit human hosts, particularly in immunocompromised individuals, to manifest diseases ranging from mild gastrointestinal upset to fatal systemic diseases. Public health implications of protozoal infections thus merit serious thought, particularly in regions with inadequate sanitation and scarce healthcare facilities. Clinical presentation of protozoal infections is highly unpredictable and can affect multiple organ systems. Some of the shared symptoms include diarrhea, abdominal pain, fever, and weakness, which are most often attributed to infections such as amoebic dysentery and giardiasis. Diarrhea, a prevalent result of some protozoan infections, is very risky, especially among susceptible populations, and contributes significantly to high morbidity and mortality rates among children. In fact, diarrheal diseases due to protozoa are major causes of mortality among children in the world, indicating the importance of determining the responsible pathogens. Against such infections, timely and proper interventions such as rehydration therapy and antimicrobial treatments play an important role in symptom control and prevention of further complications associated with delayed disease (Caramia et al., 2015). Moreover, the environmental context of protozoan infections shows a multiplicity of environmental drivers, host susceptibility, and successful transmission dynamics. For example, soil habitats support different protozoa, which can also be opportunistic pathogens when human beings are exposed to these infected resources. Soil's role in supporting such pathogenic microorganisms is evidence of interdependency between human and environmental health and thus the necessity for an integrated approach in disease control. Additionally, public health interventions aimed at improving sanitation, pure water for drinking, and proper education can help curb the incidence of protozoan infection. With more research ongoing to unveil the complexities of protozoan biology and transmission, it is imperative that targeted interventions and strategies are used to treat these infections successfully, subsequently reducing their incidence and impact on global health (Jeffery & Van Der Putten , 2011) (Figure 8.1).

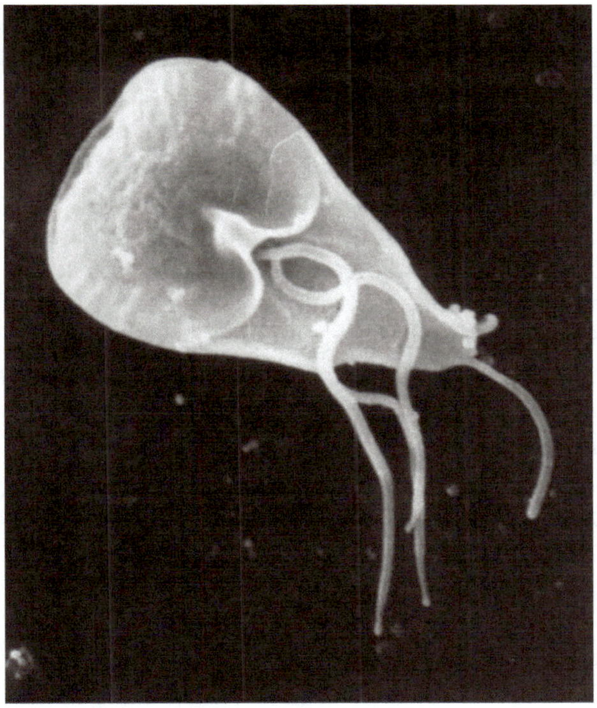

Figure 8.1. *Giardia lamblia*, an infectious protozoan.

Source: https://upload.wikimedia.org/wikipedia/commons/0/08/Giardia_lamblia_SEM_8698_lores.jpg.

Importance of Studying Protozoan Infections

The research of protozoan infections takes first precedence in public health and epidemiology due to their comprehensive influence on human health. Protozoa such as *Toxoplasma gondii* and malaria species carry repercussions greater than the emphasis of the single disease. It is clear from the typical patterns of *Schistosoma* spp. and other intestinal protozoal infections, the burden of disease may vary significantly depending on geographic and socioeconomic factors, necessitating the need for tailored public health initiatives (Coulibaly et al., 2012). An understanding of the prevalence of these pathogens in different populations can assist health practitioners in organizing sufficient prevention and control measures. Moreover, the investigation of protozoan infections deepens our knowledge of vector dynamics and host relationships within ecosystems and offers insights for environmental health programs and human-animal-environment interconnectedness. Furthermore, the significance of learning from protozoan infections is also stressed due to the ability of protozoan infections to cause morbidity and mortality not only in humans but also in domestic and wild animals (Shapiro et al., 2019). This protozoan zoonotic nature of protozoan pathogens necessitates a multi-disciplinary research and control strategy that integrates veterinary sciences, environmental science, and human health perspectives. Because protozoan diseases can endure in changing environments — e.g., *T. gondiis* survival in different foodstuffs and ecosystems — their transmission patterns must be known (Shapiro et al., 2019). Through explaining infection routes, researchers can identify points of intervention, thereby preventing outbreaks. The intricate interplay between environments and transmission vectors also underscores the necessity for immense research in the field. Lastly, protozoal infections represent an important public health issue exacerbated by globalization, urbanization, and changed environmental conditions. Such research enables disease officials to anticipate and prepare for emerging threats from protozoan pathogens that are expected to evolve to new hosts or host environments as the global dynamic remains in flux. The co-infection patterns described here, particularly within rural settings, demonstrate the sophistication of disease management and the importance of ongoing surveillance programs that account for localized variation in rates of infection (Coulibaly et al., 2012). This vigilance is critical to the maintenance of the health and welfare of at-risk populations. Accordingly, the significance of learning about protozoan infections cannot be overemphasized, as it provides us with the information and the tools necessary to contend with an ever-changing panorama of infectious illness.

8.1. Types of Protozoan Infections

The protozoan infections can be grouped into several types, which are broadly differentiated based on their transmission patterns and systems affected. The flagellates represent a significant group identifiable by whip-like appendages responsible for locomotion. *Trypanosoma cruzi*, the causative agent of Chagas disease, is an example that is transmitted through the feces of triatomine insects. This infection progresses from an acute and subsequently chronic phase, affecting several body systems, most significantly the cardiovascular, gastrointestinal, and nervous systems, emphasizing the substantial health burden of this neglected tropical disease. The Centers for Disease Control and the World Health Organization emphasize the effect of Chagas disease, which infects millions of individuals while illustrating gaps in research in its treatment and epidemiological surveillance (Sherman, 2019). Another significant group of protozoan infections involves the amoebae, namely *Entamoeba histolytica*, responsible for amoebic dysentery. The organism is primarily spread by the fecal-oral route, predominantly by contaminated food and water, causing widespread gastrointestinal upset. Individuals infected with *Entamoeba histolytica* manifest from mild diarrhea to fulminating dysentery, which can be life-threatening if left untreated. The life cycle and pathogenicity of amoebae are complex and challenge public health programs, especially where sanitation and healthcare facilities are poor. Effective intervention strategies for amoebic infections depend on a proper understanding of their epidemiology, and thus need better hygiene practices and awareness in the risk population. Ciliates are less frequently encountered with respect to human disease, but contribute to protozoan infections as well. Balantidium coli is a good illustration that occurs primarily in pigs and can be transmitted to man to cause balantidiasis. The infection typically results from human contact with contaminated water or food areas, particularly where pigs are reared close to human beings. The signs range from no disease at all to severe colitis, thus the imperative for prevention to involve controlling livestock and having clean water supplies. The life cycle of *Balantidium coli* that involves both animal and human hosts is challenging to control and needs further investigation into its pathogenic process and environmental reservoirs (Sherman, 2019). It is therefore crucial to have an understanding of the different forms of protozoan infections in a bid to devise effective public health interventions.

8.1.1. Amoebic Infections

Amoebic infections, particularly caused by the protozoan parasites *Entamoeba histolytica* and *Acanthamoeba* species, are significant worldwide public health problems. *Entamoeba histolytica*, the causative agent of amoebic dysentery, infects millions of individuals yearly, primarily from developing countries where sanitation facilities are poor. Its life cycle involves fecal-oral transmission through gastrointestinal tract contamination with manifestations of severe diarrhea and abdominal pain. High-risk populations, including children under the age of five, demonstrate heightened susceptibility to such infections due to poor hygiene conditions, environmental sanitation difficulties, and high population concentration (Unasho, 2013). Besides affecting the health of individuals, these infections are also economically burdensome to healthcare systems, necessitating increased efforts towards community education regarding preventive measures. Acanthamoeba infections, while being less frequent, pose special challenges, including among contact lens wearers. The usual disease syndrome, *Acanthamoeba keratitis,* emphasizes the hazards of unsatisfactory lens hygiene and exposure to contaminated environments. Acanthamoeba can also induce severe systemic infection in immunocompromised individuals, making the requirement for knowledge of the virulence factors and transmission routes of the pathogens central. Infectious agents like *Acanthamoeba* thrive and multiply in various habitats, e.g., soil and freshwater, making outbreaks challenging to contain (Khan, 2004) (Figure 8.2).

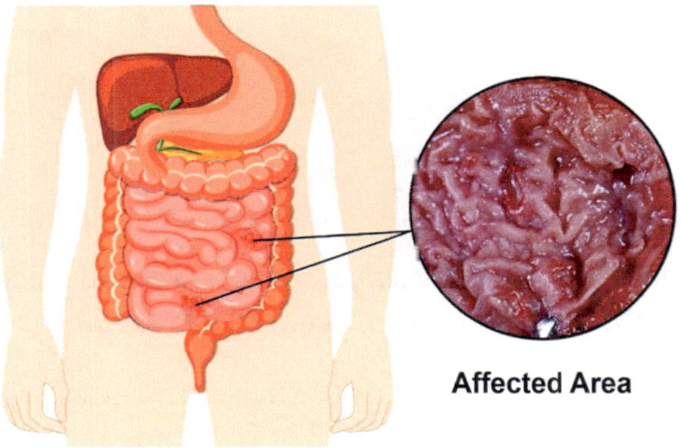

Figure 8.2. Amoebiasis.

Source: https://assets.truemeds.in/tm-cms-prod/what_is_amoebiasis_3d0467de23.jpg.

The complex interaction between the parasites pathogenic process and host variables accounts for the disease's unpredictability, making its treatment difficult and highlighting the need for further research to determine effective therapy. An understanding of the interaction between ecological, biological, and social determinants involved in amoebic infection is essential to effective control strategies. Systematic deworming, infection life cycle knowledge, hygiene behavior, and improved access to clean water are all included in preventing such protozoan infections (Unasho, 2013). Furthermore, the growing occurrence of *Acanthamoeba keratitis* requires targeted measures of prevention, particularly the correct handling of contact lenses. Through public education of these infectious dangers, communities can better become capable of reducing the incidence of amoebic infection and ultimately improve the overall public health status. The combination of study-based interventions and public education will be crucial in addressing the disease burden of amebiasis (Figure 8.3).

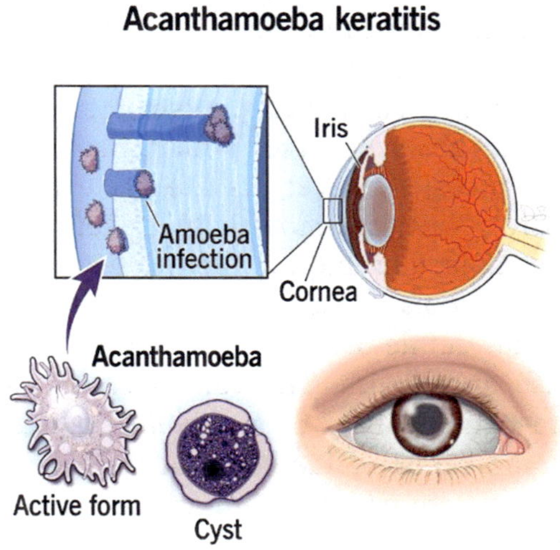

Figure 8.3. *Acanthamoeba keratitis.*

Source: https://my.clevelandclinic.org/-/scassets/images/org/health/articles/acanthamoeba-keratitis.

8.1.2. Flagellate Infections

Flagellate infections represent a broad category within the overall group of protozoan infections, but one that is recognized principally for its flagella, which both permit locomotion as well as fixation within various host environments. A typical example would be the genus *Trypanosoma*, which itself is also recognized for notorious pathogens that induce diseases such as *African trypanosomiasis*, or sleeping sickness, and American trypanosomiasis or Chagas disease. The complexity of such infections is further added to by the adaptability of *Trypanosoma* species within their hosts, leading to long-term infections that can evade immune detection. Current studies report that Treg cells play a central role in controlling immune responses such that parasites survive without weakening the hosts' global homeostasis. These observations support potential avenues for future therapeutic interventions, which demonstrate the intricate balance between pathogen survival and host immunological integrity (Domingos et al., 2015). Another of interest in flagellates is *Dientamoeba fragilis*, whose complexity renders it difficult to understand human protozoan infection due to its relatively obscure biology and questionable pathogenicity. The parasite exists in the human bowel and has been linked with gastrointestinal disturbances; however, its life cycle remains obscure. New technological developments in the molecular biology field have put new diagnostic tools on the horizon that are required to further define the role of *D. fragilis* in human disease and health. The controversial nature of the pathogenicity of *D. fragilis* emphasizes the importance of further research aimed at elucidating its clinical significance, as well as establishing successful paradigms for treatment. As the scientific community continues to grapple with this organism's multifaceted behaviors and transmission dynamics, it creates a compelling situation to explore the host-parasite interaction dynamics within the framework of flagellate infections (Barratt et al., 2016). In the prevention and control of flagellate infections, there is also a call to integrate greater public health measures. Treating such protozoan infections is not only about understanding their immunological and biological characteristics but also requires interventions that touch on the environmental etiology and allow early detection. In endemic regions for diseases like leishmaniasis, combined control interventions that include vector control and community awareness play an important role in reducing the transmission rates. Additionally, ongoing research is critical in efforts to come up with new therapies to combat resistant populations of parasites. The intricate interaction among immune responses in the host and parasite adaptation indicates a critical focus of study, which generates a demand for teamwork among researchers, health practitioners, and public health administrators to properly respond to the public health threat of flagellate infections (Barratt et al., 2016; Domingos et al., 2015) (Figure 8.4).

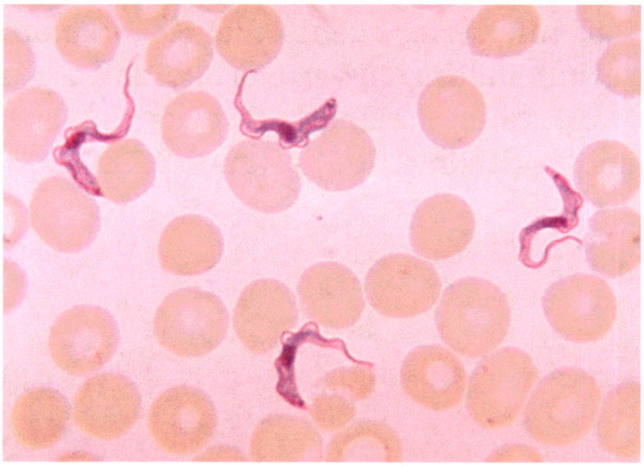

Figure 8.4. *Trypanosoma* forms in a blood smear from a patient with *African trypanosomiasis.*

Source: https://upload.wikimedia.org/wikipedia/commons/2/23/Trypanosoma_sp._PHIL_613_lores.jpg.

8.1.3. Ciliate Infections

Ciliate infestations are a significant but often underestimated component of protozoan infestations, occurring in a broad spectrum of hosts, from animals and humans to plants. Ciliates, with their hair-like appendages called cilia, are significant members of aquatic communities and can function as opportunistic pathogens. For instance, certain free-living ciliate species have been recovered in systems where the organisms are under the influence of microbial contamination, such as dishcloths in food handling. A recent study highlighted that 47% of these cloths were ciliate-positive, indicating their prevalence in conditions where the pathogens can propagate. This finding supports the vulnerability of ciliate infection to serve as a carrier for disease spread, particularly when food or water sources become infected with them, where such organisms may thrive together with more conventional bacterial pathogens, amplifying the risk of infection (Chavatte et al., 2014). The relationships between ciliates and other microorganisms can have elaborate ecological impacts, especially if one considers their involvement in the microbial food web. As predators, ciliates tend to prey on bacteria, such as harmful pathogens, with possible regulation of the population dynamics of these bacterial populations. This situation, however, may change when environmental conditions are in favor of ciliate growth, as is the case when ciliates find themselves in nutrient-dense waters or polluted environments. The case of *Pseudomonas aeruginosa* illustrates this dynamic, in which pathogenic life adaptations could impact their protist interactions, including with ciliates. Experiments illustrate that host adaptation in the long term may confer trade-offs in environmental robustness, proving that although ciliates are capable of predating on pathogenic bacteria, their increasing populations under some circumstances can initiate unintended consequences, such as the augmentation of pathogenic transmissions between hosts (Buckling et al., 2013). While infections with ciliates are regarded as highly important, their clinical significance and epidemiology are far from understood. Investigation of the prevalence of ciliate infections can give insights into their potential activities as opportunistic pathogens, particularly when the immune status of the host is depressed. Certain ciliates, such as Colpoda, have been increasingly highlighted outcomes of studies on environmental samples, but this has not yet been investigated in terms of implications of their occurrence in human health. The association of ciliates with evidence of contamination, as earlier suggested in studies involving dishcloths, means that efforts to minimize foodborne disease should account for the activity of such protozoans. In summary, ciliate infection is one of those specialized research fields of protozoan infections in need of a more sophisticated study aimed at revealing their ecological roles and impacts on human health.

8.2. Transmission of Protozoan Infections

Protozoan infections are transmitted through various channels, and the public health impact is huge around the world. One of the largest channels is transmission via the water source, where protozoa grow and infect the human population. Using or drinking contaminated water is one such mode, leading to protozoan-induced gastrointestinal illness such as *Giardia lamblia*. Apart from that, environmental factors such as poor hygiene practices and unsanitary conditions increase the chances of transmission. Enhancing water purifying technology and promoting hygiene procedure awareness are measures that need to be developed to avoid such hazards. Such an anticipatory policy is of the greatest importance in developing nations where access to clean water is limited, thus making citizens susceptible to protozoan infections, which lead to severe health problems. Essential mode transmission with vector organisms is also of utmost importance, as vector organisms play a crucial role in spreading protozoan pathogens. Mosquitoes, for instance, carry *Trypanosoma* parasites that cause sleeping sickness and Chagas disease. The life cycle in many cases of these protozoa comprises complex vector-host interactions wherein the parasites adapt to survive in different environments. Not only does this complicate disease control, but it also means that a multidisciplinary approach must be adopted to understand these interactions as a whole. Population control interventions such as the use of insect repellent or environmental modification have been shown to decrease the incidence of these infections. As a result, vector transmission is still a cornerstone of public health measures aimed at controlling protozoan infections. An underappreciated but significant pathway of transmission involves direct contact with infected patients, particularly relevant in the immunocompromised host. *Acanthamoeba keratitis* is a classic example of this route, where the organism typically enters via the cornea, often via contact lens use. Poor hygiene practices, such as the use of infected water for lens cleansing, facilitate this transmission and cause severe eye complications. Host susceptibility and environmental factors are the common factors leading to this infection. Awareness of the pathophysiology of *Acanthamoeba* infections, as described by contemporary research, may inform preventive interventions and individualized treatment protocols essential in reducing the associated risks. Promoting interest in lens care and hygiene would place health authorities at the forefront of arresting the incidence rate among vulnerable populations (Khan et al., 2004).

8.2.1. Waterborne Transmission

The waterborne transmission phenomenon is at the forefront of the global dispersal of protozoan infections, with water being a key vector for disease. Protozoan parasites such as *Giardia lamblia* and *Cryptosporidium parvum* are notorious for their induction of acute gastrointestinal disease that's most commonly transmitted through waterborne pollution. The pathogens persist in water for quite a long period and account for outbreaks in settings where there is poor sanitation. Also, climatic fluctuations can exacerbate the spread of such infections, with rising temperatures and altered precipitation patterns impacting the frequency and severity of waterborne diseases. Appreciation of the mechanisms of waterborne transmission will allow public health agencies to develop more efficient strategies to avert impending health risks from protozoan infections, particularly in vulnerable locales where access to clean water is limited. Other than the direct waterborne contamination of drinking water, the environmental stability of protozoan pathogens in water also poses other public health challenges. The oocyst phase of protozoa such as *Toxoplasma gondii* is highly resistant to environmental stress, and this allows for the widespread distribution of the parasite using surface water and sediment. These oocysts not only contaminate water sources, but also seep into food supplies, becoming encapsulated within shellfish and other aquatic organisms consumed by humans. This versatility attests to the importance of comprehensive monitoring in order to find and isolate sources of *T. gondii* and other similar pathogens within soil and water. Resolution of the transmission issue of oocysts would significantly minimize the prevalence of related diseases, thus emphasizing the need for stronger regulatory control in aquaculture and agriculture to safeguard public health effectively (Shapiro et al., 2019). With escalating global climate change in the alteration of the topography of waterborne diseases, the importance of ongoing surveillance and intervention becomes increasingly crucial. Through research, it has been observed that population displacement, intensified flooding, and water infrastructure disruption lead to the formation of waterborne pathogens and hence aggravate the situation for protozoan infection (Nichols et al., 2018). In most developing countries, where the capacity for rapid response is typically weak, the consequences of this shift are particularly devastating. Therefore, efficient management tactics, for example, better monitoring of water quality and hygiene practice training, need to be implemented. Enhanced coordination between governments and health organizations can also strengthen efforts to reach vulnerable populations, ensuring access to clean water and averting the adverse impacts of climate variability on waterborne transmission-related health outcomes (Figure 8.5).

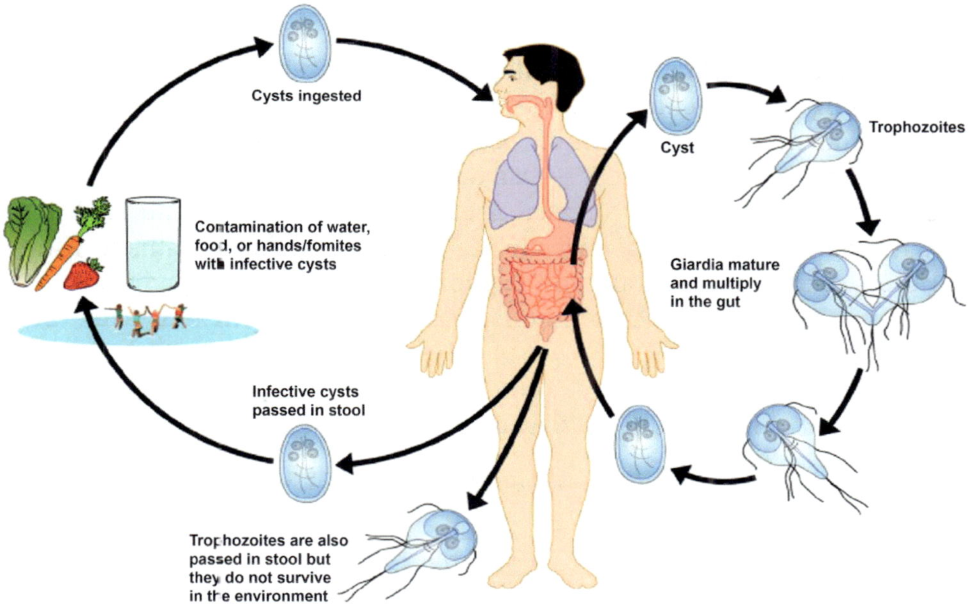

Figure 8.5. Protozoan parasites in drinking water.

Source: https://www.mdpi.com/ijerph/ijerph-15-00495/article_deploy/html/images/ijerph-15-00495-g002.png.

8.2.2. Vector-Borne Transmission

Vector transmission is of critical significance in the spread of protozoan infections, where certain groups of insects are vectors for the pathogens that can pose severe health issues to human populations. One such notable example is Chagas disease, caused by the protozoan parasite *Trypanosoma cruzi*. The disease is prevalent in 21 endemic countries of Latin America and is primarily transmitted by the feces of the triatomine insect. The insect, also referred to as the kissing bug, is adapted to be able to thrive in human habitats, and, hence, control of such vectors is essential in the process of preventing the transmission of the disease. Despite the advances in understanding more about the biology of *T. cruzi*, there are vast lacunae in Chagas disease management and control for acute and chronic infections, exposing millions to both versions, particularly affecting important organ systems such as the cardiovascular and nervous systems (Sherman, 2019). The impacts of climate change add to the vectors' dynamics of protozoan infections. More frequent and warmer temperatures, as well as changing regimes of precipitation, can directly affect vector habitats and activities, altering the dynamics of transmission to shift and extend into new geographic locations. In others, especially those with poor water supply and sanitation systems, these areas are extremely vulnerable to epidemics since they will not be able to put effective public health measures in place. The relationship between climatic changes and vector distribution may exacerbate existing health challenges, further complicating the already complex epidemiological landscape. Forecasting and surveillance become imperative within this intricate setting, allowing public health professionals to foresee probable increases in vector counts and the diseases they transmit, including Chagas and others (Nichols et al., 2018). Preventive measures would therefore need to include both vector control programs as well as other public health programs to tackle the issues of vector-transmitted protozoan infections. Programs focused on ensuring that there are effective surveillance systems that can provide valuable information regarding the distribution and prevalence of vectors and their associated pathogens can enable timely epidemiological interventions to outbreaks. Also, controlling the environmental determinants of vector amplification — i.e., progressing infrastructure, sanitation practices, and public awareness — can decrease risk of transmission. Emphasis on a One Health approach that accepts the interconnectedness of human, animal, and environmental health is needed to create comprehensive responses to the protozoan infections linked with vector-borne transmission. Herein, global cooperation and support are important to guarantee that vulnerable populations are provided with proper protection and resources (Nichols et al., 2018; Sherman, 2019) (Figure 8.6).

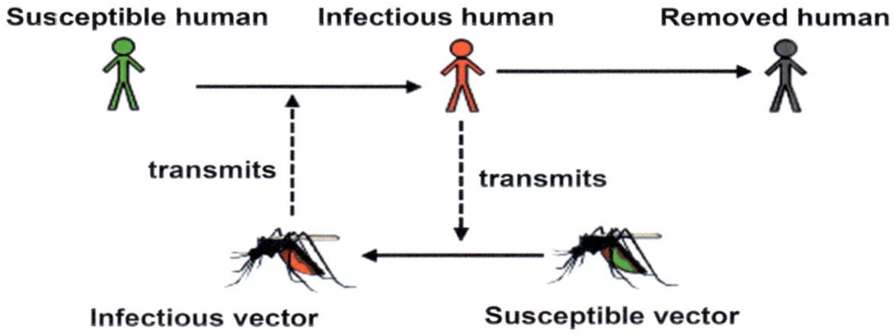

Figure 8.6. Vector-borne transmission.

Source: https://andreashandel.github.io/IDEMAbook/images/vectorborne-schematic.png.

8.2.3. Direct Contact Transmission

Direct contact transmission is the process that is part of the comprehension of the spread of the protozoan infection, particularly in light of the large number of infective agents. Acanthamoeba is an excellent example, as it is an opportunistic pathogen that causes keratitis in contact lens wearers primarily. The transmission mode of this protozoan is typically through contaminated surfaces, water, or hands. Inadequate hygienic habits in the management of contact lenses provide a route from the environment into the cornea for the amoebae, and they initiate a cascade of inflammation and, worst case, cause blindness. Pathogenesis of Acanthamoebas is further complicated by the combination of host susceptibility, environmental conditions, and virulence of the parasite. Better knowledge of these factors is needed for the development of beneficial prevention strategies and therapeutic interventions against *Acanthamoeba keratitis*, which has risen with the growth in the population of contact lens users (Khan et al., 2004). *Toxoplasma gondii*, a zoonotic parasite with a multifaceted transmission process, is also a significant agent of direct contact transmission of protozoan diseases. While passed mostly orally through ingestion of oocysts in contaminated food or water, direct contact with contaminated objects — such as soil and cat litter — is also a significant mode of transmission. Its highly durable oocyst form is well-suited to live in all types of environments, infecting numerous intermediate hosts, including humans. The organism's very resistant oocyst wall enables it not only to live within the habitat but also to invade water supplies and food, thereby guaranteeing its spread. The lack of specificity of definitive hosts, whose mainstay is domestic and wild cats, further underscores the zoonotic nature of *T. gondii* and public education on the risk of direct contact (Shapiro et al., 2019). Understanding the dynamics of transmission by direct contact of protozoan infections is key to public health interventions aimed at reducing prevalence. Health education among high-risk populations, such as those involved in agriculture or animal husbandry, can reduce the incidence of such infections as those caused by *T. gondii*. Proper hygiene practice in places such as the kitchen, garden, and those where pets visit is also the cornerstone against such infections. Incorporation of scientific information into community outreach programs can empower individuals to recognize and manage risks of direct contact transmission. Given that the environment continues to develop and human-wildlife interaction continues to increase, managing such protozoan transmission channels through the uptake of well-educated public health interventions and personal health practices will be crucial in combating the disease burden caused by these protozoa.

8.3. Symptoms and Diagnosis

Clinical features of protozoal infection are extremely varied according to the species of the protozoan as well as the location of the infection in the host. *Trypanosoma cruzi*, the causative agent of Chagas disease, for instance, has both acute and chronic phases with their respective specific clinical presentations. The acute phase can manifest with mild symptoms such as fever, weakness, and local inflammation at the site of entry, whereas the chronic phase can lead to hazardous complications on the cardiovascular system, gastrointestinal tract, and nervous system, illustrating the parasite's systemic effects on the human body (Sherman, 2019). Detection of the symptomatology is critical to the early diagnosis of these infections because it provides the first clue to potential underlying protozoan disease that would otherwise remain undiagnosed in endemic regions. Diagnosis of protozoan infection is complex and can be prevented by the unpredictability of presentation and the superimposition of symptoms on other illnesses. In optimal therapy and infection control of intestinal protozoa infection, such as *Giardia intestinalis* and *Entamoeba histolytica*, accurate diagnostic methods are required. Previously, the diagnostic methods included stool examination via direct fecal smears and concentration techniques, but are less sensitive, leading to underdiagnosis (Albonico et al., 2013). Modern developments, such as the mini-FLOTAC method, are offered with enhanced sensitivity to detect intestinal parasites in resource-limited settings and hence improve diagnostic yields and aid the detection of co- or dual-infections, which could complicate clinical presentations. The role of adequate symptoms and diagnosis in the management of protozoan infections cannot be overemphasized. Pre-early diagnosis has the potential to radically alter disease trajectory and allow for early intervention of treatments that may prevent severe health morbidities associated with long-term chronic infection. In the case of Chagas disease, for example, early diagnosis during the acute stage allows for more effective therapeutic intervention, perhaps reducing the long-term burden on health systems in endemic regions (Sherman, 2019). Furthermore, innovations in sophisticated diagnostic techniques can allow for epidemiologic study and public health interventions aimed at interrupting protozoan infections, and reducing transmission and improving patient outcomes in high-risk groups. Consequently, ongoing research and investment in diagnostics are critical components of the struggle against the scope of protozoal infections worldwide.

8.3.1. Common Symptoms of Protozoan Infections

Protozoal infections have a very diverse group of symptoms that can have a significant impact on the health of infected patients. Protozoal infections usually manifest as gastrointestinal distress in the form of diarrhea, cramps, and nausea. Infections with *Entamoeba histolytica*, for instance, the infective parasite of amoebic dysentery, are characterized by prolonged and bloody diarrhea accompanied by cramping and fever. Additionally, some of the protozoan infections can cause systemic symptoms, such as fatigue and weakness, as a result of the body's response to infection. In most instances, such symptoms can be mistaken for other conditions, making diagnosis difficult and treatment delayed, hence increasing the severity of the infection. Being aware of these common symptoms is not only important for early diagnosis but also for the formulation of effective therapeutic regimens when treating protozoan infections. Another notable aspect of protozoan infections is the potential for neurological presentation, particularly in infections with parasites like *Trypanosoma brucei*, which cause African sleeping sickness. During the initial phase, patients may experience headache, joint pain, and different forms of fever; however, if the disease is allowed to develop, there may be more dramatic neurological presentation in the form of confusion, changes in behavior, or even coma.

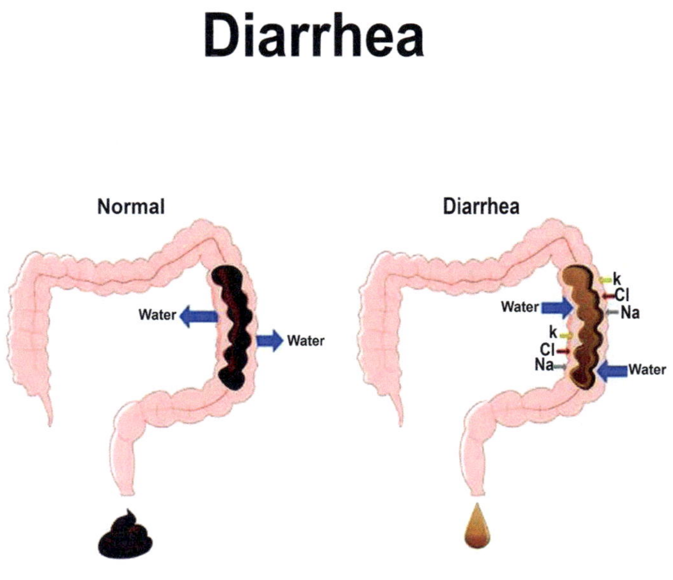

Figure 8.7. Diarrhea.

Source: https://content.health.harvard.edu/wp-content/uploads/2024/05/4c33864b-8374-4028-9351-302873e7dc40.jpg.

This progress emphasizes the seriousness of protozoan infections and the necessity of timely medical intervention. Furthermore, parasitic infections like Toxoplasmosis, caused primarily by *Toxoplasma gondii*, can lead to neurological deficits, especially among immunocompromised individuals, where the central nervous system is widely affected. Care for these differential symptoms is necessary for the worldwide control of protozoan infections and their impact on public health. In some instances, protozoan infections can result in a variety of symptoms affecting several body systems, thereby a multifaceted clinical picture. For example, in Chagas disease caused by *Trypanosoma cruzi*, the symptoms range from an asymptomatic acute febrile illness to a more complex presentation in the chronic phase, with the cardiovascular and gastrointestinal systems involved. The patients may also have cardiomyopathy, arrhythmias, or gastrointestinal illnesses that require widespread healthcare measures (Sherman, 2019). Similarly, *Cytauxzoon felis*, the protozoan parasite of the domestic cat, presents with signs that range from fever to lethargy and anemia, indicating the enormous health implications for both the cats and their owners (Hickman et al., 2010). Thus, the variation of symptoms due to protozoan infections emphasizes the need for greater knowledge and awareness among the healthcare professionals to facilitate early diagnosis and treatment strategies (Figure 8.7).

8.3.2. Diagnostic Methods Used

The diagnosis of protozoan infection employs various methods specific to the causal organism and habitat. Traditional methods include microscopy, where parasites are viewed directly in patient specimens. For instance, the Kato-Katz method is extensively used for the diagnosis of *Schistosoma mansoni* by examining stool samples; the method is also capable of estimating the intensity of infections from quantitative egg measurements of the parasite. In addition, the formol-ether concentration method enhances the recovery of intestinal protozoa by concentrating eggs and cysts in fecal samples and also the precision of diagnosis. These methods are pillars in disease-endemic settings where an understanding of the prevalence of infections informs treatment and public health measures (Coulibaly et al., 2012). With developments in diagnostics, the need for alternatives that can differentiate among multiple pathogens concurrently becomes increasingly significant. In recent years, the advancements in the diagnosis techniques have revealed more sensitive and effective techniques. The mini-FLOTAC technique, for instance, has generated interest due to its better efficacy in the diagnosis of intestinal parasitic diseases, such as protozoa. In Indian and Tanzanian studies, mini-FLOTAC provided a sensitivity of 90% for helminth infection, much greater than the traditional methods like direct fecal smear and formol-ether concentration for certain infections (Albonico et al., 2013). Mini-FLOTAC is a novel method that allows examination of many samples by a single test, thus greatly useful in low-resource environments. Moreover, the use of rapid diagnostic tests (RDTs) in the field has reduced the detection process to become a faster one, enabling quicker identification of infection. These technologies show an enhancement in the trend towards utilization of more efficient diagnostic modalities that tackle complexities of parasitic infections. The implications of selecting specific diagnostic methods have consequences far outside laboratory environments, affecting public health interventions and control measures for protozoan infections. Diagnostics are valuable in assisting in tailoring treatment protocols and in the use of surveillance strategies in areas of endemicity. For instance, the use of a rapid screening method in Côte d'Ivoire facilitated the identification of varying endemic levels of *Schistosoma* spp. across varied settings, which later informed targeted intervention strategies (Coulibaly et al., 2012). Furthermore, the discovery of co-infections among a population, as exemplified through the case of schoolchildren's double infections, underscores the significance of multivariable diagnostic techniques. Using various methods, health officials are in a better position to correctly establish patterns of infection, assess the efficacy of treatments, and sufficiently distribute resources, thereby maximizing the effectiveness of public health intervention towards controlling protozoan infections (Figure 8.8).

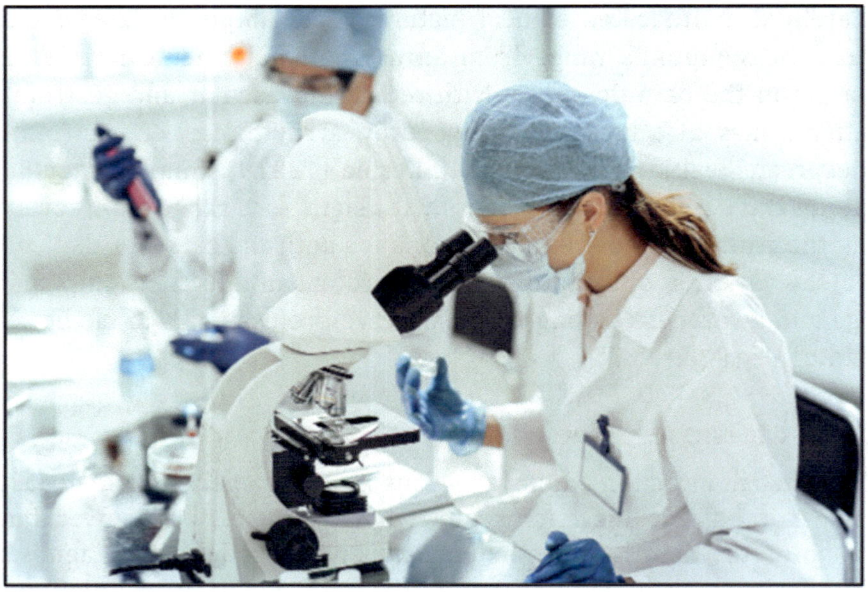

Figure 8.8. Diagnosis of protozoan infections.

Source: https://nl-lab.nl/wp-content/uploads/2023/09/stocklabfoto.png.

8.3.3. Challenges in Diagnosing Protozoan Infections

Diagnosis of protozoan diseases is extremely difficult due to intricate life cycles as well as diverse manifestations of the parasites. For instance, the parasite *Trypanosoma cruzi*, responsible for Chagas disease, is contracted in two stages: acute and chronic. This variability of presentation is likely to make it difficult to diagnose early because the acute stage may be absent or manifest in a mild form and the chronic stage may only be seen years later, and healthcare providers end up missing potential infections. Moreover, the lack of sufficiently sensitive and specific diagnostic methods prevents effective identification because standard methods may not detect the sophistication in infection stages, leaving millions of untreated disease exposure (Sherman, 2019). Increased protozoan infection rates among other host species, like livestock, also prevent diagnostic efforts. Dairy buffalo, for instance, are prone to intestinal protozoa like Giardia and Eimeria, which can mask clinical signs of infection and potentially result in misdiagnosis or the delay of treatment. These infections could be caused by environmental factors, like polluted water sources, making outreach for correct diagnosis challenging. Moreover, the current methods of diagnosis hardly detect carriers who are not affected, enabling parasites to remain undetected in populations. Thus, understanding the epidemiological status of infections among non-human hosts, in combination with novel detection techniques and technology, emerges as a top priority in addressing these diagnostic issues (Morgoglione, 2021). Finally, the emergence of drug resistance among protozoan pathogens adds another layer of complexity to the diagnosis and management of infections. Conventional prophylactic treatments have been instrumental in infection control, but their misuse has generated the risk of developing resistance, rendering some remedies less effective in the long term. This is a trend that requires ongoing epidemiological surveillance and research on new diagnostic techniques that will be able to match the evolving nature of protozoan infections. By using advanced technologies such as molecular diagnostics and immunoassays, healthcare practitioners can enhance the accuracy of protozoan infection diagnosis, resulting in more specific treatment and prevention measures in both human and animal medicine (Sherman, 2019; Morgoglione et al., 2021).

8.4. Treatment Options

Protozoan infection treatment needs to be multi-component and consider both public health actions and pharmacologic measures. Antimicrobial agents, such as antiparasitic or antimalarial therapy, remain mainstays in the treatment of most protozoan infections by specifically targeting pathogens like *Plasmodium* species and *Giardia lamblia*. For example, the use of medication such as artemisinin-based combination therapies has been shown to be effective for the treatment of malaria and for reducing levels of morbidity and mortality associated with the disease. Nevertheless, drug resistance calls for continued surveillance and research on new therapeutic agents. Additionally, preventive and supportive therapy in the guise of vaccination campaigns, where they exist, plays a significant role in limiting protozoan infection effects. Treatment, apart from relief of symptoms, also prevents interruption of transmission, thus contributing to total public health interventions in controlling such infections. Furthermore, sanitation and environmental upgrading are of the highest priority in reducing risks of protozoan infection, especially those through sources of water contamination. Irrigation with wastewater, as common practice in most developing nations, is an ongoing public health issue due to the risk of transferring pathogens, such as protozoan parasites. The risk to health in eating vegetables irrigated by untreated sewage is emphasized through evidence indicating exposure to contaminated water sources as a factor for increased disease rates. Techniques to enhance wastewater management and treatment, as recognized in recent epidemiological studies, are of utmost importance in reducing such risks. Through safer irrigation practices and effective wastewater treatment systems, communities can actually decrease the burden of protozoal diseases, resulting in improved food safety and public health gains, particularly in agriculture-based regions. Finally, preventive treatment and health education that target the community can play a crucial role in the prevention of protozoan infections. Practice habits such as good hand washing, proper cooking of food, and avoiding the consumption of untreated water can be propagated through education campaigns to promote healthier practices that significantly lower rates of infection. Additionally, health education interventions among populations at risk of infection, particularly where protozoan infections are endemic, can instill confidence to adopt preventive strategies against transmission in a proactive manner. Additionally, health education coupled with environmental management policies can help enable a synergistic effect, which enhances the overall effectiveness of procedures for treatment available. By tackling the biological as well as socioeconomic determinants of protozoan infections, a holistic public health model arises that enhances disease control while supporting sustainable health behavior in communities.

8.4.1. Antiprotozoal Medications

The treatment of protozoan infections is mostly a matter of treatment with antiprotozoal medications, which target various stages of the life cycle of the parasite to minimize their impact on human health. Some of the most visible infections, such as those caused by *Giardia intestinalis* and *Entamoeba histolytica*, are easily eliminated through properly defined pharmaceutical agents like metronidazole. But the efficacy of these conventional medicines has been increasingly threatened by the impending deluge of drug resistance. There are reports that several protozoan species are evolving resistance mechanisms against antiprotozoal agents, which render conventional medicines less effective. Resistance is most alarming in low-income countries where access to healthcare is constrained, exerting further pressure on the need for alternative therapeutic strategies that can complement or replace conventional drugs (Ojuromi & Ashafa, 2020). Elaborating further on our understanding of resistance patterns and exploring new lines of drug development are crucial in order to combat the growing healthcare costs of protozoan infection. The topic of antiprotozoal drugs is also fraught with complications due to the heterogeneity of the protozoan diseases and the variability of the pharmacology of existing drugs. An individual disease can potentially require targeted therapy that considers the specific protozoan involved as well as the specific host. For example, leishmaniasis, caused by transmission via the *Leishmania* species, needs specific antiprotozoal medications such as amphotericin B or miltefosine. Such treatments have their shortcomings, though, such as potential toxicity and the need for parenteral administration, so they are not easy to administer in endemic regions (Jada, 2024). Since researchers desire more accessible and less toxic materials, the study of natural products is now a viable option. Extracts of medicinal plants can yield bioactive compounds possessing antiprotozoal activity, which can contribute towards the holistic management of protozoan infections in different populations. Furthermore, the development of new antiprotozoal drugs is extremely necessary to transcend the shortcomings of the existing therapies as well as to treat emergent strains that are resistant. Studies in recent years that have considered natural product-derived compounds have been encouraging, as they combat infections such as visceral leishmaniasis. The best example is the alkaloid peganine, which possesses selective activity against intracellular *Leishmania donovani* and is of low toxicity against host cells. This is an exhibition of how bioactive products can be applied to create new therapeutic avenues, particularly in previously underfunded and neglected diseases (Ojuromi & Ashafa, 2020). The thrust for new drug discovery is characterized by systematic screening and optimization of such compounds to ensure maximum efficacy with minimal side effects. In the face of the ongoing menace presented by the diarrheal disease burden of protozoan infections on healthcare systems globally, interventions in the form of improved drug formulations and secondary treatments are needed to bring about better outcomes among infected populations (Figure 8.9).

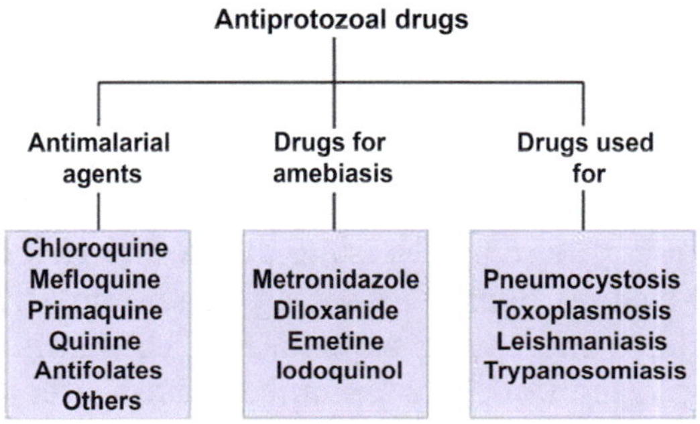

Figure 8.9. Antiprotozoal drugs.

Source: https://doctorlib.org/pharmacology/pharmacology-examination-board-review/pharmacology-examination-board-review.files/image219.jpg.

8.4.2. Supportive Care and Management

In the management of protozoan infections, supportive care and management are key determinants of improved patient outcomes. The infections are often multidimensional in nature that extending beyond conventional antimicrobial therapy. Supportive care encompasses management of symptoms, nutritional rehabilitation, and psychosocial interventions, which collectively enhance the quality of life for the infected patient. For instance, symptomatic malaria patients may require more than the antimalarial drugs, but also fluids and electrolytes for the management of dehydration and re-establishment of metabolic equilibrium. By the process of considering the total needs of the patients, healthcare providers can empower patients with an improved ability to withstand the physical and psychological stress that protozoan infections impose on them, thereby increasing prospects for recovery and reducing complications from such infections. In addition, successful management plans for protozoan infections must encompass prevention and education. As emphasized by the ongoing burden of sexually transmitted infections (STIs), prevention and behavior change remain central to the efforts against transmission and burden of such infections. World health systems must invest in the development of affordable and culturally acceptable diagnostic tests and treatment protocols. For instance, for non-HIV STIs, benefiting from what has been gained in HIV treatment and prevention can be very gratifying.

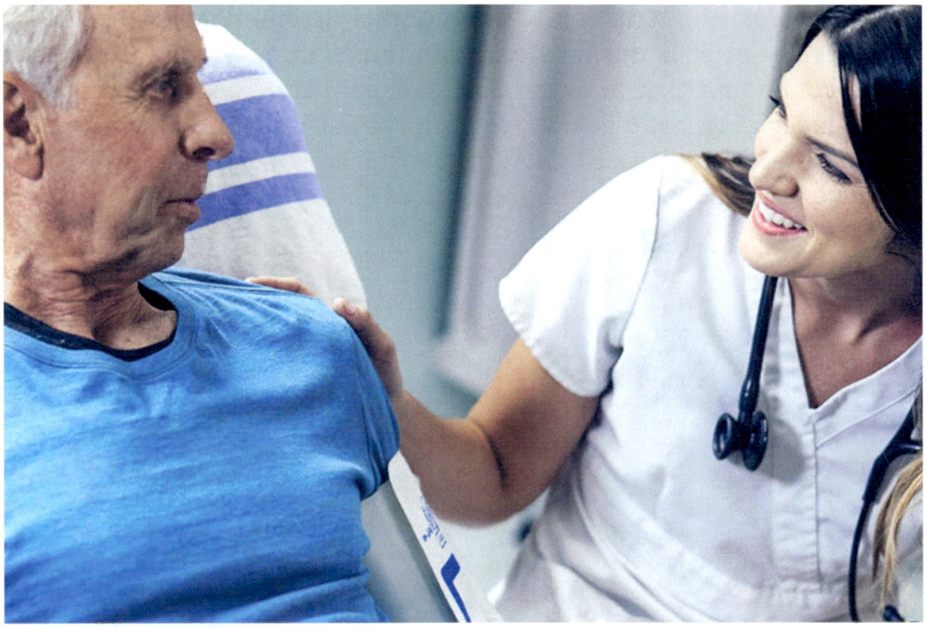

Figure 8.10. Supportive care.

Source: https://healthcare.ascension.org/-/media/healthcare/national/service-lines/hero/infectiousdisease.jpg?h=800&iar=0&w=1200&hash=7A6D937E7B38A148BE491F93FDA0DD36.

Rapid testing and point-of-care services have been successful in STI control and can be adapted to manage protozoan infections more efficiently. Such a proactive strategy for prevention and management helps to bring to the fore the pivotal intersection of supportive care in propelling health care systems to be responsive and resilient to these public health concerns (Ortayli et al., 2014). Lastly, the integration of supportive care under the broad umbrella of management of protozoan infection necessitates the collaboration of various stakeholders, including governments, healthcare workers, and populations. By developing partnerships, stakeholders can facilitate ease in sharing best practices and resources crucial to the effective delivery of care. Further, awareness of socio-economic and cultural challenges that may afflict patients can assist in maximizing intervention efficacy. Against the backdrop of ongoing protozoan infection complications, training healthcare workers and strengthening local health systems is now a pressing issue. The inclusion of behavior change interventions and a guarantee of prioritization of patient education are also imperative components of this framework, whereby it is possible to arrest the ailing socio-economic impacts of such infections (Coulibaly et al., 2012). This collective effort ultimately paves the way for enhanced health status among protozoan infection-affected persons, testifying to the importance accorded by healthcare systems to supportive care and management (Figure 8.10).

8.4.3. Emerging Treatments and Research

The production of new pharmaceuticals and investigation into protozoan diseases has become increasingly more significant, with the potential for drug resistance and a lack of an effective vaccine. New therapies are aiming towards therapies that use advanced technologies to disrupt the life cycles of protozoan diseases. Recent research has highlighted the role of extracellular vesicles (EVs) in host-parasite interaction, with potential as biomarkers and therapeutic agents. EVs, released by a variety of cells during stress and infection, may contain proteins and nucleic acids that allow for communication between host and parasite. This dynamic release of EVs can be harnessed to engineer diagnostic devices to improve early diagnosis and treatment regimens for protozoa-induced infectious diseases, thereby transforming current therapeutic approaches in translational medicine applications (Gavinho et al., 2019).

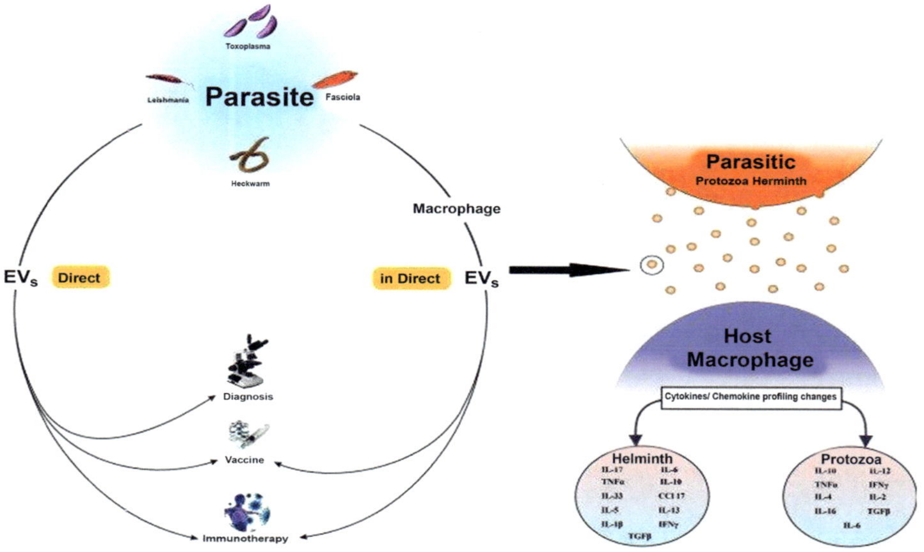

Figure 8.11. Extracellular vesicles (EVs) extracted directly from parasites or indirectly from host cells, sensed by parasites.

Source: https://www.researchgate.net/publication/340957842/figure/fig1/AS:11431281256190017@1719514471284/Extracellular-vesicles-EVs-extracted-directly-from-parasites-or-indirectly-from-host.jpg.

Another promising area in the research on protozoan infections is in the application of systems biology to the understanding of parasite-host interactions. Genomic technology advances, including next-generation sequencing, have opened up new avenues to investigate the biological mechanisms of parasitic diseases. The technologies allow researchers to acquire high-throughput omics data, which can be probed for identifying the intricate networks that are accountable for host response to protozoan infection. By integrating this information, scientists can select major routes that are prospective targets for intervention and consequently, design new drugs that can circumvent established pathways of resistance. As more progresses are made in the area, improved understanding of such intricate biological processes may set the stage for new antiparasitic therapies (Swann et al., 2015). Finally, an important aspect of new treatments for protozoan diseases is the identification and synthesis of new compounds to attack resistant parasites simultaneously. More research involves the screening of existing libraries of compounds for activity against protozoan pathogens, as well as synthesis from natural origins. Cooperative research programs, particularly those utilizing international collaborations, are essential for bringing these compounds to the world and providing equal access to effective therapy in the endemic regions. Furthermore, exploration of adjuvant treatment, which enhances the activity of drugs already available, may further enhance treatment outcome and reduce parasitic burden. With collaborative attempts towards understanding and overcoming the issues presented by protozoan infections, the potential for significant patient treatment and public health breakthroughs is promising (Figure 8.11).

8.5. Prevention Strategies

Prevention of protozoal infections includes a comprehensive approach that integrates public health interventions, education, and environmental management to control transmission. Expansion of coverage of clean water and sanitation facilities is among the most appropriate interventions. In areas where protozoal infections, such as those caused by Giardia and *Entamoeba histolytica*, are endemic, inadequate treatment of water exacerbates the situation. Educating communities to be empowered with knowledge on safe water practices and enforcing hygiene can also significantly reduce infection levels. Environmental context at the local level must be considered for public health interventions, as seen in settings where high endemic *Schistosoma* infection levels exist, where prevalence is highly variable by setting based on sanitation and availability of water (Coulibaly et al., 2012). This implies that focused prevention interventions responding to conditions in the location are essential in disease control. In addition to infrastructure improvements, faster diagnostic methods are increasingly significant in protozoan infection surveillance and management. Highly effective diagnostic methods allow better infection and prevalence detection in communities, allowing more targeted intervention programs. For instance, the establishment of rigorous diagnostic approaches drastically transformed the understanding of infection rates among schoolchildren residing in endemic areas (Coulibaly et al., 2012). These shifts in data underscore the importance of integrating technological innovation in epidemiology into interventions in public health to enable timely intervention. Moreover, continuous surveillance through community health programs can allow earlier detection of outbreaks and improve response activities, hence overall public health resilience to protozoan infections. Vector control is also crucial in preventing protozoan infections, particularly those transmitted by mosquitoes and other arthropods. Interventions such as insecticide-treated bed nets, larviciding, and environmental alteration to eliminate vector breeding sites are crucial. In regions like

Lake Kainji in Nigeria, where anthropogenic pressures have influenced the population of both fish and parasites, ecological processes play an important role in effective prevention campaigns. Integrated management of vectors that considers ecological health not only reduces disease transmission but also promotes sustainable ecosystems. With advertising of interdisciplinarity of work between ecologists, doctors, and residents, prevention methods can be significantly increased, ultimately resulting in fewer protozoan infection burdens and enhancing public health gains.

8.5.1. Hygiene and Sanitation Practices

The importance of sanitization and hygiene practice in the prevention of protozoan infection cannot be overemphasized. Good hygiene practices, such as frequent hand washing with soap and good handling of foods, are the main methods of prevention of the transmission of a range of protozoan pathogens. Substandard sanitary facilities, particularly in poor-resource environments, facilitate the transmission of infections like Giardia and *Entamoeba histolytica*, which thrive maximally in contaminated foods and water sources. Thus, minimum sanitation practices — like availability of safe, clean drinking water and adequate sewage disposal — are essential. Evidence shows that infection prevalence rates of protozoa are found to be high in places with poor sanitation, further emphasizing the need for proper public health intervention regarding hygiene and environmental sanitation, particularly in vulnerable groups (Coulibaly et al., 2012). The role of education and community participation in the facilitation of improved hygiene practices should not be overemphasized. The success of information campaigns towards raising awareness of the modes of transmission of protozoan infections and application of sanitation has been revealed through evidence of a decline in infection rates. By educating populations about the need to properly dispose of waste, boiling water, and personal hygiene protocols, all communities can avoid the risk of infection. In addition, participatory processes involving residents' engagement in sanitation activities enhance ownership and responsibility for ensuring hygiene is more sustainable. There is a need for public health practitioners to apply epidemiological approaches to assess the effectiveness of such interventions as they develop guidelines and policies to enhance hygiene levels across different areas with high susceptibility to protozoan disease outbreaks (Blumenthal et al., 2001).

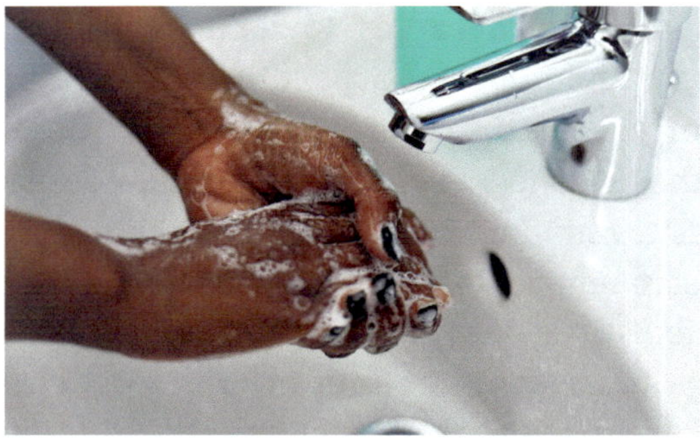

Figure 8.12. Personal hygiene.

Source: https://www.food-safety.com/ext/resources/2021/06/20/Sanitize_Img01_900.jpg?1629294586.

Knowing the challenges caused by protozoan infections, strict practice and maintenance of hygiene and sanitation are important to public health. Regular monitoring of water quality, particularly of recreational and drinking water supplies, is necessary in identifying contamination before incidents of widespread health concern can arise. Moreover, it is essential to be multidisciplinary in style and incorporate social, environmental, and health sciences into intervention development with a view to targeting protozoan pathogens efficiently. Not only does it assist in controlling the burden of disease, but it also enhances the quality of life in general among affected populations. As protozoan disease remains a public health problem of concern, the continued emphasis on sanitation and hygiene practices holds the key to leveraging impressive progress in disease prevention and control measures in the coming times (Coulibaly et al., 2012) (Figure 8.12).

8.5.2. Vaccination Efforts

The interface of vaccination and protozoan infection is a very important area to research, particularly in light of the burden of disease caused by *Trypanosoma* and *Leishmania* infection. The protozoa are a range of neglected tropical diseases with profound destructive impacts on the health system, particularly in the developing world. New genomics has disclosed the complex biology of these pathogens and given a glimpse into their genealogical relatedness as well as the broad gamut of clinical impacts they elicit. These results pave the way for targeted vaccination regimens, which are desperately needed. Toward this end, the integration of immunological treatments with molecular and clinical treatments is more critical, as discussed in recent reviews of the subject matter. The rapid advances in our understanding of these protozoan diseases present challenges like never before to reinvent drug, diagnostic, and vaccine design to combat these conditions effectively (Stuart et al., 2008). Immunization against protozoan diseases has particular issues, including compromised immunity accompanying chronic parasitic infections. Recent findings indicate that individuals with neglected tropical diseases are capable of generating diminished immune responses to conventional vaccination. Experiments in the impact of chronic trematode, nematode, and protozoan infections reveal that such infections interfere with conventional vaccination regimens, particularly in risk groups such as pregnant women and children. The immunomodulatory effect of parasitic infections has been shown to suppress the immune system's efficacy to respond to vaccines, leading to suboptimal protection responses. Therefore, the innovation of better vaccination programs requires a two-faceted approach that not only develops effective vaccines but also incorporates antiparasitic drugs to boost immunity and overall public health (Labeaud et al., 2009). To boost the efficacy of vaccination activities against protozoan diseases, comprehensive strategies must be adopted. It involves not only enhancing vaccine research but also having tight public health controls to stem the spread of these infections. The treatment of chronic parasitic infections with antiparasitic drugs can enhance vaccine effectiveness and overall health outcomes in infected populations. Future research needs to be geared towards establishing how various protozoan genera interact with the immune response, particularly in high-burden settings. Moreover, intervention strategies should consider socio-economic constraints in local epidemiological contexts that restrict vaccination coverage. By prioritizing combined measures with both parasite control and immunization, health authorities can increase the effectiveness of immunization campaigns and ultimately reduce the incidence of protozoan infections (Labeaud et al., 2009).

8.5.3. Public Health Initiatives

Public health programs are essential to controlling the transmission of protozoan diseases, particularly in low-income areas where the infections pose a significant health risk. Preventive care mechanisms such as health education campaigns and community health programs can play a major role in enhancing people's knowledge about the modes of transmission and symptoms of protozoan diseases such as giardiasis and amoebiasis. For example, incorporating hygiene education into school lessons can empower the children to promote healthier habits that decrease the risk of infection. Further, these efforts usually come with the active involvement of the surrounding communities, a factor that is important for them to be sustained and effective. Through the provision of affordable healthcare and direct engagement of members from the community, public health programs establish an environment that fosters preventive care and, in the process, slows down the prevalence of these infections over time. The challenge of treating protozoan infections is not only in the treatment itself, but also in facing the socio-economic factors that contribute to transmission. It has been evidenced that lower socio-economic status plays a significant role in the risk of intestinal parasitic infection among children in rural settings, particularly in places such as Mexico, where there are poor sanitation practices. The National Deworming Campaign and the Opportunities program reveal how organized public health interventions can mitigate such risks by reaching vulnerable groups.

By focusing on women's education and increased access to healthcare, such programs target the social determinants of health that are most directly responsible for disseminating protozoan infection. Monitoring such interventions is crucial in measuring their efficacy and how best to target them so they reach the populations that require them most, which brings about improved health outcomes. Finally, an integrated strategy that unites therapy with robust public health interventions can effectively reduce the disease burden of protozoan diseases. For instance, the integration of antiretroviral therapy programs in India is paralleled by efforts to control intestinal parasitism using combined prevention and therapy measures. These initiatives demonstrate the need for a holistic public health strategy that addresses not just the direct medical problem but also the larger systemic problem of education and clean water. As the battle against protozoan infections continues, the importance of sustained funding, community engagement, and interdisciplinarity cannot be overstated. With these investments in public health, the potential for long-term reductions in protozoan infection rates is greater, ultimately leading to healthier populations and improved quality of life for those afflicted (Quihui et al., 2006; Coulibaly et al., 2012) (Figure 8.13).

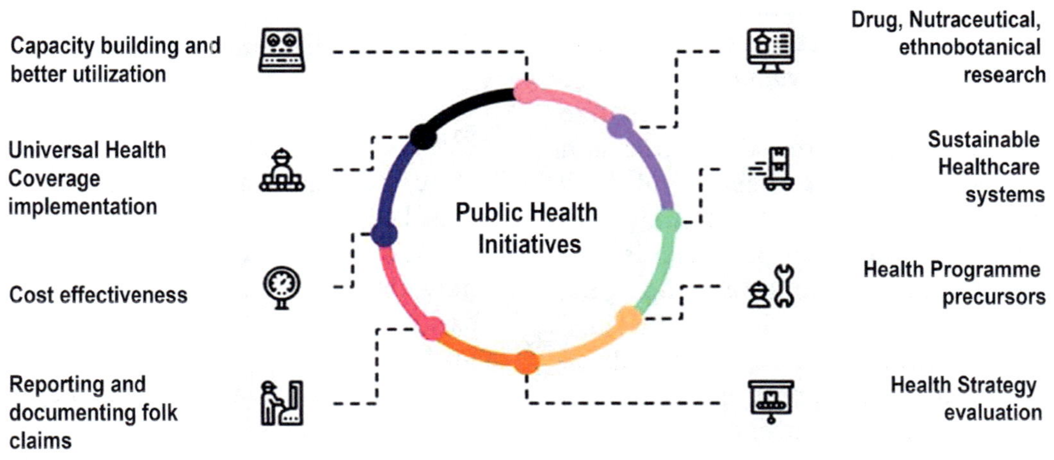

Figure 8.13. Public health initiatives.

Source: https://www.researchgate.net/profile/Karthik-K-P-3/publication/374583836/figure/fig3/AS:11431281197315779@1696963234932/Need-of-public-health-initiatives-in-Ayush.ppm.

8.6. Impact on Global Health

The impact of protozoan infections on global health is considerable, particularly in low- and middle-income countries where the socioeconomic determinants are preponderant in influencing health. An example is intestinal parasitic infections that continue to affect communities in Mexico. It has been established that schoolchildren in rural areas have a high prevalence of polyparasitism and protozoan infections, which indicates the relationship between socioeconomic determinants and health hazards. Specifically, employment and maternal education have been associated with increased rates of infection of giardiasis (*Giardia duodenalis*) and amoebiasis (*Entamoeba histolytica*). The findings highlight the necessity to urgently incorporate health programs into community development initiatives in order to address such disparities and improve public health (Quihui et al., 2006). Public health policy can promote education and sanitation to reduce the health burden of protozoan infection, ensuring a healthier future for at-risk populations. Except for parasitic disease, sexually transmitted disease is a significant health burden worldwide, and its effects are felt by numerous demographic groups. The United Kingdom has made immense strides in STI monitoring and control, yet inequalities between groups such as men who have sex with men and young adults persist. The historical trends in the epidemiology of STIs demonstrate the dynamic nature of public health problems and the necessity of adaptive intervention. The advancement of testing technologies, coupled with a changing environment for service provision, underscores the complexity of effective STI control. Current public health initiatives have to consider shifting behavior and population demographics to align programs that satisfy individualized needs of high-risk groups in an effort to promote equal health outcomes (Hughes & Field, 2015). In the end, management of STIs is based on a coordinated worldwide effort that prioritizes education, access to healthcare, and integration into society. The convergence of protozoan diseases and public health issues considers the interconnectedness of health outcomes worldwide. These infections must not only be tackled on the clinical front but also require an overarching understanding of the social determinants of health. Intestinal parasitism in Mexico, for instance, and its contributing factors — socioeconomic status, education, and practices regarding hygiene — demonstrate the need for an integrated understanding of public health. Concurrently, the STI disease burden reveals sexual health education and care access gaps that persistently disproportionately affect marginalized groups. Thus, global health responses need to embrace multi-dimensional approaches, recognizing the complex interdynamics of biological, social, and economic factors influencing health. Since health inequities persist, interdisciplinary collaborations and targeted interventions are necessary to decrease the global burden of protozoan diseases and attain healthier results in all populations (Quihui et al., 2006; Hughes & Field, 2015).

8.6.1. Prevalence in Developing Countries

Infections with protozoa are very high in developing countries, which signifies a public health problem of great seriousness. Infections with protozoa are typically caused most frequently by poor hygiene, no access to clean water, and low socio-economic status. As an illustration, parasitism by intestines was found to have an important role in school children, whose prevalence of infection with protozoa was 65% among the population studied. This figure emphasizes the high incidence of infection, particularly in the context of low income and low educational level of mothers, which has been linked to higher exposure to intestinal parasitism (Quihui et al., 2006). Furthermore, hygiene practices such as open defecation aggravated the situation, showing the need for comprehensive public health interventions that address both environmental and educational aspects of disease prevention. The recurring protozoan infection burden in developing nations is not limited to rural communities alone and includes significant prevalence in urban communities, too, due to water source contamination. A study on the Angke River in Jakarta highlighted the detection of eggs of *Ascaris lumbricoides* and *Entamoeba histolytica* cysts, which indicates severe fecal contamination of the water resources (Subahar & Sutanto, 2008). This is a manifestation of a broader issue where industrialization and urbanization have led to improper waste disposal and contamination.

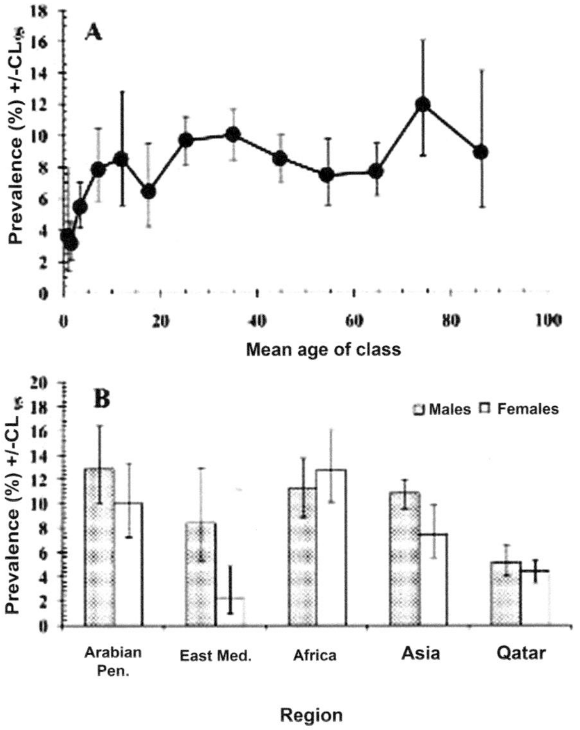

Figure 8.14. Prevalence of all protozoan infections.

Source: https://www.researchgate.net/profile/Marawan-Abu-Madi/publication/47428222/figure/fig2/AS:202530198953986@1425298370265/Prevalence-of-all-protozoan-infections-combined-For-the-goodness-of-fit-of-the-minimum.png.

As a result, individuals whose livelihood relies on such contaminated water bodies are in greater danger of contracting protozoan infections, rendering improvement in public health even more difficult. Remedy of such water quality issues is vital, considering that access to clean potable water is essential in keeping pace with controlling the spread of such infections. Interventions that reduce the prevalence of protozoan infection in developing countries must be holistic and include community health education, better sanitation facilities, and effective water quality testing. Public health education programs focusing on maternal education are particularly urgent, as statistics show that educated mothers are likely to implement improved hygiene practices and therefore reduce rates of child infection (Quihui et al., 2006). Additionally, expanded facilities for water treatment and waste disposal can go a long way in minimizing the risk of water-borne protozoal disease. Collaboration with local governments as well as non-profit organizations to promote health education and the application of sustainable sanitation systems will form the core of combating the widespread prevalence of protozoan infection in these countries. Through this large-scale approach, interruption of the cycle of infection will be facilitated, as well as overall improvement of public health in developing countries (Figure 8.14).

8.6.2. Economic Burden of Protozoan Infections

The economic burden of protozoal infections in developing nations is significant, impacting infected people's health and productivity. The prevalence of such infections, particularly where there is no good healthcare infrastructure, causes significant healthcare expenditures to governments and households. Households in affected communities with endemic protozoan infections, for instance, *Giardia duodenalis* and *Entamoeba histolytica*, end up spending recurring medical costs on treatment and consultation. In addition, repeated costs of preventive measures, such as sanitation improvements and public health programs, once more present extra burdens on limited economic resources. In the case of rural Mexican communities, socio-economic factors provide a higher number of infections, thereby increasing healthcare needs that further increase the economic burden on these vulnerable populations. The reappearance of protozoan infections, therefore, represents the ongoing problems for public health systems to address socioeconomic disparities. The impact of protozoan infections extends beyond the direct cost of medical care to encompass a broader economic dimension, such as lost productivity and lowered earnings. Such patients with chronic infection have severe symptoms that debilitate their ability to work and consequently affect their input toward family earnings and overall economic productivity. In endemic areas, the workforce is immediately impacted because parents have to stay home and care for sick children, adding to economic instability in the home. Furthermore, cases of polyparasitism — where infection occurs concurrently — are prevalent and have greater significance on the public health level as well as for economic stability. For instance, it has been shown that children in low-income families are not only more likely to be exposed to infections, but these illnesses also have a detrimental effect on their education, generating cycles of poverty and health inequality (Coulibaly et al., 2012). When calculating the economic burden of protozoan infections, it is important to consider how multifaceted interventions must be created to work against their impact. Investment in comprehensive public health interventions has the potential to stem the tide of such infections while also contributing to socio-economic development simultaneously. Improving sanitation, access to clean drinking water, and hygiene education can significantly reduce infection rates. Integrating health interventions into socio-economic development initiatives, such as Mexico's National Deworming Campaign, can also enhance overall reach and sustainability. By engaging the communities and addressing the causes of vulnerability, it is possible to not only reduce the short-term economic burden but also enhance long-term health benefits. Lastly, in order to address the economic burden of protozoan infections, there must be an effort that realizes the relationship between health and socio-economic status within the infected populations (Coulibaly et al., 2012).

8.6.3. Role in Public Health Policy

Public health policy plays an important role in the prevention and control of protozoan infections, especially in low- and middle-income countries where such diseases have a notable impact on population health. Appropriate policy environments can enable the provision of targeted interventions that address the health's socioeconomic determinants, which are at the heart of the development of such infections. Sanitation, education, and health literacy programs, for instance, are an integral component of any effective public health intervention. In Mexico, the National Campaign to Deworm and programs like Opportunities for maternal care are fine examples of interventions against intestinal parasitism. The fact that such programs fail to be coordinated with each other restricts the overall strategy, in the long term, to delivering even in protozoan infection burden prevention, as indicated by a study that links socio-economic status to the rates of prevalence among children in poor communities (Quihui et al., 2006). Moreover, public health interventions must be informed by high-quality epidemiological studies that identify unique infection patterns across different demographic groups. In *Côte d'Ivoire*, for example, identification of *Schistosoma* species and other protozoan infections prevalence within school settings outlined high heterogeneity (Coulibaly et al., 2012). This highlights the importance of differential interventions that recognize local endemicity and contextual forces shaping transmission patterns. Policies that establish routine screening schemes and augment diagnostic facilities are instrumental in the prevention and control of transmission of such infections. Increasingly, as empirical evidence accrues, it can be assimilated into policy decision-making so that resources may be utilized maximally and applied to those who are at greatest risk so as to utilize intervention strategies optimally. Lastly, successful public health policies must encourage multi-sectoral collaboration between government organizations, non-governmental organizations, and communities. In the management of protozoan infections, ensuring an aligned effort from healthcare, education, and sanitation sectors in tackling the determinants of infection is a matter of urgency. Community participation in health activities, coupled with empowerment through education, can be reflected in immense health benefits, particularly for disadvantaged groups. By prioritizing public health policy based on evidence-driven data and community needs, society can create sustainable measures that not only successfully combat outbreaks present but also enhance the health infrastructure in place to combat future public health issues caused by protozoan infections.

SUMMARY

Examination of protozoan infection holds significant public health, ecological, and veterinary medicine implications. The parasites are often overlooked when the infectious diseases are under consideration, but represent a heterogeneous group with the ability to inflict undesirable health effects in both animals and humans. As demonstrated in current research, for example, *Eimeria* spp. protozoan parasites display circadian rhythms in their life cycles that could make control efforts challenging. The ongoing research on these organisms, their biology, and the way they interact with hosts is critical if efficient countermeasures against their impact are to be developed. Without such data, disease management of protozoan disease may be lacking, and the need for research and investment in this subject, especially with conservation measures taken by birds as vulnerable as the brown kiwi, is particularly exacerbated with such susceptibility to such pathogens (Taylor, 2017). The problems of protozoan infections are also poignantly brought into focus by diseases such as Chagas disease caused by *Trypanosoma cruzi*. This public health neglected tropical disease affects millions, mostly in endemic areas of Latin America, where the interplay between socio-economic determinants and health is particularly evident. Even with advances in the understanding of the disease's pathology and diagnostic methods, gaps continue to exist in treatment access and epidemiological information. Such shortages drive the cycle of transmission and infection, and it would indicate that a concerted effort — of greater public health interventions, education, and research into prevention modalities — is necessary to check such infections effectively. These are not only a health requirement but a moral one, with the needs of affected populations addressed with the compassion they so desperately need (Sherman, 2019). Lastly, the inference of the study on protozoan infections is the need for interdisciplinary collaboration among researchers, clinicians, and policymakers. This collaboration is crucial to developing integrated, long-term approaches to combat the threats of these pathogens. The interplay among environmental factors, host immunity, and protozoan life cycles has to be better comprehended to devise effective measures, particularly in endemic regions. The integration of scientific research with community health initiatives can result in robust paradigms for combating protozoan infections to realize not only short-term health benefits but also long-term sustainability in the control of the diseases. New research should go on to explore these facets while addressing the socio-economic disparities that exacerbate the impact of protozoan infections, ultimately realizing healthier communities (Taylor, 2017; Sherman, 2019).

The protozoan diseases are a significant public health issue due to their advanced life cycles and extensive variety of interaction mechanisms with hosts. The most significant among the protozoan pathogens in them are species of the genera *Plasmodium* and *Trypanoplasma*. *Trypanoplasma borreli*, which infects cyprinid fish, is one of the advanced interactions between a protozoan and a host that induces nitric oxide (NO) synthesis with an impact on immune responses. This immune modulation could have detrimental effects on the host, including when NO synthesis inhibitors-treated carp had improved survival. *Trypanosoma carassii*, however, takes a different strategy, blocking NO production in infected hosts, which shows the diverse strategies of survival adopted by protozoan pathogens to combat host immunity. Yet another protozoan of public health significance is *Plasmodium*, the agent of malaria, spread primarily through the bite of an infected mosquito. Of interest in the interaction of *Plasmodium* with its vector mosquito is the observation that speculations regarding its origin suggest that such a parasite might have emerged from non-parasitic forms and even potentially from algal forms, thus rendering its ecological role in the system complicated to interpret. The life cycle of *Plasmodium* is also defined by mechanisms through which it escapes host immune responses, another characteristic of protozoan pathogens. Apart from enabling the parasite to survive, such an ability also renders it treatment-resistant, placing malaria among the most challenging diseases in the world to control. The evolutionary tracks and the immune evasion mechanisms of the protozoa must be elucidated for interventions to be effectively developed. The study of protozoan infections, therefore, is not only identification and cure but also understanding evolutionary biology and host-parasite interactions. Study of the immune modulation processes of protozoan parasites like *T. borreli* and *T. carassii* inspires key lessons on survival strategies and impacts on host health. In comparison, the study of *Plasmodium* origins and adaptations points to the forces of evolution affecting disease occurrence. Data obtained through such research can inform public health policy and improve therapy interventions, thereby making interdisciplinary research critical to combating protozoan infections. With the evolving epidemiology of infectious diseases, the takeaways from such points are critical to informing holistic and efficient health responses.

CLOSER LOOK

ENTAMOEBA HISTOLYTICA

Entamoeba histolytica is a unicellular anaerobic protozoan parasite that causes amoebiasis, which is an intestinal and extraintestinal infection. The parasite belongs to the phylum Amoebozoa. The infection is prevalent where hygiene and sanitation are poor, and predominantly in developing countries. Transmission is predominantly by the fecal-oral route, often via contaminated food or water (Figure 8.15).

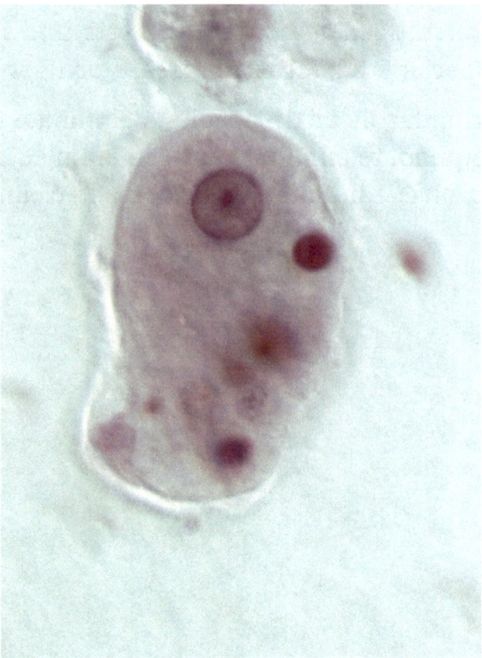

Figure 8.15. Microscopic image of *Entamoeba histolytica*, a protozoan parasite responsible for amoebiasis, showing its characteristic nucleus and ingested red blood cells.

Source: https://upload.wikimedia.org/wikipedia/commons/thumb/9/93/Entamoeba_histolytica.jpg/960px-Entamoeba_histolytica.jpg.

The two-phase life cycle of *E. histolytica* includes the trophozoite and the cyst. The infective cyst is a stable, quadrinucleated cell able to resist gastric acidity and survive extracellularly in the environment outside of the host. Excystation in the small intestine is achieved upon ingestion, releasing trophozoites that migrate to the colon. The trophozoite is the active, mobile phase responsible for tissue invasion and disease. It is characterized by the presence of a single nucleus with a centrally located karyosome and fine peripheral chromatin, and it may be identified microscopically by its ability to phagocytoze red blood cells.

Once they have entered the colon, trophozoites bind to the colonic mucosa via surface lectins, the Gal/GalNAc lectin, which enables them to adhere to epithelial cells. They secrete enzymes such as cysteine proteases and amebapores that kill host tissue, resulting in the development of ulcers.

These flask-like ulcers may result in symptoms such as abdominal pain, diarrhea, and dysentery (bloody stools). In severe cases, intestinal perforation and peritonitis may ensue.

In other people, trophozoites invade the bloodstream and migrate to extraintestinal sites, most commonly the liver, to create amoebic liver abscesses. This may present as right upper quadrant pain, fever, and hepatomegaly, and rupture at times to result in such complications as peritonitis or pleuropulmonary infection. The lungs, brain, and skin are other rare extraintestinal sites.

Diagnosis of infection with *E. histolytica* is established by microscopic examination of stool specimens for the detection of cysts or trophozoites, but this is not specific because it cannot discriminate between *E. histolytica* and the non-disease-producing intestinal amebas *Entamoeba dispar* or *Entamoeba moshkovskii*. Antigen detection, PCR tests, and serology are therefore normally used to make the diagnosis, especially for invasive disease or liver abscess.

Treatment is typically metronidazole or tinidazole to eliminate the trophozoites and a luminal agent like paromomycin or iodoquinol to eliminate any remaining cysts in the intestine and prevent relapse. Preventive treatment involves sanitation improvement, clean drinking water, food handling, and personal hygiene.

References

1. Stuart, K., Brun, R., Croft, S., Fairlamb, A., Gürtler, R. E., McKerrow, J., Reed, S., & Tarleton, R. (2008). Kinetoplastids: related protozoan pathogens, different diseases. *The Journal of clinical investigation, 118*(4), 1301–1310. https://doi.org/10.1172/JCI33945(accessed on 16th July 2025).
2. Gondard, M., Delannoy, S., Pinarello, V., Aprelon, R., Devillers, E., Galon, C., Pradel, J., Vayssier-Taussat, M., Albina, E., & Moutailler, S. (2020). Upscaling the Surveillance of Tick-borne Pathogens in the French Caribbean Islands. *Pathogens (Basel, Switzerland), 9*(3), 176. https://doi.org/10.3390/pathogens9030176(accessed on 16th July 2025).
3. Albonico, M., Barda, B. D., Clementi, M., Cringoli, G., et al. (2013). *Mini-FLOTAC, an innovative direct diagnostic technique for intestinal parasitic infections: Experience from the field.* https://core.ac.uk/download/pdf/20046407.pdf (accessed on 16th July 2025).
4. Ojuromi, O. T., & Ashafa, A. O. (2020). An overview of some medicinal plants and isolated active compounds with potential antiprotozoal activity. *Tropical Journal of Pharmaceutical Research, 19*(7), 1551–1563. https://doi.org/10.4314/tjpr.v19i7.30(accessed on 16th July 2025).
5. Shapiro, K., Bahia-Oliveira, L., Dixon, B., Dumètre, A., de Wit, L. A., VanWormer, E., & Villena, I. (2019). Environmental transmission of *Toxoplasma gondii*: Oocysts in water, soil and food. *Food and waterborne parasitology, 15*, e00049. https://doi.org/10.1016/j.fawpar.2019.e00049(accessed on 16th July 2025).
6. Bahri, A., Drechsel, P., Raschid Sally, L., Redwood, M., et al. (2025). *Wastewater irrigation and health: Assessing and mitigating risk in low-income countries.* https://core.ac.uk/download/pdf/6405282.pdf (accessed on 16th July 2025).
7. Chavatte, N., Baré, J., Lambrecht, E., Van Damme, I., Vaerewijck, M., Sabbe, K., & Houf, K. (2014). Co-occurrence of free-living protozoa and foodborne pathogens on dishcloths: implications for food safety. *International journal of food microbiology, 191*, 89–96. https://doi.org/10.1016/j.ijfoodmicro.2014.08.030(accessed on 16th July 2025).
8. Barratt, J., Chan, D., Ellis, J. T., Stark, D., et al. (2016). *Dientamoeba fragilis, the neglected trichomonad of the human bowel.* https://opus.lib.uts.edu.au/bitstream/10453/87542/1/Clin.%20Microbiol.%20Rev.-2016-Stark-553-80%20%282%29.pdf (accessed on 16th July 2025).
9. Bhat, R., Maheshwari, S. K., & Saha, S. (2004). *Treating HIV/AIDS patients in India with antiretroviral therapy: A management challenge.* https://www.iima.ac.in/sites/default/files/rnpfiles/2004-06-03rbhat.pdf. https://core.ac.uk/download/pdf/6443480.pdf (accessed on 16th July 2025).
10. Blumenthal, U., Esrey, S. A., Fleisher, J. M., Peasey, A., et al. (2001). *Epidemiology: A Tool for the Assessment of Risk.* https://core.ac.uk/download/13110839.pdf (accessed on 16th July 2025).
11. Buckling, A., Casadevall, A., Folkesson, A., Jousset, A., Kunert, A., Zaborin, A., et al. (2013). *Pseudomonas aeruginosa adaptation to lungs of cystic fibrosis patients leads to lowered resistance to phage and protist enemies.* https://core.ac.uk/download/19503793.pdf (accessed on 16th July 2025).
12. Quihui, L., Valencia, M. E., Crompton, D. W., Phillips, S., Hagan, P., Morales, G., & Díaz-Camacho,

S. P. (2006). Role of the employment status and education of mothers in the prevalence of intestinal parasitic infections in Mexican rural schoolchildren. *BMC public health, 6*, 225. https://doi.org/10.1186/1471-2458-6-225(accessed on 16th July 2025).

13. Caramia, G., Coman, M. M., Silvi, S., Verdenelli, M. C., et al. (2015). *Treatment of acute diarrhea: Past and now.* https://core.ac.uk/download/pdf/54655355.pdf (accessed on 16th July 2025).
14. Ortayli, N., Ringheim, K., Collins, L., & Sladden, T. (2014). Sexually transmitted infections: progress and challenges since the 1994 International Conference on Population and Development (ICPD). *Contraception, 90*(6 Suppl), S22–S31. https://doi.org/10.1016/j.contraception.2014.06.024(accessed on 16th July 2025).
15. Domingos, A., Domingues, N., Ferrolho, J., Santos-Gomes, G., et al. (2015). *An Overview.* https://core.ac.uk/download/187231188.pdf (accessed on 16th July 2025).
16. Hughes, G., & Field, N. (2015). The epidemiology of sexually transmitted infections in the UK: impact of behavior, services and interventions. *Future microbiology, 10*(1), 35–51. https://doi.org/10.2217/fmb.14.110(accessed on 16th July 2025).
17. Gavinho, B., Combes, V., Dlugonska, H., Hart, E., Evans-Osses, I., Rossi, I. V., Inal, J., et al. (2019). *A new landscape of host–protozoa interactions involving the extracellular vesicles world.* https://core.ac.uk/download/287580982.pdf (accessed on 16th July 2025).
18. Gillen, A. L., & Sherwin, F. (2013). *The genesis of malaria: The origin of mosquitoes and their protistan cargo, Plasmodium falciparum.* https://core.ac.uk/download/223029211.pdf (accessed on 16th July 2025).
19. Groeneveld, A., van Muiswinkel, W. B., Saeij, J. P. J., et al. (2002). *Immune modulation by fish kinetoplastid parasites: A role for nitric oxide.* https://core.ac.uk/download/pdf/29297473.pdf (accessed on 16th July 2025).
20. Nichols, G., Lake, I., & Heaviside, C. (2018). Climate Change and Water-Related Infectious Diseases. *Atmosphere, 9*(10), 385. https://doi.org/10.3390/atmos9100385(accessed on 16th July 2025).
21. Hickman, E., Kreider, D., Powell, J., Reynolds, D., et al. (2010). *Studies into cytauxzoon and helminth infections of bobcats (Lynx rufus) of Northwest Arkansas.* https://core.ac.uk/download/148340648.pdf (accessed on 16th July 2025).
22. Jada, S. (2024). *Scaffold hopping for the lead optimization of the orally active antileishmanial pyrrolo-quinazoline alkaloid natural product peganine.* https://core.ac.uk/download/603978348.pdf (accessed on 16th July 2025).
23. Swann, J., Jamshidi, N., Lewis, N. E., & Winzeler, E. A. (2015). Systems analysis of host-parasite interactions. *Wiley interdisciplinary reviews. Systems biology and medicine, 7*(6), 381–400. https://doi.org/10.1002/wsbm.1311(accessed on 16th July 2025).
24. Khan, N. A. (2004). *The pathogenesis of Acanthamoeba infections: Current status and future implications.* https://core.ac.uk/download/7518.pdf (accessed on 16th July 2025).
25. Labeaud, A. D., Malhotra, I., King, M. J., King, C. L., & King, C. H. (2009). Do antenatal parasite infections devalue childhood vaccination?. *PLoS neglected tropical diseases, 3*(5), e442. https://doi.org/10.1371/journal.pntd.0000442(accessed on 16th July 2025).
26. Jeffery S, Van Der Putten W. Soil Borne Human Diseases. EUR 24893 EN. Luxembourg

(Luxembourg): Publications Office of the European Union; 2011. JRC65787(accessed on 16th July 2025).

27. Morgoglione, M. E. (2021). *Ozonated water for parasitic control in buffalo farms (OZO-PAR).* https://core.ac.uk/download/574199266.pdf (accessed on 16th July 2025).
28. Okaeme, A.N. & Olufemi, Ben & Obiekezie, A.. (2001). Parasites and non-fish predators of tilapia with particular reference to the sustainable management of fisheries of Lake Kainji Nigeria. https://core.ac.uk/download/11019315.pdf (accessed on 16th July 2025).
29. Sherman, E. (2019). *Review of Chagas Disease and Treatment Obstacles to Eradication.* https://core.ac.uk/download/213464293.pdf (accessed on 16th July 2025).
30. Coulibaly, J. T., Fürst, T., Silué, K. D., Knopp, S., Hauri, D., Ouattara, M., Utzinger, J., & N'Goran, E. K. (2012). Intestinal parasitic infections in schoolchildren in different settings of Côte d'Ivoire: effect of diagnostic approach and implications for control. *Parasites & vectors, 5,* 135. https://doi.org/10.1186/1756-3305-5-135(accessed on 16th July 2025).
31. Subahar, R., & Sutanto, L. (2008). *Ascaris lumbricoides eggs and human-intestinal protozoan cysts found in river water of Angke River, Jakarta.* https://media.neliti.com/media/publications/148041-EN-ascaris-lumbricoides-eggs-and-human-inte.pdf (accessed on 16th July 2025).
32. Taylor, H. S. (2017). *The Eimeria species affecting brown kiwi: Host-parasite interactions and conservation implications: A thesis presented in partial fulfilment of the requirements for the degree of Master of Science in Conservation Biology at Massey University, Manawatu, New Zealand.* https://core.ac.uk/download/186668377.pdf (accessed on 16th July 2025).
33. Unasho, A. (2013). *An investigation of intestinal parasitic infections among the asymptomatic children in Southern Ethiopia.* https://core.ac.uk/download/544387414.pdf (accessed on 16th July 2025).

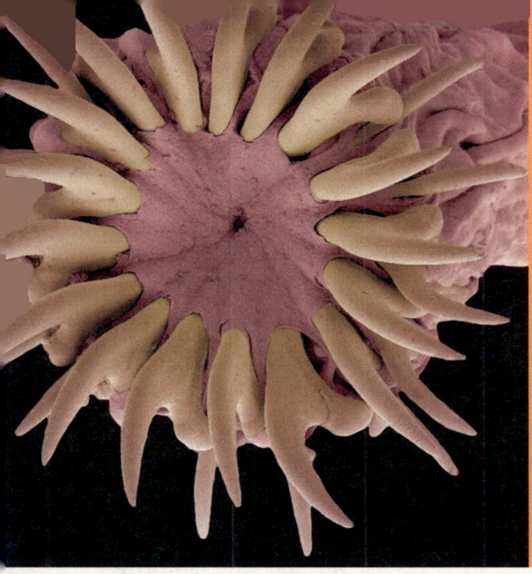

Chapter 9
HELMINTHIC INFECTIONS

Contents

Introduction

Helminthic infections, particularly intestinal helminths, are very significant public health problems, particularly in the Third World. The parasitic infestations are mostly due to poor environmental sanitation and low socio-economic status, which create a ground for easy transmission. High prevalence rates among vulnerable groups, particularly school children, are revealed by statistics as being most exposed, given their limited health education and poor hygiene habits. For instance, a study from rural India reported that 17.8% of school children were infected, and poor hand hygiene and untrimmed nails were leading risk factors for infection (Dongre et al., 2008). These findings suggest the necessity of targeted intervention to increase levels of hygiene and education to lower the disease burden of helminth infections among such groups. In those regions where helminthic infection is the prevailing problem, public health considerations are far-reaching. General infection prevalence not only causes direct health complications like malnutrition, anemia, and compromised intellectual ability among infected children, but also contributes to general socio-economic disadvantages. For example, a study in Ethiopia found an intestinal helminth rate of 13.8% among schoolchildren and stressed the necessity for continuous health information supply and treatment to offset such infections (Tefera et al., 2015). Without control, the infections lead to cycles of poverty and health inequities. Hence, projecting effective interventions involving medical treatment and participatory educational approaches is vital to break this cycle and enhance the general health of the populace. Hygiene education alongside medical intervention is a key approach in avoiding helminthic infections. Practices employed in mobilizing the community towards involvement and focusing on individual hygiene can significantly reduce the prevalence of the infections within vulnerable populations. The aforementioned study in India showed the potential of child-to-child hygiene education in promoting improved practices, with an impact on change towards hand washing and nail care among school-aged children (Dongre et al., 2008). Thus, integrating these educational activities along with routine preventive therapy is critical in sustaining health gains. This dual-track strategy can substantially lower infection levels, improve the health status of children, and indirectly contribute to helminth-infected communities' socio-economic development.

Definition of Helminthic Infections

Helminthic disease is an infection with parasitic worms, which can be grouped into broadly three classes: nematodes (roundworms), cestodes (tapeworms), and trematodes (flukes). The intricate life cycle of such organisms is usually more than one host and habitat, and hence is particularly well suited to transmission in most environments. *Ascaris lumbricoides*, *Schistosoma* species, and *Taenia solium* are certain helminths that each cause significant morbidity in infected communities. Infections tend to occur by means such as intake of contaminated food or water, skin penetration, or vectors such as insects. Awareness of the diverse modes of these parasites in colonizing a host becomes relevant in effectively tackling public health problems as well as utilizing preventative measures against such infections, especially where socioeconomic circumstances contribute to increased prevalence. The toll of helminthic infections is felt most starkly across the globe in developing countries, where inadequate healthcare infrastructure and sanitation only serve to speed up transmission.

The rates of infection are most starkly revealed in children, who are most susceptible to infection due to poor hygiene and a lack of proper nutrition. As discovered in public health research, the majority of such infections occur among children below five years and those in primary school age, emphasizing the necessity of targeted interventions (Amanda et al., 2023). Effective control of helminthic disease normally demands education at the level of the community and promotion of hygienic measures and administration of prophylactic drugs. It is essential to understand the target population infected by helminths so as to develop strategies that can tackle transmission risks and health outcomes for high-risk individuals. Recent epidemiological research has shed new insights on how helminthic infections interact with other disorders, namely, allergic disorders. Although helminths have long been viewed as being deleterious, new evidence suggests that they may have a multifunctional role in modulating the immune system. For example, some evidence for a protective effect of helminth infection on the incidence of allergic disease has existed, however, with nonuniform results and ongoing investigation (Arrais et al., 2020). This double perspective regarding helminths as pathogens and alleged controllers of immune health underscores the importance of complete comprehension of their biological and ecological actions. As researchers continue to examine this intricate relationship, it is vital that they consider the implications of the public health strategy and intervention for controlling helminthic infection with a knowledge of their broader implications for human well-being (Figure 9.1).

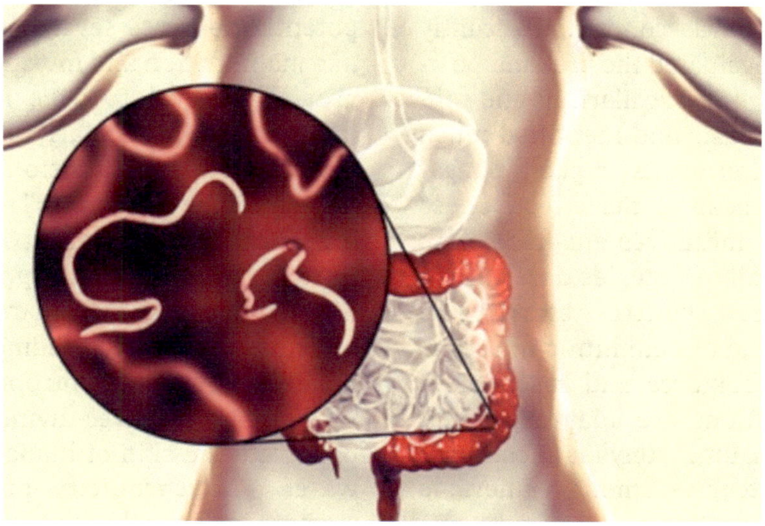

Figure 9.1. Helminthic infection.

Source: https://www.shutterstock.com/image-illustration/helminths-nematodes-enterobius-gut-threadworm-260nw-1039928545.jpg.

Importance of Studying Helminthic Infections

It is essential to learn about helminthic infections from the perspective of public health and disease control, particularly in low- and middle-income countries where the parasites are endemic. Helminth studies could reveal the complex interplays between environmental factors, human behaviors, and disease prevalence. Not only do such infections influence the individual's health, but they also have significant social and economic consequences. Where the level of sanitation is poor and access to healthcare is limited, helminthic infections can drive down productivity and educational achievement, creating a vicious cycle of poverty. Through knowledge of the prevalence and distribution of helminthic infections, researchers can develop targeted interventions and health policies that drive up health gains and reduce the burden on the health system. Moreover, the investigation of helminthic infections offers a way into the immune system and the evolutionary mechanisms that regulate it. Research has established that certain helminths have the potential to be therapeutic in the modulation of immune responses and the attainment of health. Hookworms, for instance, which were previously viewed as pathogenic parasites, are being researched for their ability to cure illnesses like autoimmune conditions and allergies. This change in the paradigm of the role of helminths in human health can lead to new treatment modalities exploiting the positive effects of the organisms. Exploring the intricate relationship between helminths and man can unveil new therapeutic opportunities, vindicating the worth of studying these infections not only from a public health perspective but also in the context of evolutionary medicine (Strosberg, 2014). In addition, studies on helminthic infections enable examining the effectiveness of public health interventions such as mass drug administration (MDA) programs. These interventions are not just meant to reduce the prevalence of soil-transmitted helminthiasis as well as its associated diseases, but also in co-endemic regions. A study that was conducted recently in Alappuzha, India, evaluated the pre- and post-MDA prevalence for lymphatic filariasis and soil-transmitted helminthiasis and identified much interesting information on its impact (Bhagat et al., 2018). Awareness of the effectiveness or shortfalls of such initiatives enables health organizations to modify strategies accordingly, leading to enhanced control efforts. By continuous monitoring of helminthic infection, the public health workforce and researchers can ensure interventions are adapted to suit the evolving scenario, ultimately manifesting as improved health outcomes among vulnerable groups.

9.1. Types of Helminths

Helminths are parasitic worms that comprise a wide variety of species grouped mainly into three major types: nematodes, cestodes, and trematodes. Nematodes, also referred to as roundworms, have cylindrical bodies with a tapering end, differentiating them from other helminth species. Some of the major human pathogens under this category are *Ascaris lumbricoides* and hookworms. Ascaris, for example, can become enormously big and can cause serious complications within the intestines, while hookworms have been known to cause anemia as a result of blood loss. Infections by these parasites are especially important in regions where there is poor sanitation and readily accessible health care, which continues to propagate poverty cycles and diseases. Cestodes or flatworms are characterized by their ribbon-like body structure and segmentation. Tapeworms, belonging to this category, inhabit primarily the intestines of their hosts and have the capacity to absorb nutrients directly from their skin and therefore are highly effective parasites. The majority of such infections in humans occur due to the consumption of undercooked or infected meat. Some species, like *Taenia saginata* and *Taenia solium,* have the potential to cause severe health-related issues like malnutrition and intestinal blockages. They are also known to have far-reaching health implications, particularly in tropical countries where proper nutritional resources are already being hindered. Trematodes or flukes are another major group of helminths with intricate life cycles and typically intermediate hosts such as snails. Schistosomes, which cause schistosomiasis, are a leading cause of morbidity in the tropics and subtropics. Infections arise when cercariae, free-swimming larval forms, penetrate the skin of humans in contaminated water. The chronicity of infection due to trematodes usually leads to long-term health effects, including liver damage and increased susceptibility to other infections. These consequences of such helminthic infections emphasize the importance of their targeting in public health efforts, particularly in co-infection-endemic regions of other disease agents, such as malaria and soil-transmitted helminths, with consequences for the interrelation among these diseases as discussed by Futagbi (2015) and Naing et al. (2017).

9.1.1. Nematodes (Roundworms)

Nematodes or roundworms represent a significant helminth group whose health significance is present across various populations, particularly in the developing world. Nematodes are multicellular parasites living in various ecosystems and infest human hosts through polluted water, soil, or food. Infection by nematodes is often associated with unhygienic sanitation and unsatisfactory hygiene conditions, lending support to their association with socio-economic status. In particular, the conditions that facilitate their transmission — such as overcrowding, improper waste disposal, and lack of access to clean drinking water — most significantly affect vulnerable groups, such as children and pregnant women. Understanding the life cycle and modes of transmission of nematodes is significant in order to develop effective public health strategies for the control of such parasitic diseases, especially in regions where such conditions are prevalent. The impact of nematode infection on health is substantial, especially when it comes to maternal and child health. Studies have shown that geohelminthiasis, which is primarily caused by nematodes, can lower cell-mediated immunity among pregnant women. This compromised immune system predisposes them to serious complications such as maternal anemia, preterm birth, and even stillbirth, making clear the gravity of the health implications of the infection (Lal et al., 2019). Also, the presence of nematodes can be harmful to the mental growth of children, causing their learning level and well-being to decline. Because infections due to nematodes have the ability to hinder physical and mental growth, efforts must be made to fight such health issues through specific interventions designed to improve sanitation and healthcare. Given the widespread health impact caused by nematodes, comprehensive prevention and control measures must be undertaken. Effective interventions include training in individual hygiene, sanitation of the environment, and community health programs to reduce the occurrence of such infections (Motran et al., 2018). Additionally, the role of public health policies in facilitating access to antihelminthic drugs cannot be overemphasized; periodic screening and treatment can also reduce the severity of the infection among vulnerable populations. By increasing awareness and education regarding the socio-economic factors behind nematode transmission, stakeholders can implement complete and sustainable strategies to address helminthic infection. Ultimately, addressing these issues will not only improve one's health outcomes but also community-wide quality of life for regions afflicted with nematodes and other helminths (Figure 9.2).

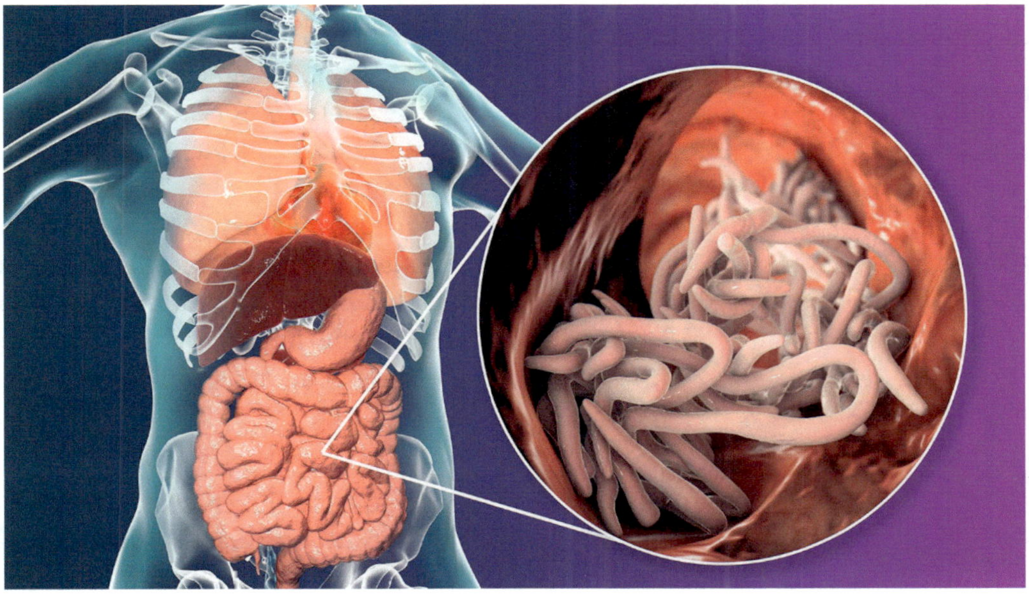

Figure 9.2. Roundworms in the human intestine.

Source: https://cdn.hswstatic.com/gif/shutterstock-1837076626.jpg.

9.1.2. Cestodes (Tapeworms)

Cestodes or tapeworms are a vast group of helminthic parasites with their flat, ribbon-like bodies and segmented look. The life forms inhabit the intestines of vertebrate hosts, humans included. They lead a myriad of health issues. Cestode life cycles are generally multihost, with eggs or proglottids being passed in the feces to be consumed as intermediate hosts like livestock or rodents. Upon reaching the intestines of the definitive host, larvae develop into adult tapeworms that are responsible for malabsorption of nutrients and lead to conditions like abdominal pain and diarrhea. Such complex life cycles are the reason why one needs to know environmental and social conditions permitting the transmission of tapeworm, which has been reported in various studies based on their prevalence in various communities. Prevalence of the tapeworm infection can vary significantly with geographical location and host species. For instance, in Ghana, a cross-sectional study reported 94.4% of goats infected with tapeworms, indicating a high parasitic burden in livestock populations (Futagbi et al., 2015).

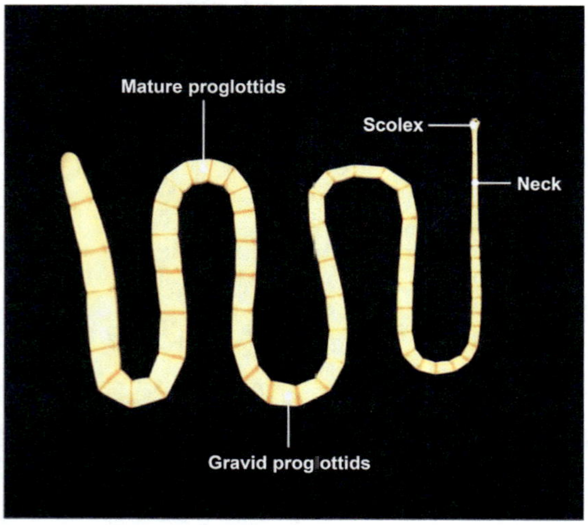

Figure 9.3. Tapeworm.

Source: https://cdn-prod.medicalnewstoday.com/content/images/articles/170/170461/the-taenia-solium-tapeworm.jpg.

The observations point to the risk to human beings who may consume undercooked or contaminated meat. Aside from domestic animals, stray dogs and cats also play important roles in the epidemiology of cestode infection. A survey in Iraq brought to light that stray cats carried high infection rates with *Dipylidium caninum*, which is responsible for zoonotic risks to human beings (Aqeele et al., 2024). Such knowledge about patterns of infection is essential for successful public health intervention and raising awareness of the potential transmission paths of tapeworms. Management of cestode infections requires an interdisciplinary approach combining veterinary practice, human health, and health education. Deworming of animals on a regular basis, pet care, and proper handling of food are essential in limiting the spread of tapeworm infections. Health education campaigns can also educate the public on signs and symptoms of helminthic infections and encourage medical care when signs and symptoms are noted. Because of the zoonotic possibility, constant surveillance of parasitic infestation of domestic and wild animals is necessary. The integration of these controls not only helps in controlling cestode infestation but also brings a broader appreciation of helminthic infections into public health. Through the collaboration of veterinarians, epidemiologists, and health officials, improvement can be achieved in reducing the impact of the parasites on the well-being of animals and humans (Figure 9.3).

9.1.3. Trematodes (Flukes)

Trematodes, or flukes, are a parasitic flatworm suborder in the class Trematoda. They are characterized by their leaf shape, soft body plan, and complex life cycle with one or more intermediate hosts, often mollusks and fish. Efforts to determine their epidemiology have yielded approximately 18,000 species, of which only a few are known to be significant human pathogens. Remarkably, these infections are more common in low-income nations where environmental and socioeconomic forces facilitate transmission. Prevalence of trematode infections highlights the need for public health interventions because they are associated with important morbidity and chronic disease, including liver and gastrointestinal disease. Moreover, some of the liver fluke species have been classified as biological carcinogens and therefore underscore the strong imperative to make people more aware and have effective control measures and prevention strategies (Harrington et al., 2017). The life cycle of trematode infections is greatly influenced by human activities, including agricultural routines and food cooking habits. Areas with irrigation can create the necessary conditions for the intermediate hosts to carry the pathogens. In addition, such habits as consumption of raw or undercooked fish have been reported to significantly elevate the risk of infestation with trematode genera such as *Opisthorchis viverrini* and *Clonorchis sinensis*. Helminthic infestations are also of concern in the global scenario because of the human mobility from endemic to non-endemic regions, which allows potential introduction of the parasites into new regions. Research indicates that understanding the complex interactions between ecological processes, human activities, and trematode life cycles is critical in the control of the burden of such infections, particularly in resource-poor settings (Teimoori et al., 2019). Trematode infections have been improved in diagnosis and management by advancements in molecular tools and epidemiological studies. Routine methods may include finding adult flukes in host material or eggs in fecal samples, but the sensitivity of such tests is typically lacking for low-burden infections. New research following the polymerase chain reaction (PCR) and sequencing of specific genetic markers has revolutionized diagnostic practice, rendering the method more reliable for the identification of previously characterized as well as newly described trematode species. For instance, molecular similarity was evident when an infection analysis of jackals with trematodes indicated cross-species transmission and complex ecological relationships (Teimoori et al., 2019). These findings not only enhance diagnostic efficacy but also highlight the importance of surveillance on a regular basis in order to control helminthic infections effectively and minimize their public health impact (Figure 9.4).

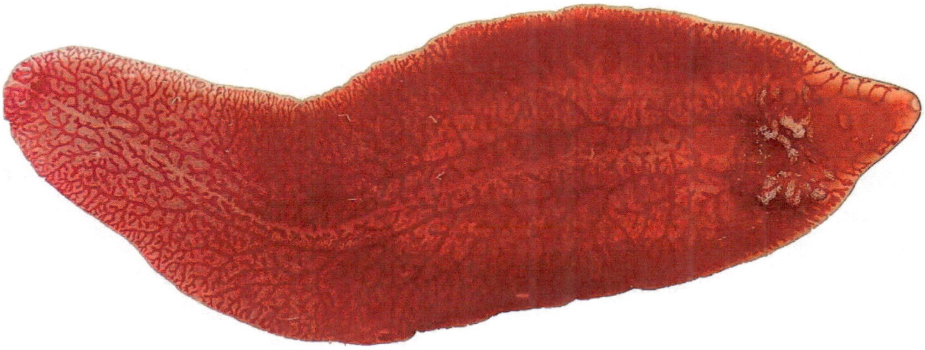

Figure 9.4. Liver fluke.

Source: https://cdn-prod.medicalnewstoday.com/content/images/articles/319/319479/liver-fluke-br-image-credit-veronidae-2013-br.jpg.

9.2. Transmission and Life Cycle

The life cycle and transmission of helminthic infection, particularly soil-transmitted helminths (STHs), are important to identify to know their high prevalence and the diseases they induce. The life cycle of STHs like *Ascaris lumbricoides*, hookworms, and *Trichuris trichiura* typically contains both human and environmental cycles. Intake of eggs through infected food or soil initiates the Ascaris' cycle, where larvae grow and move through the host's body, ultimately developing into adults in the intestines. Hookworm larvae, however, penetrate the skin, enter the bloodstream, and reach the lungs to migrate to the gastrointestinal tract. All such complex interaction between man and nature emphasizes the importance of sanitation and hygiene in controlling incidence levels. Preventive measures like the development of public health infrastructure can interrupt such life cycles, ultimately reducing infection rates. Phases during the life cycle of helminths also reflect their survival and reproductive strategies. Internally, these parasites, once within the host, can survive for years, utilizing the nutrients of the host while parrying the immune system. In *Ascaris lumbricoides*, adult worms can produce thousands of eggs per day, ensuring their multiplication in endemic populations. Of note is also their geographical distribution since transmission-favoring conditions like poor sanitation and restricted access to healthcare are prevalent in the majority of developing nations. Environmental factors like soil type and moisture content also play significant roles in the survival of helminth eggs outside the host. As highlighted in the literature, greater investments in research are needed to enhance knowledge on these dynamics and develop effective interventions for transmission reduction and its health impacts (Lamberton & Jourdan, 2015). Effective control strategies rely on a robust knowledge of both transmission dynamics and life cycle intricacies. While preventive therapy has been shown to reduce helminth disease burden, there are still challenges in accessing drugs, particularly among the vulnerable (Jourdan et al., 2018). The impact of mass deworming programs remains in question, with concerns about their potential to eradicate extreme forms of helminthiasis without parallel shifts in environmental and socio-economic conditions. To counteract these issues, the betterment of diagnostic tools and public health interventions is paramount. Developing highly sensitive diagnostic methods for helminth infection and creating greater awareness of hygiene are essential to ultimately impact the transmission rate and lifecycle of the parasites towards bettering global health.

9.2.1. Modes of Transmission

Transmission modes for helminthic infestations are diverse and have substantial effects on public health. One prominent route is the intake of contaminated food or water, particularly in areas where sanitation is lacking. For instance, those with limited access to safe drinking water are predisposed to helminth infections such as *Ascaris lumbricoides* and *Trichuris trichiura*. Inadequate hygiene among food handlers raises the risk because the contaminated food can serve as a vehicle for transmission. Studies have confirmed that food handlers play a critical role in the transmission of intestinal parasites, and the prevalence of 6.6% among food workers who are carriers of helminths has been observed based on pathogen prevalence studies. Identification and control of these transmission pathways, therefore, become crucial to successful intervention efforts. Direct contact with contaminated soil or surfaces is another critical mode of transmission of helminthic infections, often referred to as soil-transmitted helminths. The route is particularly prevalent in the tropics and subtropics due to supportive environmental conditions for survival and infectivity of helminth eggs or larvae. Young children playing on contaminated soil or engaging in farming without proper protective measures are at higher risk of infection. Environmental contamination can be attributed to fecal waste in unhygienic conditions, where the transmission of helminths such as hookworms and whipworms is increased. Moreover, studies have established that seasonal changes such as increased rainfall can influence the prevalence of helminth infestation due to increased soil and water source contamination (O'Brien et al., 2008). Hence, successful public health interventions should focus on hygiene and sanitation practices to avert this route of transmission. Vector-borne transmission of helminthic infection, even though lesser in frequent, is another important mode, particularly for specific species that incorporate an intermediate host or vector in their life cycle. Certain helminths, like the schistosomes, employ freshwater snails to complete their life cycle and can be transmitted to humans on contact with infected water bodies. Prevalence of such infections can be especially high in groups that participate in fishing or bathing in infested water. On the other hand, migrants and travelers may be differently exposed to danger from host populations, as demonstrated in a study establishing the lower risk of helminthic infections for those coming back from travel compared to immigrants and refugees who will be exposed more in the endemic areas (O'Brien et al., 2008). Solutions to these unique modes of exposure require special preventative and educational interventions, especially among high-risk populations (Figure 9.5).

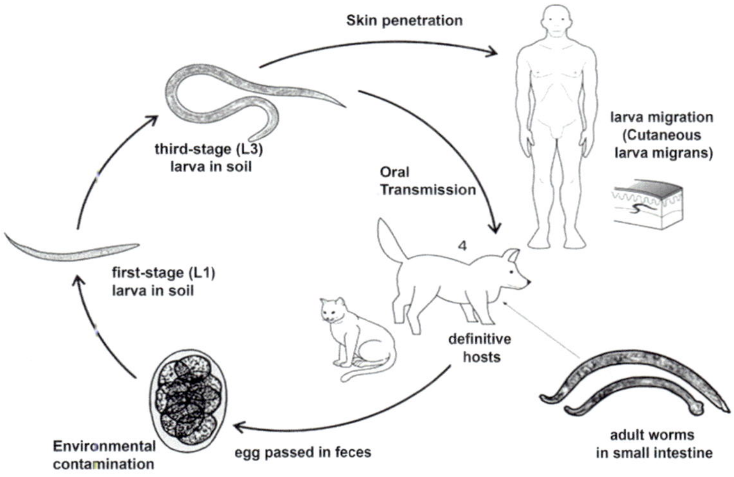

Figure 9.5. Transmission of helminthic infections in humans.

Source: https://api.intechopen.com/media/chapter/19390/media/image3.png.

9.2.2. Life Cycle Stages of Helminths

Life stages of helminths are significant to establish their transmission and their impact on human health. Helminths are intricate organisms with relatively intricate life cycles involving several developmental phases that can employ intermediate and definitive hosts. First and foremost, transmission is affected by external environment conditions because most of the helminth eggs or larvae are passed in the feces of the host. These life cycles can endure in the soil or water before being ingested by a new host. An example is soil-transmitted helminths (STHs) like *Ascaris lumbricoides* that require favorable atmospheric conditions for their survival and completion of their life cycle, hence capturing the intricate interaction among such parasites with their environments. Understanding these life cycles illuminates their existence and endurance, ultimately informing public health interventions in managing helminthic infections. Once ingested, helminth larvae continue to develop in the host body, leading to a number of growth stages as well as maturity. The process often involves migration through a number of body systems, where parasites become lodged in their particular niches. For example, while *Ascaris* larvae migrate first through lung tissues, mature worms develop in the intestinal tracts, where they exhibit fine adaptability to the host immune system. These adaptations, such as evading immune detection and modulating host responses, form the cornerstone of helminth survival for extended periods of time (Motran et al., 2018). Additionally, the excretory-secretory products released by the parasites throughout the stages of their life cycle possess the capacity to influence the immune response of the host, inducing a Th2-type response prone to promoting the survival of the helminths within the host. Transmission dynamics also differ among different helminth species. For instance, transmission of soil-transmitted helminths occurs primarily via infected food and soil, with infection rates being extremely high in unhygienic conditions (Lamberton & Jourdan, 2015). Others, such as those with secondary hosts, experience more dynamic transmission interactions that might involve other vectors for transmission. By separating the various phases of the life cycle, researchers can apply precision control techniques, including drug therapy and improved sanitation procedures whose aim is to reduce the rate of transmission. Proper knowledge of these phases of the life cycle not only enhances our knowledge of helminth biology but also assists greatly in developing successful public health programs to combat helminthic infections (Figure 9.6).

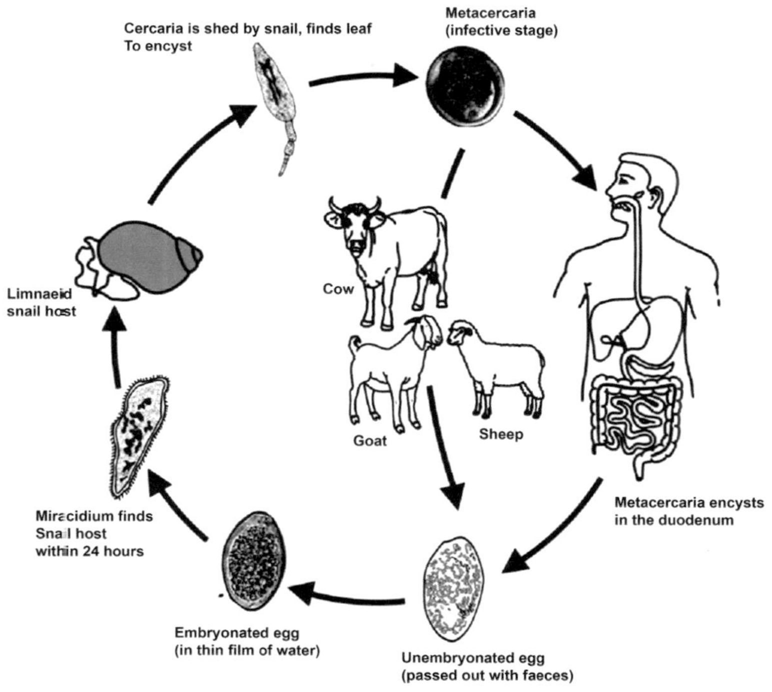

Figure 9.6. Life cycle of liver flukes.

Source: https://www.researchgate.net/profile/Omotosho-Lawal/publication/343718557/figure/fig1/AS:933791040274435@1599644541583/Life-cycle-of-liver-flukes.png.

9.2.3. Environmental Factors Affecting Transmission

The dynamical spread of helminthic diseases is motivated by an intricate interrelation with some environmental determinants that affect the prevalence and also the distribution of parasites. Climatic characteristics are critical in the determination of the lifecycle of the helminths as well as their intermediate host. For instance, optimal survival for soil-transmitted helminths (STH) occurs at warm temperatures and humidity, which are often prevalent within tropical and sub-tropical environments. These conditions result in increased rates of infection for susceptible groups, like children from rural areas who are exposed to contaminated soil and water sources. Understanding the specific environmental conditions that enable helminth transmission is thus central to informing effective intervention policies meant to minimize their impact on public health and economic well-being (Ajjampur et al., 2014).

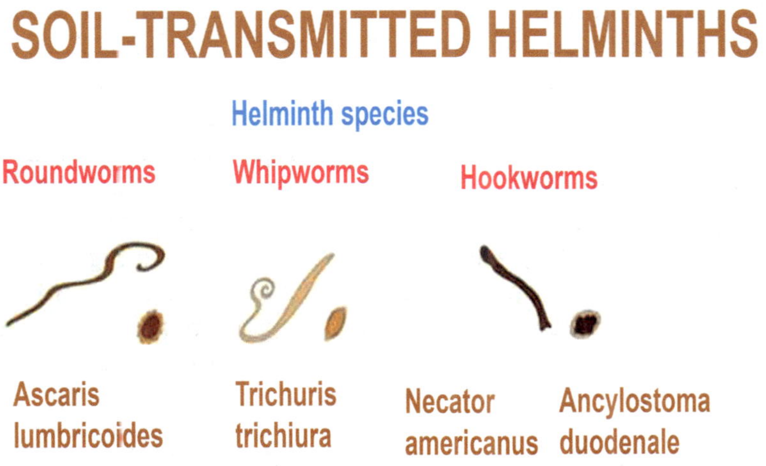

Figure 9.7. Soil-transmitted helminths (STH).

Source: https://www.who.int/images/default-source/departments/ntd-library/soil-transmitted-helminthiases/soil-transmitted-helminths-deadly-worms.tmb-549v.jpg?Culture=en&sfvrsn=f06cc6e0_2.

Socio-economic conditions cross over with environmental conditions, further adding complexities to the helminthic infection transmission dynamics. Most places, in most cases, have socio-economically disadvantaged communities that have a high rate of infections due to poor sanitary conditions and hygiene practices. For example, rural coastal Kenya has been described as having co-infections prevalent in communities, explained by sharing of common risk factors such as overcrowding within the home and inadequate access to clean water (Ajjampur et al., 2014). These risks are exacerbated by environmental degradation by deforestation and the misuse of waste, which facilitates parasite transmission. Thus, addressing the socio-economic determinants of health and the environmental factors becomes the need of the hour in designing integrated public health interventions against helminthic infections. Furthermore, spatial analysis has been a useful aid in determining the environmental determinants of helminth transmission. It has been shown through research that spatial aggregation of infection is prevalent in single villages and hence the requirement of localized interventions based on unique environmental characteristics. For instance, a study in coastal Kenya established certain clusters of single and co-infections that correlated with environmental and socio-demographic risk factors, reflecting a prevalence landscape heterogeneity across different ecosystems (Bisanzio et al., 2014). This local strategy can guide the health policy makers on where to direct the resources and prioritize the intervention measures effectively. Consequently, the incorporation of spatially aware strategies offers a precise response to the complexity of helminthic infections, ultimately enhancing the efficacy of public health action in managing these endemic diseases (Figure 9.7).

9.3. Symptoms and Diagnosis

The signs and symptoms of helminthic infections are often very unreliable, commonly dependent on the particular helminth involved and the host's immune response. Abdominal pain, diarrhea, and nausea are typical gastrointestinal upsets in infected individuals and are often replicated by other intestinal conditions. Specifically, infections caused by *Ascaris lumbricoides* can lead to serious complications, one of them being intestinal obstruction that can arise when there is intussusception due to an overwhelming worm burden. This sort of obstruction can be extremely painful and can require surgery, making the detection and management of infections early an imperative, especially in highly endemic regions where burdens of helminths are rather high (Pecorella et al., 2016). Therefore, the distinction between chronic gastrointestinal illnesses and those resulting from helminthic infections is crucial for early therapy and prevention of late complications. Laboratory examination of feces is the primary diagnostic tool for helminthic infections, by which ova, larvae, or adults are identified.

The method is still the best for diagnosing several intestinal helminths like hookworms, tapeworms, and pinworms. However, not all helminthic infections yield eggs in stool specimens during their acute phase, and a few are of restricted diagnostic manifestations the requiring serological tests for the diagnosis of some parasites. For example, schistosome infections can be confirmed by determining characteristic antibodies in blood, allowing broader application of diagnostic methods particular to the suspected helminth. Due to the nonspecific presentation of such infections, the clinician should be highly suspicious and possess a good working familiarity with the symptomology of different helminths (Pecorella et al., 2016). Even in the case of international travel, diagnosis of helminthic infection presents an added level of complexity to clinical assessment. Visitors from endemic countries also present symptoms that are easily attributed to other conditions, such as traveler's diarrhea or respiratory infections. Importantly, it is worth noting that travelers have been known to be less frequently diagnosed with helminthic infection compared to immigrants and refugees, the latter of whom are likely to present a higher prevalence due to prolonged exposure to infected environments (Pecorella et al., 2016). This difference emphasizes the importance of the use of travel history in the diagnostic process, along with pretravel medical consultation to reduce risks through preventive measures such as vaccinations and prophylactic drugs. Finally, a complete understanding of symptoms, diagnostic practices, and exposure history enhances helminthic infection care, leading to better patient outcomes.

9.3.1. Common Symptoms of Helminthic Infections

Helminthic infections caused by parasitic worms are most commonly presented in the form of a diverse spectrum of symptoms that can be quite heterogeneous based on the causative helminth and host immune response. Commonly encountered symptoms include abdominal pain, gastrointestinal disturbance, and weight loss. Patients present with episodic diarrhea and constipation, most often because of intestinal obstruction secondary to the mass effect of the worms. Specifically, *Ascaris lumbricoides* is implicated in acute infections leading to intestinal intussusception as a case of the highly deleterious effects of helminthic infection on gastrointestinal disease. In addition, resultant nutritional deficits by helminthic parasitism will support symptoms and greater health consequences, particularly among healthcare and sanitation-deficient populations. With the increasing load of worms, the severity of symptoms increases, highlighting the significance of effective prevention and treatment strategies (Pecorella et al., 2016). Apart from gastrointestinal symptoms, helminthic infections could cause systemic responses that worsen the overall health status of a person. Systemic symptoms like fever, weakness, and malaise are some common manifestations, showing the immune response of the body to the parasites. Certain helminth infections, particularly those affecting *Schistosoma* species, may cause more serious sequelae like hepatosplenomegaly and anemia resulting from blood loss.

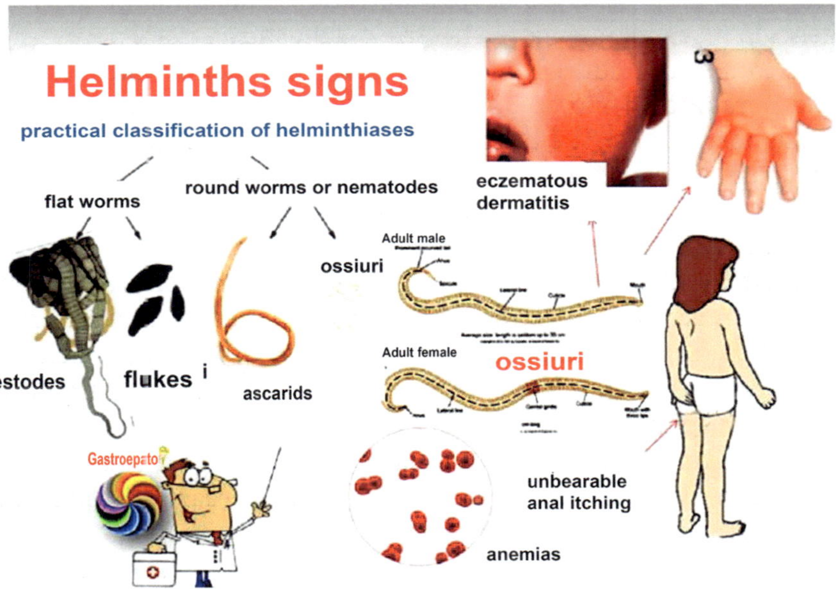

Figure 9.8. Helminths signs.

Source: https://www.gastroepato.it/en_helminths-signs.webp.

The systemic manifestations of these infections may also occur in the form of complications like eosinophilia, wherein the elevated eosinophil count may indicate an inflammatory reaction to the body's presence of the helminth. Helminthic infection patients may also present with symptoms of other diseases that overlap, complicating diagnosis. Being aware of the varied symptoms of these infections is thus crucial to enable health workers to provide proper and timely treatment (Pecorella et al., 2016). The social significance of these infection symptoms extends beyond individual health to public health outcomes and the health system, particularly where the prevalence of helminth infection is high. The chronic course of helminthic infections often results in chronic health complications, growth and cognitive impairment in children, and absenteeism from school and work. The resultant socioeconomic effects can perpetuate cycles of poverty and inhibit community development. Hence, health interventions aimed at sanitation improvement, education, and access to medical care are important not only to reduce the helminthic infections but also for overall community health. Helminth infections require a multi-caused approach that includes medication, health education, and strengthening of public health infrastructure to counteract the symptoms and the long-term sequelae of helminthic infections (Pecorella et al., 2016) (Figure 9.8).

9.3.2. Diagnostic Methods Used in Identifying Infections

Helminthic infection detection demands a multi-angle approach, using several diagnostic methods that can effectively identify helminths. The traditional methods, such as the Kato-Katz thick smear, are pivotal in the diagnosis of ascariasis infections. Although this method is a standard for detection, its sensitivity is not ideal. Increased stool sampling has the potential to enhance this sensitivity; however, it is still less sensitive compared to alternative microscopy techniques, such as FLOTAC, with higher diagnostic capability. Kato-Katz application is still prevalent for mapping and evaluating national control programs, and this underscores the value of the strategy despite its deficiencies. Therefore, investments in research into more effective diagnostic tests are necessary because current methods must evolve to improve addressing the difficulties of helminthic infection (Lamberton & Jourdan, 2015). Besides traditional microscopy, serologic tests on the basis of antibody detection have emerged as useful diagnostic tools. The tests offer the benefit of enhanced sensitivity, particularly in assessing transmission dynamics in environments focused on elimination programs. However, their worth is typically restricted by their inability to provide a definite diagnosis, thus limiting their use in clinical practice. Molecular diagnostics are yet one step further, assuring a new era of specificity and sensitivity in the identification of helminthic infections. Although the application of molecular methods is currently constrained by cost, they have unprecedented potential for individual diagnosis, drug testing, and specific identification of specific species of helminth, e.g., *Ascaris suum*. These advances in diagnostic methods are key to control of helminths and alleviation of human suffering caused by these parasitic diseases (Lamberton & Jourdan, 2015). The presence of zoonotic helminths such as *Baylisascaris procyonis* brings additional challenges in the domain of diagnostic methods. With raccoons increasingly inhabiting urban areas, environmental contamination leading to human infection is a rising public health concern. *B. procyonis* eggs can remain viable in the environment for extended periods, posing a heavy risk to unsuspecting persons, especially toddlers who might unwittingly ingest them. Early and accurate diagnosis of this infection is critical because it can lead to severe complications, including neurological damage. More advanced diagnostic methods to detect *B. procyonis* infections are therefore required to inform public health policy and prevent the dangers of this emerging zoonosis. As the field of helminthic infections expands, so must the diagnostic capabilities applied to manage them effectively.

9.3.3. Challenges in Diagnosing Helminthic Infections

Diagnosis of helminthic infections is plagued by challenges stemming from a combination of circumstances that influence the sensitivity and access to diagnostic tests. Traditional methods of diagnosis, such as the Kato-Katz test, remain prevalent but low in sensitivity, particularly in the identification of infections due to soil-dwelling helminths such as *Ascaris lumbricoides*. Although this test finds widespread application in public health surveys, its limitations necessitate other sampling and testing procedures to raise detection levels. Additionally, the overlap of symptoms with other gastrointestinal infections complicates clinical diagnoses, even more pressing the search for more accurate diagnostic methods. The dire need for more sensitive diagnostic tests has therefore become all the more pressing, particularly in regions severely impacted by helminthic infections (Lamberton & Jourdan, 2015). Molecular diagnosis advances are a landmark in the war against helminth infections and techniques hold more promise of higher sensitivity and specificity than conventional methods. For instance, PCR assays have proved very promising; however, their cost tends to restrict usage to research laboratories instead of clinical practice. Besides, antibody-based diagnostics, while potentially sensitive for detecting infections, are of practical limitations, especially in assessing transmission dynamics in areas aspiring to eliminate such infections. The cost-effectiveness versus diagnostic accuracy is still debatable, and it complicates the efforts to combat these prevalent infections at a global scale (Lamberton & Jourdan, 2015). It is necessary to understand the economic forces at play to develop effective diagnostic techniques that are grounded in public health. Furthermore, epidemiological studies for helminthic infections typically struggle with inconsistencies of prevalence data, as is illustrated in studies focused on subsets of populations. An example includes a cross-sectional study that showed a low prevalence of intestinal helminths among children who presented with diarrhea and emphasized the importance of having rigorous data collection strategies. Environmental factors, such as hygiene practices and sanitation, are also paramount determinants of infection rates, making it challenging to make accurate diagnoses and intervention strategies. The interconnectedness of these factors makes identifying populations at risk challenging and imposes effective control measures. It is thus imperative to address these issues of diagnosis through a multilateral effort that accommodates technological advancements as well as extensive field studies prioritizing environmental contexts and individual health trends.

9.4. Treatment Options

The management of helminthic infections is mainly based on effective treatment regimens, which are of utmost value in the control of the disease burden of parasitic infections. Anthelmintic medications such as albendazole and mebendazole have emerged as first-line drugs for soil-transmitted helminthiasis with significant efficacy in worm burden reduction and alleviation of clinical symptoms. However, even in the presence of such efficacious and safe drugs, treatment inequalities continue to exist even in places where they are available, particularly in infected zones. Statistical data indicate that fewer than half of exposed children were treated in 2016, and this points to a gigantic gap in public health efforts in treating these infections within vulnerable groups (Jourdan et al., 2018). Thus, increasing access to anthelminthic treatment in addition to raising awareness regarding the need for treatment is important to reducing morbidity and ultimately improving the quality of life of the infected. In addition to standard pharmacologic therapy, other forms of treatment have been researched and are an exciting area of research for helminthic infection treatment. The evolving paradigm of molecular medicine encompasses new approaches, including the identification of druggable targets with cutting-edge bioinformatics and omics technologies. The technologies have the potential to lead to the development of personalized medicine, which can optimize therapeutic impacts tailored to each patient. With the development of our understanding of genomics and pathophysiological underpinnings of helminthic infections, the healthcare community is poised to institute more targeted and effective treatment regimens, beyond existing modalities not effective for all patients (Singh, 2020). As such studies are further developed, they will be utilized to enhance existing systems of care, resulting in a better overall management of helminthic disease. Public health policies should also supplement clinical interventions with the promotion of prevention and control strategies as much as treatment. Large-scale deworming campaigns have gone a long way to limit the impact of helminthic infestations in some of the endemic areas, but such programs need to have an integrated scope that entails sound diagnostics coupled with community awareness. It is crucial that not only treatment is provided by health professionals but also patient and community education on hygiene behaviors, dietary modifications, and environmental control to prevent reinfection. Equally crucial will be the sharpening of diagnostic methods in identifying individuals who can benefit from treatment as well as reinforcing the efficacy of public health interventions to prevent helminthic infections (Jourdan et al., 2018). By adopting an all-embracing strategy comprising prevention and treatment, the health field can finally work towards safeguarding risk groups and drastically minimizing the role of helminthic infections in global health.

9.4.1. Anthelmintic Medications

The anthelmintic drugs are of key importance in the treatment of helminthic infection, which is caused by many parasitic worms. The infections, being significant public health problems, chiefly present themselves within the vulnerable population, particularly in developing nations where socio-economic conditions are unsupportive. Anthelmintic drugs constitute a primary defense against helminths such as flukes, tapeworms, and nematodes that inhabit human hosts. Drugs like albendazole and mebendazole are widely used for their effectiveness against soil-transmitted helminths, demonstrating the huge impact these medicines can have in reducing morbidity due to such infections. Treatment of helminthiasis not only has health benefits but also promotes economic development through productivity and improved quality of life among the affected, since the infections have been associated with stunted growth, anemia, and mental disabilities in children, according to Lamberton & Jourdan (2015). However, the excessive reliance on a limited arsenal of anthelmintic drugs is highly problematic, particularly due to the resistance to drugs. The routine use of drugs such as albendazole and mebendazole is among the contributory reasons for the trend, most notable in veterinary medicine and causing alarm regarding similar trends occurring in human health. The World Health Organization highlights the imperative to combat neglected tropical diseases but concedes that the possibility of resistance is one that deters their attempt at helminthic infection control and eradication. Thus, it becomes necessary to research new lines of treatment and introduce novel compounds that have a wide range of activity against various helminthic strains. Drug repurposing and discovery of new pharmacological agents from nature are of critical importance in the quest for alternatives, as presented by Tewelde & Tadesse (2022). Moreover, vaccine development against helminthic infections is a promising avenue for a long-term solution. The concept of a pan-anthelmintic vaccine is a novel approach to attempting to provide broad protection against multiple helminth species, thus reducing drug dependency and avoiding the chance for resistance. With intimidating challenges to vaccine creation, including complexity in helminth biology and immune avoidance mechanisms, innovations in research provide hopeful possibilities. Utilization of strategies like optimizing advanced immunological techniques and implementing recombinant technology can enhance the effectiveness of vaccines. Interdisciplinary collaboration between health care workers, researchers, and international health organizations is essential to accomplish these goals, ultimately to maximize the global health significance of helminthic infections, as outlined in the ongoing debate regarding the need for new anthelmintic interventions by Tewelde & Tadesse (2022) (Figure 9.9).

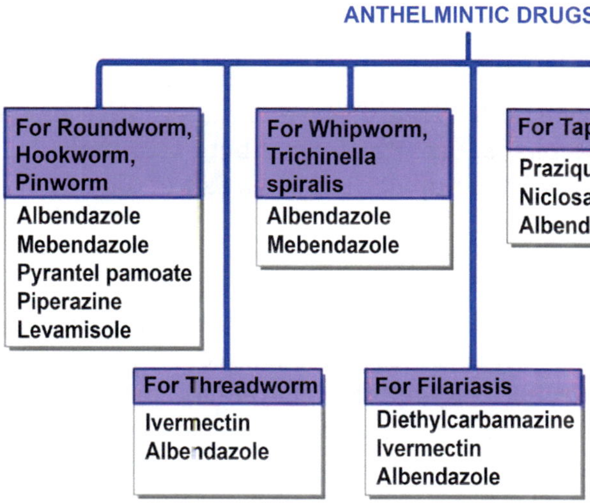

Figure 9.9. Anthelmintic drugs.

Source: https://pharmacyfreak.com/wp-content/uploads/2025/05/CLASSIFICATION-OF-ANTHELEMETIC-DRUGS.jpg

9.4.2. Alternative Treatment Approaches

The search for alternative therapy approaches to helminthic infections has gone a long way, especially with a consideration of the limitations of conventional pharmacological treatments. Effective as they are, conventional anthelmintics have the disadvantages of offering partial coverage of endemic areas, being costly, and posing risks of resistance build-up. In reaction to this, researchers have explored other methodologies such as food-based therapies, probiotics, and immunomodulatory treatments that rely on the immune system of the host instead of chemical compounds. These are not only promising in meeting current gaps in drug availability but also in reducing the damage caused by chemical drugs. Exploring these options is relevant to at-risk groups, particularly children living in areas where helminthic disease is most prevalent and often left unaddressed for logistical reasons in the provision of care (Jourdan et al., 2018). Immunotherapy, which uses the body's own immune response mechanisms, is a very promising candidate for the treatment of helminthic infections. The highly polarized immune responses associated with helminth infestations, for instance, increased levels of IgE, may provide hints about potential therapeutic approaches. For instance, some immunotherapies directed against the Th2 immune response, usually increased in co-infected individuals with malaria and helminthiasis, are under research. Current studies indicate that co-infections with helminths can potentially augment total serum IgE significantly, suggesting a mechanistic correlation between helminthic infection and immune modulation in co-infective settings (Belyhun et al., 2014). Based on this knowledge, it may be possible to develop focused interventions that can reverse the effect of both malaria and helminthic infections, with a doubled advantage through an augmented modulation of the immune response. Another potential alternative treatment approach involves the use of traditional and native medication therapies that have been in use for centuries across cultures. Many communities have relied on herbal medicines and plant therapies to eliminate helminthic infections, which are subsequently passed from generation to generation. Recent ethnopharmacology has begun investigating the viability of these traditional treatments when combined with mainstream medication. Such integrative approaches not only might offer efficient treatment modalities but also increase patient compliance and acceptance. As public health systems continue to seek cost-effective and socially acceptable answers to helminthic infection, it is necessary to carry out systematic research on such alternative modalities so that their effectiveness and safety can be established and thus contribute to a more holistic strategy for the control of helminthic disease in endemic populations (Jourdan et al., 2018).

9.4.3. Importance of Proper Treatment Adherence

The importance of following proper treatment for the control of helminthic infection cannot be overemphasized, particularly given the morbidity that these infections confer to vulnerable population groups such as children. Not only is the relief of symptoms guaranteed by proper treatment, but also prevention of the long-term health consequences of untreated infection. Where the prevalence of helminthic infection is high, particularly among children five years and below, it is especially important that treatments be followed to the letter. A study of mothers from Kuwaluhan Village highlights the correlation between knowledge and rates of adherence to helminthic drug intake. The study revealed that most of the mothers had medium rates of adherence despite their sufficient level of knowledge on treatment protocols, something that signifies special education intervention for enhanced compliance. This variance suggests that even with sufficient information, socioeconomic status and healthcare access may hinder uniform treatment protocols, which can exacerbate the public health impact of helminthic infections (Amanda et al., 2023). Adherence to proper treatment is also underscored by the negative consequences of untreated helminthic infections, which can result in severe health complications, including anemia and stunted growth. The pathogenesis between helminths and anemia in postpartum women depicts the intricate relationship between parasitic infection and overall wellness.

Research in Mbarara Regional Referral Hospital indicates that non-compliance with hematinic treatment has a great contribution to postpartum anemia, apart from factors such as helminthic infestations (Anwar et al., 2016). The advantages of this information apply to children's health, too; failure to treat helminthic infections can contribute to cognitive disabilities and malnutrition, also contributing to disease cycles and poverty. Proper compliance therefore, not only cures the immediate health problem of helminthic infection but is also a necessary step in improving long-term health status and breaking the disease cycle of disease spread in the affected communities. Public health programs aimed at the control of helminthic infections need to incorporate treatment adherence as a central component of their strategies. This needs to involve an integrated, multi-component approach which includes education, drug availability, and community involvement in promoting good health behavior. All parties involved need to get together and formulate overall programs which target the socioeconomic and cultural determinants of adherence. Regular follow-up and supportive treatment can also facilitate adherence by reminding the patient of the importance of maintaining treatment regimens. Encouraging an adherence culture, communities are in a position to reduce the prevalence and burden of helminthic infections greatly, resulting in improved quality of life among the affected populations. Compliance from medical professionals, governments, and communities will be paramount in ensuring that treatment guidelines are followed uninterrupted, paving the way to healthier lives and the relief of helminthic disease burden (Amanda et al., 2023).

9.5. Prevention and Control

Prevention and management of helminthic infections are important both for public health and socioeconomic advancement in the affected regions. Effective interventions also rely on community participation and education, emphasizing respect for hygiene and sanitation measures. One of the simple interventions is promotion of hand washing with soap, which has been found to have considerable effectiveness in reducing rates of transmission of gastrointestinal pathogens, including helminths. Research in low- and middle-income countries highlights the protective function of handwashing, with repeated adherence and behavior change playing a role in improved population health when faced with these infections. Addressing hygiene-related behavior is therefore a key component within the broad context of helminthic infection prevention (Jourdan et al., 2018). Vaccination is also a priority among preventive measures for helminthic infections, with implications that necessitate coordinated healthcare approaches. For example, in managing cervical cancer risk due to human papillomavirus (HPV), evidence indicates that young girls' vaccination is discouraged by a number of barriers, including access-related challenges. Low-resource environments tend to experience barriers, for example, travel distance to a healthcare facility, and this tends to have a profound impact on the rate of completion of vaccinations (Mabeya et al., 2018). Thus, new delivery approaches and educational interventions among children and their parents are crucial in dismantling barriers to vaccination. By making vaccines both accessible and supported by extensive education about their benefit, the likelihood of isolating younger generations from preventable illness increases greatly. Moreover, the instatement of routine deworming programs is another critical intervention in the prevention and control of helminthic infections. These interventions are particularly beneficial in school children, who are also the most prone to these parasites. Deworming on a routine basis, if accompanied by health education, can lead to improved physical well-being, mental growth, and scholastic performance. Systematic approaches towards deworming have been supported by the World Health Organization for the endemic regions on the basis of its effectiveness in reducing the rate of infection and attendant morbidities. Ongoing monitoring and assessment of the programs are also important to keep them sustainable and scalable, which can ultimately reduce helminth burdens in communities to a drastic level (Mabeya et al., 2018). Thus, an integrated multi-pronged approach involving hand hygiene, vaccination, and deworming interventions can immensely enhance the prevention and control of helminthic infections globally.

9.5.1. Public Health Strategies for Prevention

Prevention of helminthic infections at the public health level requires a multifaceted intervention involving vaccination, education, and enhanced access to healthcare. The use of preventive vaccines, particularly where helminthic infection and other infectious diseases are endemic, has far-reaching benefits to public health. For instance, the introduction of HPV vaccinations into general health programs may be taken as a case study to highlight both success and challenge. In Africa's sub-Saharan area, where cervical cancer cases caused by HPV are incredibly high, unavailability based on geography and others' misinformation are the main hurdles for vaccination coverage. This has been demonstrated in one study, whereby only 39.1% of schoolgirls were given the third dose as advised due to logistical challenges and inadequate health education, according to the findings of the study (Mabeya et al., 2018). Avoiding such failures through the use of new delivery strategies is critical to enhancing public health outcomes in general. In addition to vaccination, promoting behavior change through organized activities of health education is a major factor in preventing helminthic infections. Hand soap-washing has already been well proven to significantly reduce the transmission of parasitic infections, such as helminths. Public health practitioners should therefore concentrate efforts on promoting hygiene awareness and practice, especially among low-resource populations. It is stated in studies carried out in this field that the effective operation of handwashing programs depends on knowing the behavior determinants and hygiene-related cultural practices (Jourdan et al., 2018). This fact highlights the importance of situating health messaging within context and adapting interventions according to the needs of particular communities. By incorporating the knowledge of local customs and practices into public health programs, campaigns have the ability to better reach populations and induce sustainable behavior change for the purposes of controlling helminthic transmission. Lastly, the strengthening of healthcare systems to ensure equal access to treatment and prevention services is the cornerstone of any effective public health intervention against helminthic disease. This involves not only upgrading physical infrastructure but also increasing healthcare personnel training and provision of resources to rural regions of nations where helminthic infections are most prevalent. Strategic partnerships between governments and non-governmental organizations can enable the dispensation of necessary medication and the implementation of regular deworming programs in schools. Through these programs, public health administrators can target vulnerable populations where the prevalence of helminthic diseases is most concentrated. Moreover, ongoing studies and surveillance are essential for evaluating the effects of such public health interventions and the necessary adjustments on the basis of emerging data. Therefore, improving the quality and availability of healthcare continues to be a top priority of an overall prevention strategy against helminthic infections (Figure 9.10).

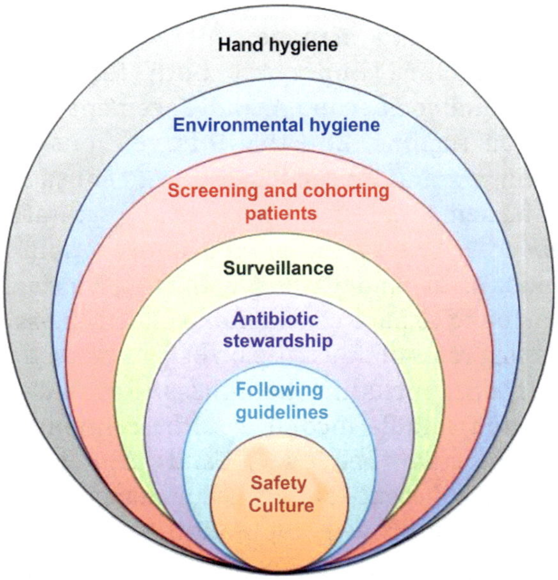

Figure 9.10. Strategies to prevent healthcare-associated infections.

Source: https://infectionsinsurgery.org/wp-content/uploads/2019/02/prevention-1.jpg?w=863.

9.5.2. Role of Sanitation and Hygiene

The interrelation of sanitation, hygiene, and helminthic infection incidence is crucial in understanding the broader public health implications of public health policy. Intestinal parasites are largely spread by poor hygiene practices and sanitation, which predominantly affect vulnerable populations, like children in developing nations. As has been recorded in a recent review of literature on hand hygiene, effective hand washing with soap has been shown to reduce levels of infection with pathogens, such as helminths, by disrupting the transmission chain (Jourdan et al., 2018). Also, communities that invest in improved sanitation facilities are seen to reduce rates of parasitic infections, indicating the importance of integrating sanitation programs into broader health programs.

The findings of research performed in rural India further explain the role of hygiene education in the prevention of helminthic infections. Research indicated that there was a high prevalence of intestinal parasites in children with poor hygienic practices, such as not washing hands and having long nails (Dongre et al., 2008). The use of specific hygiene education effectively changed habits of behavior, significantly improving the incidence of proper handwashing after defecation and enabling the practice of nail care. This double approach of providing drug treatment alongside participatory hygiene education was considered essential to reduce parasite loads among infected groups, demonstrating that education can be a highly viable tool in fighting helminthic disease. Overall, the development of a sanitation and hygiene culture is fundamental to public health and disease prevention. Incorporation of serious practice of hygiene into daily life can significantly decrease the burden of helminth infection and other infectious illnesses. Additional actions to address basic infrastructure in terms of access to pure water and appropriate sanitary facilities should accompany education campaigns as well. By targeting these interventions initially, societies can establish a healthier environment that promotes the health and well-being of their members, breaking the cycle of infection and ushering in the doors to enduring health gains in the long term.

9.5.3. Education and Awareness Programs

Education and awareness campaigns play a key role in combating helminthic infections, particularly in regions where the parasitic infections are endemic. The infections thrive in environments with limited resources, where socio-economic levels hinder the ability to gain access to healthcare as well as sanitation. Initiatives geared towards educating community members on hygiene behavior, such as the frequent washing of hands with soap, have a significant capacity to hinder the helminths and other pathogens. Evidence indicates that behavioral modification by evidence-based interventions directly translates to decreased disease prevalence; in one instance, a comprehensive analysis of handwashing practices noted uniform findings in the reduction of infections in low- and middle-income countries, highlighting more intense focus on outreach and education as a crucial intervention (Jourdan et al., 2018). With outreach to communities and implementing certain programming, one can promote a culture of health promotion, focusing on the importance of hygiene in the control of helminthic infection. In addition to promoting general hygiene practice, campaigns must also inform about the specific health risks posed by helminthic infections, particularly among vulnerable populations such as school-age children. Malnutrition and impaired physical and mental growth are potential outcomes of such infections, thus having a significant impact on school performance. Awareness schemes, particularly in Sub-Saharan Africa, have set the premise for access to prevention interventions, i.e., sanitation facilities and healthcare services, which are crucial in averting helminthic disease burden. Acknowledgement of these linkages can empower communities to call for better public health policy and resource allocation. One Kenyan research detected significant barriers to HPV vaccination of girls as directly related to accessibility to health care and therefore reiterating the symbiotic relationship between health education and public health goals in the early general (Mabeya et al., 2018). Secondly, the integration of educational campaigns in vaccination campaigns also encourages better health outcomes among helminthic infection-at-risk individuals. A collaborative effort of health authorities and communities towards disseminating information regarding both hygiene and vaccine practices can help produce an integrated approach towards the prevention of diseases. Effective strategies include conducting workshops, school-based health education, and engaging local leaders to facilitate community acceptance. All these can lead to high levels of vaccination program participation and increased coverage rates and community health. As emphasized in cervical cancer awareness and HPV immunization campaigns, informed populations are more likely to de-stigmatize health interventions and follow practice guidelines. Therefore, successful health education and awareness interventions are essential to reversing the implications of helminthic infection and creating healthy, aware populations.

SUMMARY

Research on helminthic infections provides relevant data on their prevalence and impact on health, particularly in resource-constrained settings. The infections not only lead to malnutrition and anemia but also complicate the treatment of diseases, particularly HIV/AIDS. Helminth infections coexisting with malaria have been documented to exacerbate the health problems of vulnerable populations, necessitating joint health interventions to treat these co-infections concurrently. The elevated infection rates of helminths within populations in Sub-Saharan Africa highlight the need for public health actions that stress education, treatment access, and prevention. Without such integrated strategies, the disease burden cycle will continue, further hindering advancements toward better health outcomes in affected areas. Furthermore, the intersection of helminthic infection and vaccine receipt, with the most striking example being HPV, indicates the role of health systems and environmental determinants in shaping health outcomes. Research indicates that high infection prevalences, i.e., for malaria and helminths, can impact immune responses to vaccines, quite possibly requiring adapted vaccination schedules in these populations. Kenyan research outcomes demonstrate that logistical barriers, including travel distance to vaccination sites, are significant predictors of vaccine completion. Groundbreaking methods for extending access and knowledge about HPV and cervical cancer screening are essential to empower communities to overcome these barriers and strengthen public health interventions. Comprehensive strategies considering both infectious diseases and immunization strategies are crucial to reducing the overall disease burden. Lastly, the treatment of helminthic infections has far-reaching consequences for world health, particularly in the prevention of comorbidities and improving health autonomy among infected subjects. Targeted deworming programs and their impact on immune status must be further researched, as indicated by studies that bring to the fore the benefits of albendazole treatment on CD4 counts and hemoglobin levels among HIV-infected patients. With the adoption of a multi-faceted strategy across prevention, treatment, and education, stakeholders can create strong health systems that can respond to the dual challenge posed by helminths and other infectious diseases. In the end, progress toward the prevention of helminthic infections will not just contribute to individualized health improvements but also supplement greater public health initiatives committed to healthier communities, as well as alleviating the socioeconomic impacts associated with infection.

The interaction with other diseases, such as malaria and HIV, is crucial in understanding the broader epidemiological picture. Co-infections, particularly in high-risk groups such as pregnant women, have been observed to compound health issues such as anemia, based on studies. For instance, a study in Rwanda revealed that significant proportions of HIV-positive expectant women were co-infected with helminths and malaria, proving the co-occurrence of the two in resource-poor settings. Such findings call for the comprehension of the interaction between such infections in order to come up with more efficient public health strategies, particularly for the targeted affected groups. With targeted interventions, such as deworming and fortified education initiatives, health in these populations would be greatly improved, and attest to the focal dependency of treating multiple infectious disease burdens simultaneously (Emil, 2017). Additionally, research on helminth infections reveals that certain parasite species, such as hookworms, have specific associations with malaria, which affect the severity and prevalence of anemia. Evidence shows that among expectant mothers, the infected hookworm-carrying women are at much higher risk of contracting malaria than uninfected women. This evidence shows the vulnerability of helminths to compromise individuals' immunity abilities so that they are susceptible to other infections like malaria (Naing et al., 2017). The exceptional nature of these interactions requires exhaustive research that not only examines the infections individually but also their co-occurrence and the subsequent health consequences. This can yield insightful findings that are instrumental in gaining a deeper understanding of how helminthic infections function within the parameters of larger infectious disease models. Finally, deworming intervention implications are specifically impressive in the management of helminthic infections in HIV-positive individuals. Research has shown that treatment with albendazole significantly affects immune indicators, with increased CD4 counts and decreased viral loads among infected populations. This effect shows the potential benefits of treating helminthic infections, particularly among those already compromising their health, such as those on antiretroviral treatment. Additionally, the untargeted or targeted deworming intervention has been equally efficient in reducing the prevalence of helminth diseases and overall improving health benefits. The interconnectedness between helminth treatment and other comorbid diseases, such as HIV and malaria, signals the necessity of integrated health measures that consider the multidimensionality of infectious disease (Emil, 2017).

CLOSER LOOK

TAENIA SAGINATA

Taenia saginata or beef tapeworm is an intestinal parasitic flatworm belonging to class Cestoda and family Taeniidae. It infects man, its definitive host, and uses cattle as its intermediate host. The parasite is endemic in the majority of the world, where beef is consumed raw or undercooked and sanitation is low.

The Taenia saginata life cycle is indirect and occurs in two hosts. Infection in man results from eating raw or undercooked beef harboring cysticerci (larval cysts). The cysticercus developed within the human gut into an adult worm that may measure up to 10 meters in length. The adult worm is made up of a scolex (head) and a long proglottid chain (body segments). *T. saginata* has a scolex devoid of hooks but four muscular suckers utilized in attachment to the intestinal wall (Figure 9.11).

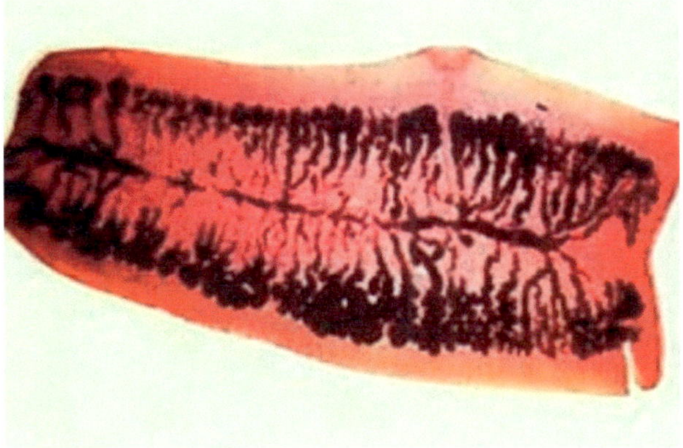

Figure 9.11. Stained image of *Taenia saginata*, also known as the beef tapeworm, showing its segmented body structure characteristic of cestodes.

Source: https://upload.wikimedia.org/wikipedia/commons/thumb/9/95/Taenia_saginataD.JPG/250px-Taenia_saginataD.JPG.

The adult proglottids are hermaphroditic, possessing the male as well as the female reproductive system. Gravid proglottids containing fertilized eggs are formed as the worm grows and detach from the worm to be passed out in the feces of the host. In the outside world, cattle become infected if they consume infected food or ingest infected water containing these eggs. The eggs are hatched in the bovine intestine, with oncospheres that infect the intestinal tissue and travel through the blood to the striated muscles, where cysticerci form.

Only humans are the final host of *T. saginata*, and infection is typically asymptomatic or is accompanied by nonspecific gastrointestinal symptoms such as abdominal discomfort, nausea, diarrhea, or excessive eating. The most noteworthy symptom is the passage of living proglottids in stools or the perianal region, which causes anxiety and embarrassment in the patient.

Diagnosis is typically confirmed by microscopic examination of stool for eggs or proglottids. Eggs of *T. saginata* and *T. solium* are not distinguishable morphologically; thus, identification in some cases requires recovery and examination of the scolex or counting the number of branches of the uterus in gravid proglottids. Imaging or endoscopy may be employed in rare cases.

Treatment involves the administration of antiparasitic medications such as praziquantel or niclosamide to destroy the mature worm. After treatment, the entire worm, including the scolex, must be evacuated to prevent recurrence. In cases involving solely proglottids passed, re-treatment is often done.

Prevention measures include the proper cooking of beef to kill cysticerci, meat inspection, sanitation control, and public health education on the risk of consuming raw or undercooked meat. Infected patients must be treated promptly to prevent environmental contamination.

References

1. Futagbi, G., Abankwa, J. K., Agbale, P. S., & Aboagye, I. F. (2015). Assessment of helminth infections in goats slaughtered in an abattoir in a suburb of accra, Ghana. *West African Journal of Applied Ecology*, *23*(2), 35-42.(accessed on 16th July 2025).

2. Jourdan, P. M., Lamberton, P. H. L., Fenwick, A., & Addiss, D. G. (2018). Soil-transmitted helminth infections. *Lancet (London, England)*, *391*(10117), 252–265. https://doi.org/10.1016/S0140-6736(17)31930-X(accessed on 16th July 2025).

3. Ajjampur, S. S. R., Kang, G., Kattula, D., Levecke, B., et al. (2014). *Prevalence & risk factors for soil transmitted helminth infection among school children in south India.* https://core.ac.uk/download/55800525.pdf (accessed on 16th July 2025).

4. Amanda, S. R., Hadi, I., Haresmita, P. P., Wardani, W., et al. (2023). *Description of mother's knowledge and adherence to use of helminthic drugs in Kuwaluhan Village, Magelang Regency, Central Java.* https://core.ac.uk/download/654628895.pdf (accessed on 16th July 2025).

5. Motran, C. C., Silvane, L., Chiapello, L. S., Theumer, M. G., Ambrosio, L. F., Volpini, X., Celias, D. P., & Cervi, L. (2018). Helminth Infections: Recognition and Modulation of the Immune Response by Innate Immune Cells. *Frontiers in immunology*, *9*, 664. https://doi.org/10.3389/fimmu.2018.00664(accessed on 16th July 2025).

6. Anwar, Z., Bulus, L. N., Chakura, A., Joseph, M., et al. (2016). *Incidence and factors associated with postpartum anemia at Mbarara Regional Referral Hospital.* https://core.ac.uk/download/234691696.pdf (accessed on 16th July 2025).

7. Aqeele, G. (2024). *Traditional detection of intestinal helminths in stray cats in Wasit Province, Iraq.* https://core.ac.uk/download/618209136.pdf (accessed on 16th July 2025).

8. Arrais, M., Brito, M., Cooper, P., Gama, C., et al. (2020). *Helminth infections, atopy, asthma and allergic diseases: Protocol for a systematic review of observational studies worldwide.* https://core.ac.uk/download/323385702.pdf (accessed on 16th July 2025).

9. Ash, L. R., Berlin, O. G. W., Morse, S. A., Sorvillo, F., et al. (2002). *Baylisascaris procyonis: An emerging helminthic zoonosis.* https://core.ac.uk/download/323062358.pdf (accessed on 16th July 2025).

10. Belyhun, Y., Elias, D., Erko, B., Kassu, A., et al. (2014). *Helminths and malaria co-infections are associated with elevated serum IgE.* https://core.ac.uk/download/pdf/50697116.pdf (accessed on 16th July 2025).

11. Jain, Sudhir Kumar. (2018). Effect of Multiple Rounds of Mass Drug Administration under Lymphatic Filariasis Elimination Program on Prevalence of Soil-Transmitted Helminthiasis in One of the Co-endemic Districts of India. Journal of Communicable Diseases. 50. 9-15. 10.24321/0019.5138.201803. (accessed on 16th July 2025).

12. Bisanzio, D., Bustinduy, A. L., King, C. H., Kitron, U., et al. (2014). *Cross-sectional study of the burden of vector-borne and soil-transmitted polyparasitism in rural communities of Coast Province, Kenya.* https://core.ac.uk/download/29469451.pdf (accessed on 16th July 2025).

13. Biwott, G. K., Ngeiywa, M. M., & Wanjala, P. M. (2014). *Prevalence of gastrointestinal parasitic infections among food handlers in Eldoret Municipality, Kenya.* https://core.ac.uk/download/234660479.pdf (accessed on 16th July 2025).

14. Dongre AR, Deshmukh PR, Boratne AV, Thaware P, Garg BS. An approach to hygiene education among rural Indian school going children. *Online J Health Allied Scs.* 2007;4:2 (accessed on 16th July 2025).

15. O'Brien, D. P., Leder, K., Matchett, E., Brown, G. V., & Torresi, J. (2006). Illness in returned travelers and immigrants/refugees: the 6-year experience of two Australian infectious diseases units. *Journal of travel medicine, 13*(3), 145–152. https://doi.org/10.1111/j.1708-8305.2006.00033.xc(accessed on 16th July 2025).

16. Pecorella, I., Okello, T. R., Ciardi, G., Ogwang, D. M., & Opira, C. (2016). Intestinal Intussusception in An Adult Caused by Helminthic Parasitosis. *Gastroenterology Insights, 7*(1), 6469. https://doi.org/10.4081/gi.2016.6469 (accessed on 16th July 2025).

17. Ekanem, E. E., Eyong, K., Ikobah, J. M., Uhegbu, R., et al. (2021). *Helminthic infestation in children aged 6 to 59 months with diarrhea in Calabar.* https://core.ac.uk/download/478392701.pdf (accessed on 16th July 2025).

18. Emil, I. (2017). *The prevalence of helminth and malaria infections and the effects of de-worming on disease progression markers in HIV-1 infected pregnant women on antiretroviral therapy in Rwanda.* https://core.ac.uk/download/188775605.pdf (accessed on 16th July 2025).

19. Harrington, D., Lamberton, P. H. L., & McGregor, A. (2017). *Human Liver Flukes.* https://core.ac.uk/download/96882191.pdf (accessed on 16th July 2025).

20. Lamberton, P. H., & Jourdan, P. M. (2015). Human Ascariasis: Diagnostics Update. *Current tropical medicine reports, 2*(4), 189–200. https://doi.org/10.1007/s40475-015-0064-9 (accessed on 16th July 2025).

21. Mabeya, H., Menon, S., Weyers, S., Naanyu, V., Mwaliko, E., Kirop, E., Orango, O., Vermandere, H., & Vanden Broeck, D. (2018). Uptake of three doses of HPV vaccine by primary school girls in Eldoret, Kenya; a prospective cohort study in a malaria endemic setting. *BMC cancer, 18*(1), 557. https://doi.org/10.1186/s12885-018-4382-x(accessed on 16th July 2025).

22. Lal, S. S., Mohan, A. J., & Upmanyu, N. (2019). *Pregnancy, children and inter-relating factors affected by geohelminthiasis.* https://core.ac.uk/download/322445222.pdf (accessed on 16th July 2025).

23. Naing, C., Whittaker, M. A., Nyunt-Wai, V., Reid, S. A., Wong, S. F., Mak, J. W., & Tanner, M. (2013). Malaria and soil-transmitted intestinal helminth co-infection and its effect on anemia: a meta-analysis. *Transactions of the Royal Society of Tropical Medicine and Hygiene, 107*(11), 672–683. https://doi.org/10.1093/trstmh/trt086(accessed on 16th July 2025).

24. Tefera, E., Mohammed, J., & Mitiku, H. (2015). Intestinal helminthic infections among elementary students of Babile town, eastern Ethiopia. *The Pan African medical journal, 20*, 50. https://doi.org/10.11604/pamj.2015.20.50.5251(accessed on 16th July 2025).

25. Singh, B. (2020). *Molecular Medicines for Parasitic Diseases.* https://core.ac.uk/download/322580845.pdf (accessed on 16th July 2025).

26. Teimoori, S., Mowlavi, G., Arimatsu, Y., Sripa, B., Mobedi, I., Sharifdini, M., Massoud, J., & Naddaf, S. R. (2019). Infection of the Jackal (*Canis aureus*) by *Haplorchis taichui* (Trematoda: Heterophyidae) in Southwestern Iran: A Clue for Potential Human Infection. *Iranian journal of parasitology, 14*(1), 120–126.(accessed on 16th July 2025).

27. Strosberg, S. A. (2014). *The human–hookworm assemblage: Contingency and the practice of helminthic therapy*. https://core.ac.uk/download/232563064.pdf (accessed on 16th July 2025).

28. Tewelde, E., & Tadesse, S. (2023). Drug Discovery and Development for Soil-Transmitted Helminthiasis: Current Anthelmentics and Compounds in the Pipeline. IntechOpen. doi: 10.5772/intechopen.106830(accessed on 16th July 2025).

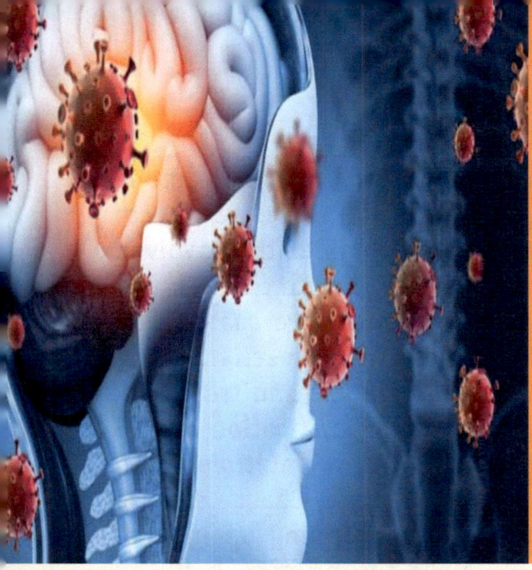

Chapter 10

CENTRAL NERVOUS SYSTEM INFECTIONS

Contents

Introduction

The central nervous system (CNS) is a key go-between between sensory input and motor output, integrating various body functions and mental activities. However, when infections break through this delicate system, the damage can be severe and permanent. CNS infections constitute a broad category of diseases caused by various pathogens, including viruses, bacteria, fungi, and parasites. These infections also have the potential to lead to diseases such as meningitis, encephalitis, and myelitis, which are characterized by specific clinical features and complications. It is important to understand the etiology, transmission, and pathophysiology of such infections in order to make an early diagnosis and treatment, reflecting the imperative for continued public health initiatives and research to combat these prevalent threats. One of the most important aspects of CNS infections is that they are capable of being caused by geographically transitory or unidentifiable pathogens, which makes them capable of surprising healthcare practitioners. The Zika virus is one such example, which has gained attention due to its association with neurological disease, in particular among returning travelers within endemic countries. Neurologists may get to deal with cases related to this virus even when there is no active transmission in certain regions. The complexities involved in dealing with CNS infections demand inter-professional collaboration among health experts, and there is a critical need to develop comprehensive guidelines to deal with such rare cases in an effective manner (Leonhard et al., 2018). By exploring the intricate relationship between infecting agents and host responses, researchers hope to uncover more effective diagnostic and treatment strategies. Furthermore, certain diseases, like Chagas disease, illustrate the sophistication of CNS infections, as they include both the acute and chronic phases of infection affecting multiple organ systems, including the nervous system. Caused by the *Trypanosoma cruzi* parasite, Chagas disease is a significant public health concern in Latin America but is increasingly cropping up in non-endemic regions through migration. The transmission mechanisms, with the primary pathway being through triatomine bugs that harbor the parasite, complicate prevention, particularly in situations of scarce resources. Continued evolution of the disease emphasizes the importance of epidemiological research and the need for far-reaching educational efforts to generate awareness and evoke immediate action. The durability of such research will advance our understanding and management of CNS infections as a central component of global health (Sherman, 2019).

Definition of Central Nervous System (CNS)

The CNS refers to the well-evolved and complex network of the brain and spinal cord that serves as the foundation for the overall performance of the human organism. The CNS also serves as the primary control center, receiving information and directing responses to stimuli, thereby making an individual interact with the environment. This structure is also protected by the blood-brain barrier, the skull, and the vertebral column, a critical structure that regulates the exchange of material between the blood and the brain. It is essential to understand the complexity of the CNS, particularly when presenting with infection because various agents may infect this sensitive area, leading to disastrous neurological consequences. The role of the CNS in homeostasis cannot be overstated; thus, the susceptibility of the CNS to infection can have extensive implications for overall health and wellness. CNS infections are a unique challenge due to the intricacy of the central nervous system's structure and function. Microorganisms such as viruses, bacteria, and fungi can infiltrate the CNS defense barrier and cause such conditions as meningitis, encephalitis, and myelitis. Upon entering the body, these causative agents may elicit dramatic inflammatory reactions, frequently leading to neuronal injury or dysfunction. For example, systemic infections affecting the CNS have been well reported, with impressive figures documenting the incidence of healthcare-associated infections (HAIs) in hospitals. One Scottish national survey found a prevalence of 9.5% of HAIs in acute hospitals, highlighting the need for careful monitoring and intervention regimes (Reilly et al., 2008) (Figure 10.1).

The intersection of infections and CNS well-being demands acute insight and perception to mitigate the impact on neurological integrity. Advances in medicine have unveiled the challenges posed by CNS infections, particularly in chronic diseases such as HIV management. The central nervous system is now a potential reservoir for HIV, which complicates its cure. This advance indicates the significance of anti-retroviral therapy (ART), which seeks to minimize neurotoxicity without compromising efficacy in infections. Moreover, various diagnostic techniques, including neuroimaging, have enhanced HIV-related neurocognitive dysfunction monitoring and shown an immense demand for an organized response to CNS infection (Ellero et al., 2017). As researchers continue to unravel the complexities of the CNS and how it is susceptible, understanding preventive treatments and therapeutic management becomes more essential in protection against the effects of infections that breach this important system.

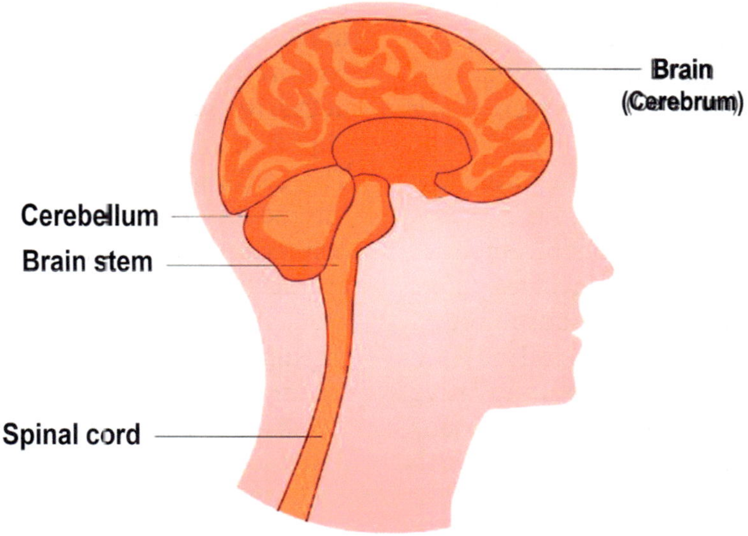

Figure 10.1. Central nervous system (CNS).

Source: https://www.simplypsychology.org/wp-content/uploads/what-is-cns.jpeg.

Importance of Studying CNS Infections

Aside from mere understanding of the pathophysiology of CNS infections, the investigation of CNS infections holds paramount significance to public health, patient care, and advancing medical knowledge. Neuroinfectious diseases such as meningitis and encephalitis have the potential to increase morbidity and mortality substantially. CNS infections usually occur in the form of acute medical urgencies or emergencies, and hence their need for prompt diagnosis and management. Left untreated, CNS infections can lead to irreversible neurological damage and death. Therefore, ongoing research to explain the mechanisms of neuroinvasion and host immune response is essential for the development of effective therapeutic approaches. As the burden of CNS infections increases worldwide, with the most vulnerable populations being affected, it is important that the challenges with the diseases be addressed as a key agenda for health systems worldwide; therefore, the need for enhanced awareness and education among healthcare providers and society. Aside from their immediate health impacts, the investigation of CNS infections makes it possible to appreciate their epidemiological trends and, consequently, contributes to preventive and control interventions. As the increasing incidence of conditions like neurosyphilis, which is a significant risk factor particularly among immunocompromised groups, has shown, ongoing observation and research are critical in monitoring these infections and instituting early public health intervention (Arvind et al., 2025). Besides, the growing incidence of healthcare-associated infections (HAIs) as revealed by recent surveys captures the complexity of managing such infections in hospital settings

(Reilly et al., 2008). Not only does the evidence of these studies inform clinical management, but also supports broader public health policy for the prevention of the occurrence of CNS infections, which eventually will improve the outcomes of patients and the quality of care provided in communities. Carrying out extensive CNS infection studies also plays an essential role in facilitating interdisciplinary coordination among policymakers, researchers, and clinicians. The multifaceted interplay between infectious and non-infectious diseases within the CNS necessitates the involvement of a multidisciplinary interface that involves public health, infectious disease, and neurobiology. Through interdisciplinary coordination, researchers are able to develop innovative diagnostic approaches and treatment regimens for specific infections and populations. Such synergy is particularly important due to the dynamic nature of CNS infections, including the discovery of new pathogens that have the ability to affect the CNS. Hence, CNS infection research not only aids in preventing current medical problems but also places the healthcare system in a better position to deal with future threats, encouraging ongoing investment in research, education, and intervention.

10.1. Anatomy and Function of the Central Nervous System

The CNS includes the brain and spinal cord and is the body's main control centre. Its anatomy comprises several regions: the cerebrum, cerebellum, and brainstem, all of which are responsible for various functions. The cerebrum regulates higher brain functions like reasoning, memory, and sensation. The cerebellum, however, regulates voluntary movements and coordination, while the brainstem regulates involuntary activities such as heartbeat and breathing. Additionally, the CNS is also enveloped by a protective membrane referred to as meninges and sustained by cerebrospinal fluid, serving to maintain intracranial pressure and deliver nutrients. It becomes crucial to understand such a complicated structure while diagnosing and treating infections that would compromise such functions, emphasizing the necessity to treat CNS infections as they are high risk to cognition as well as overall health. The CNS's operation is reliant on the complex interaction of its diverse cellular components, primarily neurons, glial cells, and supporting extracellular matrix. The structural building blocks are neurons, which carry electrical impulses, convey information to other neurons or target tissues by transmitting signals via synapses. Glial cells, astrocytes, oligodendrocytes, and microglia have specialized supporting roles such as homeostasis maintenance, formation of myelin sheaths, and participation in the immune system. This tripartite relationship between glia, neurons, and the extracellular environment allows for proper communication and protects the CNS from infection. In the setting of infection, as described in recent literature, disruption of this environment can lead to many neurologic complications. For instance, a pathological immune response can exacerbate conditions rather than help them, showing the importance of thorough knowledge of the cellular dynamics of the CNS in making effective therapeutic interventions against CNS infections. From various studies, it was established that the CNS is susceptible to infection by all types of infections, from viruses, bacteria, to more complex pathogens, each with a varying effect on it. The unique anatomy and function of the CNS make it an ideal target for infectious pathogens, which may induce inflammation, neuronal cell death, and ultimately lead to disruption of critical cognitive and motor functions. Prior research has shown that activation of the NLRP3 inflammasome plays a significant role in the inflammatory response of the CNS to infection (Smith, 2024). While inflammation may be of benefit in defending against microbial infections, overzealous responses may result in damaging sequelae that undermine the integrity of neural tissue and cause long-term neurological dysfunction. Understanding of the balance of the immune response in the CNS deconstructs critical insight into both the pathophysiology of CNS infections and potential therapeutic paths to mitigate their impact on human health (Smith, 2024).

10.1.1. Structure of the Brain and Spinal Cord

The structure of the spinal cord and the brain is at the heart of understanding CNS infections. The brain holds varied parts, including the cerebrum, cerebellum, and brainstem, all enveloped by protective coats known as meninges. These defenses, along with the cerebrospinal fluid (CSF), provide critical protection against pathogens. Nevertheless, there are some viruses that have been able to penetrate these covering tissues. For instance, the MHV-4 strain of the mouse hepatitis virus exhibits widespread neurovirulence, infecting specific neuroanatomical areas and propagating through the CSF. This serves to establish the vulnerability of the CNS infrastructure towards infectious organisms. Hence, the difference in infection patterns — like the high-speed movement of MHV-4 as opposed to its variant — illustrates the compelling risks to brain health and function during debilitating infectious events (Fazakerley et al., 1992) (Figure 10.2).

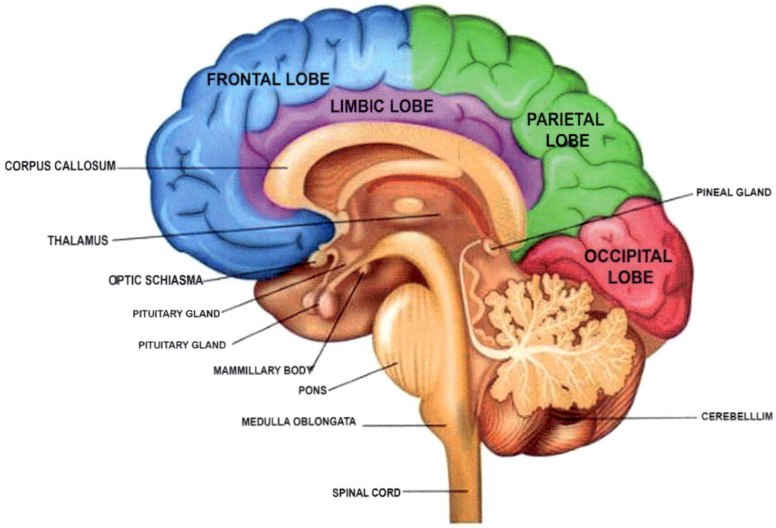

Figure 10.2. Anatomy of the human brain.

Source: https://www.news-medical.net/image-handler/picture/2020/10/shutterstock_284175866.jpg.

Understanding the anatomy of the spinal cord also helps to elucidate the impact of CNS infections. A conduit for neural impulses between the peripheral nervous system and the brain, the spinal cord is composed of segments aligned with various parts of the body and both gray matter and white matter used for the transmission of sensory and motor impulses. It is also protected by cervical and lumbar enlargements, which have nerve roots extending to the limbs. Infections targeting these neural tracts have the ability to disrupt the exchange of information between the brain and body, leading to severe neurological impairment. For example, protein expression changes induced by spinal cord injury highlight the dynamic character of the response of the spinal structures to trauma and subsequent infections, leading to neuropathic pain and other conditions, which are caused by viral infections attacking the CNS (Coronel et al., 2016). The interplay of the brain, spinal cord, and processes of infection raises important questions about the approaches to treatment and results of recovery. The distinctive structural features of the central nervous system allow certain pathogens to escape immune reactions, complicating the therapeutic scenario. For example, the differential neurovirulence of diverse viral strains, as demonstrated by MHV-4, indicates that all infections are not of an equivalent risk for neural architecture. The spinal cords' alteration in neurosteroid expression on injury also indicates the potential for localized biological response to infection that varies with time. Understanding these complex dynamics of infection with brain/spine structure is paramount in developing effective interventions aimed at minimizing the impact of CNS infections on patient recovery and well-being (Fazakerley et al., 1992; Coronel et al., 2016) (Figure 10.3).

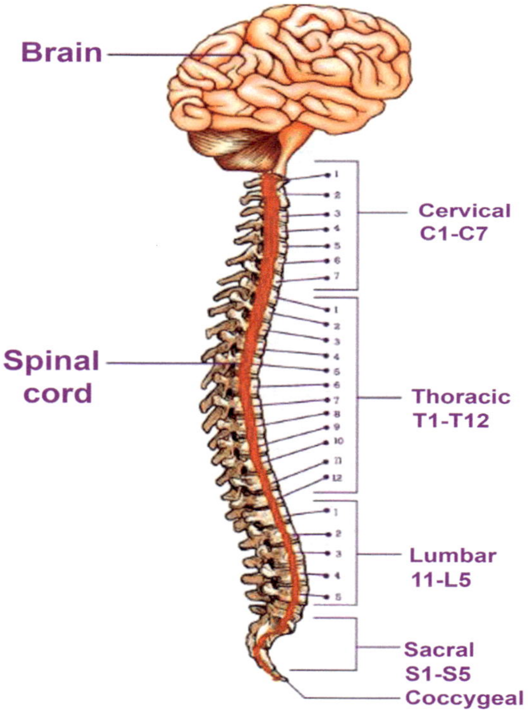

Figure 10.3. Structure of the spinal cord.

Source: https://cdn1.byjus.com/wp-content/uploads/2020/11/spinal-cord-diagram-updated.png.

10.1.2. Role of the Blood-Brain Barrier (BBB)

The blood-brain barrier (BBB) is a critical interface between peripheral circulation and the CNS, regulating the passage of substances in order to maintain homeostasis in the nervous system. Formed primarily by the endothelial cells forming the brain's capillaries, the barrier is supported by tight junctions that restrict permeability to possibly harmful pathogens and toxins. With central nervous system infections, BBB integrity is important; any compromise can facilitate the invasion of pathogenic organisms into the brain, which advances neurological damage. As the infection progresses, the selective permeability of the BBB is compromised, and immune cells and inflammatory mediators penetrate, leading to increased susceptibility of neural tissues. This dynamic equilibrium between the immune response and the BBB is in accordance with the delicate balance that the body must attain to fight infections while preventing the brain from being over-damaged. The role of some immune mediators, e.g., interferon-gamma (IFN-γ), is also pivotal in understanding how infections subvert the BBB. Recent studies identify differential impacts of individual trypanosome genotypes on central nervous system infections and their severity, showing that variations in systemic IFN-γ responses are capable of determining the courses of diseases like human *African trypanosomiasis*. Notably, infections by certain genotypes are associated with a notable elevation in plasma levels of IFN-γ, which correlate with an enhanced probability of subjects acquiring meningoencephalitic conditions. This would suggest a complex interaction in which the immune response not only serves to prevent infection but actually induces pathogen transmigration through the BBB by error. The consequences of this discovery would be that tailored therapeutic intervention in the immune system may need to be employed to maintain BBB integrity during infection stages to prevent the development of severe neurological diseases (Cooper et al., 2007) (Figure 10.4).

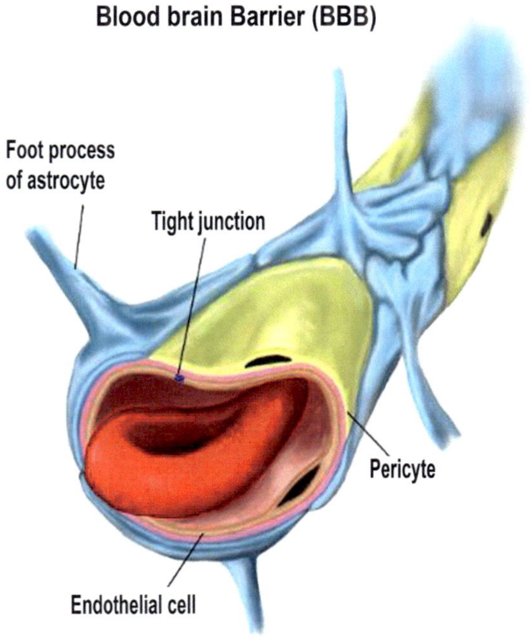

Figure 10.4. The blood-brain barrier.

Source: https://altoida.com/wp-content/uploads/2022/07/shutterstock_1933594793-1-scaled.jpg.

Furthermore, neuroinflammation, often an aftermath of BBB injury, poses an extreme threat to neuronal health and overall CNS function. Astrocytes, which are the primary glial cells of the brain, play a role in modulating inflammatory processes. Once activated, they secrete various pro-inflammatory cytokines that may exacerbate the inflammatory environment and cause neurodegenerative processes. The BBB that is broken down during such attacks of inflammation can increase its permeability, facilitating increased penetration of immune cells and sustaining a vicious cycle of inflammation and damage to the neurons. Repeated activation of astrocytes can lead to deleterious consequences, affecting regular neural circulation and inducing hypoxia in brain tissue. This cycle of neuroinflammation-BBB impairment highlights the importance of investigating how systemic infection controls astrocyte function and, in turn, CNS general well-being (Anis et al., 2022).

10.1.3. Functions of the CNS in Overall Health

The CNS plays a crucial role in the general wellness of people by regulating many physiological processes and responding to environmental stimuli. Present literature shows that neurodegeneration, a process that occurs naturally and is often associated with aging, has a significant influence on health outcomes. For instance, genetic redundancy loss in the CNS would contribute to neurodegenerative conditions such as Alzheimer's, reinforcing the importance of metabolic stability and robust immunity for optimal CNS function. Disturbances in metabolism or chronic immunity against infection deepen neurodegeneration in this perspective (Zhang, 2011).

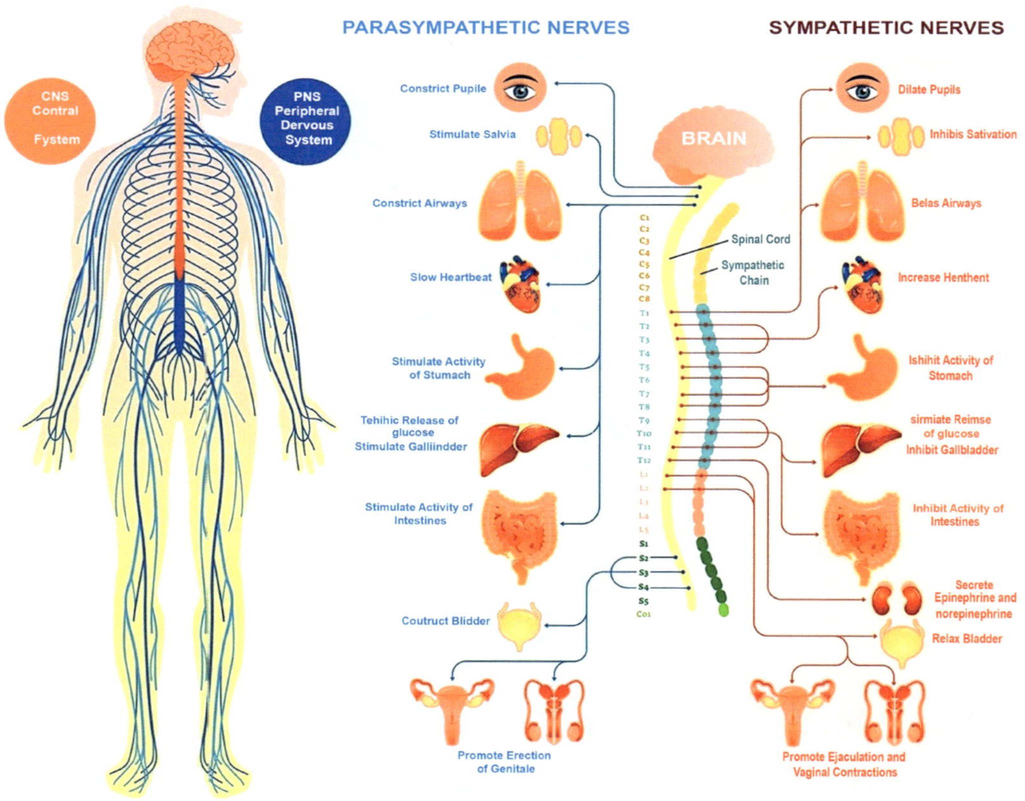

Figure 10.5. Functions of the CNS in overall health.

Source: https://www.news-medical.net/image.axd?picture=2018%2F10%2Fnervous-system-big.jpg.

Hence, understanding the processes of the CNS, including homeostasis and reaction to challenges, becomes of extreme importance in designing preventative strategies as well as therapeutic interventions for cognitive maintenance. The intricacies of the workings of the immune system also relate directly to the lateralization of the hemispheres of the brain that decide the body's overall resistance to infections. Studies portray a relationship between hemispheric lateralization (HL) and immune function, with variation in the strength of the brain hemisphere impacting the efficiency of the immune system. Specifically, decreased left hemisphere functioning is correlated with poorer immune function, and greater right hemisphere functioning appears to be correlated with enhanced immune response (Gidron et al., 2011) (Figure 10.5).

Such linkage indicates that the CNS is not only pivotal in cognition but also in immunomodulation, especially in the context of infection. Increased understanding of this interaction will perhaps reveal new directions in the treatment of CNS infection with improved patient outcomes through integrated models of care. With CNS infections, CNS functions other than the specific immediate neurological problem involve broader implications on immunity and health. The interface between the CNS and the immune system will determine the severity and direction of infections. Chronic infections lead to chronic activation of the immune system, once more influencing neurodegenerative processes within the CNS and ultimately causing irreversible cognitive impairment. With the necessity to modulate both immune and metabolic processes identified as crucial for lessening neurodegenerative effects, researchers now direct their interest toward the design of interventions that impact such processes (Zhang, 2011). This accentuates the significance of adopting a holistic perspective of the CNS's function and role in contributing to overall health, especially in the context of infections compromising its fine balance.

10.2. Types of CNS Infections

The heterogeneity of CNS infections can be categorized broadly into viral, bacterial, and fungal infections, each with distinct pathophysiologies and clinical presentations. Viral infections, such as those caused by the herpes simplex virus (HSV) and varicella-zoster virus (VZV), are increasingly being found to be capable of producing severe neurological sequelae in the form of encephalitis and meningitis. The host immune response complexities are significant in the determination of susceptibility, particularly in the case of HSV, which has been linked to known innate immune deficiencies. For instance, scientists have shown that those with defects in the Toll-like receptor 3 pathway are predisposed to herpes simplex encephalitis, indicating that an interaction of host defense and virus is critical in the pathogenesis of such diseases. Infections of the CNS by bacteria, especially meningitis, represent significant threats to health according to their violent course and potential for serious sequelae. Commonly incriminated bacterial pathogens include *Streptococcus pneumoniae* and *Neisseria meningitidis*, both of which tend to produce an inflammatory response that, if not promptly identified and treated, can lead to significant morbidity and mortality. Compared to viral infections, bacterial meningitis is usually associated with more prominent systemic findings, such as fever, headache, nausea, and confusion, necessitating prompt medical intervention. Furthermore, complications like intracranial hypertension and chronic neurological disability are possible, adding to the public health burden of these infections. The development and application of new diagnostic tools, including PCR and culture tests, are crucial for the early identification and treatment of bacterial CNS infections (Lewandowski et al., 2024). Fungal infections, although less common than viral and bacterial infections, pose severe dangers, particularly in immunocompromised hosts. Diseases such as cryptococcal meningitis, which are chiefly seen in patients with AIDS or other states of immunosuppression, reflect the susceptibility of some groups to fungal infections. *Cryptococcus neoformans* is the responsible organism and can cause fatal meningoencephalitis if not treated, causing high rates of morbidity. Diagnosis is usually by serology and examination of cerebrospinal fluid, and treatment is often with long-term regimens of antifungal agents. Particularly, the identification of the spectrum of CNS infections, such as fungal infections, is crucial to clinicians, especially in expanding susceptible populations via immunosuppression or environmental exposure (Lewandowski et al., 2024). Finally, this relates to ongoing research and surveillance towards maximizing outcomes with respect to CNS infection in different patient groups.

10.2.1. Meningitis

Meningitis, an inflammation of the brain and spinal cord covering membranes, is a formidable challenge in the area of central nervous system infection. Meningitis can result from various etiologic causes like bacteria, viruses, and fungi and thus presents variable clinical manifestations and therapeutic intervention.

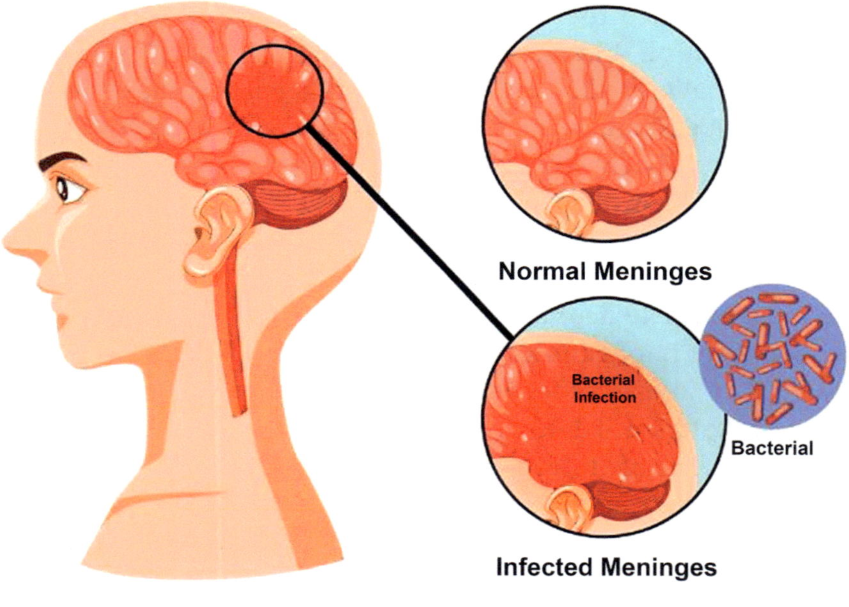

Figure 10.6. Meningitis.

Source: https://www.fortishealthcare.com/drupal-data/2024-08/y5zj_iwgh_220217.jpg.

Bacterial meningitis, particularly, is for its rapid onset and high rate of complications, often leading to chronic neurological dysfunction if not treated early. Vaccination strategies against major pathogens like *Neisseria meningitidis* and *Streptococcus pneumoniae* have dramatically remapped the epidemiologic landscape of this disease, focusing preventive interventions as the mainstay for reducing the public health burden of meningitis. Meningitis pathogenesis involves complex host-pathogen interactions and host response. More recent research emphasizes the human microbiome's role in infection susceptibility, suggesting that microbial community disturbances increase the risk of bacterial meningitis. For example, the use of intrapartum antibiotic prophylaxis among pregnant women colonized with *Streptococcus agalactiae* has altered the course for neonates at risk of early-onset meningitis. These advancements underscore the interaction between prevention measures, microbial ecology, and clinical manifestations of meningitis. Understanding these interactions is core to developing targeted interventions and optimizing patient outcomes in groups at risk of the acute disease (Janowski et al., 2017) (Figure 10.6).

Aside from the direct medical effects of meningitis, psychological considerations can influence infection outcomes. Adjustment disorders have been found to be linked with increased rates of infection, possibly due to the modulation of immune status by stress. In individuals with adjustment disorder, increased hospitalization rates for infection have been seen, reinforcing the mind-body relationship. These observations mean that relief from psychological stress is essential not only for improving mental health outcomes but also for reducing the risk of secondary infection, like meningitis. This convergence of mental health with infections underscores the significance of an integrated process of paying attention to patient care in the treatment of central nervous system infection (Smith et al., 2020).

10.2.2. Encephalitis

Encephalitis, or inflammation of the brain, is a serious problem in the spectrum of central nervous system infections. It may occur as a result of several etiological agents such as viruses, bacteria, and parasites. The most common cause of encephalitis is viral infection, and the viruses such as herpes simplex virus (HSV), varicella-zoster virus (VZV), and West Nile virus are the leading among the causative agents. These infectious pathogens have the capacity to enter the central nervous system, leading to neurological damage, complicating their presentation clinically. Clinical presentation is typically characterized by fever, seizures, mental status change, and focal neurological deficits, necessitating prompt diagnosis and intervention.

The pathology of encephalitis is not only infectious in nature but also the resultant inflammatory response generated due to it, which may exacerbate neuronal damage even after the removal of the original infection. Improvements in medical diagnostic techniques have facilitated an easier identification of the causative pathogens of encephalitis. Polymerase chain reaction (PCR), serology, and imaging tests permit rapid detection and viral etiology differentiation. Early detection is critical because the therapeutic window for effective intervention may be brief. For example, prompt acyclovir therapy can significantly alter the prognosis in herpes simplex encephalitis. In certain cases, supportive care forms the mainstay of management, bearing in mind that specific antiviral treatments are not available for all etiological pathogens. Ultimately, innovation in the detection of newly emergent pathogens is critical, considering the ever-changing infectious disease situation. Thorough understanding of such pathogens, coupled with progressive preventive measures, is important to improve patient outcomes in encephalitis cases (Ludlam et al., 2006) (Figure 10.7).

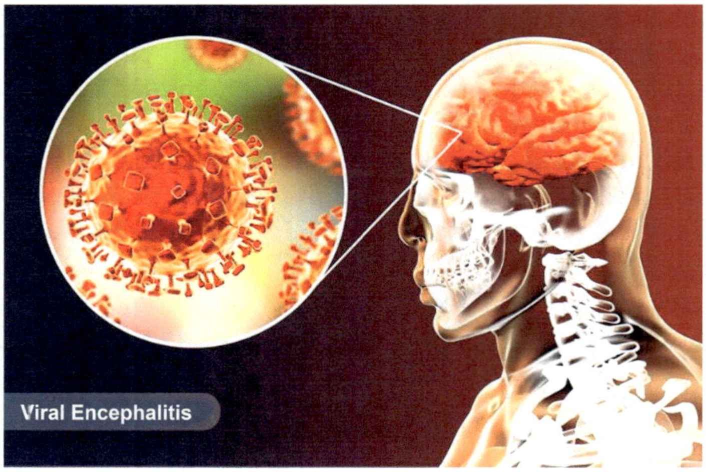

Figure 10.7. Viral encephalitis.

Source: https://img.lb.wbmdstatic.com/vim/live/webmd/consumer_assets/site_images/article_thumbnails/BigBead/encephalitis_bigbead/1800x1200_encephalitis_bigbead.jpg.

The effects of encephalitis extend beyond the direct clinical effect, affecting public health and health care resources. As a result of the potential for outbreaks by vector-borne viruses, such as those transmitted by mosquitoes, surveillance and prevention are relevant to reduce the frequency of encephalitis. Public health initiatives should aim information campaigns on preventive interventions, such as vaccination initiatives and control of vectors. Secondly, rising threats posed by pathogen resistance to standard methods of intervention underscore the need for ongoing research and monitoring. Based on recent overviews, there are zoonotic transmission concerns and genetic modification of pathogens that have the potential to result in chronic recurrence of encephalitis, thus the need to be prepared to fight infectious diseases (Coronel et al., 2016). The intricate interaction between these emerging pathogens and encephalitis constitutes a necessity for sustained multidisciplinary collaboration and creativity in public health responses.

10.2.3. Brain Abscesses

Brain abscesses present an acute issue in central nervous system infection, characterized by the accumulation of localized collections of pus within the brain parenchyma. They most commonly occur as a direct result of infection at distant sites, with the causative agents entering the body via the bloodstream and traveling eventually through the blood-brain barrier. Among the most common aetiologies are bacterial, i.e., odontogenic or sinus infections, and fungal, particularly in immunocompromised patients. Presentation can include headache, fever, and focal neurological findings, which can mask the underlying infection. The correct diagnosis of brain abscesses matters because improper diagnosis can lead to serious neurological outcomes and added morbidity, mirroring the significance of early diagnosis and treatment of cases of central nervous system infection (Dobosz et al., 2024). Brain abscesses typically need high-tech imaging techniques such as CT or MRI, which can detect the characteristic features of abscess formation. The inflammatory process is marked by a central zone of necrosis, often with pericentral oedema. Imaging is valuable for diagnosis, but microbiological evidence is most valuable where certain pathogens are implicated and empirical treatment is instituted. For example, a case was highlighted to show the necessity of proper diagnosis and treatment in a child with central nervous system infection due to *Aspergillus fumigatus*, detailing the good outcome that followed as a consequence of early treatment with antifungal therapy and surgical drainage (Green et al., 1991) (Figure 10.8).

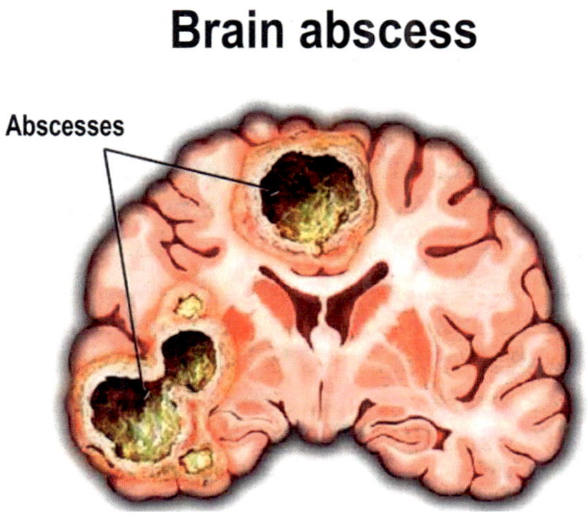

Figure 10.8. Brain abscess.

Source: https://cdn.medizzy.com/TCOCczxnppREodMqdHJJl0fYXpk=/800x621/img/posts/5659e3e5-7ff1-47d5-99e3-e57ff1d7d510.

Thus, an integrative method incorporating laboratory and imaging is imperative in successfully treating brain abscesses. Brain abscess management protocol is dependent upon both medical and surgical methods, the latter being largely determined by the abscess etiology, size, and also the patient's clinical condition. Initial therapy typically involves empirical antibiotics, with adjustment of the therapeutic regimen according to identified pathogens once microbiological data are obtained. Surgical intervention is necessary in the presence of large abscesses with significant mass effects or unresponsiveness to antibiotic therapy by itself. Neurosurgical procedures such as aspiration or resection of the abscess carry a double benefit: decompression of intracranial pressure and the scope to send specimens for further microbiological culture. When combined, these strategies enhance the outcomes of patients with brain abscess, highlighting the need for being vigilant in diagnosing and treating central nervous system infections effectively and promptly (Dobosz et al., 2024).

10.3. Causes of CNS Infections

The cause of CNS infections can most frequently be linked to numerous different pathogens, from bacteria, viruses, and fungi to parasites. These bacterial infections, such as *Streptococcus pneumoniae* and *Neisseria meningitidis*, are well-known culprits behind encephalitis and meningitis, both of which impair neurological function and entail extreme long-term consequences. These infections are most frequently spread by respiratory droplets or, in a select number of cases, direct contact with contaminated surfaces. It is worth mentioning that immunocompromised individuals, including those with significant comorbid illnesses and other psychiatric disorders, may be at increased risk of these infections, with a concerning overlap between mental and physical states, as suggested by the increased susceptibility to infection in adjustment disorders (Smith et al., 2020). It is thus necessary to learn about the intricate microbial environment that leads to CNS infections to develop efficient prevention and treatment strategies. Viral infections also share a significant contribution to CNS infections, and the herpes simplex virus and human immunodeficiency virus (HIV) are among the frequentist pathogens. HIV, in particular, is characterized by more than mere viral load difficulties because it targets the central nervous system through the formation of reservoirs that complicate cerebrospinal fluid (CSF) management and the onset of neurocognitive disorders. Despite the advances of antiretroviral therapy (ART) that have significantly reduced HIV-associated dementia in cases, milder forms of HIV-associated neurocognitive disorder (HAND) remain clinically significant (Ellero et al., 2017). This reflects the intricacy of the treatment of CNS infections on the basis of viral etiology, wherein not merely pathogen load, but even neurological effect must be treated. Neurological sequelae have the possibility of significantly influencing the quality of life of such individuals and require continued research into the effectiveness of targeted therapies that address both the viral and neurocognitive aspects of HIV infection. Environmental and socio-economic factors are pivotal within the etiology of CNS infections, creating heterogeneity in infection rates between disparate populations. Homelessness, malnutrition, and poor sanitation enhance the vulnerability of populations to infectious pathogens, thereby enhancing the transmission of pathogens capable of penetrating the CNS. Furthermore, psychiatric illnesses and psychological distress, such as adjustment disorder, have been associated with an increased risk of infections, suggesting a complex relationship between physical and mental health (Smith et al., 2020). This social-ecological perspective on CNS infections highlights the importance of public health interventions to improve living circumstances and mental illness care, as both play critical roles in the prevention of not only infection but also chronic disease from neglected illness. These determinants need to be targeted for a combined effort to decrease the burden of CNS infections across different populations.

10.3.1. Bacterial Pathogens

The frequency of bacterial pathogens as etiologic factors of central nervous system infections is a matter of concern for medical microbiology. *Neisseria meningitidis* and *Streptococcus pneumoniae* are some of the primary causes of bacterial meningitis in children. The changing dynamics of these pathogens necessitate ongoing observation and study. The epidemiology of bacterial meningitis has changed dramatically as a result of vaccination measures to stop the illnesses caused by these organisms. Vaccination against *Streptococcus pneumoniae* has significantly decreased the rates of incidence, making it possible to achieve better clinical outcomes. The ongoing evolution of bacterial strains represents a challenge requiring ongoing upgrading of public health protection to counter possible outbreaks and offer protection to the community, particularly the vulnerable population, such as children and older adults, who have a higher chance of contracting severe complications and death (Janowski et al., 2017). Understanding of the pathogenesis of bacterial pathogens infecting the central nervous system permits comprehension of the mechanisms through which the bacteria infect the host. Pathogenesis entails complex relationships between bacteria and host immune systems with effects on disease susceptibility and severity. The ability of *Neisseria meningitidis* to interfere with the blood-brain barrier is significant to its pathogenicity, for instance. This bacterial invasion triggers inflammation that exacerbates the manifestation of meningitis. Moreover, current human microbiome research indicates that the balance between bacterial and viral populations may dictate the risk of acquiring bacterial meningitis. These observations create avenues for the use of microbiome-directed therapies and prevention interventions towards the improvement of host resistance against such infections, therefore underscoring the need for intensive investigation into bacterial host interactions (Janowski et al., 2017) (Figure 10.9).

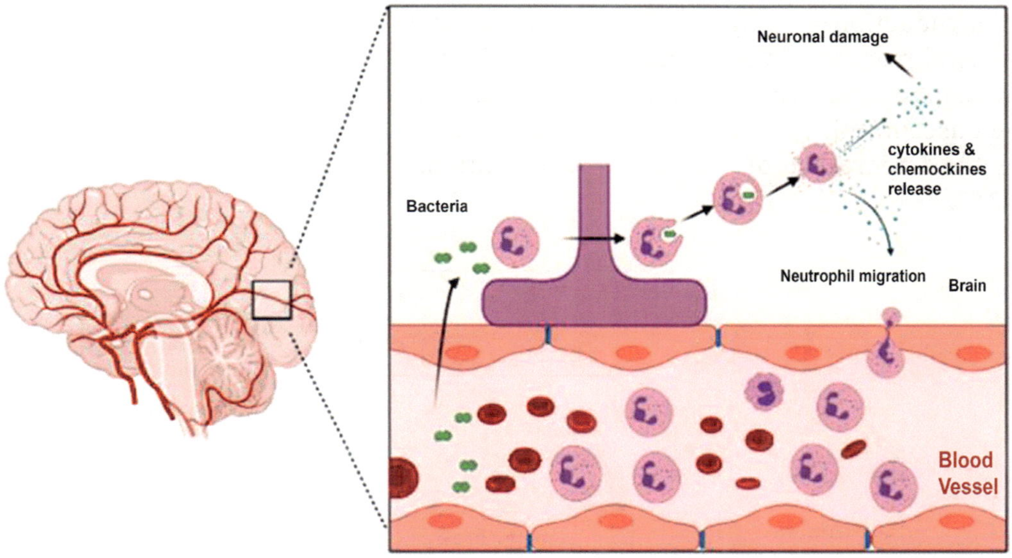

Figure 10.9. Pathophysiology of neuronal damage due to bacterial meningitis.

Source: https://www.mdpi.com/microorganisms/microorganisms-09-00535/article_deploy/html/images/microorganisms-09-00535-g001.png.

Preventive protocols continue to play the lead role in the fight against central nervous system infections caused by bacterial pathogens. Use of intrapartum antibiotic prophylaxis among pregnant women colonized by *Streptococcus agalactiae* is a measure that has significantly reduced the incidence of meningitis among neonates. In addition, vaccination implications not only reduce the rate of disease but also aid in herd immunity, hence protecting non-immunized individuals through suppression of pathogen circulation among populations. Evidence of the changing epidemiological trend of bacterial meningitis has been provided by studies, which have hugely impacted disease transmission patterns and mortality. With increased efforts to combat bacterial pathogens, a highly iterative strategy using vaccinations, public health policy, and enhancing therapeutic interventions will be significant towards lessening the disease burden of central nervous system infection. These ongoing issues need to be addressed effectively by the combined efforts of health workers, researchers, and policymakers.

10.3.2. Viral Pathogens

Virology of viral pathogens has relevance in CNS infections since such pathogens are capable of causing serious neurological complications. These viruses, such as herpes simplex virus (HSV), West Nile virus (WNV), and enteroviruses, are known to infect the CNS, leading to infections like meningitis and encephalitis. For instance, HSV has been known to produce recurrent as well as severe neurological disease, particularly in immunocompromised persons. The ability of such viral pathogens to cross the blood-brain barrier not only complicates diagnosis but also poses severe challenges for treatment strategies. Hence, understanding the mechanisms by which such viruses infect neuronal tissue is of prime importance to effective therapeutic programs. In addition, the epidemiology of viral CNS disease has dramatically changed throughout the decades. Greater vigilance and the new technology of diagnostics have identified more viral pathogens. For instance, the recent introduction of polymerase chain reaction (PCR) technology has revolutionized the detection of viral nucleic acid from cerebrospinal fluid (CSF). This has improved clinical outcomes because clinicians are now in a position to rapidly confirm diagnoses and treat patients accordingly. The vaccine susceptibility of viral pathogens, e.g., with varicella-zoster virus and influenza virus, emphasizes the importance of prevention interventions in the regulation of viral CNS infections (Figure 10.10).

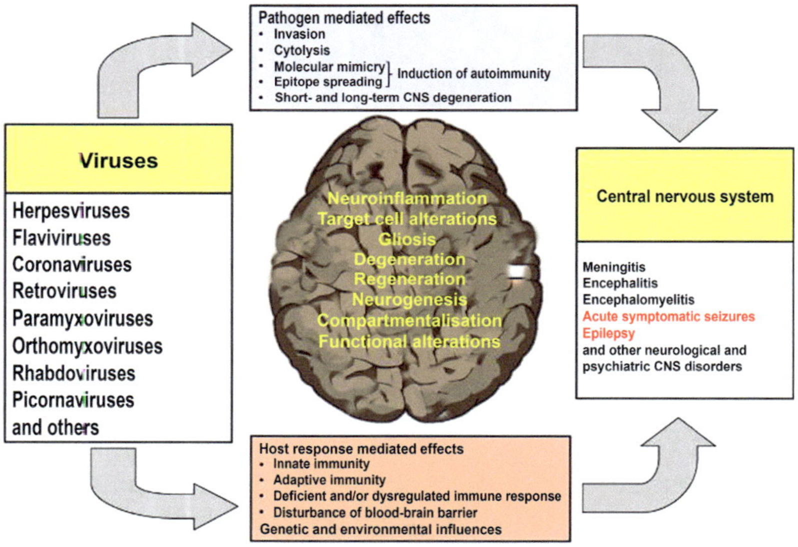

Figure 10.10. The viral pathogens are critical in understanding central nervous system (CNS) infections.

Source: https://external-content.duckduckgo.com/iu/?u=https%3A%2F%2Fwww.frontiersin.org%2Ffiles%2FArticles%2F870868%2Ffnmol-15-870868-HTML%2Fimage_m%2Ffnmol-15-870868-g001.jpg&f=1&nofb=1&ipt=c02a22a828e4180db4e89f18a052b0cde606083955a812022304c46c9eea7f93.

Nevertheless, the emergence of new viral threats strains public health infrastructure and demands constant surveillance and research to adapt vaccination strategies in response accordingly. It has been proven that the complex interplay between viral pathogens and immune response from the host might yet further complicate infection in the CNS. Janowski et al. (2017) believe that the most recent research into the human microbiome illustrates dynamic interactions between viral and bacterial communities influencing susceptibility to viral infection. For example, dysbiosis can lead to immune dysregulation, which enhances the vulnerability to CNS diseases. Further, the ongoing health crisis worldwide, as observed by Relich & Abbott (2018), indicates the manner in which newly arisen viruses can suddenly impact neurological health at the population level. It is thus important to understand these intricate interactions not just for the development of successful vaccines and therapy but for the establishment of guidelines that can decrease the likelihood of CNS infection by viral pathogens. The intersection of virology, immunology, and public health is thus critical in addressing the problem created by these infections.

10.3.3. Fungal and Parasitic Infections

Fungal and parasitic infections are a severe challenge to the CNS which often leads to severe neurological compromise and complications. These infections can be due to various sources, including opportunistic fungi and parasites that are otherwise non-pathogenic in healthy individuals but can lead to life-threatening conditions in immunocompromised hosts. For instance, the organism *Cryptococcus neoformans* can cause cryptococcal meningitis, particularly in immunocompromised hosts, for instance, HIV/AIDS patients. The presentation of such infections can be nonspecific, ranging from headache to alteration in mental status, and hence potentially delayed diagnosis and management. Thus, recognition of the risk factors and clinical syndromes of fungal and parasitic infections is quite crucial for healthcare workers because early treatment can reduce morbidity and mortality rates among infected patients. Systemic inflammation and immune response are crucial in the management of fungal and parasitic CNS infections. Some immune responses, particularly those mediated by cytokines like interleukin-17 (IL-17), are critical in the restriction of these pathogens. Although IL-17A and IL-17F are involved in the activation of protective immunity against various infections, such as fungal and parasitic infections, they might also be involved in pathological side effects, such as excessive inflammation, and thus exacerbation of CNS tissue damage. The duality of IL-17 function argues for the complexity of the host response to infections and the delicate balance between protective immunity and damaging inflammation. This information underlines the need for accurately engineered therapeutic interventions to enhance immune defenses with little risk of inflammatory damage to neural elements, resulting in a more effective defense against CNS infection. Furthermore, the intersection of mental health disorders and infectibility adds one further level of complexity in the case of fungal and parasite-caused CNS infections. It has been revealed by research that disorders such as adjustment disorder can raise the risk of infections caused by stress-induced immune imbalances, which contribute to increased rates of complications caused by these pathogens It is established by studies that people with adjustment disorders exhibited higher rates of infection, showing how psychological tension can have a negative effect on physiological responses to pathogens (Smith et al., 2020). This affiliation is pertinent inasmuch as it draws attention to the need for a holistic response that is both for mental health as well as handling the physical impact of infections. Effective treatment of CNS infections could thus include not just antimicrobial treatment but also psychosocial interventions to optimize resilience and immune function, thus working towards better health outcomes for the affected individuals.

10.4. Symptoms and Diagnosis

Clinical manifestations of CNS infections are extremely pathogen-dependent and localizing sign-dependent in brain and spinal cord infection. Preadministration fever, headache, nuchal rigidity, alteration in mental status, and neurologic deficit (e.g., seizure or focal weakness) are the frequent presentations. It is important that healthcare professionals distinguish these symptoms from other neurological disorders because timely diagnosis can have significant implications for the outcome of patients. For example, differentiation between bacterial and viral infections is important because bacterial infections are usually treated with immediate intervention using antibiotics, whereas viral infections are often treated conservatively. The variability of the presentation of symptoms emphasizes the importance of proper clinical evaluations to establish the etiology of CNS infections to guide further testing and treatment. Laboratory procedures for the diagnosis of CNS infections are wide and two-targeted, addressing both the clinical and the laboratory examinations. The basis for the diagnosis commonly begins with an excellent history and physical exam, and then imaging of the brain, such as magnetic resonance imaging (MRI) or computed tomography (CT) scans, to establish structural changes. Cerebrospinal fluid (CSF) examination by venipuncture or lumbar puncture is also an essential diagnostic tool in determining diagnoses. An abnormal number of some biomarkers in the CSF can indicate particular infections. For example, recent studies have demonstrated that the chemokine CXCL13 is significantly elevated in CSF in patients with neuroborreliosis, relative to other neurological conditions in diagnostic performance (Brettschneider et al., 2009). This highlights the rationale for the application of CSF analysis not only for diagnosis but also for the monitoring of disease course and response to treatment. Furthermore, the inclusion of novel biomarkers in the diagnostic algorithm for CNS infections is enhancing clinical practice. Outside traditional methods, novel research indicates that CXCL13 can be both a diagnostic marker of neuroborreliosis and a predictor of therapeutic success, demonstrating its use in clinical practice (Brettschneider et al., 2009). The two-sided activity of CXCL13 defines its role in disease activity determination and patient-tailored treatment programs. With expanding awareness of the pathophysiologic mechanisms underlying CNS infection, there is an expanding opportunity for application of advanced diagnostic methods in clinical decision-making. Ultimately, the interface between the clinical syndrome and emerging diagnostic technologies will be central to improved patient outcomes in these infections.

10.4.1. Common Symptoms of CNS Infections

CNS infection manifests with a broad range of symptoms based on its underlying pathology. Most commonly, patients develop fever, headache, and stiff neck, which may be early manifestations of meningitis or encephalitis. The headache associated with CNS infection is characteristically different, being severe and prolonged, as opposed to the normal tension or migraine headache. Additionally, the presentation of consciousness changes from confusion to coma sharply accentuates the severity of infections and their impact on neurological functioning. These are best seen in such as meningococcal meningitis, with development of fulminant clinical course. Overall, symptomatology of CNS infection demands quick clinical evaluation in order for proper intervention to be initiated prior to being too late. Neurological impairment is another concerning aspect of CNS infections and is responsible for considerable morbidity. Infections with pathogens such as *Borrelia burgdorferi*, for instance, may lead to *Lyme neuroborreliosis* with syndromes manifesting as encephalitis, cranial nerve infection, and peripheral neuropathy (Figure 10.11).

These cases are characterized by symptomatology that may include weakness in motor function, sensory loss, and deficits in cognitive function, with some patients experiencing difficulties with balance and coordination. According to Di Domenico et al. (2018), the rate at which such neurological symptoms develop may also be unpredictable, with some patients quickly developing severe symptoms. Of particular note is the awareness of the spectrum of neurological deficits that follow

CNS infections because this assists clinicians in guiding therapeutic management more effectively and monitoring disease progression, with early supportive care and rehabilitation interventions. Another important characteristic in the realm of CNS infections is the development of secondary symptoms that may indicate systemic disease, such as gastrointestinal distress or cutaneous manifestations. For example, in human *African trypanosomiasis* by *Trypanosoma brucei* rhodesiense, the patient will present with early symptoms that mimic a flu-like syndrome and then more severe neurological manifestations like ataxia and abnormal mental status, as seen in the more acute forms of the disease (MacLean et al., 2010). Identification of such peculiar presentations is very significant to clinicians as they are typically of diagnostic significance in diagnosing the organism causing the CNS symptoms. The interface between systemic and neurological presentation highlights the multifaceted nature of CNS infections, mandating a combined approach in diagnosis as well as in treatment to achieve the maximum possible outcome for the patient.

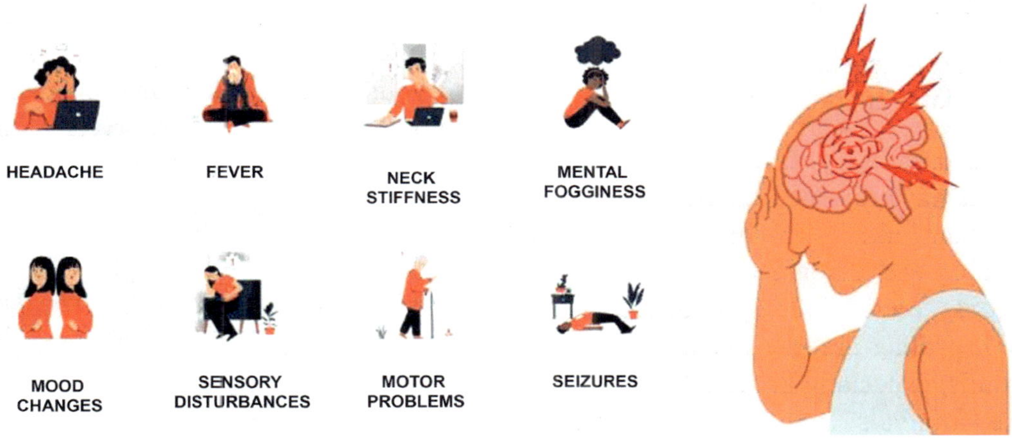

Figure 10.11. Common central nervous system symptoms.

Source: https://lonestarneurology.net/wp-content/uploads/2024/09/2-Symptoms-of-Central-Nervous-System-Inflammation.jpg.

10.4.2. Diagnostic Methods (e.g., Lumbar Puncture, Imaging)

The diagnostic tests employed in infections of the central nervous system are critical to establishing a correct and timely diagnosis, thereby directly influencing the prognosis of treatment. Among the tests employed, lumbar puncture (LP) is a critical method to obtain cerebrospinal fluid (CSF) for analysis. It can be employed to analyze various constituents of CSF, including cell count, protein, and glucose. Of particular importance, LP findings can confirm infection by revealing elevations in cell count suggestive of a disorder such as bacterial meningitis or viral illnesses. These will be variable based on when the sample is obtained and the clinical status of the patients, attesting to the necessity for skilled operators to achieve maximal diagnostic sensitivity. As LP is a significant diagnostic route, it usually makes decisions on additional imaging tests in accordance with the initial results in the examination of fluid (Tang et al., 2025) (Figure 10.12).

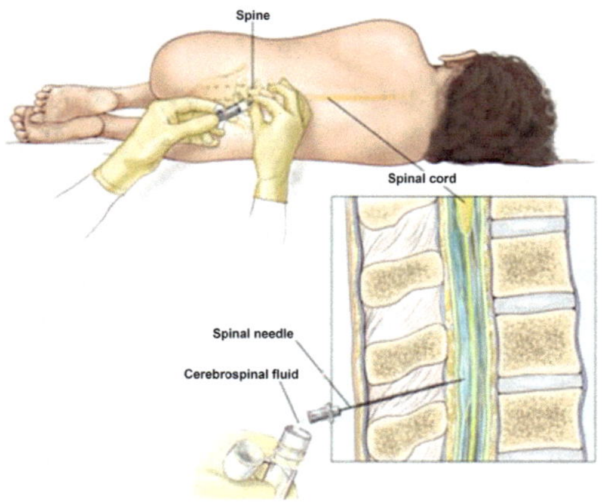

Figure 10.12. Method of lumbar puncture.

Source: https://curesearch.org/wp-content/uploads/Lumbar-Puncture-Web.jpg.

Over the past few years, developments in metabolomics have revealed further diagnostic value in CSF. Using ultra-high-performance liquid chromatography with tandem mass spectrometry, investigators have found characteristic metabolomic profiles associated with individual CNS infections, especially bacterial meningitis. Metabolite analysis has shown excellent diagnostic accuracy, outperforming conventional techniques that are based only on CSF leukocyte counts. For example, certain metabolites such as glucose and lactate reveal profound variations in infected patients so that CNS infections can be discriminated from other neurologic conditions more effectively. It is a novel method that complements the traditional diagnostic methods, further improving the sensitivity and specificity of diagnosis. The integration of metabolomic profiles with standard LP findings has the potential to transform clinical practice in terms of enhancing diagnostic precision and management of patients with suspected central nervous system infections (Steven et al., 2025). Other imaging modalities including magnetic resonance imaging (MRI) and computed tomography (CT) are also critical in the diagnosis of central nervous system infections. While not specifically imaging CSF, these modalities are valuable for the imaging of the structural and functional impact of infection on the spinal cord and brain. MRI is particularly well-suited to showing edema, abscesses, and other pathological changes secondary to infection. Together with LP results, imaging may provide a full understanding of the nature and degree of infection. For instance, MRI can validate the diagnosis from LP, or signal complications that need treatment adjustment. Therefore, with LP complemented by the application of advanced imaging techniques, there is a multi-faceted approach to diagnosing and treating central nervous system infections, ensuring that the patient is treated appropriately and in time (Tang et al., 2025) (Figure 10.13).

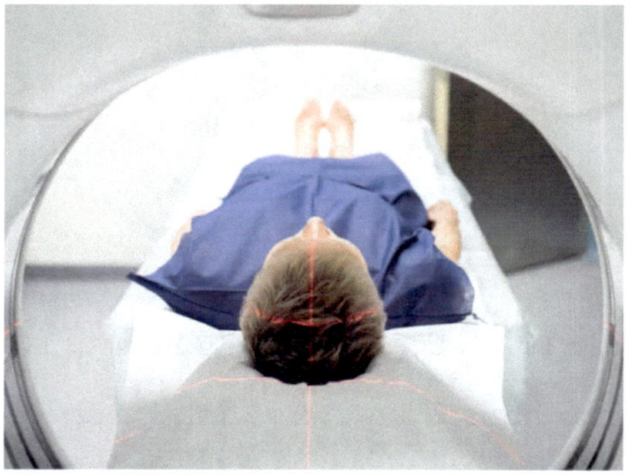

Figure 10.13. Cranial CT scan.

Source: https://media.post.rvohealth.io/wp-content/uploads/2020/08/cranial-ct-scan_thumb.jpg.

10.4.3. Importance of Early Diagnosis

Recognition of CNS infections at an early stage is critical in avoiding morbidity and mortality from these infections. Early detection enables the patient to be treated immediately, which can dramatically alter the prognosis of patients with severe infections like meningitis, brain abscess, and subdural empyema. Treatment is effective based on the timely use of empiric antibiotic therapy, as the etiologic pathogens of these infections are capable of spreading fast and leading to irreparable complications. Delays in diagnosis were associated with higher rates of neurological sequelae based on research, and this emphasizes the importance of clinicians having a high index of suspicion, particularly in high-risk individuals such as those who are undergoing neurosurgery (Dobosz et al., 2024). Also, early diagnosis allows for appropriate management strategies tailored to the identified pathogen. As indicated in the literature reviewed, the types of pathogens infecting the CNS differ with the patient group and comorbidities. For instance, healthcare-associated infections are common among post-neurosurgery patients and need to have such pathogens detected early. Early intervention not only includes antibiotic treatment but may also include surgical procedures in such complicated infections as brain abscesses and subdural empyemas. The early initiation of appropriate diagnostic modalities and therapeutic approaches underlines the emergent nature of early clinical intervention with CNS infections (Dobosz et al., 2024). Furthermore, the application of standard protocols for early diagnosis of CNS infections in health facilities is essential. Hospitalized patients, especially those with compromised immune status or recent surgery, are at greater risk for nosocomial infection that can have substantial impacts on recovery trajectories. By designing environments in which early detection is prioritized, health facilities can minimize the adverse consequences of delayed treatment. Routine training and education of personnel on the detection of CNS infection symptoms and risk factors also increase the prospects of early treatment and diagnosis. These are important measures, especially because CNS infections are high-stakes, involving serious dangers of death and permanent impairment (Dobosz et al., 2024).

10.5. Treatment Options

The treatment of central nervous system infections is multidimensional and predominantly founded on the etiologic pathogens, drug resistance profiles, and the patients' clinical conditions. Particularly, multi- and pan-drug resistant bacterial infections, such as *Acinetobacter baumannii*, are problematic. The bacteria are increasingly becoming known causes of serious central nervous system infections, particularly in intensive care settings, with high rates of mortality among infected patients. Treatment approaches can include long-term courses of systemic antibiotics, but their effectiveness is frequently impaired by a lack of penetration through to the cerebrospinal fluid. Novel approaches are thus needed, and these include the use of intraventricular delivery of antibiotics, which has been found in certain instances of resistant infections to be effective, as evidenced by successful treatments of neonatal meningitis and ventriculitis using polymyxin B (Piparsania et al., 2012). The second important area of management of central nervous system infections is the prevention of the inflammatory response, which typically follows as a result of such infections. Inflammation has the potential to aggravate neuronal damage and also impede recovery. Therefore, management can be aimed at modulating the immune response to minimize neuronal damage. Current hypotheses suggest that infection-induced neurodegeneration can be predetermined to a great extent by immune responses and metabolic regulation. For instance, conditions like Alzheimer's disease, whose causes can lie in prolonged infection, indicate the type of therapies that would address both metabolic and immunologic factors. Addressing these factors through applied treatments might improve the prognosis for patients with neurodegenerative alterations resulting from central nervous system infections (Zhang, 2011). New therapy for central nervous system infections aims to not only eradicate pathogens but also restore neurological function. A number of research studies are also exploring adjunctive treatments, including the administration of anti-inflammatory drugs, immunomodulators, and neuroprotective treatments. The rationale for these treatments is to target both infectious causes and inflammatory mechanisms responsible for long-term damage. Future directions might include personalized medicine strategies, which would again further individualize treatment regimens to patient-specific profiles, including genetic susceptibilities and distinct pathogen characteristics. Lastly, the approach will involve a coordinated strategy inclusive of antimicrobial therapy in addition to supportive treatment and neuroprotection measures in order to promote improvement in prognosis and quality of survival life among survivors of serious central nervous system infections (Figure 10.14).

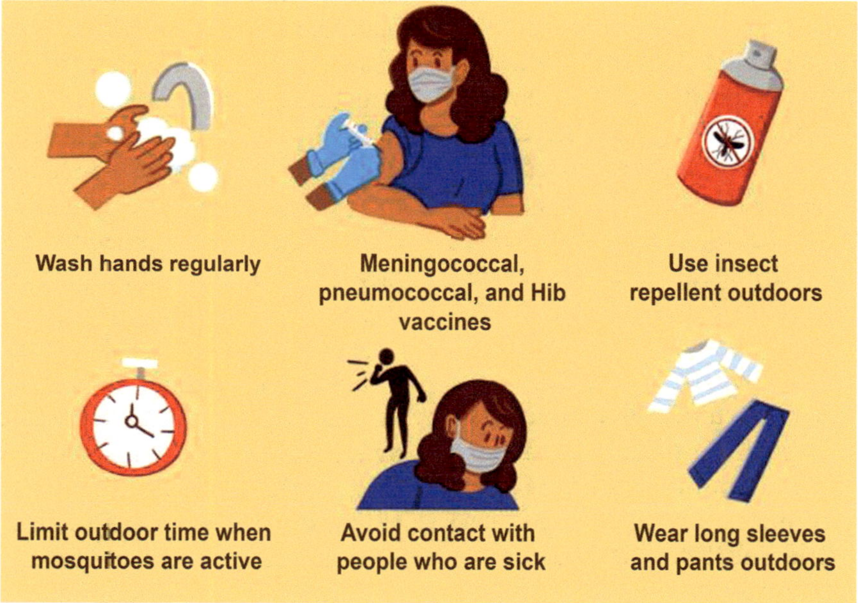

Figure 10.14. Preventing brain infections.

Source: https://www.verywellhealth.com/thmb/5cUFTs-b1uqpFrA4Qybw9fTVRDo=/1500x0/filters:no_upscale():max_bytes(150000):strip_icc()/VWH_Illustration_Brain-Infection_Illustrator_Sydney-Saporito_Final-08cd4a9c5e22483683d1fa6e984afcc6.jpg.

10.5.1. Antibiotic and Antiviral Therapies

Management of CNS infection typically calls for advanced management, with antibiotic and antiviral therapies playing central roles. Antibiotics are typically employed against bacterial infections such as meningitis and brain abscess, with broad-spectrum activity against a wide range of pathogens. The correct antibiotics to use depend on the type of bacterial strain and its resistance pattern, as resistance patterns may determine the success of treatment. For instance, the increasing incidence of resistant organisms requires strict control and potential therapeutic adjustment. Particular infections caused by *Staphylococcus aureus* and certain gram-negative bacteria require individualized antimicrobial treatment. The increasing complexity of therapy in these instances necessitates a similar overall problem for clinicians: sustaining the individual necessity to eradicate resistance while maintaining tolerability and preventing resistance. Antiviral therapy, on the other hand, plays a critical role in the management of viral CNS infections, such as those caused by HSV and CMV. These infections may be accompanied by severe neurological manifestations requiring effective and prompt management. The use of drugs such as acyclovir and ganciclovir has changed the fate of these patients. For instance, the efficient therapy of herpes simplex encephalitis with acyclovir has been associated with reduced morbidity as well as improved survival. Moreover, the addition of antiviral therapies in the treatment of children, especially in the case of congenital infections, demonstrates the possibility of significant long-term neurological complications. As indicated by advancing progress, the use of antiviral therapies at early stages has the potential to reverse permanent injury and thereby improve the quality of life in infected patients, as an indicator of the pivotal role played by these therapies in treating CNS infections. The future prospects of antibiotic and antiviral therapy for treating CNS infections rely upon ongoing research and progress in drug and treatment regimen formulations.

As new pathogens emerge and resistance patterns evolve, it is essential to incorporate an adaptive response that incorporates the latest scientific data. New technologies, like fast diagnostic devices and genome sequencing, are enhancing pathogen identification velocity and quality, which allows for more targeted therapies. Moreover, the development of novel antimicrobial agents and research into adjunctive treatments, such as immunotherapies, are research areas with potential. Integration of these advances into clinical care can lead to increased survival and reduced long-term repercussions among patients who are fighting CNS infections. With advancement in the field, it is necessary to implement antibiotic stewardship and infection control methods to combat resistance and safeguard the efficacy of existing treatments (Backere et al., 2013; Kenneth, 2017).

10.5.2. Supportive Care and Management

In the management of CNS infection, supportive care plays an important role in determining patient outcomes. Effective supportive care aims at stabilizing the general health of the patients and treating the specific neurological deficits resulting from infection. For instance, in bacterial meningitis (BM), the onset of major complications such as stroke or cerebral hemorrhage requires instant action. Empiric broad-spectrum antimicrobial therapy is essential, but equally important is the control of secondary complications, such as elevated intracranial pressure. Physicians use of adjunct therapy, such as corticosteroids to reduce inflammation and prevent further neurological damage, is widespread. The importance of close monitoring of vital signs and neurological status allows for early detection of deterioration, which is essential to preventing morbidity from these infections. This multi-disciplinary approach emphasizes the point that supportive care is not a secondary aspect but a cornerstone of successful treatment regimens for CNS infections. Moreover, the particular challenges posed by individual pathogens require individualized supportive care interventions. Naegleria fowleri, for example, while an uncommon isolate, presents particular challenges of management in terms of its rapid and often fatal course. The recent experience with a child with fulminant myocarditis due to *N. fowleri* infection emphasizes the role of supportive care in atypical presentations of CNS infections. Early commencement of chemotherapeutic agents such as Amphotericin B in combination with supportive measures such as ECMO emphasizes aggressive treatment protocols and the need for early intervention. The case emphasizes that while direct treatment of the infection is paramount, management of secondary complications is crucial to stabilize the patients and improve survival rates. Thus, the convergence of innovative and supportive care interventions is highly critical in addressing the multifaceted character of CNS infections. Lastly, the evolving profile of CNS infections demands ongoing research and enhancement of supportive management protocols. The creation of treatment guidelines, which is fueled by outcomes of current cases and clinical trials, aims to optimize patient care. For instance, ongoing studies on the efficacy of adjunct therapies alongside standard antimicrobial therapy are vital to maximizing outcomes in complicated meningitis patients. Additionally, analysis of genetic heterogeneity among infectious pathogens, as with new detection methods on cases like *N. fowleri*, might have relevance to more optimal treatment strategies and surveillance practices. In total, management and supportive care must be adapted to deal with the complex needs presented by CNS infections, utilizing both current evidence and emerging knowledge to optimize survival and quality of life in infected patients. Addressing these issues comprehensively is all part of refining the standard of care in this central area of medicine.

10.5.3. Role of Vaccination in Prevention

Vaccination is now the cornerstone in the prevention of central nervous system infection, and most importantly, infections caused by bacterial causes such as *Neisseria meningitidis* and *Streptococcus pneumoniae*. Prevention through vaccination has led to a significant decline in the incidence of bacterial meningitis among various populations. For instance, evidence has confirmed that routine immunization can actually limit not only the prevalence of disease but also the morbidity and mortality rates of disease among infected adults and children. These strategic health measures underscore the importance of inducing herd immunity, which subsequently protects vulnerable populations who are not necessarily likely to reap direct benefits from vaccination. With the continued evolution of epidemiology for meningitis, the role of vaccination remains pivotal to shaping clinical outcomes and in reducing the cumulative burden of the disease, marking a milestone in infectious disease prevention (Janowski et al., 2017). The campaign of vaccination has also remained pivotal to averting the transmission of viral infections that affect the central nervous system. Rabies vaccine is a perfect example of how well proactive immunization can work in the prevention of fatal outcomes. As rabies is primarily transmitted by dog bites, large-scale dog vaccination is necessary to eliminate canine rabies while at the same time protecting human health. It not only makes it possible to decrease the number of human cases of rabies, but also addresses the public's attitude towards keeping pets and adequate vaccination. By integrating vaccines into community health interventions, as happens in the Western Hemisphere, we can make a big reduction in the transmission risks of rabies and accomplish more general public health targets. The common campaign for vaccination of dogs shows the articulation between human and animal health regarding central nervous system disease (Velasco-Villa et al., 2017) (Figure 10.15).

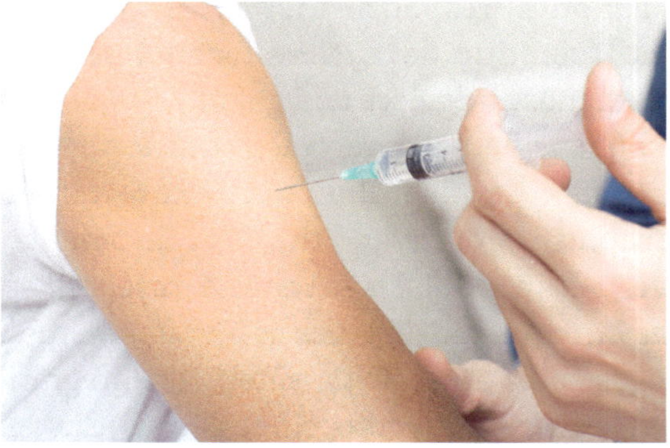

Figure 10.15. A common method for vaccine delivery.

Source: https://www.aidsmap.com/sites/default/files/styles/aidsmap_medium_crop/public/2019-07/VACCINE%20%20.png?itok=p2ffKU4q.

The interaction between central nervous system infection prevention and immunization programs represents an engaged public health strategy requiring frequent refinement and is financially supported via study and investment. Constant issues such as public resistance and the variable availability of vaccines all contribute to underscoring the need for mass education campaigns aimed at these barriers. Ensuring fair access to immunization not only increases individual immunity but also strengthens collective resilience to infectious epidemics capable of leading to severe neurological complications. As we further advance our understanding of the human microbiome and how it interacts with pathogens, the role of vaccines will remain critical to safeguarding public health and reducing the burden of central nervous system infections. Finally, an adaptive response to the vaccine strategy, grounded in good scientific evidence and effective policy intervention, will become essential in curbing the effects of these potent health threats (Janowski et al., 2017).

SUMMARY

As a whole, infections of the CNS are of the greatest concern within the overall context of infectious disease. These infections, caused by an array of pathogens including viruses, bacteria, and fungi, are extremely difficult to diagnose and treat. The complex structure of the CNSs, combined with the fragility of neural tissue, renders it an area requiring innovative approaches to be able to successfully manage such infections. As medicine continues to enhance diagnostic capability and therapeutic intervention, there is a growing need to comprehend the pathogenic mechanisms responsible for such infections, particularly in the context of immunocompromised hosts. Further insight will only serve to offer new avenues towards treatment and vastly improve patient outcomes. Recent advances in antiviral therapy have also instilled renewed interest in the dynamics between HIV and CNS infections, particularly glioblastoma multiforme. Research indicates that HIV-related glioblastoma patients enjoy improved survival rates due to highly active antiretroviral therapy (HAART), although the precise mechanisms are unknown. The identification of such correlations highlights the requirement for holistic management strategies in consideration of both viral load as well as complications arising as a result of nervous system infections, such as tumor formation. These findings underscore the importance of current research that not only deepens our understanding of CNS infection pathophysiology but also informs clinical approaches towards improving patient care over time (Bui et al., 2016). Moreover, ongoing research into barriers to HIV cure strategies also suggests the challenging nature of the CNS in managing infections and accompanying neurological complications. While anti-retroviral therapy has reduced the incidence of HIV-associated dementia by a considerable margin, milder forms of HIV-associated neurocognitive disorder (HAND) are still present and remain of clinical interest. The CNS, a probable reservoir for HIV, presents treatment difficulties and underscores the need for the development of new approaches that can cross the blood-brain barrier without creating excessive neurotoxicity. As diagnostic imaging technologies and biomarker research advance, they have the ability to continue our understanding and management of HAND, eventually assisting in the fight against CNS infections (Ellero et al., 2017). This is a constantly evolving situation that demands concerted efforts, with ongoing research, new therapies, and an interdisciplinary approach to understanding CNS infection complexities.

CNS infections are a significant area of research due to their complex pathophysiology and impact on patient well-being. Among the many organisms that cause infections, *Trypanosoma brucei* spp. stands out due to its causation of sleeping sickness, a critical public health problem in certain regions of Africa. The appreciation of its transmission and impact on the CNS has progressed, particularly with modern imaging. For instance, contrast-enhanced MRI studies have contributed to an understanding of how the parasite degrades the BBB and results in neuroinflammatory responses that may worsen with time. Despite this parasite's past identification, the intricacies of its migration into the CNS and pathogenesis are still topics of much controversy in the scientific literature, which underscores the importance of ongoing research in advancing our understanding of these deadly infections (Bradley et al., 2017). Also, how CNS infections relate to mental health has become increasingly significant as scientists and practitioners have come to realize that infection impact includes more than mere physiological expression. In particular, conditions such as HIV have much broader implications for mental health, prompting holistic treatment strategies. Sylvia Kaaya and others' work highlights the preeminent significance of incorporating mental health interventions into HIV care systems. This is especially relevant in light of the potential neurological sequelae present in the context of HIV, generally further compromising CNS integrity. Recognition of mental health as a central component to be added to comprehensive care is crucial, indicating a shift towards more integrated treatment for CNS infections and their impacts. Such integrative practice not only improves individual outcomes but also those of more extensive-scale public health strategies (Creese et al., 2013). Generally, the review of key points regarding central nervous system infections illustrates the complexity of infection caused by these diseases. The ever-changing interaction of infectious agents like *Trypanosoma brucei* with the CNS illustrates the need for new diagnostics and treatment to avert serious repercussions. Further, the incorporation of mental health care into disease management aimed at diseases against the CNS, e.g., in HIV infection, provides a window for an integrated care approach to both the physiological and psychological aspects of such infections. With acknowledgment of the intricate interconnections between infection, neuroinflammation, and mental health, health care professionals can structure more focused interventions for individuals affected. Thus, continued research and incorporation of care will be the main factors in the future of CNS infections, ultimately towards improved health outcomes and quality of life for the patients.

CLOSER LOOK

HERPES VIRUSES

Herpes viruses are the most common viral etiology of CNS infection in immunocompromised hosts and can cause acute infection, latent infection, and reactivation in the setting of immunodeficiency. Cell-mediated immunodeficient immunocompromised hosts (HIV infection, transplant recipients, recipients of corticosteroids or lymphocyte-depleting regimens) are at greatest risk of herpes virus infections of the CNS, which in many cases are naturally neurotropic in the latent state. The herpes viruses that are most closely associated with CNS infections include herpes simplex viruses (HSV-1 and HSV-2), VZV, EBV, CMV, and human herpes virus 6 (HHV-6).

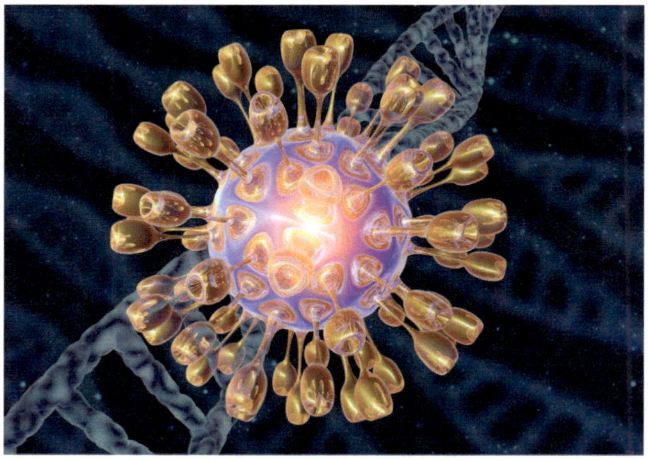

Figure 10.16. 3D illustration of a herpesvirus particle, depicting its envelope glycoproteins, capsid structure, and associated genetic material.

Source: https://scitechdaily.com/images/Herpes-Virus-Genetics.jpg.

HSV is one of the major causes of encephalitis, meningitis, and myelitis in both immunocompetent and immunocompromised host. The host with impaired cell-mediated immunity is at higher risk for developing disseminated disease compared to the immunocompetent host. HSV-1 is the most common cause of endemic encephalitis in the United States. HSV-1 encephalitis in the immunocompetent host is bilateral or unilateral temporal lobe disease. However, clinical presentations in immunocompromised patients may be atypical, leading to treatment delay and unnecessary mortality. Whole-brain irradiation is likewise a newly emerging risk factor for HSV-1 encephalitis. On the other hand, HSV-2 is a rather infrequent cause of encephalitis but likewise is responsible for both meningitis and myelitis. Identification of HSV DNA in the CSF is the gold standard for diagnosing herpetic neurologic disease. HSV PCR of CSF is approximately 95% sensitive and almost 100% specific for diagnosing encephalitis, although in the early course of disease false-negative results are seen (Figure 10.16).

VZV is a neurotropic herpes virus responsible for the clinical syndromes of chickenpox, seen with acute illness, and of zoster, seen with reactivation of latent virus. Immunocompromised hosts, particularly those with impaired cell-mediated immunity, are at greatest risk for disease. CNS infection with VZV most commonly presents as encephalitis but also may be seen as varicella cerebellitis, meningitis, myelitis, or vasculopathy in unusual instances. CSF analysis shows a mononuclear pleocytosis, and diagnosis is made by identification of VZV by PCR or by intrathecal antibodies.

EBV is a ubiquitous herpesvirus that can cause CNS infection as a result of acute infection or reactivation of the latent virus. Individuals with impaired cell-mediated and humoral immunity, both the HIV and transplant recipients, are particularly at risk for reactivation illness. Acute CNS EBV infection can present as nonspecific meningitis, encephalitis, or myelitis. However, EBV reactivation is also observed following infection with a second pathogen and therefore a positive result must be interpreted cautiously. For example, in two retrospective studies that characterized the neurologic clinical syndromes of positive CSF viral PCR, merely 20 to 37% of positive EBV PCR were associated with a clinical syndrome compatible with neurologic infection. The other 63 to 80% of the positive specimens were not related to viral neurologic infection and were thought to be subclinical reactivation of the virus in the setting of immunosuppression or noninfectious neurologic disease, for example, malignancy, multiple sclerosis, and stroke. EBV-associated lymphoma is an HIV-associated complication and typically presents as an intracerebral mass lesion. Definitive diagnosis of EBV-associated lymphoma is made by hematopathological examination of a tissue biopsy specimen, but the observation of an abnormal EBV PCR in the spinal fluid can be suggestive of this diagnosis. Particularly, an EBV CSF viral load of >10,000 in the setting of a CNS mass lesion has been said to have 96% specificity and 50% positive predictive value for CNS lymphoma in one small series.

CMV may cause reactivation disease and acute primary infection in patients with impaired cell-mediated immunity, including HIV-infected patients. Encephalitis, which is expressed by periventricular white matter alterations, and lumbosacral myelitis, which is acute, is the clinical presentation in these patients. The diagnosis is made by PCR detection of CMV from spinal fluid in a clinically relevant neurologic syndrome. Like EBV and HHV-6, CMV also reactivates with immunosuppression.

HHV-6 is a neurotropic herpes virus that, once recognized, has been found to cause encephalitis and myelitis with an aggressive propensity for neurologic infection in hematopoietic stem cell transplant patients. HHV-6 achieves latency in monocytes and brain tissue and reactivates in the setting of compromised cell-mediated immunity. Clinically, its most helpful CNS presentation is posttransplant acute limbic encephalitis (PALE), presenting with anterograde amnesia, seizures, and an otherwise mild lymphocytic pleocytosis of the spinal fluid. The risk period for infection is highest at 15 to 60 days from transplantation. The diagnosis is made by the detection of HHV-6 in spinal fluid through PCR. Detection of HHV-6 must be interpreted cautiously because HHV-6 DNA was also found in the cerebrospinal fluid of symptom-free patients because of viral DNA integration into chromosomes of the host. Without viral DNA integration, a positive HHV-6 CSF PCR can only be considered equivalent to CNS infection and not reactivation in the presence of a clinical syndrome of encephalitis that cannot be explained by another causative pathogen.

References

1. Relich, R. F., & Abbott, A. N. (2018). Syndromic and Point-of-Care Molecular Testing. *Advances in Molecular Pathology, 1*(1), 97–113. https://doi.org/10.1016/j.yamp.2018.07.007(accessed on 16th July 2025).
2. Coronel, M. F., Sánchez Granel, M. L., Raggio, M. C., Adler, N. S., De Nicola, A. F., Labombarda, F., & González, S. L. (2016). Temporal changes in the expression of the translocator protein TSPO and the steroidogenic enzyme 5α-reductase in the dorsal spinal cord of animals with neuropathic pain: Effects of progesterone administration. *Neuroscience letters, 624*, 23–28. https://doi.org/10.1016/j.neulet.2016.04.067(accessed on 16th July 2025).
3. Aimoni, C., Busi, M., Calzolari, F., Castiglione, A., et al. (2015). *Cochlear implant outcomes and genetic mutations in children with ear and brain anomalies.* https://core.ac.uk/download/53523126.pdf (accessed on 16th July 2025).
4. Reilly, J., Stewart, S., Allardice, G. A., Noone, A., Robertson, C., Walker, A., & Coubrough, S. (2008). Results from the Scottish National HAI Prevalence Survey. *The Journal of hospital infection, 69*(1), 62–68. https://doi.org/10.1016/j.jhin.2008.02.019(accessed on 16th July 2025).
5. Anis, Z., Baig, A. A., Bano, S., Islam, S., et al. (2022). *Impact of Hypoxia on Astrocyte Induced Pathogenesis.* https://core.ac.uk/download/539671319.pdf (accessed on 16th July 2025).
6. Dobosz, M., Arciszewska, K., Bogoń, A., Buczkowski, J., Pieniążek, J. M., Padkowska, A., ... Laskowska, A. (2024). Infections of the Central Nervous System. *Quality in Sport, 20*, 53865. https://doi.org/10.12775/QS.2024.20.53865(accessed on 16th July 2025).
7. Arvind, N., Parimala, S., & Rahil, S. A. P. (2025). *Neurosyphilis: A comprehensive review of clinical manifestations, diagnosis, and treatment.* https://core.ac.uk/download/655802352.pdf (accessed on 16th July 2025).
8. Bamiou, D. E., Barajas, J., Brechmann, A., Callimachou, A., et al. (2017). *A European perspective on auditory processing disorder: Current knowledge and future research focus.* https://core.ac.uk/download/144472883.pdf (accessed on 16th July 2025).
9. John, C. C., Carabin, H., Montano, S. M., Bangirana, P., Zunt, J. R., & Peterson, P. K. (2015). Global research priorities for infections that affect the nervous system. *Nature, 527*(7578), S178–S186. https://doi.org/10.1038/nature16033(accessed on 16th July 2025).
10. Piparsania, S., Rajput, N., & Bhatambare, G. (2012). Intraventricular polymyxin B for the treatment of neonatal meningo-ventriculitis caused by multi-resistant Acinetobacter baumannii--case report and review of literature. *The Turkish journal of pediatrics, 54*(5), 548–554. (accessed on 16th July 2025).
11. Fazakerley, J. K., Parker, S. E., Bloom, F., & Buchmeier, M. J. (1992). The V5A13.1 envelope glycoprotein deletion mutant of mouse hepatitis virus type-4 is neuroattenuated by its reduced rate of spread in the central nervous system. *Virology, 187*(1), 178–188. https://doi.org/10.1016/0042-6822(92)90306-a(accessed on 16th July 2025).
12. Bogner, J. R., Goebel, F. D., Junge-Hülsing, B., Kronawitter, U., et al. (1992). *Expansion of neopterin and beta2-microglobulin in cerebrospinal fluid reaches maximum levels early and late in the course of human immunodeficiency virus infection.* https://core.ac.uk/download/12168947.pdf (accessed on 16th July 2025).

13. Di Domenico, E. G., Cavallo, I., Bordignon, V., D'Agosto, G., Pontone, M., Trento, E., Gallo, M. T., Prignano, G., Pimpinelli, F., Toma, L., & Ensoli, F. (2018). The Emerging Role of Microbial Biofilm in Lyme Neuroborreliosis. *Frontiers in neurology*, *9*, 1048. https://doi.org/10.3389/fneur.2018.01048(accessed on 16th July 2025).

14. Ludlam, C. A., Powderly, W. G., Bozzette, S., Diamond, M., Koerper, M. A., Kulkarni, R., Ritchie, B., Siegel, J., Simmonds, P., Stanley, S., Tapper, M. L., & von Depka, M. (2006). Clinical perspectives of emerging pathogens in bleeding disorders. *Lancet (London, England)*, *367*(9506), 252–261. https://doi.org/10.1016/S0140-6736(06)68036-7(accessed on 16th July 2025).

15. Bradley, B., Kennedy, P. G. E., & Rodgers, J. (2017). *Delineating neuroinflammation, parasite CNS invasion, and blood-brain barrier dysfunction in an experimental murine model of human African trypanosomiasis*. https://core.ac.uk/download/83960572.pdf (accessed on 16th July 2025).

16. Brettschneider, J., Ludolph, A. C., Pfister, H. W., Rupprecht, T. A., et al. (2009). *The chemokine CXCL13 in acute neuroborreliosis*. https://core.ac.uk/download/19450594.pdf (accessed on 16th July 2025).

17. Ellero, J., Lubomski, M., & Brew, B. (2017). Interventions for Neurocognitive Dysfunction. *Current HIV/AIDS reports*, *14*(1), 8–16. https://doi.org/10.1007/s11904-017-0346-z(accessed on 16th July 2025).

18. Broenen, E., Brüggemann, R., Kamphuis-van Ulzen, K., Mavinkurve-Groothuis, A., et al. (2014). *Screening of the central nervous system in children with invasive pulmonary aspergillosis*. https://core.ac.uk/download/131024764.pdf (accessed on 16th July 2025).

19. Brown, B., Simms, M., & Smith, S. C. (2018). *Would You Recognize Lupus?* https://core.ac.uk/download/215483268.pdf (accessed on 16th July 2025).

20. Bui, T. T., Choy, W., Lagman, C., Lee, C., et al. (2016). *Impact of human immunodeficiency virus in the pathogenesis and outcome of patients with glioblastoma multiforme*. https://core.ac.uk/download/323076887.pdf (accessed on 16th July 2025).

21. Cairns, S., Gibbons, C., King, H., Llano, M., et al. (2018). *Results from the third Scottish National Prevalence Survey: Is a population health approach now needed to prevent healthcare-associated infections?* https://core.ac.uk/download/293863931.pdf (accessed on 16th July 2025).

22. MacLean LM, Odiit M, Chisi JE, Kennedy PGE, Sternberg JM (2010) Focus–Specific Clinical Profiles in Human African Trypanosomiasis Caused by *Trypanosoma brucei rhodesiense*. PLoS Negl Trop Dis 4(12): e906.(accessed on 16th July 2025).

23. Cooper, A., MacLeod, A., Bakhiet, M., Bancroft, G. J., Cattand, P., Hertz, C. J., Hunter, C. A., et al. (2007). *Spatially and genetically distinct African trypanosome virulence variants defined by host interferon-g response*. https://core.ac.uk/download/89760.pdf (accessed on 16th July 2025).

24. Creese, A., Jaquet, A., Van Rie, A., Thota, A. B., Owe-Larsson, B., Sherbourne, C. D., Gilks, C. F., et al. (2013). *Grand challenges: Improving HIV treatment outcomes by integrating interventions for co-morbid mental illness*. https://core.ac.uk/download/pdf/16666900.pdf (accessed on 16th July 2025).

25. Velasco-Villa, A., Escobar, L. E., Sanchez, A., Shi, M., Streicker, D. G., Gallardo-Romero, N. F., Vargas-Pino, F., Gutierrez-Cedillo, V., Damon, I., & Emerson, G. (2017). Successful strategies implemented towards the elimination of canine rabies in the Western Hemisphere. *Antiviral*

research, 143, 1–12. https://doi.org/10.1016/j.antiviral.2017.03.023(accessed on 16th July 2025).

26. Das, S., & Khader, S. (2017). *Yin and yang of interleukin-17 in host immunity to infection [version 1; referees: 2 approved]*. https://core.ac.uk/download/84911322.pdf (accessed on 16th July 2025).

27. De Backere, F., De Leenheer, M., De Turck, F., Keymeulen, C., et al. (2013). *NEOREG: Design and implementation of an online neonatal registration system to access, follow and analyze data of newborns with congenital cytomegalovirus infection*. https://core.ac.uk/download/55764362.pdf (accessed on 16th July 2025).

28. Smith, M. L., Farkas, D. K., Sumner, J. A., Jiang, T., Lash, T. L., Galea, S., Sørensen, H. T., & Gradus, J. L. (2020). Associations between adjustment disorder and hospital-based infections in the Danish population. *Journal of psychosomatic research, 132*, 109976. https://doi.org/10.1016/j.jpsychores.2020.109976(accessed on 16th July 2025).

29. Leonhard, S. E., Lant, S., Jacobs, B. C., Wilder-Smith, A., Ferreira, M. L. B., Solomon, T., & Willison, H. J. (2018). Zika virus infection in the returning traveller: what every neurologist should know. *Practical neurology, 18*(4), 271–277. https://doi.org/10.1136/practneurol-2017-001789 (accessed on 16th July 2025).

30. Gidron, Y., Kishore, U., Nowicky, A. V., Parton, M., et al. (2011). *Hemispheric lateralization and immune function: A systematic review of human research*. https://core.ac.uk/download/20496329.pdf (accessed on 16th July 2025).

31. Green, M., Starzl, T. E., Todo, S., Tzakis, A., et al. (1991). *Aspergillosis of the CNS in a pediatric liver transplant recipient: Case report and review*. https://core.ac.uk/download/12204611.pdf (accessed on 16th July 2025).

32. Janowski, A. B., & Newland, J. G. (2017). *From the microbiome to the central nervous system: An update on the epidemiology and pathogenesis of bacterial meningitis in childhood [version 1; referees: 3 approved]*. https://core.ac.uk/download/80495074.pdf (accessed on 16th July 2025).

33. Lewandowski, D., Toczyłowski, K., Kowalska, M., Krasnodębska, M., Krupienko, I., Nartowicz, K., Sulik, M., et al. (2024). *Varicella-zoster disease of the central nervous system in immunocompetent children: Case series and a scoping review. Vaccines, 12*. https://www.semanticscholar.org/paper/51c528c40ba3b5b72a9b7cb30cd4317e98dfda83 (accessed on 16th July 2025).

34. Lin, L., Luo, L., Wu, M., Chen, J., Liao, Y., & Zhang, H. (2024). *Utilizing metagenomic next-generation sequencing and phylogenetic analysis to identify a rare pediatric case of Naegleria fowleri infection presenting with fulminant myocarditis. Frontiers in Microbiology, 15*. https://www.semanticscholar.org/paper/599027ab05d69f6be7a10cb985b63b2ca06851e9 (accessed on 16th July 2025).

35. Pelton, T. (2009). *Bad water 2009: The impact on human health in the Chesapeake Bay region*. https://core.ac.uk/download/80510793.pdf (accessed on 16th July 2025).

36. Radke, J., Meinhardt, J., Aschman, T., Chua, R., Farztdinov, V., Lukkassen, S., Ten, F. W., et al. (2023). *The central nervous system's proteogenomic and spatial imprint upon systemic viral infections with SARS-CoV-2*. https://www.semanticscholar.org/paper/771f1738ad50999e64e8381e1cb985ce9cd595da (accessed on 16th July 2025).

37. Rolston, K. V. I. (2017). *Infections in Cancer Patients with Solid Tumors: A Review.* https://core.ac.uk/download/pdf/81700368.pdf (accessed on 16th July 2025).

38. Sherman, E. (2019). *Review of Chagas Disease and Treatment Obstacles to Eradication.* https://core.ac.uk/download/213464293.pdf (accessed on 16th July 2025).

39. Shirani, K., Khorvash, F., Karamshahi, A., & MaghamiMehr, A. (2025). *Investigating outcomes and treatment of long coronavirus disease 2019 in patients with multiple sclerosis treated with rituximab: A case series study. Journal of Research in Medical Sciences: The Official Journal of Isfahan University of Medical Sciences, 30.* https://www.semanticscholar.org/paper/fda266ab90793e543fb6a1c52e764abb3ea7b75a (accessed on 16th July 2025).

40. Skouboe, M. K., Werner, M., & Mogensen, T. (2023). *Inborn errors of immunity predisposing to herpes simplex virus infections of the central nervous system. Pathogens, 12.* https://www.semanticscholar.org/paper/dd9624e3632ff7d2fd542c9e1fb71127296c7a24 (accessed on 16th July 2025).

41. Smith, J. K. (2024). *The effects of microgravity on cellular elements of the central nervous system: Astrocytes, microglia, neurons, oligodendrocytes, and oligodendrocyte precursor cells. International Journal of Frontline Research and Reviews.* https://www.semanticscholar.org/paper/da55cd69ffe0bfb5c94402e3f6214a94e4818822 (accessed on 16th July 2025).

42. Staal, S. L., Olie, S. E., van Weeghel, M., Schomakers, B. V., Vaz, F. M., van de Beek, D., & Brouwer, M. (2025). *Cerebrospinal fluid metabolome in central nervous system infections: A study of diagnostic accuracy. Annals of Neurology.* https://www.semanticscholar.org/paper/78ed90829e6ee1b7309abf5505f67eb179e9b8ef (accessed on 16th July 2025).

43. Tang, Y., Xu, H., Liu, D., Lin, T., Zuo, F., Wen, D., Liao, Y., et al. (2025). *Comparative study on the sensitivity of lumbar puncture and external ventricular drainage cerebrospinal fluid in the diagnosis of central nervous system infections after craniotomy. Frontiers in Neurology, 16.* https://www.semanticscholar.org/paper/0606a96a05d6899d8ff76466ece876cdf15195 6d (accessed on 16th July 2025).

44. Wong, S., Gee, A., Bazzi, Y. T., Hamby, M., Zheng, J., Henderson, H., Schaar, M., et al. (2024). *Current patient management for bacterial meningitis simultaneously affected by stroke. Cureus, 16.* https://www.semanticscholar.org/paper/db3b63a4c984664acf44cd7057ea3135333eed6d (accessed on 16th July 2025).

45. Zhang, L., Tang, Y., Huang, P., Luo, S., She, Z., Peng, H., Chen, Y., et al. (2024). *Role of NLRP3 inflammasome in central nervous system diseases. Cell & Bioscience, 14.* https://www.semanticscholar.org/paper/537644106d7cd391eed27a07ae747637aba4ffcd (accessed on 16th July 2025).

46. Zhang, Z. (2011). *Neurodegeneration: Potential causes, prevention, and future treatment options.* https://core.ac.uk/download/pdf/290265.pdf (accessed on 16th July 2025).

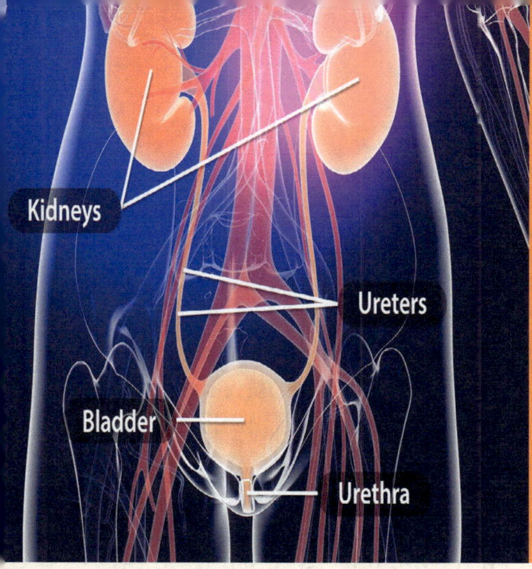

Chapter 11

URINARY TRACT AND GENITAL INFECTIONS

Contents

Introduction

Urinary tract and genital infections are a tremendous public health issue prevalent among populations around the world, particularly among women and individuals with certain predisposing conditions. The infections, caused by a variety of pathogens that include bacteria, fungi, and viruses, have a tendency to cause a variety of clinical presentations from asymptomatic infections to severe, life-threatening conditions. Effective prevention and treatment of such infections improve individual outcomes as well as reduce the economic burden on healthcare systems. Understanding mechanisms for such infections, such as transmission of pathogens and resistance, is vital to developing effective prevention and treatment regimens. Therefore, research on the etiology of urinary tract and genital infection prevalence, causes, and options for prevention remains significant for enhancing patient care as well as public health in general. Analysis of urinary tract and genital infection shows a variety of risk factors that contribute to their occurrence, including anatomical, behavioral, and environmental factors. For example, anatomical variations predispose to recurrent urinary tract infection, while habits of hygiene determine the risk of genital infection. Female vulnerabilities are especially heightened owing to anatomical as well as hormonal variations. Lifestyle factors such as sexual behavior, contraceptive exposure, and individual hygiene habits also play important roles in infection. It is vital to educate patients and clinicians on these determinants since awareness thereof may inform optimal prevention. It is most necessary to tackle infections in pregnancy because they are likely to lead to serious complications unless tackled; thus, it is necessary to learn comprehensively about optimum nursing interventions in treating such infections (Shen, 2017). Moreover, the implications of urinary tract and genital infections extend beyond individual health to influence the well-being of society in a large way by contributing to healthcare costs and impairing efficiency. For instance, the cost of repeated infection often involves additional consultations with clinicians, laboratory examinations, and antimicrobial treatment. Besides, infection by such pathogens as those in Ajani et al. (2010) can lead to increased health hazards and systemic consequences, requiring effective public health interventions. Early detection, treatment, and increased awareness will mitigate these impacts, enhance both health and saving costs. Thus, a multi-faceted approach to tackling education, preventive measures, and early interventions is called for to effectively combat urinary tract and genital infections, ultimately to the gain of both individual health and social health.

Definition of Urinary Tract Infections (UTIs)

Urinary tract infections (UTIs) are infections within any part of the urinary system, including the kidneys, ureters, bladder, and urethra. They most commonly arise from bacterial invasion, with *Escherichia coli* as the etiologic pathogen in approximately 80–90% of all UTIs. Prevalence is particularly notable in women, who have a higher rate of developing UTIs than men due to anatomical reasons, such as having a shorter urethra, which makes them susceptible to bacterial entry. It can manifest as increased frequency of urination, urgency, painful urination (dysuria), and, in more severe infections, potential systemic signs such as fever or shivering when the kidneys are infected. This greater prevalence in women underlines the need for information about risk factors, preventive measures, and treatable complications in the overall context of urinary tract and genital infections. In addition to gender-specific anatomical risks, some other conditions, such as age, sexual activity, and certain medical conditions, may increase the risk for UTIs. In particular, postmenopausal women are susceptible due to low estrogen levels that can lead to altered urinary tract flora. Diabetics or individuals with a history of urinary catheter use are also susceptible, as both make the body immunocompromised and provide potential entry points for bacterial colonization. Research has shown that frequent UTIs have the ability to significantly impact the quality of life of a person, causing healthcare spending and necessitating effective control measures. Understanding these factors is crucial for effective treatment and diagnosis of UTIs, which form a significant aspect of managing urinary tract infections and genital infections in a holistic way. The diagnosis of UTIs is most often made by clinical examination and laboratory tests, such as urinalysis and urine culture, to confirm the presence of pathogens. Choosing the appropriate antibiotic is a significant aspect of the treatment of UTIs due to the rising issue of antibiotic resistance as a public health concern. Empirical treatment may be founded on local resistance profiles, necessitating clinical professionals to keep themselves informed about the evolving situation of the efficacy of antibiotics. Furthermore, preventive practices like educating the patient about hydration, personal hygiene, and sexual activity are essential factors in the reduction of recurrent UTI occurrences. As ongoing research is always refining, elucidating the processes of bacterial infection and host response can reveal new avenues for intervention and thus enhance general urinary tract and genital infection management, e.g., UTIs (Clar et al., 2012; Hamid & Losco, 2014) (Figure 11.1).

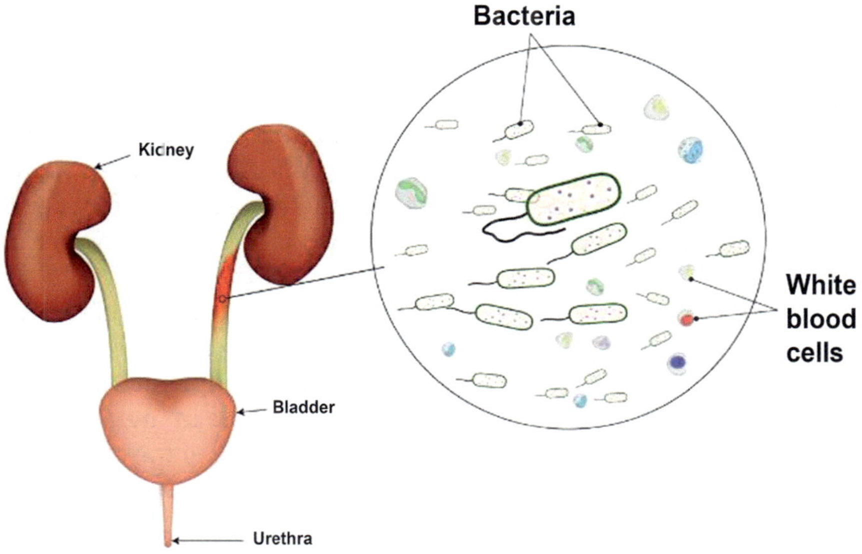

Figure 11.1. Urinary tract infections (UTIs)

Source: https://external-content.duckduckgo.com/iu/?u=http%3A%2F%2Flittlespurspedi.com%2Fwp-content%2Fuploads%2F2019%2F04%2Fsign-symptoms-urinary-tract-infection-children.jpg&f=1&nofb=1&ipt=e7929dcc0084122c325927639ff17e0f8c2523d74fd4ef140d6ede2df96474f1.

Definition of Genital Infections

Genital infections are a broad term referring to conditions affecting the genital and reproductive system. Genital infections can be caused by various pathogens, including bacteria, viruses, fungi, and parasites, which can lead to severe health consequences if left untreated. Sexually transmitted infections (STIs) like chlamydia, gonorrhea, syphilis, and herpes are examples of genital infections, which have symptoms like abnormal discharge, itching, and inflammation. The complexity of such infections necessitates interdisciplinarity of diagnosis and care for effective management, considering that they may also have systemic symptoms and long-term complications such as infertility, chronic pain, and ectopic pregnancy. Genital infections, if left untreated early, not only pose individual health threats but also raise broader public health concerns through high transmission rates in the community. The consequences of genital infections extend beyond the immediate physical complications, potentially affecting mental health as well as interpersonal relationships. For instance, STI patients often experience stigma and anxiety, which can be a deterrent to seeking expert attention. Psychological outcomes of genital infections can result in social isolation, particularly among those who fear judgments from peers or partners. In addition, integrating education and awareness about safe sexual behavior is necessary to prevent the spread of such infections. Population education programs on the risks of unsafe sex can lower the rate of genital infection as well as promote healthier attitudes. Such multi-faceted interventions will encompass not just clinical but also community-based interventions, further emphasizing the necessity of a public health approach to this issue. Also, some communities of people, such as women who have undergone female genital mutilation (FGM), will probably experience complications regarding genital infections. Research by organizations like AkiDwA suggests the need for healthcare access for such communities since FGM may cause anatomical changes as well as an increased risk of infections (Green et al., 2008) (Figure 11.2).

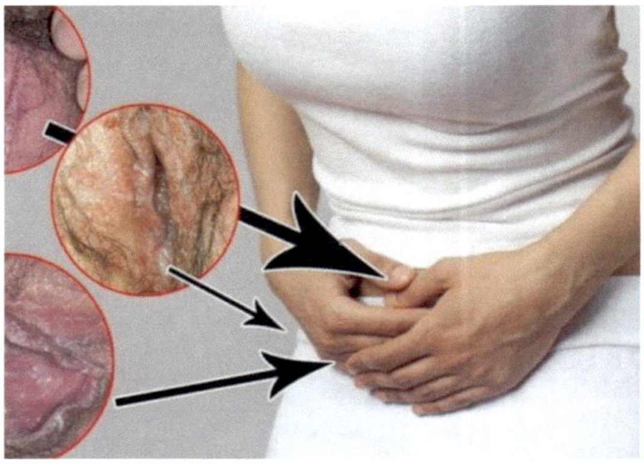

Figure 11.2. Genital infections.

Source: https://www.nirujahealthtech.com/wp-content/uploads/2020/09/vaginal-yeast-infection-in-women-8.jpg.

Healthcare workers need to be able to address such specific requirements through culturally sensitive and informed care. It is critical that there is recognition of the fact that the intersection of genital infections with broader health issues necessitates ongoing study and investment in healthcare access and outcomes for risk groups. Furthermore, proper training of health workers in identification and treatment of such conditions is necessary in order to promote an inclusive practice in healthcare that addresses the diverse needs of all patients with genital infections (Clar et al., 2012).

11.1. Anatomy of the Urinary and Genital Systems

The anatomy of the urinary system is the basis for understanding urinary tract infections (UTIs), among the most common bacterial infections in individuals worldwide. The kidneys, ureters, bladder, and urethra are the main parts of the system, and they all work together to filter blood, excrete waste, and regulate fluids. The kidneys, whose intricate nephrons filter blood to form urine, are complemented by the ureters that carry this urine to the bladder to be stored. The muscular walls of the bladder enable it to dilate and contract, hence aiding in the voiding process through the urethra. Yet, the vulnerabilities of the anatomy, especially in women whose urethra is shorter, expose them to infection. It is crucial to learn about these anatomical organs to realize how infections can occur, thus the importance of coming up with efficient prevention and treatment while managing UTIs that are usually predisposed by conditions like diabetes (Sayied et al., 2021). Beyond the urinary system, genital system anatomy is equally vital to take into consideration when dealing with urinary tract and genital infections. The female genital system contains structures such as vagina, cervix, uterus, and ovaries, whereas the male genital system contains penis, scrotum, and testicles. These physical structures are not only responsible for reproduction but also overlap the urinary system, particularly in the females. The proximity of the urethra to the vaginal and anal openings exposes the organism to infections since bacteria can easily move from the genital tract into the urinary tract. This anatomical arrangement highlights the importance of hygiene practices in the prevention against infection. For example, awareness of the need for hygiene before and after sexual intercourse can reduce the risk of UTIs, especially in populations that have higher frequencies because of unsafe habits of personal hygiene (Sayied et al., 2021). Yet another important factor that is also intricately connected to the anatomy of such systems is the increasing case of antimicrobial resistance, which complicates the treatment of urinary and genital infections. The most prevalent uropathogen, *Escherichia coli*, has evolved mechanisms allowing it to survive antibiotic therapy, leading to treatment failure and increased morbidity in infected patients. The anatomical characteristics of the urinary system favor colonization and infection, which is enhanced by structural abnormalities or dysfunctional voiding. Existing evidence emphasizes the need to understand the pathogenesis of UTIs in depth and also how anatomical vulnerabilities interact with the process of microbial resistance. As infections become increasingly resistant to traditional therapy, it is essential that integrated approaches considering both the anatomical realities and evolving realities of microbial resistance be applied to ultimately guide more successful therapeutic interventions.

11.1.1. Overview of the Urinary System

The urinary system is a significant organ system that controls all the various physiological functions, including urine production and excretion. The system includes kidneys, ureters, bladder, and urethra. The primary function of this system is to filter blood, remove waste products, control electrolytes, and give overall homeostasis of body fluids.

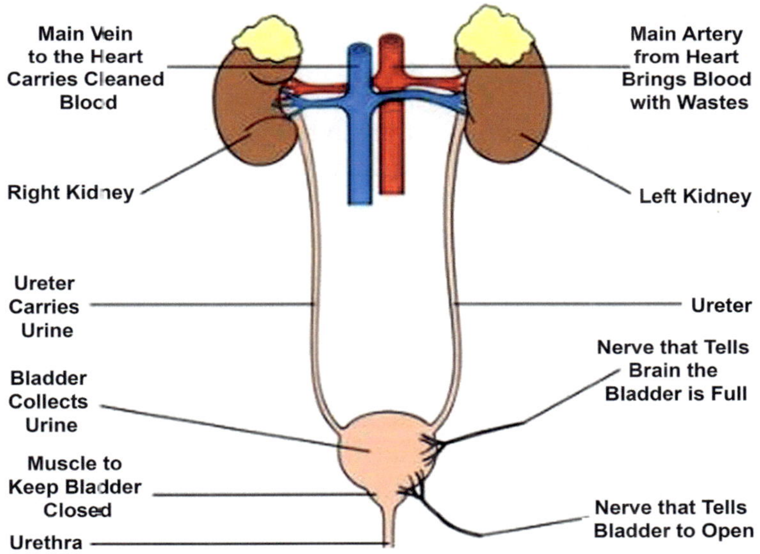

Figure 11.3. Urinary system.

Source: https://cdn.mos.cms.futurecdn.net/v2/t:35,l:0,cw:500,ch:375,q:80,w:500/sFBn3sxD8797R4H2yCMFRE.jpg.

The kidneys are crucial, as they carry out nephron filtration, where toxins and excess substances are filtered from the blood. The result of this process is urine, which is conveyed via the ureters into the bladder, where it is stored temporarily until voluntary elimination via the urethra. This effective functioning underscores the role of the urinary system in maintaining the body's internal milieu, having a direct bearing on infection susceptibility within this system. Urinary tract infections

(UTIs) usually occur when causative infectious microorganisms infect the urinary system, leading to inflammation and severe complications if left untreated. Among the numerous pathogens associated with UTIs, *Staphylococcus saprophyticus* stands out, especially in young women. Study indicates that this bacterium is responsible for a high percentage of UTI among this group, and it causes 7.4% of the infection among 16- to 24-year-old women (Adeghate et al., 2016) (Figure 11.3).

The frequency of this infection specifies the necessity of learning this organism's behavior and resistance to some antibiotics. As seen in the case study, antibiotic resistance rates vary greatly, which suggests the need for regular surveillance and targeted treatment approaches. It is important information for healthcare professionals who are trying to minimize the impact of UTIs on patients' health. Apart from being familiar with urinary infections, the health of the urinary system is particularly significant during pregnancy. Pregnant women are more susceptible to urinary infections, which can become a complicating factor in pregnancy and lead to unfavorable outcomes both for the fetus and the mother. Incorporating preventive measures into nursing practice can go a long way in assuring better patient outcomes by decreasing the incidence of severe infection during this vulnerable phase. Effective measures such as surveillance for signs of early infection and proper hydration are core components of treatment (Shen, 2017). When the need for remedial intervention becomes evident, the healthcare community must highly prioritize urinary system education in an effort to equip patients, increase awareness of the potential for infection, and promote active engagement with health management.

11.1.2. Overview of the Genital System

The genital system, a crucial component of the human body, comprises reproductive and regulatory structures of sexual characteristics. In men, the primary structures are the testes that secrete sperm and testosterone and the penis that performs the act of delivering the sperm during intercourse. Women have a more complex system comprised of the ovaries, uterus, fallopian tubes, and vagina, all crucial in reproduction. The ovaries also secrete ova and hormones such as progesterone and estrogen, which regulate the menstrual cycle and reproductive function. An understanding of the physiological functions and anatomical organization of these organs is relevant because they are prone to various infections that make reproductive and urinary health difficult and complicated, thus influencing fertility and general health. The genital system, besides facilitating reproduction, is responsible for protective and regulatory functions that maintain health. The female genital tract, for example, is comprised of the vagina and cervix that are shielded from infection by the secretions of mucus and a proper healthy microbial flora. In men, however, the urethra passes through the penis, presenting a pathway for sperm and urine. Since both urinary and genital systems are interrelated, infections can appear as double whammy, typically complicating genital or urinary tract infections (UTIs). The complexity of these interactions necessitates the significance of an awareness and knowledge base pertaining to the anatomy of genital systems, especially with considerations for prevention against infections and treatments (Figure 11.4).

New research has also revealed how certain infections may target the genital tract in particular, with dramatic effects. Such as Zika virus infection, which has been shown to be mosquito-borne but also sexually transmitted, proving a unique ability to replicate in the female reproductive tract outside normal mechanisms. This duality justifies the susceptibility of sexual transmission to transmit diseases that emerge in the genital system and, as such, cause reproductive health and fetal impacts during pregnancy (Busch et al., 2017). In addition, the impact of female genital mutilation (FGM) on reproductive health is a good example of how culture may significantly impact the anatomical health of the genital system with a variety of physical and mental health problems (Green et al., 2008). Therefore, an overall understanding of the genital system, particularly infection management and prevention that could negatively impact individual and public health, is required.

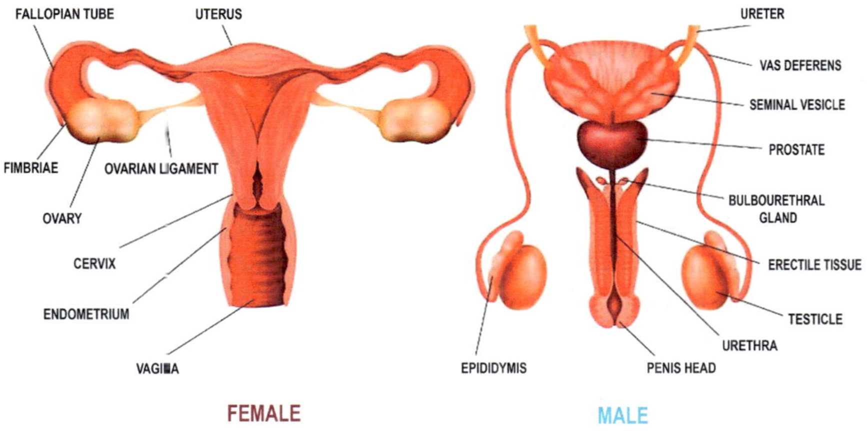

Figure 11.4. Reproductive system.

Source: https://lh7-rt.googleusercontent.com/docsz/AD_4nXeAjEroq6d_hQexvaOiLhnwDnfNibO_O-RMnnHRFce89TU3saWdXAFw41y_hyUrNG-vorwYqoGasqKwwKL34Bu1V_6uVGGIIVE6hsdnr4dhUlsO atWHyTD-XbhZ5DjM_oYe_CYWnljr1jFq2zqEk9w?key=T2ACAExqnqUPLi54sRmolqkk.

11.1.3. Interconnection Between the Two Systems

The interaction between the urinary and genital tracts shows a complex interdependence that predominantly influences infection patterns and overall reproductive well-being. The urinary tract image has been updated by new studies, recognizing the presence of a rich microbiota, which was previously believed to be sterile. This new vision brings with it the potential for resident urinary bacteria to have a function in the modulation of susceptibility to infection, particularly from uropathogens. For instance, research has established that interactions within the urinary microbiota can suppress or activate the pathogenicity of causative bacteria of UTIs. Therefore, it is an essential area of research in understanding how the urinary tract microbiome functions together with pathogenic microorganisms to influence health outcomes in infected patients (Brons et al., 2021). Also, the interactional effect between genital and urinary infections highlights that both systems have to be considered in concert in the clinical setting. For example, bacterial vaginosis (BV), which is primarily a genital infection, significantly impacts urinary health. In pregnant women, BV has also been linked with infertility and fetal mortality. The microbiota responsible for BV may lead to the formation of biofilms, enhancing antimicrobial resistance and complicating treatment. Notably, the presence of genital mycoplasmas, which are typically associated with BV, further reinforces the interconnectedness of both systems, with a significant risk during pregnancy (Redelinghuys, 2014). Therefore, identification of the interaction between urinary and genital tract infection is necessary for more successful prevention and treatment of the infection. Furthermore, the implication of this interaction for public health extends beyond the individual into the general public health approaches. Co-occurrence between urinary and genital infection complicates diagnosis and highlights the necessity for the unification of healthcare strategies. For instance, infections have a lot of overlapping symptoms, hence it is hard to determine the precise causative organism without comprehensive testing. There is hence an increasing need for affordable point-of-care testing that verifies these infections accurately, enabling proper interventions in a timely manner that can cut the risks of uncontrolled infections. With studies continually revealing the microbial communities within the urinary and the genital tract, public health interventions must adapt to incorporate these findings so that interventions are intersectional and are tailored to reverse the impact on both maternal and fetal health at critical stages such as pregnancy (Redelinghuys, 2014).

11.2. Common Types of Urinary Tract Infections

Urinary tract infections (UTIs) are one of the most common bacterial infections and affect millions of individuals annually. The types of UTIs generally bifurcate into two groups: lower urinary tract infections, which predominantly consist of the bladder (cystitis), and upper urinary tract infections, which include the kidneys (pyelonephritis). Cystitis has frequent urination and painful urination with lower abdominal pain as a common presentation, while pyelonephritis can have a more serious presentation with fever, chills, and costovertebral angle pain. This distinction not only is crucial for diagnosis but also for therapy choice because upper UTIs can need more severe therapy due to their complications. The most common etiologic agents of UTIs are *Escherichia coli*, which cause approximately 80% of the infections, though other bacteria, such as *Klebsiella*, *Proteus*, and *Enterococcus* species, can also be culprits. Cystitis occurs most frequently in females, particularly due to anatomical reasons leading to susceptibility to infection. In addition, coitus, the use of certain modes of contraception, and menstrual hygiene also influence the frequency of UTIs in women. Furthermore, men acquire UTIs less frequently; however, when they do, the infections could be more indicative of anatomical abnormalities or underlying diseases, and thus differential diagnosis is paramount in such populations (Smith et al., 2020). Another notable aspect of UTI epidemiology is the interplay of psychological illness, such as stress and adjustment disorders, with infectious susceptibility. It has been established through evidence that adjustment disorder patients can experience higher infection rates, including UTIs, reflecting the relationship between psychological status and immune response (Smith et al., 2020). Sexual health is also a very important aspect, particularly in young adults, where STIs and UTIs happen to coexist, thereby complicating treatment. Identifying the most common types of UTIs, causative microorganisms, and contributing factors can really enhance clinical practice, lower recurrence and improve outcomes in patients with genital and urinary tract infections.

11.2.1. Cystitis

Cystitis, or inflammation of the bladder, is a symptomatic urinary tract infection (UTI) that predominantly affects women but may also affect men. Symptoms are dysuria, frequency, urgency, and pelvic pain, and cystitis can severely impair the quality of life for the afflicted patient. Cystitis is most commonly caused by bacterial infection, most commonly *Escherichia coli*, responsible for approximately 80–90% of cases. Diagnosis of cystitis is usually carried out by urine culture and sensitivity, and this aids in the individualization of the appropriate antibiotic therapy and provision of adequate management. Mismanagement of UTIs may lead to recurrent infection, and additional investigation might be necessary, particularly in individuals with persistent or complicated infection, which might require more extensive analysis and management (Bonnici, 2014). Apart from bacterial etiology, cystitis may be due to non-infectious causes such as chemical irritants, radiation therapy, or presentation of interstitial cystitis. The latter, indicative of chronic pelvic pain and urgency, is associated with an entity known as central sensitization (CS). This is heightened nervous system sensitivity to stimuli, typically characteristic of chronic pain disorders. Research indicates good evidence of correlation between the duration of bladder pain syndrome (BPS) and CS, emphasizing the importance of early diagnosis and intervention to prevent symptom worsening. Treatment in patients suffering from interstitial cystitis or chronic cystitis has to extend beyond the general use of antibiotics to incorporate multidisciplinary treatments that target physical symptoms and psychological aspects prevalent in the disorders (Cambieri et al., 2016) (Figure 11.5).

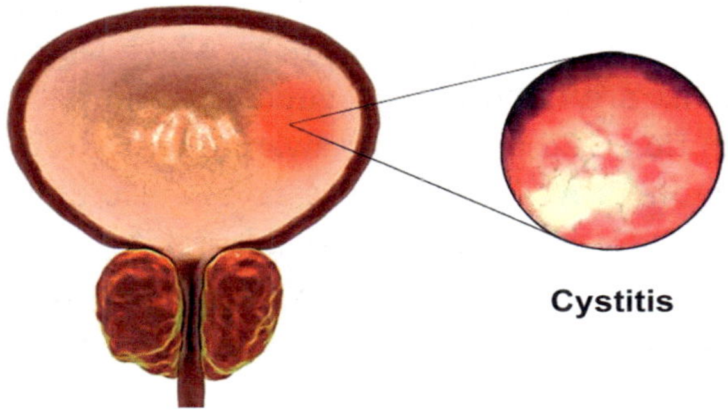

Figure 11.5. Cystitis.

Source: https://urocarechennai.com/wp-content/uploads/2024/07/cystitis.jpg.

Preventive methods are crucial in managing cystitis and inhibiting its recurrence. The methods may include an increased fluid intake, urine dilution, and elimination of bacteria, and cranberry products that inhibit bacterial adhesion to the urinary tract. Other methods include proper hygiene, urination after intercourse, and avoidance of irritants such as alcohol and caffeine. For those with recurrent cystitis, medical practitioners can speak with patients about prophylactic antibiotic therapy or non-antibiotic alternatives. Appropriate education with these options must be done to promote patient awareness and patient empowerment in active decision-making about urinary tract health. Finally, overall care that addresses both the physiological and lifestyle aspects of cystitis will create improved outcomes for those enduring this common but uncomfortable disease.

11.2.2. Pyelonephritis

Pyelonephritis is an inflammatory renal illness that is a severe disruption of renal function, typically due to ascending urinary tract infections (UTIs). Pyelonephritis results when bacteria, in this case most frequently *Escherichia coli*, migrate from the lower urinary tract to the kidney and begin bacterial colonization and inflammation. It is an acute or a chronic illness, and acute pyelonephritis includes abrupt fever, chills, and flank pain, while chronic pyelonephritis will lead to scarring and progressive kidney destruction. The risk factors of pyelonephritis are usually urinary obstruction, anatomical defects, and a prior history of UTI, which highlights its connection with general urinary tract health. Hence, pyelonephritis treatment is essential to prevent severe renal impairment and optimize patient outcomes for recurrent UTIs. Laboratory work should support clinical diagnosis in order to treat pyelonephritis, which usually constitutes clinical evaluation combined with laboratory data. Dysuria or frequency can be mimicked by lower UTIs and represent a challenge to the diagnosis. In acute presentations, clinical presentation supported by urinalysis and urine culture are essential for diagnosis, but chronic infections may need to include imaging studies to assess renal function and structure. Further, it is necessary to remove the predisposing risk factors that lead to recurrent infection. Effective antibiotic treatment, depending on culture and sensitivity, is necessary to eradicate the infection and avoid complications. Today's guidelines in favor of narrow-spectrum antibiotics emphasize the need to individualize treatment to reduce the chances of antibiotic resistance, ultimately enhancing patient safety and efficacy in urinary infection management (Beveridge et al., 2011) (Figure 11.6).

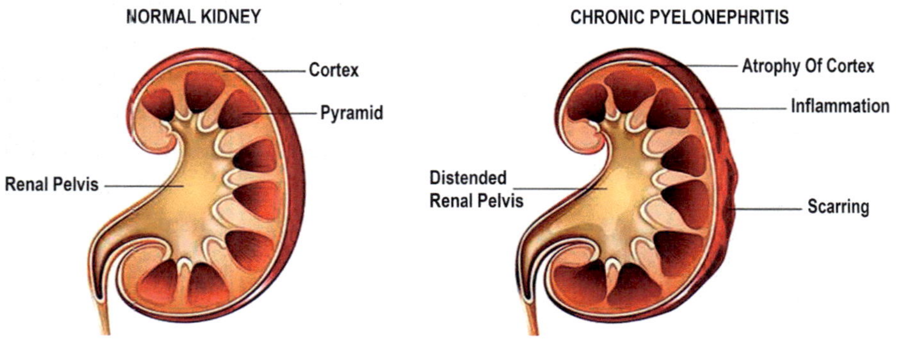

Figure 11.6. Kidney pyelonephritis.

Source: https://www.apexhospitals.com/_next/image?url=https%3A%2F%2Fbed.apexhospitals.com%2Fuploads%2Fkidney_pyelenephritis_828eed07ff.png&w=1920&q=75.

Aside from acute clinical manifestations, the effects of pyelonephritis are multifarious. Pyelonephritis has significant effects in pregnancy, such as severe maternal and fetal consequences for untreated pyelonephritis. Pregnant patients are also susceptible to complications because they are going through some physiological alterations predisposing them to UTIs, which calls for more attention and intervention. Nursing interventions are important in educating the patient regarding prevention measures, proper fluid consumption, and early signs awareness to prevent risks. Incorporation of such preventive work not only improves individual care but also aids in supporting public health interventions that aim to decrease the rate of pregnancy-related severe infection (Shen, 2017). Hence, it is important to understand and address pyelonephritis in the broader perspective of genital and urinary tract infections with implications for future studies and enhanced clinical practice.

11.2.3. Urethritis

Urethritis, which is the urethral inflammation, is a central element of urinary tract and genital infections. Urethritis can be caused by numerous etiologic agents, including sexually transmitted infections caused by causative agents like *Chlamydia trachomatis* and *Mycoplasma genitalium*. Symptoms of urethritis can include dysuria, urethral discharge, and, in more serious forms, urethral stricture. A correct diagnosis is not only necessary for effective treatment but also to prevent future sequelae such as infertility and chronic pelvic pain. It can be challenging to identify etiologic organisms since standard diagnostic tests might be less specific and sensitive, and thus more sophisticated methods must be sought in the clinic. Emerging diagnostic tools such as automated urine flow cytometry (AUFC) have emerged as promising choices for the measurement of urethral infection. The method is more specific in detecting infections by quantifying white cells in first-void urine specimens, much superior to traditional point-of-care methods such as Gram-stained urethral smears. For example, research shows that AUFC has a diagnostic sensitivity of 81.5% and specificity of 85.8% for the detection of *M. genitalium* and *C. trachomatis* infection and could potentially be an improved diagnostic test (Green et al., 2008) (Figure 11.7).

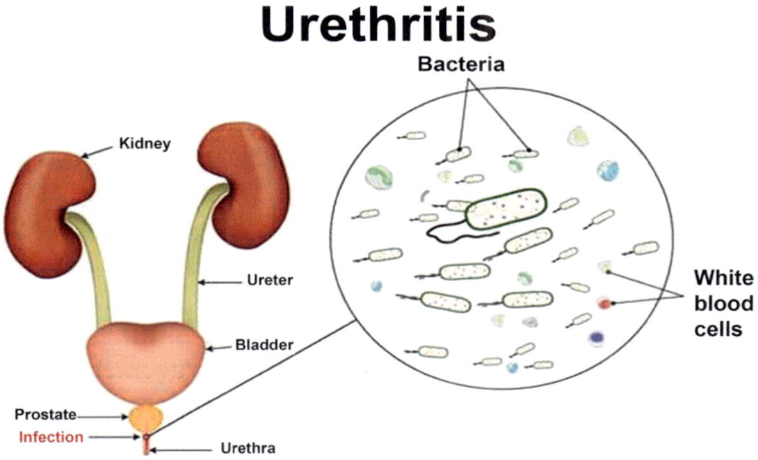

Figure 11.7. Urethritis.

Source: https://www.pristyncare.com/blog/wp-content/uploads/2019/08/urethritis.jpg.

Further, AUFC uses the potential that exists in the detection of asymptomatic patients who otherwise may go untreated. The practice would revolutionize the direction of urethritis diagnosis and treatment, with beneficial impacts on patient outcomes. Evolving non-conventional pathogens also necessitate an adapted conception of the management of urethritis. The studies have confirmed that bacteria such as *Aerococcus* spp. and *Streptococcus bovis* increasingly play more specific roles in genitourinary infection, and thus patient history and clinical presentations must be evaluated more intensively. Most notably in men, variables of rising age and urinary catheter use have been linked to an elevated incidence of these organisms as a pathogen. Adjustment of treatment protocols to include effective antibacterial therapy against these new agents, along with conventional therapies for STIs, will be essential in optimizing patient care for urethritis. As the understanding of urethral pathogens continues to evolve, so must the frameworks for proper diagnosis and tailored treatment plans for urgent care and primary care.

11.3. Common Types of Genital Infections

Genital infections are a public health concern, infecting millions of individuals worldwide and requiring proper medical treatment to prevent complications. Among the most common genital infections, sexually transmitted illnesses (STIs) such as chlamydia, gonorrhea, and syphilis are the most prevalent. Chlamydia, an infection caused by the bacterium *Chlamydia trachomatis*, is especially concerning due to its frequent lack of symptoms and resulting serious reproductive complications if left untreated. Gonorrhea, which is caused by *Neisseria gonorrhoeae*, is indicative of this silent invasion, with a higher risk of disseminated infection. Syphilis, which has several stages, has devastating systemic effects if left untreated. Therefore, periodic screening and education about preventive measures are necessary to reduce the incidence of these infections as well as their corresponding health outcomes. In addition to STIs, other genital diseases such as yeast infection and bacterial vaginosis are of critical significance in genital health pathogenesis. Bacterial vaginosis resulting from the imbalance of vaginal flora normally presents with abnormal discharge and odor. Although an STI , it increases susceptibility to STIs and can cause reproductive damage. Yeast infections, typically caused by *Candida* species overgrowth, can be a source of discomfort with symptoms of itching and abnormal discharge. Both conditions highlight the importance of recognizing the specific etiologies that affect genital health. Additionally, cultural and social influences play a significant role in how individuals manage such infections, further solidifying the importance of public health interventions to be targeted specifically towards awareness and treatment modalities. Psychological factors have also been linked by research to the greater risk of infections, making the genital health situation even more complicated. Adjustment disorder, for instance, has been linked with increased incidences of a range of infections, including STIs, as evidenced in recent research that investigated the relationship in different populations (Smith et al., 2020). Depression and anxiety have also resulted in the engagement in dangerous behaviors, speeding up STI transmission. It is important that healthcare professionals understand these interactions in terms of developing good prevention and treatment plans. Furthermore, addressing the psychological aspect of health can assist in generating better outcomes for patients who are afflicted with these infections, emphasizing the intersection of physical and mental wellness with respect to treating genital infections successfully (Hussein et al., 2014).

11.3.1. Bacterial Vaginosis

Bacterial vaginosis (BV) is a highly prevalent infection in most women and is a significant component of the epidemiology of urinary tract and genital infections. It is linked with a disturbance of the normal vaginal flora, which results from a decrease in *Lactobacillus* species — these are the good bacteria that are otherwise dominant in the vagina — and multiplication of other groups of microorganisms. This alteration influences not just vaginal well-being but also has other implications, as BV is associated with other complications like pelvic inflammatory disease and sexually transmitted disease risk. The condition is usually asymptomatic, and therefore, its diagnosis and effective control become challenging. Understanding of the causation of BV is crucial, as alterations in hormone levels, sexual behavior, and douching behavior predispose an individual to its development. The linkage of bacterial vaginosis with postpartum purulent-septic complications (PPSC) further points towards the management of this condition within health clinics. Research has identified that there is a linkage between a history of gynecological disease, for example, BV, and the onset of PPSC, which has significant potential to impact maternal health outcomes (Figure 11.8).

These are the complications in postpartum intervals that are associated with severe outcomes like elevated morbidity and mortality. Hence, the identification of BV as a risk factor for PPSC is a sign of the need for preventive and early interventions. Effective treatment of BV in pregnant and postpartum women has the potential to reduce the incidence of these severe complications, highlighting the importance of routine screening and education about vaginal health. Emerging studies suggest that probiotics may be an effective tool for the prevention and treatment of bacterial vaginosis and thereby improve women's urogenital health. Probiotics, and notably *Lactobacilli* species, have been demonstrated to possess the capacity to restore healthy vaginal microbiome equilibrium, reversing the dysbiosis that characterizes BV. By augmenting populations of good microorganisms, such microorganisms could potentially alleviate symptoms and incidence of BV. Careful selection criteria need to be adhered to; however, for probiotics to work, selected organisms need to deliver genuine benefits to health. Clinical trials to evaluate the effectiveness of probiotic interventions are required because they will establish the most effective applications for the rejuvenation of vaginal health and the prevention of the risks imposed by bacterial vaginosis and its complications (Nader-Macías & Tomás, 2015; Feyta & Pyrohova, 2018).

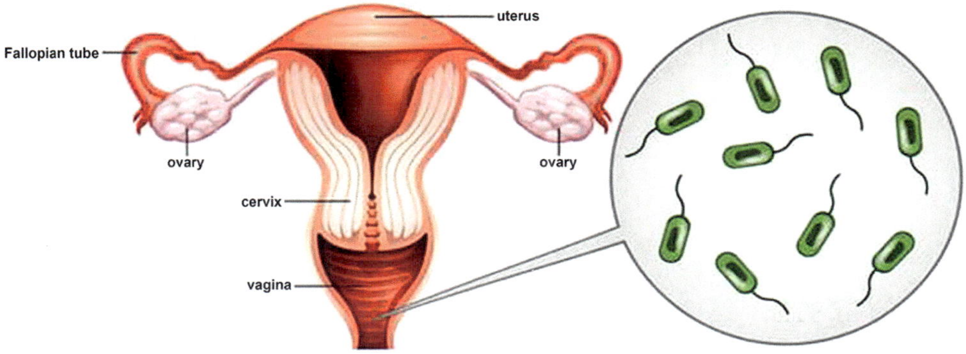

Figure 11.8. Bacterial vaginosis.

Source: https://dam.upmc com/-/media/upmc/services/womens-health/images/conditions/bacterial-vaginosis.jpg?rev=3472a0c4e6a64b619ed40f37d7df200e&la=en&h=323&w=640&hash=890A0AFD79C42A72C9C6753E0DEE8B62.

11.3.2. Sexually Transmitted Infections (STIs)

Sexually transmitted diseases (STIs) are a significant public health concern, particularly as they relate to genital and urinary tract infections. The majority of STIs, like *Chlamydia trachomatis* and *Mycoplasma genitalium*, if not detected or treated, can lead to severe complications. For instance, they lead to urethritis, which is an inflammation of the urethra, producing dysuria and abnormal discharge. As the number of asymptomatic STIs is increasing, diagnosis and treatment become more complex, and there is a need for good screening tests. Another study revealed that the performance of the automated urine flow cytometry provides superior specificity for predicting infection compared with existing diagnostic tests like Gram-stained urethral smear (GSUS) which may be operator-dependent and less sensitive. This underlines the necessity of utilizing advanced diagnostic tools in an integrated approach to cure STIs, particularly in populations where symptoms are not evident or not perceived correctly (Green et al., 2008). The interconnectedness between UTIs and STIs is generally not given much heed since UTIs are thought to be related to bacterial infections. Nevertheless, in women who are sexually active, approximately 50% of the cases with urinary symptomatology can be attributed to STIs. Such overlapping in symptoms makes healthcare providers have a high index of suspicion in the presence of STIs in the treatment of UTIs. Sadly, most providers have inadequate knowledge of the intersection of these infections, which hampers screening opportunities for vulnerable populations. A quality improvement project targeting providers within a walk-in clinic setting successfully demonstrated that expanded education on sexual health history and the importance of STI screening could maximize patient outcomes. Such an education intervention could expand screening practice among healthcare providers, thus maximizing STI detection rates in populations otherwise missed (Mendez, 2022) (Figure 11.9).

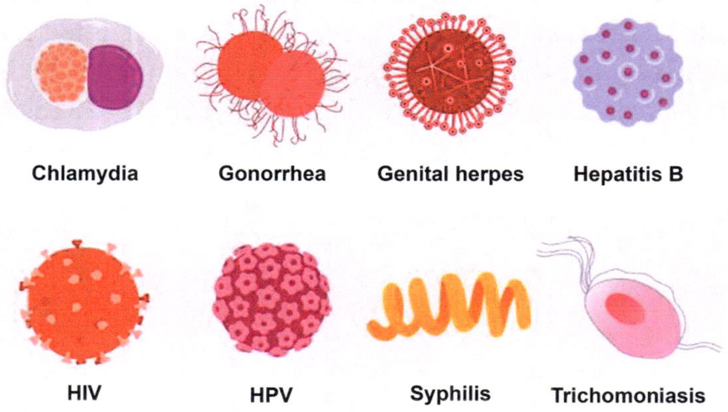

Figure 11.9. Types of STIs.

Source: https://flo.health/cdn-cgi/image/quality=85,format=auto/uploads/media/sulu-1000x-inset/08/7358-sexually-transmitted-infections-types-10_1006x755.jpg?v=1-0.

Since the epidemiology of STIs continues to be dynamic, it impacts public health in profound ways. Increased awareness and education about screening for STIs and urinary symptoms linked to them would have a considerable effect on decreasing the disease burden from these infections. Enhanced screening programs, as has been demonstrated through the quality improvement project outlined here, illustrate how provider education can alter clinical practice and enhance rates of detection among sexually active individuals. Additionally, the use of new diagnostic technologies like automated urine flow cytometry can enable non-invasive approaches to detecting asymptomatic STIs, enabling early treatment and correct intervention. By focusing on the convergence of STIs and urinary tract infections, health systems are able to adopt a more integrated sexual health plan that not only manages present symptoms but reduces infection transmission among populations (Green et al., 2008; Mendez, 2022).

11.3.3. Fungal Infections

Fungal infections constitute a significant problem among genital and urinary tract infections, having a tendency to lead to complications that can significantly affect patient health and well-being. Among the most prevalent fungi causing such infections is *Candida albicans*, a species of yeast able to grow at many different body sites, including the urinary tract. The growth of *Candida* is not limited to immunocompromised hosts; it may also occur in healthy hosts, particularly under conditions where there is facilitation for fungal growth, such as when antibiotics are administered or there is an alteration in hormone levels. Being an opportunistic pathogen, fungal infections necessitate a good understanding of their pathophysiology and factors that predispose them to their occurrence, which eventually aids in establishing effective prevention and treatment regimens. The challenges that are faced while diagnosing the mycotic infections are that the majority of symptoms are shared by bacterial infections and therefore accurate identification is necessary, but becomes challenging. For instance, candidiasis may present with a variety of symptoms like burning, itching, and abnormal discharge that may be similar to bacterial cystitis or vaginitis. Significantly, the increasing incidence of these infections promotes an awareness of their multifactorial cause and the necessity for increased clinical suspicion and diagnostic acumen. Observing that preventive measures can be more effective than simply relying upon antifungal treatment following an established infection, scientists point out that eradication of the fungus does not preclude re-emergence. This pre-emptive approach to management plays a vital role in reducing the overall risk of fungal infections in genitourinary health (Figure 11.10).

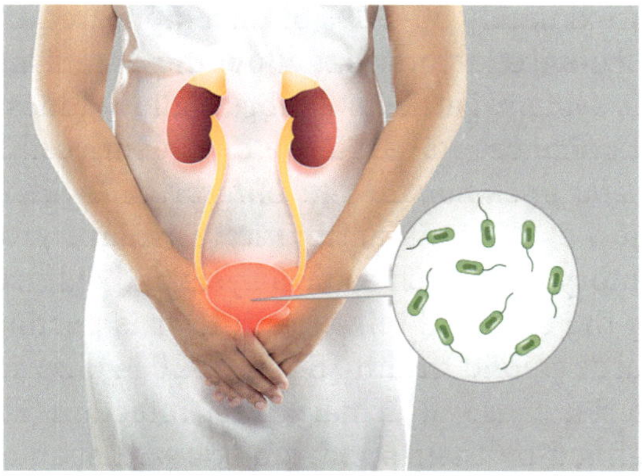

Figure 11.10. Fungal infections of genital infections.

Source: https://www.rghospitals.com/assets/admin/images/blog/1746009293_efa87bafb5d5b50c9b9f.png.

New treatment and research strategies are being developed, not just directed against the eradication of fungal pathogens but also against the understanding of the predisposing environmental and physiological factors leading to these infections. Understanding the multifactorial etiology of candidiasis, researchers emphasize that the disease is predisposed to by various predisposition factors such as diabetes, use of antibiotics, and alteration in immune status. This intricacy necessitates both the strategy of comprehensive treatment when infection occurs as well as aggressive preventive practice with the aim of risk factor minimization. In another perspective, previous studies suggest that integrative models of care could enhance patient outcomes via the facilitation of better screening and management of comorbid conditions, ultimately facilitating the holistic approach of infection control as it pertains to urinary tract as well as genital infection (Legido-Quigley et al., 2012; Sher et al., 2014).

11.4. Causes and Risk Factors

The multifactorial pathogenesis of urinary tract and genital infections (UTIs and GIs) complicates the prevention and treatment of such infections. The presence of pathogenic microorganisms, e.g., bacteria *Escherichia coli*, responsible for the majority of UTIs, is one of the primary reasons for UTIs and GIs. Anatomical and physiological characteristics of the reproductive and urinary systems are primarily risk factors for UTIs and GIs. Women, for instance, are predisposed due to their short urethras through which bacteria can more easily travel up to the urinary bladder. The use of some types of contraceptive methods, poor hygiene, and frequent use of antibiotics are other habits that predispose one to disruption in normal flora, thereby increasing susceptibility to infection. An understanding of these underlying causes allows health workers to develop certain methods of prevention and cure. In addition to anatomical and behavioral factors, several medical conditions are liable to significantly enhance the risk of genital and urinary tract infections. Conditions such as diabetes mellitus compromise the immune system, making one prone to infection. Even more so, individuals with extragenital pathologies, i.e., cardiovascular and pulmonary diseases, typically tend to be at greater risk since they tend to have poorer health status. As reported by recent studies, women with a history of gynecological disease — e.g., chronic inflammatory conditions or bacterial vaginosis — have a greater chance of developing postpartum purulent-septic complications (PPSC) after childbirth. Analysis of anamnestic information in women reveals that such obstetric complications are intrinsic predictors of postpartum infection risk (Feyta & Pyrohova, 2018). The results highlight the necessity of careful screening and prevention in high-risk populations. The contribution of behavioral factors cannot be ruled out when it comes to urinary and genital infections. Sexual habits, habits and sexual activity can significantly shape the possibilities of contracting such infections. For instance, poor genital wiping after urination can enable bacteria to flow through the urethral entry in females. In addition, sexual intercourse can infect the urinary tract with disease-causing organisms, with having numerous new sex partners contributing to the risk. In addition, systemic factors like stress and diet can weaken the immune system and hence lower the body's resistance to infections. Synthesis of research that classifies patients based on behaviors recorded can enhance the understanding of such risks, leading to more effective public health interventions in halting urinary tract and genital infections (Hussein et al., 2014). All of these elements are critical in the broader arena of infection susceptibility and demonstrate the importance of individualized care policies.

11.4.1. Bacterial Causes of UTIs

Bacterial urinary tract infections (UTIs) are caused primarily by some uropathogens, with *Escherichia coli* (*E. coli*) being the single most common culprit. Approximately 80–90% of uncomplicated UTIs are due to *E. coli*, an organism that possesses several virulence factors that allow the organism to attach to uroepithelial cells and escape the host's immune system. Pathogen fimbriae allow adhesion to the urinary tract, while the production of hemolysin enhances its virulence by causing cellular lysis in host tissue. *E. coli* is not the only cause; *Klebsiella pneumoniae* and *Enterococcus faecalis* are some other bacteria that contribute to the formation of UTIs. As antibiotic resistance grows among these pathogens, accurate diagnosis using laboratory tests such as urinalysis and culture is necessary for effective treatment. Hence, understanding the bacterial universe in UTIs is pertinent to minimizing the contribution of these infections towards public health (Bonnici, 2014). Besides *E. coli*, the *Proteus* genus is also another primary bacterial cause of urinary tract infection. Such species as *Proteus mirabilis* and *Proteus vulgaris* are defined by their opportunistic pathogenicity, especially among patients with underlying illness. Proteus bacteria are characterized by their unique swarming phenotype through which they can travel and colonize surfaces effectively, particularly troublesome in catheterized patients. Urea in the urinary tract results in proteus growth due to its urease enzyme that hydrolyzes the urea, thus producing an alkaline environment favorable for bacterial growth (Figure 11.11).

Proteus-mediated struvite stone formation in the urinary bladder is an additional problem for patients. An understanding of *Proteus* spp. is necessary for planning targeted therapeutic measures in the play complicated UTIs (Różalski et al., 2013). In addition, the interaction between virulence factors of the bacteria and the immune response of the host plays an important role in the pathogenesis of UTIs. Biofilm presence and iron acquisition are some of the conditions that immensely enhance uropathogen persistence and survival within the urinary tract. The uropathogens can settle on the surface of the urinary tract and form biofilms upon which they can survive host immunity as well as antibiotic treatment. This characteristic is highly prevalent in species like Proteus, whose production of biofilms can complicate therapy and lead to chronic infections. In addition, the host's immune response may be impaired as a result of anatomical or functional impairment, which predisposes the host to infection. Thus, a comprehensive knowledge of both the bacterial cause of UTIs and the host defense mechanism is important to plan effective prevention and therapy (Bonnici, 2014).

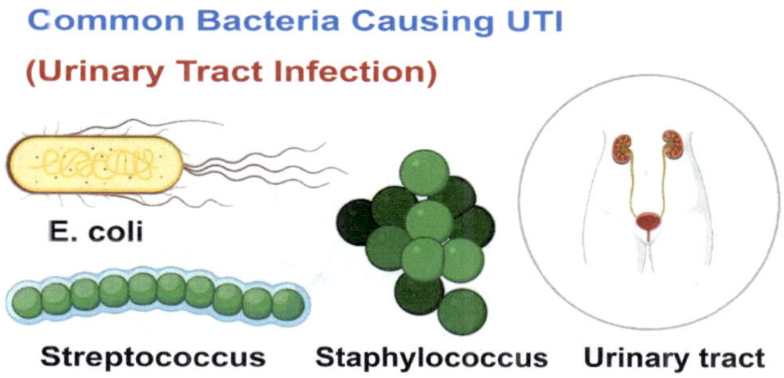

Figure 11.11. Common bacterial causes of UTIs.

Source: https://microbenotes.com/wp-content/uploads/2022/05/Common-Bacteria-Causing-UTI-Urinary-Tract-Infection.jpeg.

11.4.2. Viral and Bacterial Causes of Genital Infections

The prevalence of genital infections is in the rich variety of viral and bacterial pathogens that have a major impact on reproductive health. The most prominent among bacterial aetiologies is *Neisseria gonorrhoeae*, the cause of gonorrhea, an infection with symptoms of dysuria and discharge. The same applies to *Chlamydia trachomatis*, another prevalent bacterium causing chlamydia, which is usually asymptomatic but can have severe complications if not diagnosed and treated. The ability of these bacteria to circumvent the host's immune response is also responsible for their persistence as well as a formidable public health burden. Besides, as pointed out by recent studies, mental factors such as adjustment disorder also engage with such infections to enhance vulnerability and severity, particularly among specific groups (Smith et al., 2020). It is hence essential to be aware of the roles of such pathogens for the development of effective treatment and prevention strategies. Genital diseases are also caused by viral pathogens, the most common ones being herpes simplex virus (HSV) and human papillomavirus (HPV). HSV can lead to recurrent genital ulcers, leading not only to physical discomfort but also to psychosocial issues. By contrast, HPV is infamous for its role in causing cervical cancer, which has led to screening and immunization programs aimed at reducing its effects. The complicating factors of the viral infections are further increased by the viruses' capacity for persistence in the body and immune evasion, complicating the course of treatment. Also, the psychological stress load from such infections can increase the susceptibility to future infections, as indicated by evidence linking psychological stress to higher infection rates of all types (Smith et al., 2020) (Figure 11.12).

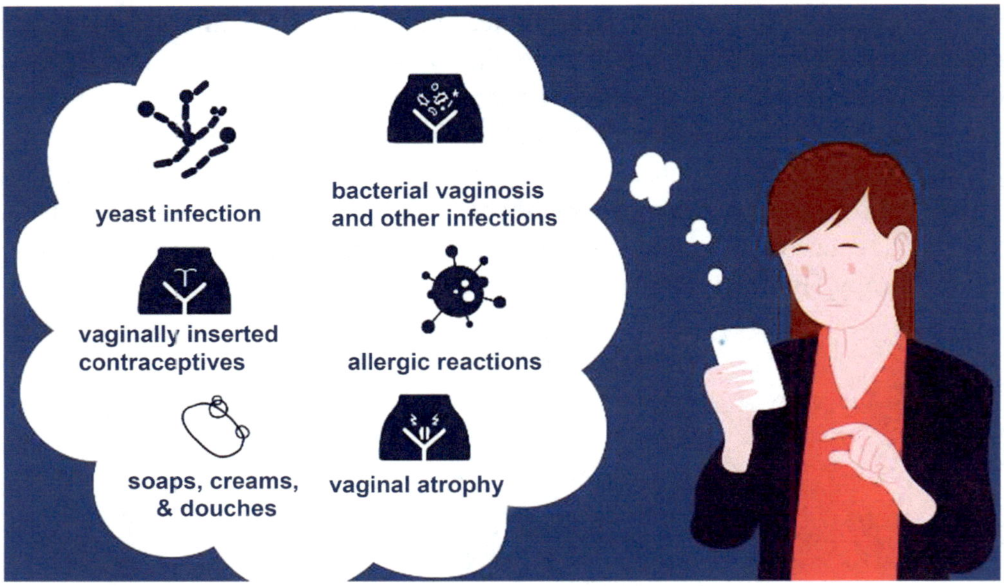

Figure 11.12. Common causes of genital infections.

Source: https://www.drarohitasgaonkar.com/wp-content/uploads/2022/11/Yeast_Infection.jpg.

So, it is necessary to incorporate integrated care that addresses the physical as well as emotional components of these viral infections. In pregnancy, genital infection concerns become particularly significant because it poses danger to mother and fetus alike. Bacterial infection, such as bacterial vaginosis or sexually transmitted infection (STI), can lead to pregnancy complications such as preterm labor and low birth weight. The research conducted on the subject of genital infections in pregnancy brings out the importance of making pregnant women and healthcare providers aware of the prevention and management of severe infection at this critical time. Furthermore, competent nursing care plays a vital role in educating pregnant women regarding signs and symptoms of genital infection, reiterating the importance of early detection and intervention. By better understanding and implementing preventive health measures, we can reduce the incidence of these infections and create healthier outcomes for both mothers and babies.

11.4.3. Risk Factors for Both Types of Infections

Understanding risk factors for urinary tract infections (UTIs) and genital infections is important for effective prevention and control. One of the risk factors for UTIs is female anatomy since females have a shorter urethra compared to males, and thus bacteria find it easier to flow to the bladder. Other predisposing factors, such as sexual activity, particularly in sexually active young females, can enhance risk with exposure of the urinary tract to pathogens. Moreover, the use of some methods of birth control, such as diaphragms or spermicides, can change the vaginal flora to enhance bacterial colonization and hence enhance the risk of UTIs. Decreasing incidence rates and women's health in general regarding urinary infections depends on resolving these risk factors related to behavior and anatomy, making targeted educational materials for high-risk groups of particular importance. Genital infections share typical risk factors with UTIs, namely in relation to socioeconomic and behavioral determinants. For instance, low socioeconomic status has been linked to limited access to health care, and this often results in delayed treatment and susceptibility to infection. Further, certain lifestyles, such as having multiple sexual partners or not using protective devices during sex, predispose one to sexually transmitted infections (STIs), which may complicate or lead to genital infection. Extragenital conditions, such as preexisting medical illnesses such as diabetes or immunocompromised status, also predispose individuals to increased susceptibility, leaving them open to both genital and urinary tract infections. Such identification of related risks can assist healthcare providers in taking preventive measures and educating the patient, so that there is a proactive element of reproductive health management and decreased infection prevalence (Figure 11.13).

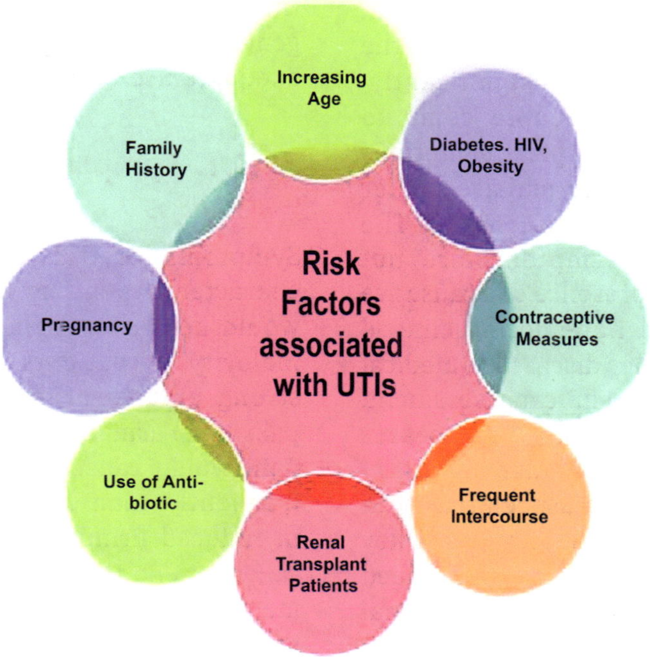

Figure 11.13. Various risk factors associated with UTIs.

Source: https://www.researchgate.net/profile/Kanika-Rani-3/publication/352864056/figure/fig2/AS:1040545342300161@1625096750541/arious-risk-factors-associated-with-UTIs.png.

In medical facilities, some risk factors for postpartum disease also need consideration. As was found in recent studies, maternal health complications during and after pregnancy can also significantly increase the likelihood of postpartum purulent-septic complications (PPSC), which are important due to the implications for maternal morbidity and mortality. Pre-existing factors like obesity and diabetes, as well as obstetric factors like prolonged labor, premature rupture of membranes, and complications in pregnancy such as preeclampsia, have been associated with an increased rate of postpartum infections. Identification of these important correlations allows healthcare professionals to formulate certain interventions that can be applied to prevent infection among postpartum patients based on extensive prenatal and postnatal care practices to rule out risks associated with urinary tract and genital infections (Hussein et al., 2014; Feyta & Pyrohova, 2018).

11.5. Symptoms and Diagnosis

Recognition and interpretation of urinary tract infection (UTI) symptoms are important for effective diagnosis and treatment. The classic presentation of UTI is dysuria, frequency of micturition, urgency, and suprapubic tenderness. For genital infection, additional symptoms such as abnormal discharge or pruritus also occur. Worth mentioning, the symptomatology of the affected population may vary significantly; thus, for instance, elderly people come to medical attention with non-typical symptoms like confusion or nonspecific malaise rather than anticipated uro-genital discomfort. The challenge is that these symptoms are not necessarily related to the presence of a causative infection, particularly in non-specific clinical signs overlapping with other diseases of medical origin, calling for adequate clinical assessment. It should be differentiated from other diseases for proper diagnosis. New-onset urinary symptoms, whether or not associated with systemic findings, in older patients are a key diagnostic criterion. Not all such symptoms need necessarily be indicated by the conventional methods, such as urinalysis, however, because asymptomatic bacteriuria is relatively common but does not require treatment (Beveridge et al., 2011). Diagnostic steps therefore, assume all the more significance. Healthcare providers are urged to employ combined laboratory findings and clinical presentation, like urine cultures, to distinguish true infections from non-disease processes. Such diagnostic rigor is required not to fall prey to overdiagnosis and overtreatment pitfalls that lead to unwarranted antibiotic exposure and resistance patterns. Implications of proper diagnosis do not end at therapeutic possibilities but reach infection control measures in the clinical setting. In urinary tract infections caused by catheters, stringent guidelines are a requirement as they contribute immensely to hospital-acquired infection (Beveridge et al., 2011). Healthcare workers are encouraged to utilize alternatives to indwelling catheters when appropriate and utilize preventive strategies that accord with local resistance patterns. Narrow-spectrum antimicrobial medications are encouraged in an effort to combat such infections more effectively, a sign of the trend towards more localized therapies (Beveridge et al., 2011). Thus, symptom stringency in evaluation and diagnostic precision becomes the key element in managing urinary tract and genital infection to guarantee patient safety and adequate use of resources.

11.5.1. Symptoms of Urinary Tract Infections

Symptoms for UTIs can vary significantly in character depending on the individual, so it would be a challenging task to diagnose. The majority of patients would present with a strong urge to urinate along with a burning pain while urinating, which is called dysuria. The pain would cause individuals to urinate more frequently than required at times, resulting in reduced urine output at times, a condition called urgency incontinence. Also, other patients may also experience urine appearance changes, where the urine becomes cloudy, dark, or even with a smell. All these are typical symptoms but often nonspecific, and that is why healthcare providers need to thoroughly check patients to ascertain diagnosis and avert misdiagnosis for other diseases or conditions with similar symptoms. In older patients, symptoms of UTIs may differ from the common symptoms one finds in younger patients. Older patients will come with generalized symptoms rather than localized urinary symptoms, and these consist of confusion or a confused mental status without a clear cause, rather than normal urinary symptoms. The generalized symptoms may lead to misdiagnosis because health care workers might redirect the causation of such changes to dementia or other cognitive illnesses. Furthermore, systemic symptoms like lymphadenopathy, fever, chills, or malaise may potentially add to the complexity of the clinical presentation. Due to the risk of overdiagnosis and overtreatment within this population, health care practitioners must emphasize prudent evaluation and treatment verification to determine the true presence of disease of a urinary tract infection, as recommended in geriatric literature (Beveridge et al., 2011) (Figure 11.14).

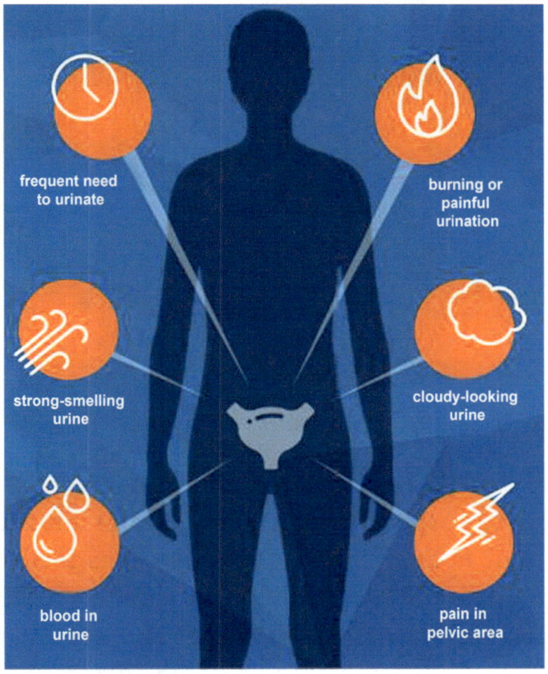

Figure 11.14. Common UTI symptoms.

Source: https://www.cxbladder.com/assets/Uploads/UTI-Symptoms.jpg.

Besides, the relationship between psychological stressors and UTI symptom worsening cannot be overlooked. Research demonstrates that individuals with adjustment disorders may experience an increased infection vulnerability, such as UTIs (Smith et al., 2020). This association might result from compromised immune function as a consequence of chronic psychological stress or maladaptive coping styles, such as poor hygiene and decreased motivation for self-care. Women, in particular, can be anticipated to experience more severe UTI symptoms as a result of anatomical and hormonal susceptibility to urinary tract infection. The relationship between psychological health and UTI symptoms is significant to know to provide holistic management and underscores the need for integrative medical practices taking into account physical and mental status.

11.5.2. Symptoms of Genital Infections

Genital infection symptoms may range very broadly depending upon the nature of the infection and its etiological factors. Pain, itchiness, or burning in the genitals are some of the typical presentations. Symptoms may also be in the form of urinary symptoms, where patients have frequency or urgency of micturition. Genital infection may also present with abnormal discharge in terms of color, consistency, or odor. These alterations are generally indicative of underlying disease, for example, bacterial vaginosis or sexually transmitted diseases (STDs) such as chlamydia and gonorrhea. These symptoms should be identified early, since untreated genital infection may lead to further severe health consequences, such as pelvic inflammatory disease or infertility, emphasizing the value of awareness and early medical assessment in individuals with these symptoms (Hussein et al., 2014). Infectious pathogens responsible for genital infection can be bacterial, viral, or fungal, with each producing different symptoms. Bacterial infection typically manifests as recurrent foul-smelling discharge accompanied by increased associated discomfort. Viral infections, such as herpes, may have painful sores or blisters, whereas fungal infections such as yeast infection may lead to itchy discharge and intense itching. This combination of symptoms can be further compounded by comorbidities, with psychological stress patients also having an increased risk of infection. Recent research has shown that psychological factors can increase infection severity, as individuals with adjustment disorder showed significantly higher infection rates of all kinds, including urinary tract infection and sexually transmitted infections (Smith et al., 2020) (Figure 11.15).

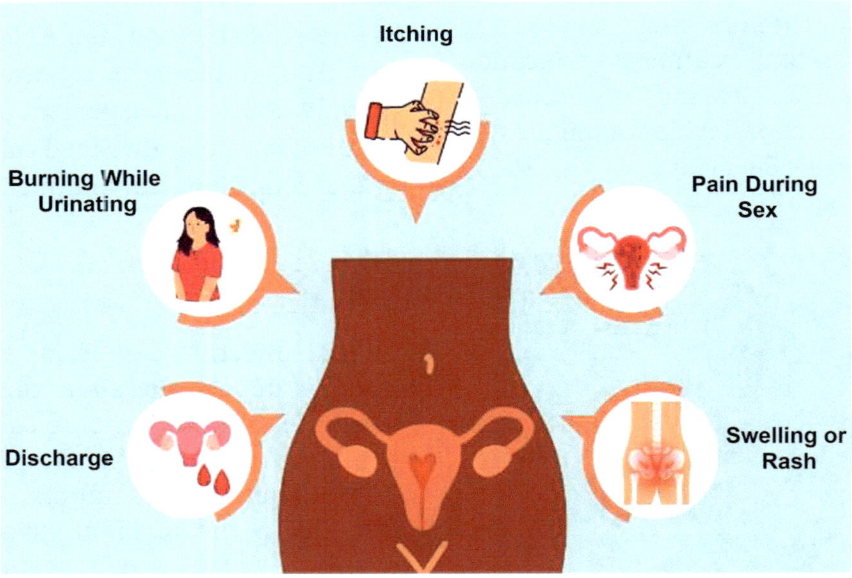

Figure 11.15. Symptoms of a vaginal yeast infection.

Source: https://www.everydayhealth.com/yeast-infection/guide/symptoms/.

Thus, understanding the multi-dimensionality of genital infection requires an integrative approach with the appreciation of physiology and psychology aspects. Diagnosis of genital infection is based on clinical examination and laboratory results; it is thus crucial that one seeks medical care upon development of symptoms. The clinician will often conduct a complete general physical examination and a comprehensive patient history to determine potential risk factors and exposures. Lab tests, e.g., culture or molecular studies, enable accurate identification of etiologic pathogens and provision of appropriate therapy. Early treatment is important, particularly in infections that have sequela in the future, i.e., infertility or chronic pelvic pain. Moreover, education on preventive measures like safe sex is needed to prevent genital infections. Symptom perception and active seeking of health care can substantially decrease individual health risk from these infections as well as overall public health impact, underscoring the mutual dependence of individual and population health status (Hussein et al., 2014).

11.5.3. Diagnostic Methods for Both Infections

The diagnostic processes of urinary tract infection (UTI) and genital infection are multifaceted, characteristic of the pathogenic complexities and the specificities of each infection syndrome. A thorough medical history and physical examination are typically the initial steps, wherein clinicians assess for manifestations of dysuria, frequency of micturition, or foul-smelling discharge. After an initial assessment, laboratory tests come into prominence. A urinalysis is usually performed to verify the existence of leukocytes, nitrites, or bacteria as an indication of a UTI. These are crucial preliminary tests that differentiate between uncomplicated and more complicated types that require other diagnostic tests. Furthermore, in infections of the genitalia, nucleic acid amplification tests and cultures serve to identify sexually transmitted pathogens, providing specificity to the diagnosis and allowing for individualized treatment of underlying conditions. Such a multi-level approach is essential in accurately diagnosing and treating infections with regard to patient-specific considerations. On the basis of initial examinations, sophisticated diagnostic modalities also enhance accuracy in detecting urinary and genital infections. For instance, if routine investigations prove to be inconclusive, imaging investigations such as ultrasound or computed tomography can be applied to investigate anatomical defects predisposing the patients to chronic infections. In cases of suspected sexually transmitted diseases (STDs), serology testing can determine the degree of antibodies against specific pathogens, thus providing valuable information regarding the patient's general risk profile (Figure 11.16).

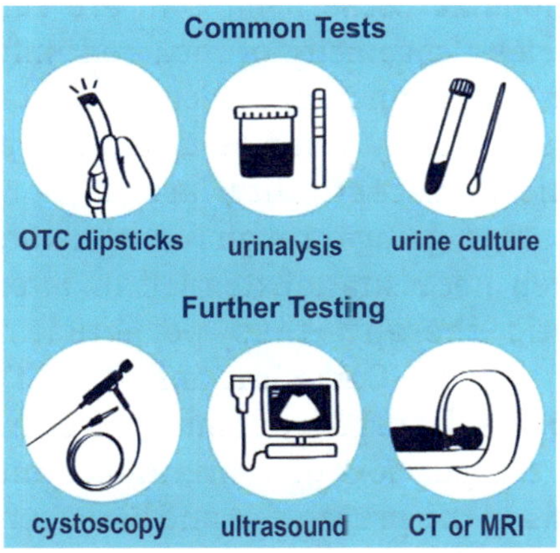

Figure 11.16. Urinary tract infections (UTIs) diagnostic.

Source: https://pbs.twimg.com/media/FboOkQpX0AAvYLU.png:large.

Besides that, molecular diagnostic methods, for instance, polymerase chain reaction (PCR) assays, have ushered in infection detection through fast, sensitive, and precise identification of pathogen DNA or RNA. This technology not only rapidly establishes the diagnosis but also assists clinicians in making highly informed decisions about the treatment regimen tailored to the individual patient. Secondly, the relevance of using such diagnostic methods extends beyond simple direct clinical practice; they are significant contributors to public health. Accurate UTI and STI detection is priceless in successful tracking of infection trends that are essential in formulating preventive strategies. For example, identification of UTI risk factors, such as anatomical and prior information, can guide community education programs on how to prevent or reduce incidence rates. Similarly, the identification of associations with psychological stress, such as adjustment disorders, and increased infection rates determines the need for a holistic patient care strategy. It is shown that even psychological comorbidities such as adjustment disorder are associated with increased infection rates, and the management of such psychological comorbidities can decrease the prevalence of infection indirectly (Smith et al., 2020). By placing strong importance on the decisive function of proper diagnostic methods, medical professionals can apply synchronized strategies that treat not just the infections as a whole but also the more generalized social and psychological elements affecting patient wellness (Feyta & Pyrohova, 2018).

11.6. Treatment and Prevention

Management of urinary tract and genital infections is often multi-modal, with the strategic use of medical therapy and lifestyle modifications. Medications especially involve the use of antibiotics that kill the offending microorganisms that cause the infection. Nitrofurantoin and trimethoprim-sulfamethoxazole are common in uncomplicated urinary tract infections; however, antibiotic resistance is a major concern for which the selection of the medication must be done cautiously. Additionally, the patients are instructed to improve hydration in order to improve the flow of urine, which can potentially flush out the bacteria and lead to relief from symptoms. Patient education is an important consideration, such as counseling regarding the importance of adherence to medication regimes and the early identification of potential complications due to infections, so that timely medical care can be instituted. Preventive measures are critical in minimizing the incidence of urinary tract and genital infections. Risk factor knowledge is the priority in the development of targeted preventive measures. For example, individuals with a history of recurrent infections can be counseled regarding lifestyle change, including continuous hydration, genital cleansing, and voiding after intercourse to reduce bacterial colonization. Furthermore, patient counseling regarding abstaining from irritants such as deodorant soap or cleansing agents can also reduce infection risk. The regular gynecological and urological checkups are also instrumental since they enable clinicians to check up on patients at risk of infection, particularly during the periods of hormonal change or after birth, which are periods of increased rates of infections as revealed by recent studies (Feyta & Pyrohova, 2018). Further, advances in preventive medicine are creating new prospects for the prevention of urinary tract and genital infections with vaccines and prophylactic treatment. Studies are underway to consider the potential for using vaccines against such pathogens, most commonly causing such infections, which would revolutionize prevention strategies entirely. These vaccines would rely on the body's immune system to confer long-term immunity, thereby drastically cutting down infection rates in vulnerable groups of individuals. Until such interventions become more universal, attention remains on the use of one-to-one prevention plans to align individual risk profiles with appropriate broad-based care. Furthermore, technology application in patient education, in the form of mobile health applications for reminding patients about medication schedules and fluid targets, are new strategies in facilitating adherence and self-management among patients who want to prevent such infections (Hamid & Losco, 2014).

11.6.1. Antibiotic Treatments for UTIs

Urinary tract infections are some of the most common bacterial infections, and in women especially, traditional therapy is virtually all antibiotics. The widespread use of antibiotics, however, has led to the alarming development of antibiotic resistance, which makes the treatment of recurrent infections challenging. Empirical treatment typically begins with the standard first-line agents such as nitrofurantoin and trimethoprim-sulfamethoxazole, to which most of the pathogens of UTI, particularly uropathogenic *Escherichia coli*, are sensitive. Nonetheless, chronicity of recurrent infections calls for an examination of factors that underlie such susceptibility. Females, as a result of their anatomical susceptibility, are at particular disadvantage, going through repeated infections that often necessitate extended or alternative antibiotic therapy, thus perpetuating the resistance cycle. Complications of such nature bring to fore the urgency of innovative strategies beyond the purview of conventional antibiotic regimens in the prevention and management of recurrent UTIs. Recent studies have reported on promising treatments that could potentially complement or even substitute for traditional antibiotic therapy. These include the application of host defense peptides (HDPs) that enhance the urogenital innate immune response. From experiments, it is evident that high levels of HDPs, like BD2, are particularly effective in combating uropathogenic infection. For instance, a connection was identified in research between low BD2 in recurring UTI women and higher susceptibility to infection. This is the interesting prospect of incorporating into treatment the increase of HDP production as a mechanism for boosting the body's natural immunity to UTIs. In addition, local treatments, like vaginal probiotics and hormonal therapy, may offer other prevention opportunities, potentially decrease the appeal of systemic antibiotics and offset the issue of resistance with long-term antibiotic therapy (Ali et al., 2017) (Figure 11.17).

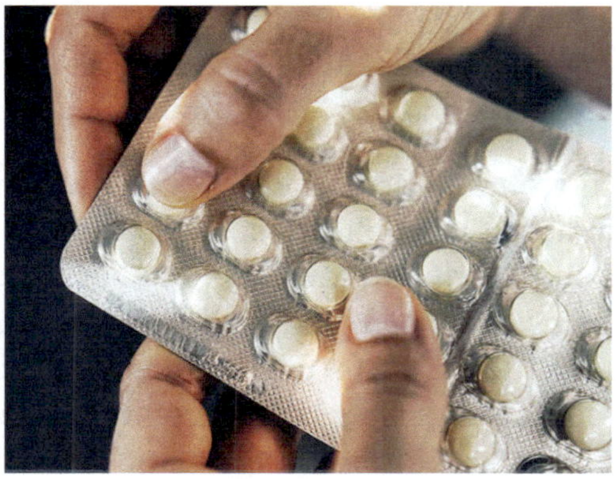

Figure 11.17. Antibiotic for UTI.

Source: https://media.post.rvohealth.io/wp-content/uploads/sites/3/2024/04/antibiotics-UTI-GettyImages-1706521204-Thumb.jpg.

Lastly, the application of probiotics as adjunctive treatment for UTIs has also been on the rise in current clinical practice. Probiotics like *Lactobacilli* strains may restore and maintain the natural urogenital microbiome, thereby ensuring a protective envelope against pathogenic bacteria. This restoration of the ecosystem may suppress infection through competitive inhibition and modulation of mucosal immunity. Clinical trials highlight the need for additional studies to identify targeted probiotic preparations for urogenital health because patient heterogeneity has the potential to undermine treatment effectiveness. In expanding our understanding of the urogenital microbiome, probiotics can potentially contribute to existing antibiotic therapy, offering a means of long-term UTI management while reducing the side effects of antibiotic excess (Nader-Macías & Tomás, 2015). By incorporating a holistic treatment plan, healthcare professionals are able to maximize the control of UTI and improve the health of affected patients.

11.6.2. Treatment Options for Genital Infections

The treatment of genital infections is diverse and also typically based on the causative pathogen. Bacterial infections, e.g., by *Chlamydia trachomatis* and *Neisseria gonorrhoeae*, can be treated with antibiotics, e.g., azithromycin or doxycycline for chlamydia and ceftriaxone or azithromycin for gonorrhea. Prompt diagnosis and treatment promotion are crucial because untreated infections will progress to serious complications like pelvic inflammatory disease and infertility. Moreover, the occurrence of antimicrobial resistance necessitates continuous monitoring of treatment efficacy and seeking alternative treatments. New technology in molecular diagnosis may assist in recognizing such infections at an early stage, which would facilitate more targeted treatment protocols and would also assist in preventing the spread among high-risk populations, especially among the young generation (Munson et al., 2016). In current research into trichomoniasis treatment, the use of commercial molecular assays has been suggested to expand screening protocols to non-traditional groups. Long regarded as a nuisance disease, trichomoniasis is rapidly being recognized to occur in the heterogeneous populations, most particularly in those who reside in clusters of sexually transmitted infection high-prevalence settings. Detection and treatment of *Trichomonas vaginalis*, and likely implications of HIV and HPV infections, are all reasons to make routine screening part of clinical practice. With the evolving treatment patterns, the importance of preventive and awareness educational campaigns stands above reducing the transmission of trichomoniasis, thereby improving overall sexual health outcomes (Munson et al., 2016) (Figure 11.18).

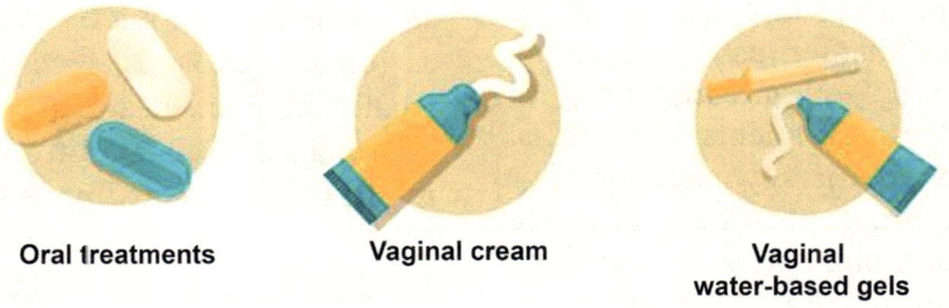

Figure 11.18. Treatments of bacterial vaginosis.

Source: https://i0.wp.com/post.healthline.com/wp-content/uploads/2023/03/2842963-7-Best-Bacterial-Vaginosis-Treatments-FAQs-and-More-1296x2213-Body-1296x2177.jpg?w=1155&h=4575.

With respect to genital infection during pregnancy, non-antibiotic prevention has been more and more emphasized owing to the problems involved with the application of antibiotics and antimicrobial resistance. Various alternative strategies like hygiene practices, cranberry juice, immunization measures, and nutritional supplements like ascorbic acid and Canephron® N have been discovered to be safe for use during pregnancy according to various studies. Although hygiene measures are currently the only recommendations supported by strong evidence, a systematic review highlights that additional investigation is needed before a better realization of prevention measures like this is achieved. By expanding the body of knowledge in this area, clinicians are better equipped to aid pregnant patients in lowering the risk of infection while contributing to solving the greater problem of antibiotic overuse in such susceptible patients.

11.6.3. Preventive Measures for Both Infections

Preventive care for urinary tract infection and genital infections is very important in minimizing risk and maximizing overall health outcomes. Regular education about hygiene habits can make a huge difference in minimizing the occurrence of such infections. An example is the wiping technique — where one needs to wipe from the front to the back — to avoid the transmission of bacteria from the anal area to the urethra, minimizing the risk of urinary tract infection (UTI). Moreover, it is important to promote the importance of proper hydration because greater fluid intake results in more frequent urination and thus flushing out probable pathogens from the urinary tract. Lastly, the use of fragrance-free and gentle personal care products may maintain the genitalia's normal flora, thus minimizing the risk of infection. Expenditure on such behavioral and educational interventions forms the foundation for effective infection prevention interventions. Control of urinary tract infection and genital infection-related risk factors highlights the role of healthful behavior. Women are particularly cautioned against irritants like douches, leading to a derangement of vaginal flora and causing infections like bacterial vaginosis. Early detection of any abnormality or infection requires regular gynecological check-ups, and they allow for timely medical intervention. Especially, pregnant women must receive personalized care to minimize the complications because chorioamnionitis can remarkably enhance postpartum infections, especially in patients who have underlying conditions such as diabetes or obesity. Directed risk assessment allows doctors to identify high-risk patients, and hence it becomes more feasible to have individualized preventive measures to achieve optimal maternal and fetal outcomes (Feyta & Pyrohova, 2018). Lastly, it is necessary to encourage vaccination and screening procedures as part of preventive measures against genital infection. Vaccines such as the human papillomavirus (HPV) vaccine are significant in the prevention of infection that could develop into more severe health complications, including cervical cancer. Second, repeated screenings for sexually transmitted diseases (STDs) should be part of the public health program, particularly among sexually active adults below the age of 25 years or those with two or more sexual partners. These screenings can identify infection at an early stage before it becomes other serious medical conditions. Public health campaigns should advocate desensitization of these diseases and implore individuals to seek early medical care. By encouraging a prevention culture, awareness, and education, it is possible to substantially reduce the prevalence of urinary tract and genital infections (Hussein et al., 2014).

SUMMARY

Briefly, genital and urinary tract infections constitute major health issues with multifaceted approaches to understanding their etiology, presentation, and management. Careful assessment shows that these infections not only impact the quality of life in single patients but also have implications for public health. The development of resistance to antibiotics serves as a strong reminder for new therapeutic methods and the judicious application of existing antibiotics. These measures are of utmost importance considering that the delay in effective intervention leads to severe complications. Public health initiatives to educate populations on prevention and early detection need priority to minimize the incidence of such infections. The role of medical professionals cannot be overstated in dealing with urinary tract and genital infections. Routine screening and risk assessment interventions can help identify high-risk groups and appropriately inform interventions. Further, newer drugs like SGLT-2 inhibitors are an area of great interest, that is, their impact on infection rates. It has been seen that while SGLT-2 inhibitors have promise in diabetes control, they carry an increased risk of mycotic infections and thus proper patient management and observation are critical (Nathan et al., 2016). This concurrent balancing of effectiveness and potential side effects is emblematic of the difficulty of managing co-morbid diseases and reflective of the need for patient care strategies that aim for a more holistic approach. Ultimately, urinary tract and genital infections are going to demand different stakeholders — researchers, physicians, and public health professionals — work together. Future research must tackle the underlying mechanisms that predispose one to infection, as well as develop therapies that target with the least amount of side effects. Moreover, patient education initiatives targeting hygiene, sexual health, and preventive practices are essential to the control of infection rates. As the epidemiology of infectious disease evolves further, vigilant and responsive clinical practice and public health policy will be essential to minimizing the burden of genital and urinary tract infection (Hussein et al., 2014).

Recognition of the complexity of urinary and genital tract infections includes regard to their etiology, clinical features, and management. Causation of urinary tract infections (UTIs) is primarily by bacterial pathogens, with the most prevalent pathogen of community-acquired UTIs being *Escherichia coli*. Female gender, sexual practices, and certain kinds of anatomical abnormalities are risk factors for the susceptibility of subjects to these infections. Symptoms typically range from dysuria and frequency to more severe presentations such as flank pain or fever. The symptoms must be detected early in order to allow proper treatment to commence and subsequent complications such as pyelonephritis and recurrent infection do not ultimately affect a patient's quality of life. Treatment of genital and urinary infections involves a wide range of both pharmacological and non-pharmacological treatments. Antibiotic therapy is the treatment of choice, though the choice should be made on the basis of local resistance patterns and patient-specific issues. Minimally invasive surgery, such as the Perigee operation in anterior vaginal wall defects, has been found in more recent studies to reduce the incidence of recurrent urinary infection by repair of the anatomy (Gojevi et al., 2008). Besides, education on proper hygiene practice, fluid intake, and post-coital voiding can be significant in preventive steps. Knowledge about these factors can help patients manage their health better and avoid such infections. Apart from this, the consequences of urinary tract and genital infection are not just immediate pain; they may continue to have long-term effects on the person's overall health, such as fertility complications and recurrent pelvic pain. Notably, the fact that clinically significant residual fragments remain after treatment, specifically in stone management, signifies the necessity for strategic follow-up and individualized patient treatment (Rassweiler et al., 2001). Further research is required to create improved management protocols and maximize patient outcomes. By focusing on a multi-disciplinary approach that includes preventive care, early diagnosis, and effective treatment regimens, medical professionals are better equipped to address the problem of urinary tract and genital infections, ensuring improved patient health in these often-overlooked areas of care.

CLOSER LOOK

IMPORTANT TLRS (TOLL-LIKE RECEPTORS) IN UGTIS

Despite the presence of strong barriers made up of urothelial cells in human UGT, uropathogenic bacteria such as UPEC can cross the barriers. Upon the entry of UPEC in UGT, the innate immune responses are triggered by the generation of particular toll-like receptors (TLRs) within the urothelial cells of the bladder and kidneys. TLR expression initiates a cascade of many components of the immune system, like chemokines, interferons, interleukins, antimicrobial peptides, and proinflammatory cytokines. The innate immunity reacts because of the event of UPEC entry, attachment and invasion. The adhesion of the bacteria to the urothelial cells is achieved by the virulence factors of FimH adhesins situated at the tip of type I fimbriae. The adhesion of UPEC cells onto urothelium cells under normal circumstances results in TLRs expression, interleukin (IL-)6 secretion and the action of programmed cell death (apoptosis; genome fragmentation), whereby apoptosis can halt the invasion process of bacteria into the UT epithelial cells and serve as a mechanism of direct bacterial clearance. The UPEC cells are typically recognized by TLRs 4 and 5.

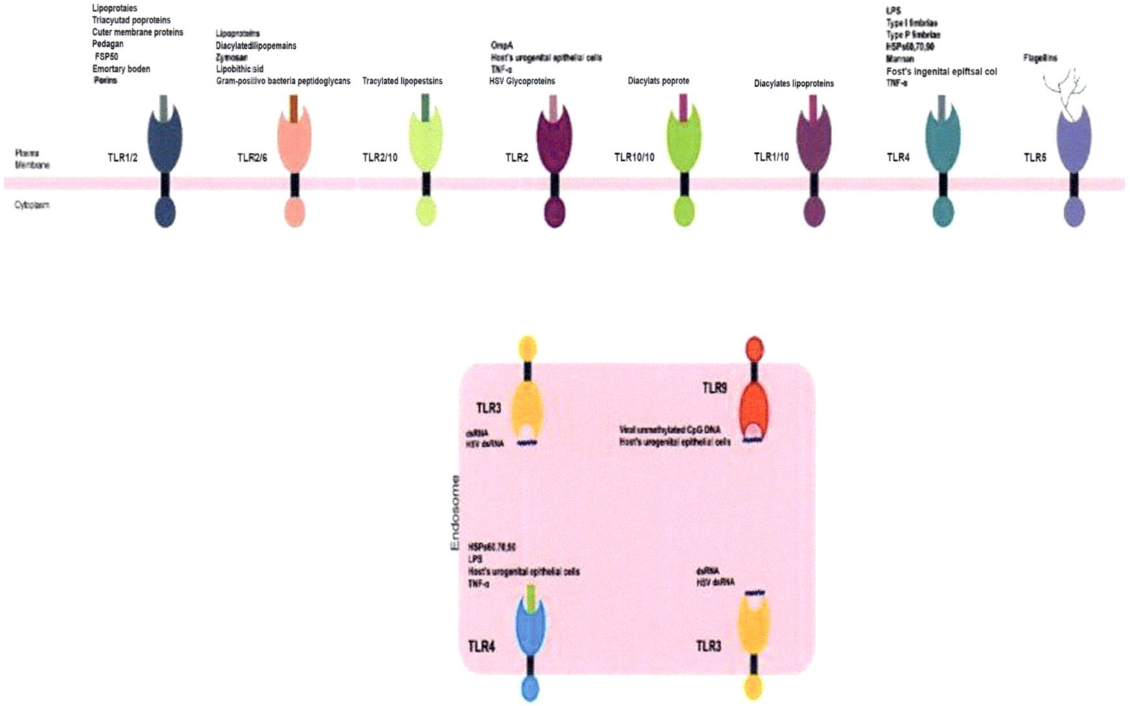

Figure 11.19. The situation, arrangement and relationship between pathogen-associated molecular patterns (PAMPs) and TLRs in UGTIs.

Source: https://pmc.ncbi.nlm.nih.gov/articles/PMC6449866/.

According to different surveys, the molecules of TLR4 are expressed by bladder and kidney urothelial cells, but the molecules of TLR5 are expressed by bladder urothelial cells. Bacterial lipopolysaccharides (LPS) or P fimbriae bind to CD14 and glycoprotein molecules (present on uroplakins/cell membrane of bladder and kidney urothelial cells), respectively, resulting in TLR4 expression, while bacterial flagella units (flagellins) induce TLR5 molecule expression in bladder urothelial cells. Activation of TLR4 may trigger IL-8 and IL-6 secretion. IL-8 and IL-6 cytokines contribute to neutrophil recruitment and secretion of mucosal antibody of IgA in situ, respectively. Apart from UPEC as a major microbial etiologic pathogen of UGTIs, fungi such as C. albicans are relevant pathogens responsible for causing UGTIs. Interestingly, C. albicans can stimulate the innate immune reactions by different types of TLRs, including TLR2/6 (zymosan) and TLR4 (neutrophil activation and mucosal IgA antibody secretion). The associations among microbial etiologic agents of UGTIs and TLRs are shown in Figure 11.19.

References

1. Green, Sioban O'Brien; Patel, Sudha; Nugent, Andrea Scharfe; Aboud, Kate; Basnet, Samjhana; Cuthill, Jane; et al. (2008): Female Genital Mutilation. Information for Health-Care Professionals Working in Ireland.. Royal College of Surgeons in Ireland. Report. https://doi.org/10.25419/rcsi.10788482.v1(accessed on 16th July 2025).
2. Adeghate, J., Juhász, E., Kristóf, K., Pongrácz, J., et al. (2016). *Does Staphylococcus saprophyticus cause acute cystitis only in young females, or is there more to the story? A one-year comprehensive study done in Budapest, Hungary*. https://core.ac.uk/download/50568914.pdf (accessed on 16th July 2025).
3. Nathan, K. T., Ahmed-Sarwar, N., & Werner, P. (2016). SGLT-2 Inhibitors: A Novel Mechanism in Targeting Glycemic Control in Type 2 Diabetes Mellitus. *The Consultant pharmacist : the journal of the American Society of Consultant Pharmacists*, *31*(5), 251–260. https://doi.org/10.4140/TCP.n.2016.260(accessed on 16th July 2025).
4. Ajani, O. O., & Nwinyi, O. (2010). *Identification, and clinical relevance of Gram–positive spore formers*. https://core.ac.uk/download/32224855.pdf (accessed on 16th July 2025).
5. Anderson, M., Bearden, R., Bekal, M., Bernat, S., Cao, D., Cerca, N., et al. (2009). *Antibiotherapy and pathogenesis of uncomplicated UTI: Difficult relationships*. https://core.ac.uk/download/55610177.pdf (accessed on 16th July 2025).
6. Ali, A.S.M., Mowbray, C., Lanz, M. *et al.* Targeting Deficiencies in the TLR5 Mediated Vaginal Response to Treat Female Recurrent Urinary Tract Infection. *Sci Rep* **7**, 11039 (2017). https://doi.org/10.1038/s41598-017-10445-4(accessed on 16th July 2025).
7. Legido-Quigley, H., Montgomery, C. M., Khan, P., Atun, R., Fakoya, A., Getahun, H., & Grant, A. D. (2013). Integrating tuberculosis and HIV services in low- and middle-income countries: a systematic review. *Tropical medicine & international health : TM & IH*, *18*(2), 199–211. https://doi.org/10.1111/tmi.12029(accessed on 16th July 2025).
8. Beveridge, L. A., Davey, P. G., McMurdo, M. E. T., Phillips, M., et al. (2011). *Optimal management of urinary tract infections in older people*. https://core.ac.uk/download/20450519.pdf (accessed on 16th July 2025).
9. Bonnici, J. J. (2014). *Urinary Tract Infections in the Community*. https://core.ac.uk/download/46603064.pdf (accessed on 16th July 2025).
10. Brons, J., de Vos, M., Halverson, T., Wolfe, M., et al. (2021). *The good and the bad: Ecological interaction measurements between the urinary microbiota and uropathogens*. https://core.ac.uk/download/519043799.pdf (accessed on 16th July 2025).
11. Busch, M., Carroll, T., Dutra, J., Fritts, L., et al. (2017). *Zika virus preferentially replicates in the female reproductive tract after vaginal inoculation of rhesus macaques*. https://core.ac.uk/download/323071269.pdf (accessed on 16th July 2025).
12. Cambieri, C., Ceccanti, M., Cervigni, M., Gori, A., et al. (2016). *Central Sensitization in the Bladder Pain Syndrome*. https://core.ac.uk/download/98348580.pdf (accessed on 16th July 2025).
13. Hussein, J., Ramani, K. V., Kanguru, L., Patel, K., Bell, J., Patel, P., Walker, L., Mehta, R., & Mavalankar, D. (2014). The effect of surveillance and appreciative inquiry on puerperal

infections: a longitudinal cohort study in India. *PloS one*, *9*(1), e87378. https://doi.org/10.1371/journal.pone.0087378(accessed on 16th July 2025).

14. Rassweiler, J. J., Renner, C., Chaussy, C., & Thüroff, S. (2001). Treatment of renal stones by extracorporeal shockwave lithotripsy: an update. *European urology*, *39*(2), 187–199. https://doi.org/10.1159/000052435(accessed on 16th July 2025).
15. Clar, C., Court, R. A., Gill, J. A., Waugh, N., et al. (2012). *Systematic review of SGLT2 receptor inhibitors in dual or triple therapy in type 2 diabetes*. https://core.ac.uk/download/9561752.pdf (accessed on 16th July 2025).
16. Derbigny, W. A., & Kumar, R. (2019). *TLR3 deficiency leads to a dysregulation in the global gene-expression profile in murine oviduct epithelial cells infected with Chlamydia muridarum*. https://core.ac.uk/download/227054227.pdf (accessed on 16th July 2025).
17. Różalski, A., Torzewska, A., Moryl, M., Kwil, I., Maszewska, A., Ostrowska, K., ... Stączek, P. (2012). Proteus sp. – an opportunistic bacterial pathogen – classification, swarming growth, clinical significance and virulence factors. *Acta Universitatis Lodziensis. Folia Biologica Et Oecologica*, *8*, 1–17. https://doi.org/10.2478/fobio-2013-0001 (accessed on 16th July 2025).
18. El Sayied, H., Hemida, S., Mohamed, H., Ragheb, A., et al. (2021). *Effect of Web Causation Epidemiological Model on preventive behaviors of diabetic females with genitourinary tract infection*. https://core.ac.uk/download/524771923.pdf (accessed on 16th July 2025).
19. Expósito Ruiz, M., Gutiérrez Fernández, J., Gutiérrez-Soto, M., Navarro Marí, J., et al. (2023). *Presence and relevance of emerging microorganisms in clinical genitourinary samples*. https://core.ac.uk/download/574719676.pdf (accessed on 16th July 2025).
20. Smith, M. L., Farkas, D. K., Sumner, J. A., Jiang, T., Lash, T. L., Galea, S., Sørensen, H. T., & Gradus, J. L. (2020). Associations between adjustment disorder and hospital-based infections in the Danish population. *Journal of psychosomatic research*, *132*, 109976. https://doi.org/10.1016/j.jpsychores.2020.109976(accessed on 16th July 2025).
21. Feyta, Y., & Pyrohova, V. (2018). ASSESSMENT OF RISK FACTORS OF SEPTIC COMPLICATIONS OF THE PUERPERIUM. *EUREKA: Health Sciences*, (3), 29-38. https://doi.org/10.21303/2504-5679.2018.00627(accessed on 16th July 2025).
22. Ghouri, F., Hollywood, A., & Ryan, K. (2018). A systematic review of non-antibiotic measures for the prevention of urinary tract infections in pregnancy. *BMC pregnancy and childbirth*, *18*(1), 99. https://doi.org/10.1186/s12884-018-1732-2(accessed on 16th July 2025).
23. Gojević, A., Kalafatić, D., Lovrić, H., Banović, M., Orešković, S., Župić, T. (2008). *Korekcija cistokele sintetskom mrežicom transobturatornim pristupom (PERIGEE sistem)*. https://core.ac.uk/download/14396416.pdf (accessed on 16th July 2025).
24. Hamid, R., & Losco, G. (2014). *Pelvic organ prolapse-associated cystitis*. https://core.ac.uk/download/29410932.pdf (accessed on 16th July 2025).
25. Nader-Macías, M. E., & Juárez Tomás, M. S. (2015). Profiles and technological requirements of urogenital probiotics. *Advanced drug delivery reviews*, *92*, 84–104. https://doi.org/10.1016/j.addr.2015.03.016(accessed on 16th July 2025).
26. Mendez, O. (2022). *Increasing knowledge of sexually transmitted infections in sexually active females reporting symptoms of UTIs at walk-in clinics: A quality improvement project*. https://core.ac.uk/download/548485968.pdf (accessed on 16th July 2025).

27. Munson, E., Munson, K. L., & Napierala, M. (2016). *Update on laboratory diagnosis and epidemiology of Trichomonas vaginalis: You can teach an "old" dog "new" trichs.* https://core.ac.uk/download/213085579.pdf (accessed on 16th July 2025).

28. Nori, A. V., Copas, A. J., Apoola, A., Bowie, C., Bradshaw, T., Broeren, J., Dupin, N., et al. (2015). *Performance evaluation of automated urine microscopy as a rapid, non-invasive approach for the diagnosis of non-gonococcal urethritis.* https://core.ac.uk/download/46166140.pdf (accessed on 16th July 2025).

29. Redelinghuys, M. J. (2014). *The association between genital mycoplasmas and bacterial vaginosis in pregnant women with or without genital symptoms.* https://core.ac.uk/download/528274327.pdf (accessed on 16th July 2025).

30. Shen, D. (2017). *Prevention of Serious Infections During Pregnancy.* https://core.ac.uk/download/161420459.pdf (accessed on 16th July 2025).

31. Martins, N., Ferreira, I. C., Barros, L., Silva, S., & Henriques, M. (2014). Candidiasis: predisposing factors, prevention, diagnosis and alternative treatment. *Mycopathologia, 177*(5-6), 223–240. https://doi.org/10.1007/s11046-014-9749-1(accessed on 16th July 2025).

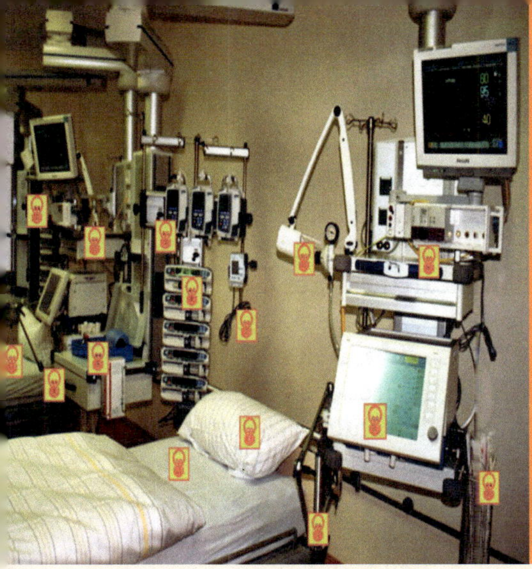

Chapter 12

HOSPITAL-ACQUIRED INFECTIONS (HAIS) AND INFECTION CONTROL

Contents

Introduction

Hospital-acquired infection cases have emerged as a cause of major concern in the healthcare sector, drawing attention from public health professionals, practitioners, and researchers alike. The infections, which are contracted by patients during treatment for other conditions, illustrate the complexities of patient safety care in various healthcare settings. HAIs impact millions of patients annually, and they add morbidity, mortality, and expenses to healthcare systems. The difficulty of managing these infections is further compounded by the development of antimicrobial resistance, thereby elevating the need for prevention and control even more. Understanding how HAIs are transmitted is indispensable to designing effective interventions and maintaining high standards of patient safety. Given the invariable issues associated with HAIs, extensive research into their causes, implications, and measures of control is essential. In addition, the role played by environmental determinants in sustaining HAIs cannot be overlooked. Hospital settings serve as reservoirs of pathogens due to a range of factors, including the presence of vulnerable patient populations and ineffective infection control measures. Proper cleaning and disinfection protocols are essential to minimizing the hazards of unclean surfaces and medical devices. Consistent with contemporary literature, proper hand hygiene protocol and disinfection practices have been vital for the prevention of HAIs in healthcare facilities. Suggestions range from frequent washing with soap and water to the use of alcohol-based disinfectants, with plain emphasis on adherence to the set protocols. Knowing the various methods practiced in infection control is, hence, of the utmost significance in developing comprehensive approaches against HAIs and ensuring patient safety. The dynamic nature of HAIs necessitates continuous research and development in the area of infection control. Modern approaches, as suggested by the Technology Strategy Board (TSB) and Department of Health (DH), are bringing attention to the application of advanced diagnostic tests for detecting HAIs effectively. Research on high-priority issues, including Methicillin-resistant *Staphylococcus aureus* (MRSA) and *Clostridium difficile*, demonstrates the economic value of point-of-care testing for early intervention and control. These advances not only contribute to current knowledge but also facilitate areas of practice and economics of new technology gaps to be identified. As healthcare facilities strive to reduce the incidence of HAIs, adopting a multi-faceted approach with extensive research, improved diagnostic methods, and efficient infection control measures becomes the hour of need in safeguarding patient health as well as ensuring the best healthcare outcomes.

Definition of Hospital-Acquired Infections (HAIs)

HAIs are a significant concern in healthcare facilities, as they refer to infections that a patient contracts during their stay in the hospital or healthcare facility, which were not present or incubating at admission. This definition encompasses a variety of infections, including urinary tract infection, surgical site infection, and bloodstream infection. The presence of HAIs emphasizes the need for sound infection control practices. For instance, the Scottish national point prevalence survey reported 9.5% of acute hospital patients had healthcare-associated infection, the most common presentations being urinary tract and surgical site infection (Reilly et al., 2008). Not only do these figures indicate prevalence, but also the intricacy of the impact they have upon patient health, an understanding that in turn necessitates the development of holistic strategies towards their prevention and management. The implications of HAIs are not only confined to the direct health consequences on the patients. They are prime drivers for increased morbidity and mortality rates, with a colossal financial cost to the healthcare systems. Control of HAIs is generally accompanied by longer hospital stays, additional diagnostic tests, and increased use of antibiotics, all of which contribute to the rising cost of healthcare provision. Moreover, HAIs are the primary force behind antimicrobial resistance, which complicates treatment and presents a challenge for public health initiatives (Protano et al., 2019). The complexity of HAIs and their relationship with healthcare economics highlights the critical significance of effective infection control practices in hospitals. Effective infection control practices are critical not only in maintaining patient health but also in the sustainability of healthcare resources. Active infection control is essential in the effective management of HAIs. Adoption of rigorous cleaning and disinfection policies, as well as rigorous hand hygiene measures, are some of the basic measures of infection prevention. Studies indicate that adoption of measures, known as bundles, applied together can reduce HAI incidents by a significant degree (Protano et al., 2019). Furthermore, the classification of medical devices according to their risk of transmitting infection informs suitable sterilization processes, thereby maximizing safety measures. The implementation of these strategies in hospitals is essential, as such facilities may be reservoirs of the pathogens that cause HAIs. Therefore, an integrated strategy focusing on prevention and education among healthcare staff is the priority in reducing hospital-acquired infection prevalence, ultimately improving patient outcomes and maintaining public health standards (Figure 12.1).

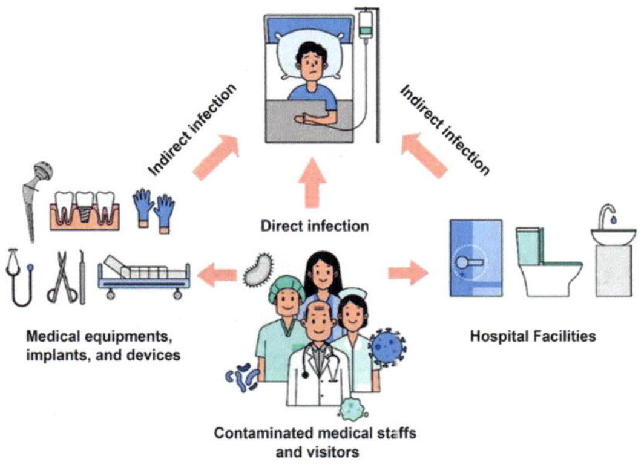

Figure 12.1. Schematic illustration of transmission routes of hospital-acquired infections (HAI) or nosocomial infection.

Source: https://www.researchgate.net/publication/360825411/figure/fig1/AS:11431281360750071@1744104123867/Schematic-illustration-of-transmission-routes-of-hospital-acquired-infections-HAI-or.png.

Importance of Addressing HAIs in Healthcare Settings

The incidence of HAIs is a significant challenge to healthcare systems, and thus, the need for effective reporting and communication mechanisms is imperative. Ensuring a safety culture in healthcare settings, as emphasized by the European Federation of Nurses Associations, is paramount in addressing HAIs. The culture of safety entails on-the-spot reporting of errors, exchange of best practices, and mutual dissemination of research findings. By promoting open communication among healthcare professionals, organizations are able to identify patterns and mitigate threats of HAIs. Moreover, enhanced knowledge through education and training supports this culture, holding all members of staff accountable for infection prevention. Such programs not only improve patient safety but also facilitate a reduction in healthcare costs associated with prolonged in-hospital stays and inappropriate treatments of HAIs, thus having a positive impact on overall community health outcomes (Smith et al., 2008). The solution to the issue of HAIs is not only crucial for patient safety but also has important implications for HCWs themselves. It has been proven that HCWs are most likely to get infected with infections through occupational exposure, especially in blood and other body fluids. Tanzania-based research highlights the danger of HIV transmission owing to needle stick injury, evoking the need for effective prevention measures in health settings (Kilale et al., 2013). However, inadequate guidelines and the absence of good health and safety instructions add to the problems further for HCWs. To address this, healthcare facilities must emphasize rigorous training in infection control practices, as well as the provision of personal protective equipment (PPE). Proper provision of resources to HCWs not only protects their health but also aids in making the environment safer for patients, which ultimately minimizes HAIs. With the multifaceted complexity of HAIs, adherence to standard infection control practices is critical. Comprehensive practices — ranging from strict hand hygiene methods to strict sterilization methods — must be present in all healthcare institutions. The incorporation of best practices of successful European practices also underscores the imperative for evidence-based interventions in combating HAIs. As well, systematic collection and review of infection data allow for the introduction of targeted interventions and continuous improvement in infection control measures. Having those measures in place does require healthcare leaders to commit to generating adequate resources for training and compliance monitoring. By prioritizing HAIP prevention through structured and highly intellectualized infection control measures, healthcare organizations can significantly maximize patient safety, reduce healthcare-associated costs, and cultivate a culture of health and safety among patients and providers (Smith et al., 2008) (Figure 12.2).

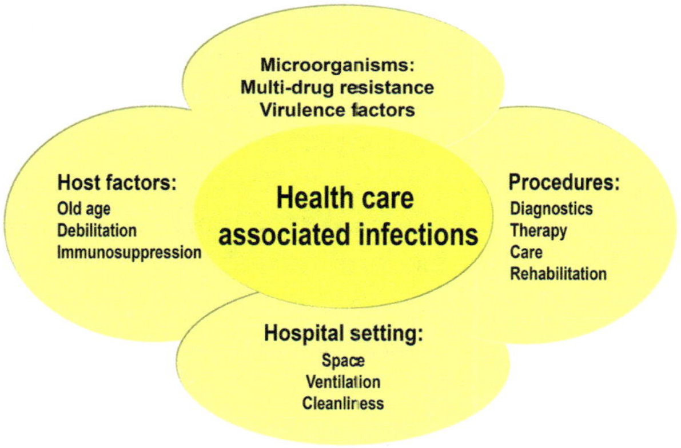

Figure 12.2. Factors determining healthcare-associated infections.

Source: https://www.researchgate.net/profile/Hans-Kolmos/publication/221925213/figure/fig4/AS:668677443690514@1536436534912/Factors-determining-health-care-associated-infections.png.

12.1. Types of Hospital-Acquired Infections

Among the various types of HAIs, urinary tract infections (UTIs) are most prevalent. The infections often occur as a consequence of catheterization, where catheters are inserted into the urinary tract offering access for microorganisms. According to research, UTIs account for approximately 17.9% of total HAIs in acute hospital patients, and this highlights the significance of monitoring catheter insertion and patient hygiene as a measure against such occurrences. The availability of fundamental preventive factors, including the implementation of aseptic practices, can significantly reduce UTI incidents. Furthermore, enhanced training and sensitization of healthcare workers are necessary since catheter handling mistakes cause increased infection rates, contributing to patient suffering as well as healthcare costs. Hence, studying some HAIs, especially UTIs, is crucial in the development of robust infection control regulations in healthcare institutions (Bocicor et al., 2016). Surgical site infections (SSIs) form another significant category of HAIs with serious patient outcomes. They can be acquired post-operatively, and usually, it is as a result of surgical process contamination; they contribute to about 15.9% of HAIs in the hospital environment. SSIs can be caused by the patient's pre-existing medical condition, the skill used in surgery, and the observance of sterile procedure. The impact of SSIs on managing hospitals is immense because, in addition to raising mortality rates, they increase hospital stays and healthcare costs. For instance, the meticulousness regarding surgical sterilization and the preventive application of antibiotics before, during, and after surgical procedures can be programmed in clinical processes to minimize the occurrence of SSIs.

The embedding of such factors improves the safety of the patient and reduces the aggregate hospital burden of HAIs (Bocicor et al., 2016). Gastrointestinal infections are another type of HAIs, and they are caused by several environmental and procedural factors that compromise the health of the patient in hospitals. They account for 15.4% of all hospital-acquired infections. The mechanisms of infection for such infections usually involve transmission of pathogens through contaminated food, water supply, or improper sanitation by healthcare workers. Hospitals can prevent the development of gastrointestinal infections by adhering to strict infection prevention practices such as frequent hand washing, disinfection of medical instruments, and monitoring of food safety in hospital kitchens. The infection disproportionately risks individuals who belong to susceptible groups, such as the aged or those with weakened immune systems, as revealed by a national survey. This underscores the necessity for precise infection control practices that match the distinct needs of diverse patient populations and promote a culture of safety among healthcare facilities (Reilly et al., 2008).

12.1.1. Surgical Site Infections (SSIs)

Surgical site infections (SSIs) are a predominant issue within the larger context of HAIs. SSIs not only contribute to the duration of hospital stay but also contribute to the incidence of morbidity and mortality among surgical patients. Pathogenesis of SSIs is usually multifactorial with interactions between patient, environmental, and surgical factors. For instance, patient comorbidities, nutritional status, and the presence of foreign material such as sutures and implants play a huge role in the development of SSIs. Additionally, surgical timing and sterilization are also of crucial importance to minimize SSIs. Adequate infection control procedures must address all these determinants in an organized manner in order to prevent the development of SSIs in the hospital, keeping in mind better patient outcomes and reduced healthcare costs. One component of foundation strategies in SSI management is the integration of detailed Infection Control Risk Assessments (ICRAs). According to recent research, the highest risk assessment among HAIs is surgical site infections, hence the important target of infection control measures within healthcare organizations (Rosa et al., 2019). This degree of specificity entails identification and questioning of possible risks associated with various surgical procedures. By stopping the chain of transmission of harmful microorganisms, health care providers can significantly reduce of SSI rates. Rational antibiotic regimens, for instance, have been demonstrated to reduce risks of bacterial infection among patients undergoing surgery. Additionally, ongoing monitoring and periodic review of infection control measures can underpin the effectiveness of prevention measures, ultimately leading to a safety culture in operating rooms. In addition to the enforcement of prophylactic precautions against SSIs, specialized teams and evidence-based practice significantly enhance infection control. Dedicated teams for the management of surgical procedures can ensure strict adherence to infection control practices, as seen in successful practices for the reduction of central line-associated bloodstream infections (Reilly et al., 2008). They can assist in tracking infection rates, sharing best practices, and providing feedback to continuously improve. Secondly, engaging surgical staff in collaborative measures encourages active infection prevention behavior. Systematic training, communication, and adherence to protocol-based care can optimize patient care and even decrease the inherent risks of surgical procedures further. Finally, addressing SSIs in HAIs and infection control environments yields a safe healthcare environment for enhanced patient safety and treatment outcomes (Figure 12.3).

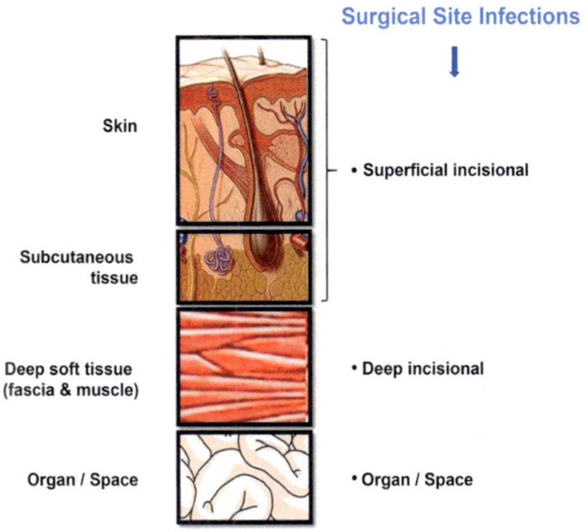

Figure 12.3. Anatomy of surgical site infections and their classification.

Source: https://www.researchgate.net/publication/339826667/figure/fig1/AS:873756780138498@1585331258606/Anatomy-of-surgical-site-infections-and-their-classification-adapted-from-CDC-1.jpg.

12.1.2. Catheter-Associated Urinary Tract Infections (CAUTIs)

Catheter-associated urinary tract infections (CAUTIs) are a serious issue in the hospital-acquired infection (HAI) continuum. With the Centers for Disease Control and Prevention (CDC) projecting that CAUTIs affect approximately 40% of all HAIs in the United States, the prevalence of the condition makes it essential to have effective infection control procedures. Indwelling catheters, employed for myriad clinical indications, by default become a route for pathogens with improper insertion or management. Due to CAUTIs' likelihood of causing increased length of stay and patient morbidity, it becomes crucial for healthcare organizations to put extra importance on education and adherence to predetermined guidelines to avoid such risks. Acquiring knowledge on determinants of CAUTI occurrence necessitates an interventional response encompassing clinician training, patient education, and stringent infection control policies to allow for efficacious management within healthcare settings (Ali, 2018).

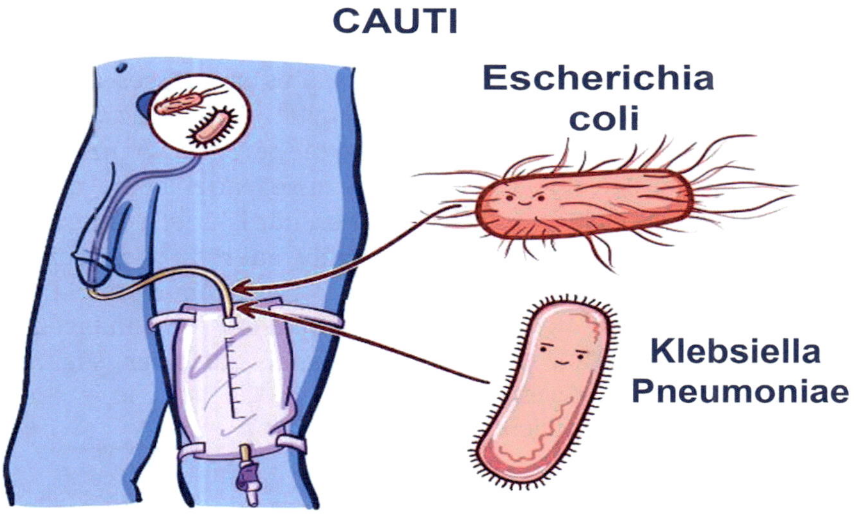

Figure 12.4. Catheter-associated urinary tract infections (CAUTIs).

Source: https://www.osmosis.org/_next/image?url=https%3A%2F%2Fd16qt3wv6xm098.cloudfront.net%2FyEaRWOZiRtudrdVBOW9jevhiSQKLgu2j%2F_.jpg&w=3840&q=75.

To effectively curb the incidence of CAUTIs meaningfully, evidence-based practices (EBPs) need to be implemented, encompassing preventive and response measures. A major determinant in this system is the Post Foley Removal Guideline (PFRG), which aims to reduce unnecessary catheter reinsertion that raises the risk of infection. Research indicates that CAUTIs are preventable in the majority of cases, and the length of use and time of catheter insertion are significant risk factors. Thus, the application of organizational systems that support the dissemination of EBPs in any clinical setting can significantly enhance the quality of care. Interventions to ensure compliance with the guidelines, coupled with comprehensive training of nursing staff on the care of catheters, have been effective in lowering CAUTI rates markedly. By prioritizing these interventions above everything else, hospitals are able to enhance patient safety and global healthcare outcomes (Gabbard, 2016). A study of the impact of organized interventions on the incidence of CAUTIs reveals the power of infection control measures. An education project aimed at reducing the incidence of CAUTIs reported that targeted educational interventions for nurses resulted in spectacular reductions in infections. With the implementation of a CAUTI maintenance tool and associated training of the staff, CAUTI reports decreased appreciably, reflecting the power of education in transforming clinical practices. These findings also suggest the necessity to empower nursing personnel in understanding the complexity that goes into the use of indwelling catheters and the associated risks. This educational approach not only encourages a safety culture within healthcare facilities but ultimately contributes towards bettering the quality of patient care, reducing hospitalization, and enhancing patients' overall quality of life. Therefore, improving the knowledge base of healthcare professionals is a critical component in the prevention of CAUTIs and in improving infection control measures (Ali, 2018) (Figure 12.4).

12.1.3. Ventilator-Associated Pneumonia (VAP)

Ventilator-associated pneumonia (VAP) is a serious complication in mechanically ventilated patients, particularly that of hospital-acquired infection (HAI). Pneumonia more than 48 hours after mechanical ventilation characterizes VAP, and this is typically due to the aspiration of the pathogens from the oropharynx or stomach. Multifactorial risk factors are mechanical ventilation for an extended duration, the use of endotracheal tubes, and patient immobility. Moreover, the immunocompromised status of most patients undergoing ventilation puts them at risk of bacterial colonization and infection. VAP prevention is not just crucial for maximizing patient outcomes but also for minimizing the overall burden of HAIs in healthcare institutions, thus depicting the significance of strict infection control practices targeted at this high-risk population. Effective prevention methods for VAP are evidence-based practice choices that aim to provide airway cleanliness and reduce exposure to pathogens. Implementation of systematic processes — designed from synergistic research — has proven helpful in fighting back against this infection. Semi-upright positioning during mechanical ventilation, for instance, can help significantly reduce the risk of aspiration, while oral care is essential for avoiding bacterial colonization. In addition, pathophysiologic knowledge is the basis for the need for aggressive suctioning regimens and strict use of antibiotics to maintain respiratory tract integrity.

The use of specialized teams to track protocol adherence demonstrates the degree to which VAP occurrence may be reduced considerably by establishing accountability among healthcare personnel for infection control practices (Reilly et al., 2008). Second, there is a lack of recognition of the role of ongoing education among nursing and medical staff in prevention against VAP, which is most essential for ongoing infection prevention. As observed in the majority of healthcare institutions, patient safety interventions are expanding, indicating the significance of experiential training paradigms for procedural error reduction involved in the etiology of VAP. Methods like simulation-based training have been promising towards establishing the expertise of healthcare workers, thereby reducing rates of VAP. Specific goal-based evidence-based practices and compliance with best practices make cultures that safeguard the patient. By collaborative effort and adherence to ongoing education, health care centers can alter their approach, ultimately minimize VAP occurrence and improve patient morbidity and mortality (McCarthy et al., 2011). This comprehensive adherence to infection prevention benefits not only individual patient care but also overall hospital-acquired infection reduction (Figure 12.5).

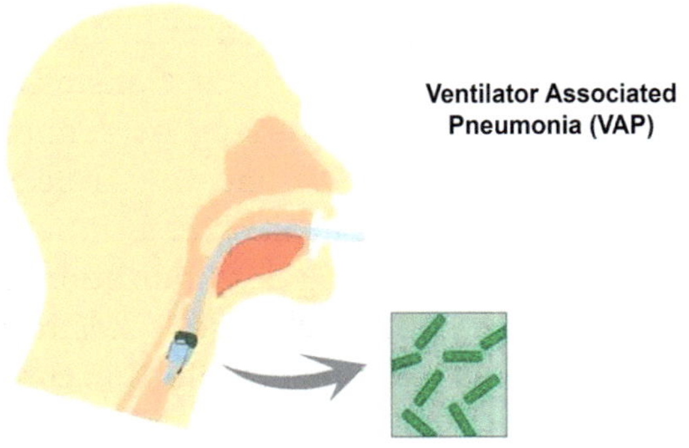

Figure 12.5. Ventilator-associated pneumonia (VAP).

Source: https://stgaccinwbsdevlrs01.blob.core.windows.net/newcorporatewbsite/blogs/June2024/2dQb3MjKXmtujgKSkoY5.webp.

12.2. Causes and Risk Factors

HAIs pose a great health problem in healthcare facilities, mostly because of their diverse causes and risk factors. Colonization of patients by pathogenic microorganisms during hospital stay is one of the major causes of HAIs. Patients could be admitted to hospitals with their own infections or colonization of soft tissues, making it easier for infectious agents to be spread. Furthermore, the invasive procedures performed on the patients, such as the intravenous catheter placement or operative procedures, subject them to greater risk by allowing the pathogens direct entry into sterile sites. Thus, understanding these pathways highlights the imperative need for proper infection control methods in hospital settings to ensure that healthcare workers consider exhaustive sterilization and cleanliness processes as prerequisites of patient safety, as advocated by the European Federation of Nurses Associations while establishing a culture of safety for averting medication errors and HAIs (Smith et al., 2008). Also adding to HAIs are risk factors that extend beyond the individual patient's characteristics to environmental and process factors within health care facilities. The presence of multi-drug-resistant organisms, as enhanced by the abuse of antibiotics and ineffective sterilization, presents a challenging environment in which to battle infections. People with compromised immune systems, either due to underlying health conditions or prolonged periods of hospitalization, are greatly at risk of contracting HAIs. The increasing healthcare spending attributable to HAIs, as reported in various studies, supports the significance of maintaining an organized infection prevention strategy.

The techniques employed to estimate excess LOS attributable to HAIs also indicate the rising cost burden for healthcare systems over the years, illustrating the essence of accurate measures in informing the efficient allocation of resources and improving patient outcomes (Giraldi et al., 2019). Lastly, infection prevention strategies and staff awareness remain a top priority in minimizing HAIs. Educational sessions that foster a culture of vigilant awareness among health workers can have a significant influence on the incidence of these infections. Encouragement by organizations of continuous education and bundle creation of best practices can enhance the capacity of healthcare workers to detect and respond to possible threats to infection. In addition, encouraging an open reporting culture for errors or near misses by healthcare professionals in a safe manner, free from intimidation, is essential in improving patient safety. This is according to the guidelines given by the EFN for creating highly reliable organizations that recognize safety as a priority value in the provision of care (Smith et al., 2008). By addressing both system and individual risk factors, hospitals can decrease HAIs to a great extent and promote a healthier setting for all patients.

12.2.1. Patient-Related Factors (e.g., Age, Comorbidities)

The effect of factors related to the patient, primarily age and comorbidities, is a key factor in the etiology of HAIs. As age advances, the immune status of the patients deteriorates, decreasing their infection-fighting capabilities and increasing their susceptibility to infection by a variety of etiologic agents. Older patients often have some comorbid conditions, such as diabetes, chronic respiratory diseases, and heart disease, which complicate treatment and increase the risk of HAIs. This age demographic trend creates a need for healthcare providers to have a comprehensive understanding of older adults, because they can benefit from specific infection control interventions to ward off risks of long-term hospital stay and heightened susceptibility to infection. As such, the combination of advancing age and comorbidities can become a recipe for disaster regarding the development of adverse consequences from HAIs, thus increasing total patient morbidity and healthcare expenditure.

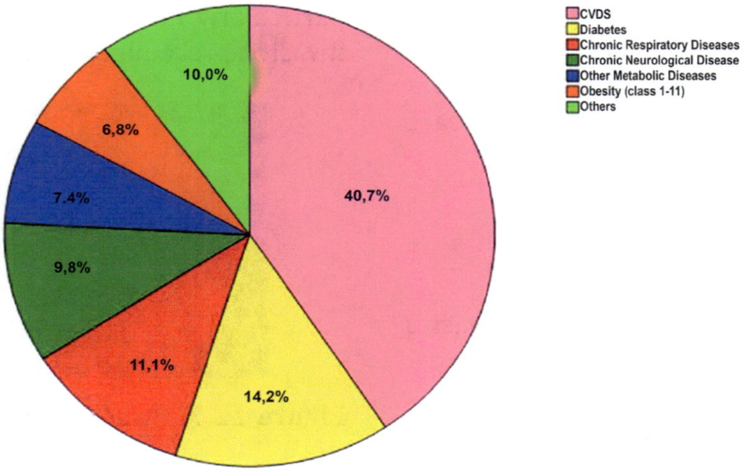

Figure 12.6. Proportions of comorbidities of patients. The pie chart shows the proportion of each comorbidity among the total of 2295 comorbidities recorded in the study population.

Source: https://www.researchgate.net/publication/372196752/figure/fig3/AS:11431281176627579@1690215230784/Proportions-of-comorbidities-of-patients-included-in-the-study-The-pie-chart-shows-the.png.

Further, inpatient comorbidities can exacerbate the risk of HAIs. Those with complex medical histories are likely to be hospitalized for extended periods due to resultant complications of their original conditions. Comorbidities are also linked with a higher prevalence of invasive procedures, such as catheterizations and surgery, which are risk factors for opportunistic infection. As highlighted by the literature, patient complexity and longer length of stay are some of the primary determinants in understanding the interactions in HAIs in healthcare settings (Hauck & Zhao, 2010). Such harmful interactions of patient health status and hospital setting only tend to accentuate the need for comprehensive infection control measures specially designed to mitigate comorbid patient vulnerabilities. To these, historical antimicrobial use can continue to complicate the HAIs' situation. The administration of antibiotics, while required for curing the infection at hand, may also unconsciously help in the process of resistance in bacterial populations, particularly in patients with complex infections. Existing literature indicates that past antimicrobials can make significant impacts on the susceptibility levels of ensuing isolates, thus undermining the effectiveness of empirical treatment policies (Wong et al., 2015). This positive feedback cycle of infection and resistance necessitates added caution among health workers regarding proper medication management, especially among vulnerable patient populations. Therefore, awareness of these patient factors becomes an important factor while formulating efficient infection control policies to reduce the incidence of HAIs, hence resulting in improved patient outcomes and preservation of healthcare resources (Figure 12.6).

12.2.2. Healthcare-Related Factors (e.g., Invasive Procedures)

The medical environment involves some invasive interventions that contribute significantly to the development of HAIs. Surgery, catheterization, and intravenous line placement, though often unavoidable in in-patient care, provide a clear pathway for the introduction of pathogens into the body. Once introduced into the sterile environments, microorganisms can proliferate and present as complications such as surgical site infection or bloodstream infection. Studies have indicated that a majority of infections attributable to these invasive procedures are caused by multi-resistant organisms, particularly in the case of patients with previous exposure history to healthcare facilities. This raises the need for continued measurement of infection rates and implementation of rigorous infection control measures unique to certain procedures to mitigate the risks of HAIs (Ceccarelli et al., 2015). In hospital settings, inappropriate and excessive use of antibiotics, particularly in patients who are undergoing invasive procedures, can exacerbate the problem of resistant infection. The emergence of multi-drug-resistant organisms poses a serious risk because empirical treatment with an antibiotic may fail, leading to treatment failure, longer hospital stay times, and increased mortality. For example, a study highlighted that empirical therapy was largely not appropriate for infections that occur in the hospital, indicating a glaring need for better diagnostic practice that enables the pathogen and its drug resistance profile to be established in due time. It emphasizes the importance of antibiotic stewardship programs that educate healthcare workers in proper and responsible administration of antibiotics, particularly in the case of infections following invasive procedures (Ceccarelli et al., 2015).

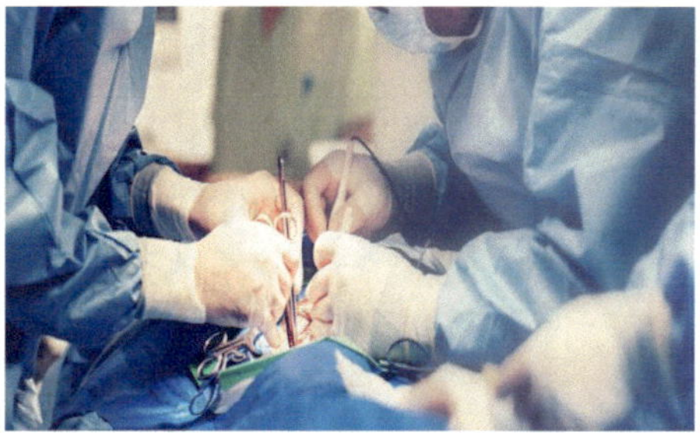

Figure 12.7. Invasive procedure.

Source: https://yashojyotfetalmedicine.com/wp-content/uploads/2020/10/AdgDr8BJ2L-768x342.jpg.

Moreover, education and training of health professionals also play a central role in the prevention from invasive procedures. The implementation of extensive educational interventions is able to significantly improve infection control practice adherence and therefore reduce the incidence of HAIs. For instance, specific training programs that combine motivation and application strategies have been found to strengthen hygiene and precautionary protocols compliance and preventive methods among healthcare professionals. These actions align with the ongoing need for hospitals to develop a safety culture and an attitude of responsibility in infection prevention. Ultimately, an accountable healthcare workforce with the knowledge and skills to prevent HAIs, most notably those that accompany invasive medical procedures, is essential to effective risk management (Figure 12.7).

12.2.3. Environmental Factors (e.g., Hospital Cleanliness)

The relationship between environmental circumstances, particularly hospital hygiene, and the occurrence of HAIs is a significant area of concern for infection control. The evidence suggests that high cleanliness standards in healthcare settings are crucial to minimizing the risk of HAIs. Hospitals with rigorous cleaning practices demonstrate lower infection rates, a situation with which there is a growing evidence base to emphasize the importance of cleanliness of the environment. However, a key deficiency exists within the assessment of cleanliness through current performance measures because visual examination is unsatisfactory. The application of such subjective observations does not provide an accurate portrayal of hospital environments. Therefore, it is necessary that health centers adopt more objective methods of verification, such as cleaning, to ensure that measures for infection control are in fact effective, as suggested in the review by May & Pitt. (2012). Secondly, public impression about cleanliness in health organizations cannot be underestimated. Individuals in the general population associate cleanliness with safety, and this factor plays a huge role in their trust in health centers. Recurring worries regarding hygienic standards may make patients avoid proper medical care, thereby worsening their health situations. Surprisingly enough, even though places in public use — public transport, for example — are usually viewed as being unhygienic, studies show that the actual risk of contracting pathogens in public spaces might be overestimated (Bernard et al., 2014). This discrepancy between expectation and experience underscores the need for hospitals not just to succeed in cleanliness but also to publicize their initiative to society. Educating employees as well as patients regarding the stringent cleaning protocol and its impact on infection prevention is a measure that can contribute to the general hospital's safety perception. Finally, hospital hygiene cannot be addressed institutionally alone; it also requires a coordination of efforts from all stakeholders, including clinical personnel and facility management. Facilities often underestimate the complex, multi-faceted nature of the environmental cleaning-infection control relationship, as per existing literature. For instance, while clinicians are aware of the significance of cleansing procedures, there is still an immediate need for official alignment with facility management staff to ensure harmonized cleansing procedures and infection prevention policies.

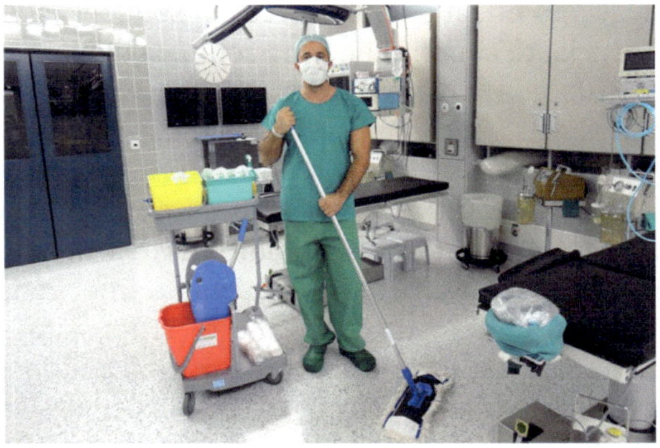

Figure 12.8. Cleanliness and hygiene in hospitals.

Source: https://miro.medium.com/v2/resize:fit:780/1*4qsj6eFGPxxjJDFDhDMcrA.jpeg.

As indicated by the findings of May & Pitt (2012), technological interventions that produce measurable knowledge on cleansing routines can foster harmonization and enhance overall infection control processes. By instituting a culture where cleanliness is emphasized and made a cornerstone of patient safety, hospitals will be able to further decrease rates of HAIs and improve patient outcomes (Figure 12.8).

12.3. Impact of HAIs on Patient Outcomes

The impact of HAIs on patient outcomes is widespread and far-reaching, having a major effect on both the health and economic consequences of healthcare systems. HAIs are the cause of increased morbidity and mortality in patients in hospitals, as populations that are at risk, such as the elderly or those with comorbidities, are the most susceptible to HAIs. The price tag for HAIs extends to influencing patients' well-being, with additional hospital days that can contribute to an estimated 90% of total HAIs costs (Giraldi et al., 2019). Thus, the need for effective infection controls is pivotal to offset such adverse consequences. It is crucial to comprehend the complex dynamics of HAIs and patient health for the purpose of designing targeted interventions that potentially enhance patient safety and overall quality of care. In addition to health impact, HAIs impose a significant economic burden on the healthcare system. Hospital-acquired infections result in additional costs due to longer stays in the hospital, additional treatments, and lost productivity due to prolonged recovery times. As indeed in the case of the National Health Service (NHS), these infections exact great economic costs not just on healthcare facilities but also on patients and society in general (Stewart et al., 2019). To the patient, these costs are added to the charge of out-of-pocket payments for further medical treatment. Moreover, the psychological effect of acquiring an HAI can manifest as diminished quality of life and increased fear of future hospitalization. Thus, the economic cost of HAIs warrants widespread acknowledgment of their impact on outcomes and the call for aggressive infection control. The measurement of HAI-related outcomes underscores the imperative for continued research and infection control practice development. Studies, such as the Evaluation of Cost of Nosocomial Infection study (ECONI), attempt to provide meaningful data regarding HAI incidence rate, costs, and broader impacts on patient health (Stewart et al., 2019). If researchers examine how patients who acquire HAIs fare in comparison to non-infected patients, it is easier for them to identify risk factors and construct stronger prevention strategies. Understanding these dynamics is essential to inform infection control practices and policies that guarantee patient safety and facilitate recovery trajectories. In the end, in refining patient outcomes due to HAIs with solid research and infection control strategies, healthcare facility care quality can be radically enhanced.

12.3.1. Increased Morbidity and Mortality Rates

The mechanism of high morbidity and mortality rates due to HAIs is a significant problem confronting the public health and healthcare delivery systems. Such HAIs, caused by infection of the patient during the period of hospitalization or shortly after discharge, can have their causative origins from surgery, medical devices, and the hospital environment. The complexity of managing these infections generally translates into longer hospital stays, increased healthcare costs, and most critically, an increased risk of severe health complications. The imperative for strict infection control measures is evident as the incidence of HAIs continues to raise concerns, necessitating elaborate action plans with emphasis on patient safety and effective treatment protocols. At the center of prevention against HAIs is understanding their epidemiology and associated health hazards, particularly among vulnerable patient populations. Evidence indicates that some infection types, such as MRSA and *Clostridium difficile*, are significant contributors to increased morbidity rates, which have appalling trends of resistance and spread in the healthcare setting. Advancements in diagnostic testing and innovative application of point-of-care testing could yield substantial economic benefits as well as improved patient outcomes by enabling timely intervention. Initiatives by organizations such as the Technology Strategy Board and Department of Health demonstrate the need for unique research and investment in developing useful diagnostic tools, eventually aiming to minimize the burden of HAIs on patient health and healthcare resources (Szczepura & Osipenko, 2009). Moreover, emerging evidence suggests a relationship between respiratory infections and increased cardiovascular events, proving the wide-ranging impacts of HAIs on general health outcomes. Studies have shown that the diseases caused by common pathogens, such as *Streptococcus pneumoniae* and influenza viruses, can lead to acute cardiovascular events, producing large numbers of myocardial infarctions and strokes among the infected group. The association is a crucial mandate for high levels of vaccination coverage and infectious disease preventive control in hospitals. Through the targeting of infection twoness and potential cardiovascular complications, healthcare professionals are better able to create and enact prevention practices that not only reduce HAIs but also increase the general health environment for patients, demonstrating that effective infection control is at the heart of reducing rates of morbidity and mortality due to such infections (Andrew et al., 2018).

12.3.2. Length of Hospital Stay and Recovery Time

Hospital length of stay and recovery time are crucial variables that are influenced by HAIs in a way that heavily impacts patient outcomes as well as healthcare costs. HAIs lead to longer stays for patients because they require additional treatments, observation, and sometimes surgery. For instance, in the case of *Clostridium difficile* infections, the use of strict antibiotic guidelines has been linked to improved outcomes, reducing overall incidence of such infections, and possibly shortening length of stay. However, evidence suggests that while mortality may be decreased following severe infection, secondary outcomes like length of stay do not change, indicating a complex association between infection control intervention and patient recovery times (Ritchie et al., 2017). Preventing HAIs through effective infection control practice is thus important in optimizing patient recovery and health facility resource utilization. Recovery times from infections acquired during the time of hospitalization can be quite varied from one individual to another, based on factors like the nature of the infection, overall condition, and the timeliness of initiating treatment. In the case of community-acquired pneumonia (CAP) cases, the time to the first antibiotic dosing has been shown to directly influence patient recuperation. One study demonstrated that the patients experienced prolonged waiting, 7 hours and 48 minutes on average, before they received their first dose of antibiotics, which can prolong recovery and complicate their in-hospital stays (Callus et al., 2012).

Proper infection control measures, for example, early diagnosis and early treatment, are essential in preventing HAIs' adverse effects on recovery time. By standardizing procedures and instituting standardized management procedures, healthcare centers can reduce hospital stay durations and also enhance patient outcomes. Ultimately, attempts at reducing hospital stay durations and speeding up recovery periods must be extended to the entire strategy for infection control procedures. That involves not just the implementation of guidelines to combat HAIs but also constant training and educating the workforce. Having stringent infection control practices implemented can promote the achievement of a safer patient environment, which lessens the risk of HAIs and associated complications. The relationship among antibiotic stewardship, infection control, and patient outcomes makes healthcare facilities invest in evidence-based practices enhancing patient safety, as well as operational effectiveness. These actions not only positively impact recovery rates and length of stay, but they also increase the efficiency of resource management in healthcare systems, emphasizing interdependence between effective infection control and quality care (Figure 12.9).

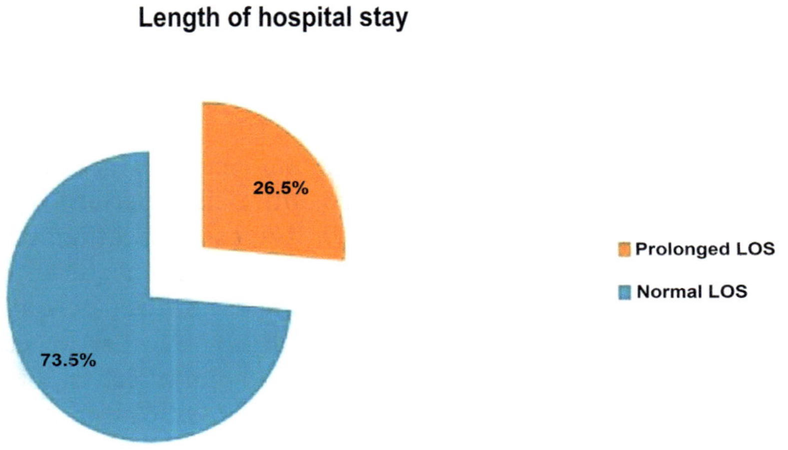

Figure 12.9. Length of hospital stay.

Source: https://www.medrxiv.org/content/medrxiv/early/2023/12/09/2023.12.07.23299680/F1.large.jpg.

12.3.3. Financial Implications for Healthcare Systems

The financial cost of HAIs is a huge burden on healthcare systems, impacting many operational and clinical aspects. Direct costs of HAIs include extended hospital stays, additional diagnostic imaging and laboratory tests, and more treatment due to infection management. HAIs can also result in severe long-term complications, leading to ongoing patient care. Medical facilities carry the cost burdens of higher readmission rates and receive penalty payments from such payers as Medicare, which have implemented fiscal penalties for high HAIs for hospitals. As there is growing emphasis on patient safety outcomes, it is evident that hospitals spend significant amounts on infection control measures to curb these expenses and comply with healthcare regulations. In addition, the implications of HAIs extend beyond immediate clinical costs to encompass broader influences on financing health and policy. For instance, the cost of HAIs annually in the United States has been projected to be in billions of dollars. Not only does the cost rise due to the high mortality and morbidity rates of the infection, but also because it absorbs hospital resources and undermines public faith in healthcare facilities. Attempts at greater infection control, from state-of-the-art sanitation technologies to the introduction of new technology, are worthwhile investments. Such systems do, however, come with substantial initial capital costs that may be hard to swallow on an upfront budgetary basis. Under these conditions, hospitals must weigh upfront costs against downstream gains since preventive measures for infection control can substantially reduce the long-term fiscal impact of HAIs and enhance overall patient outcomes. Antibiotic resistance also contributes to the fiscal situation of the healthcare organizations that are treating HAIs. Overuse of antibiotics has led to the emergence of resistant strains of bacteria, which complicate treatment regimes and push the cost upwards. When it comes to HAIs, infections caused by resistant organisms tend to be more expensive and take longer to treat. This can lead to extended hospitalization, increased intensive care usage, and a higher risk of adverse health consequences. With the increasing threat of antibiotic resistance, healthcare systems must budget for research, education of healthcare professionals, and implementation of effective antibiotic stewardship interventions to counter this acute threat. Successful control of HAIs and resistant infection not only has the potential to save lives but will also significantly cut the financial cost to the healthcare system in the long term, i.e., by reducing the costs associated with prolonged hospital stay and complicated treatment protocols (D'Alessandro et al., 2016; Lillestolen, 2018).

12.4. Infection Control Strategies

Adoption of effective infection control practices is at the core of preventing HAIs in health care facilities. Among such practices, fostering a safety culture is a core activity. According to the European Federation of Nurses Associations (EFN), health services must establish a culture in which mistakes can be reported safely and from which lessons are derived, thus maintaining improvement in patient safety and infection control (Smith et al., 2008). This approach encourages healthcare workers to report cases without fear of retribution, required for determining which areas of improvement are necessary. Furthermore, applying best practices grounded in research and peer exchanges has the ability to codify the infection control process into an improved means of HAIP prevention. Another distinguishing aspect of infection control interventions is the implementation of Antimicrobial Stewardship Programs (ASPs). As the recent study has noted, these interventions have an important impact on pediatric populations by reducing the use of inappropriate antibiotics and related risks (Donà et al., 2020). The evidence supports that when ASPs are introduced in hospitals, not only are they reducing the use of unnecessary antibiotics but are also preventing the emergence of antimicrobial resistance — an emerging risk in hospitals. By taking on a systematic approach to antibiotic prescribing, hospitals are able to improve outcomes of treatment without reducing the adverse effects associated with the misuse of antibiotics.

Figure 12.10. Logo of the U.S. Centers for Disease Control and Prevention since 2024.

Source: https://upload.wikimedia.org/wikipedia/commons/thumb/7/71/CDC_logo_2024.svg/800px-CDC_logo_2024.svg.png.

Ultimately, ASPs are an essential element in effective infection control, consistent with overall strategies for enhanced patient safety and quality of care. In addition, improving hand hygiene among healthcare workers stands as an important infection control strategy. The Centers for Disease Control and Prevention (CDC) identifies hand hygiene as a first defense in avoiding the spread of HAIs. Consistent washing with soap and water, along with the use of alcohol-based hand sanitizers, noticeably reduces the spread of pathogens in healthcare environments. Education and enforcing compliance with optimal hand hygiene practices can drastically reduce infection rates. Based on several studies and reports, even minimal increases in hand hygiene compliance are correlated with dramatic decreases in HAIs, thereby underlining the efficacy of this simple yet effective intervention. Thus, complementing stringent hand hygiene training with universal infection control practices increases the effectiveness of hospital-acquired infection reduction endeavors, delivering enhanced results and patient safety (Figure 12.10).

12.4.1. Hand Hygiene Practices

Proper practice of hand hygiene is inevitable in prevention against HAIs and goes a long way in enhancing patient safety in health facilities. The World Health Organization emphasizes that proper handwashing decreases the transmission of pathogens and thus reduces the incidence. Various practices, such as hand cleaning with soap and water, antiseptic alcoholic rubs, and surgical hand scrubs, are practiced based on clinical conditions. This multidimensional approach allows health professionals to select appropriate hand hygiene procedures tailored to specific situations, thereby maximizing infection control interventions. Notably, integrating these procedures into standard care practices fosters a culture of safety and a sense of responsibility among healthcare professionals, which is essential in minimizing HAIs' risk factors and ultimately improving patients' outcomes. The complexity of hand hygiene extends beyond just compliance; it is about constructing a safe environment for patients and healthcare staff. Healthcare facilities are known to be significant reservoirs for cross-transmission of infection, and this explains the strict application of disinfectants. Evidence indicates that high reliability organizations apply extensive hand hygiene programs that involve not only direct handwashing but also surface and equipment disinfection aimed at diminishing the risk of infection further. These approaches address evidence of the necessity of a multifaceted strategy for infection control, consisting of monitoring hand hygiene adherence and serially revising guidelines based on emerging research. Based on literature, the use of "bundles" consisting of more than one evidence-based practice is an especially helpful method of HAIs control and promoting an environment of patient safety (Protano et al., 2019). Apart from that, education and training are crucial to ensuring that hand hygiene practices remain effective in healthcare environments.

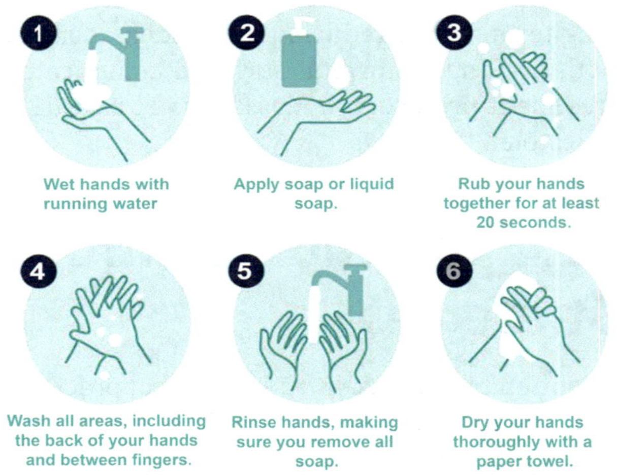

Figure 12.11. Six steps of hand hygiene.

Source: https://i.pinimg.com/736x/ae/5f/b5/ae5fb5e5c395cfd84285e526e5e156b9.jpg.

Through research, healthcare workers' functions in misinterpreting guidelines and ignoring infection control importance were established as common experiences (Smith et al., 2008). Efforts in continuous professional development in making healthcare workers aware and enforcing proper application of hand hygiene practices can significantly increase compliance rates. By forging a culture that is infection prevention-focused, healthcare administrators not only improve patient safety but also reduce the HAIs' burden, which has the potential to carry weighty clinical and financial impacts. Consequently, incorporating hand hygiene training into the overall plan for infection control highlights its pivotal function in affecting organizational practice, with the net effect that patient safety will always be on top of the agenda in health care (Figure 12.11).

12.4.2. Use of Personal Protective Equipment (PPE)

The use of personal protective equipment (PPE) is a key measure in hospital-acquired infection (HAI) prevention that ensures healthcare workers are protected while treating vulnerable populations. PPE serves to create a barrier that does not allow for the passage of pathogens between healthcare workers and patients, especially in high-risk areas. This notwithstanding, there remain problems with the non-adherence to prescribed PPE guidelines among healthcare workers. A study at St. Mary's Hospital Lacor, revealed that few of the participants were aware of the purpose of PPE, and even fewer had appropriate methods in donning and doffing the gear. These results point to gaps in training and awareness as central to improving compliance and, by extension, infection control within healthcare units (Okello et al., 2017). Besides, the supply and accessibility of PPE are essential for effective infection control in hospitals. Research conducted at Queen Elizabeth Central Hospital revealed extreme diversities in the availability of various PPE types in wards. For instance, whereas the fundamental glove was stocked in every ward, critical items such as goggles were not available in most wards. This gap is dangerous, as medical staff can resort to inappropriate protection in the case of potentially infectious situations. Enhancing supply chain management to ensure the timely availability of PPE is critical. Not only does it support healthcare workers in their work, but at the same time, it reinforces the overall process of infection control within the facility (Madziatera et al., 2020). Training and continuing education are vital in the promotion of compliance with PPE use among health care providers. It is evident that health care workers who undergo concentrated training have improved adherence to PPE guidelines, hence reducing the occurrence. Implementation of stringent training schemes in professional training, as well as continuing in-service training, can significantly improve the knowledge base for proper use of PPE. Furthermore, the support of institutions, including management control and the provision of quality PPE, contributes to a safety culture among health institutions. Through education prioritization and budgeting, hospitals can enhance their infection control processes, thereby improving patient outcomes and reducing the burden (Okello et al., 2017; Madziatera et al., 2020) (Figure 12.12).

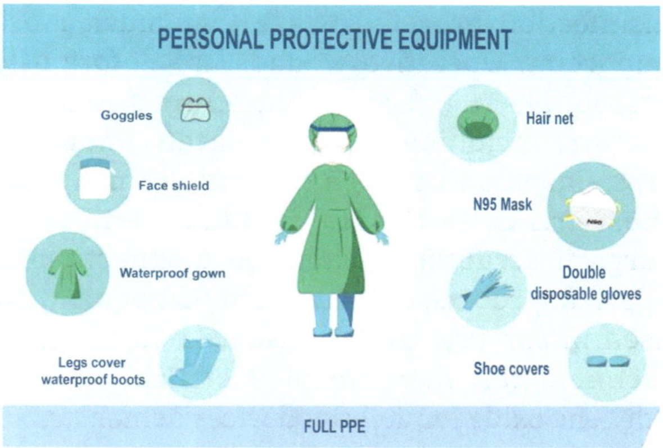

Figure 12.12. Personal protective equipment (PPE).

Source: https://www.netmeds.com/images/cms/wysiwyg/blog/2021/05/1620809350_PPE_big_2.jpg.

12.4.3. Sterilization and Disinfection Protocols

Proper sterilization and disinfection procedures are critical components in combating HAIs, a persistent threat in the healthcare environment. Not only do these infections have an impact on the outcome of patients, but they also impose significant logistical and financial pressures on healthcare systems. Careful implementation of sterilization and disinfection protocols is required so that microbial transmission is avoided, particularly in high-stakes environments such as operating theaters and intensive care units. Interventions such as aggressive hand hygiene, surface disinfection, and environmental cleaning have been able to significantly reduce infection rates. The addition of repetitive and harsh sterilization measures helps in building a safety culture in healthcare facilities, which empowers employees with the necessary equipment to effectively fight HAIs rise. As highlighted by hospital hygiene studies, consistent emphasis on such infection control procedures is essential to maintaining patient health and best results for the provision of medical care (Mohamed & Ali, 2023). In surgeries, rigorous sterilization and disinfection procedures are that much more important. Operative wounds are notoriously susceptible to infection, caused by a range of vectors, including direct medical contact or cross-infection between patients. To minimize these risks, practices include meticulous surgical scrubbing, extensive disinfection of operating rooms, and sterilizing all equipment used in surgery. Use of advanced sterilization technologies like steam sterilization and ethylene oxide for delicate devices demonstrates the necessity of adapting practices to suit unique clinical needs. Additionally, training programs for surgical staff are a requirement, ensuring that members of staff understand how to prepare and use disinfectants as well as the sterilization process. Combined, these practices form an efficient infection control framework, in the long term yielding lower levels of HAIs in operating rooms (Singh & Alam, 2024). In addition, technological advancements in sterilization technology continue to occur, providing improved infection control within healthcare. Emerging technologies such as ultraviolet light disinfection and cold plasma technology represent promising supplements to traditional methods, potentially providing speed and efficiency in deactivating infectious agents. Advanced modalities such as these can complement traditional measures to enhance the overall effectiveness of sterilization. Given that hospitals are facing not only antibiotic-resistant infections but also chronic HAIs, the integration of emerging disinfection technology into practice is more important than ever. By promoting an environment in which conventional as well as cutting-edge sterilization methods are of utmost importance, healthcare facilities can promote better health outcomes and patient safety. Lastly, observance of strict sterilization and disinfection protocols is the cornerstone of effective infection control strategies, at the heart of the fight against HAIs (Mohamed & Ali, 2023) (Figure 12.13).

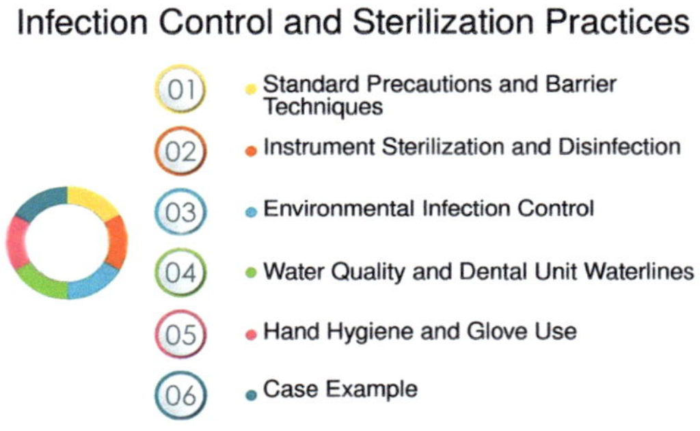

Figure 12.13. Infection control and sterilization practices.

Source: https://fastercapital.co/i/Dental-quality-assurance-Ensuring-Dental-Excellence--Quality-Assurance-Strategies-for-Dental-Entrepreneurs--Infection-Control-and-Sterilization-Practices.webp.

12.5. Role of Healthcare Professionals

The responsibility of healthcare practitioners in preventing HAIs is to safeguard patient safety and enhance healthcare outcomes. Healthcare practitioners form the primary barrier against infection with their training and expertise, and screen for, prevent, and treat HAIs. Their responsibilities go beyond direct patient contact; healthcare practitioners play a part in instigating evidence-based practice, adhering to rigorous infection control protocols, and inculcating a culture of safety within healthcare facilities. This involves constant training and education to stay up-to-date with the latest guidelines and practices of infection control, which are essential in minimizing the risks of HAIs. Moreover, cooperation among healthcare staff is essential in compiling an extensive infection control plan. Interdisciplinary communication and collaboration among nurses, physicians, pharmacists, and infection control specialists are essential in identifying potential infection threats and taking effective interventions. These professionals participate in multidisciplinary rounds and committees to discuss infection cases and share ideas. Institutions like the European Federation of Nurses Associations (EFN) with a focus on a culture of safety also point towards the reporting of errors on time as well as sharing best practices between health workers (Smith et al., 2008). This team-based model not only ensures improved patient outcomes but also creates a solid learning culture and quality improvement. As antibiotic resistance continues to build, with mounting pressure on healthcare providers, practitioners must be adequately informed with knowledge and interventions to treat this condition efficiently. Inadequate use of antibiotics has enabled resistant bacteria to develop, making HAIs harder to treat and contributing to a rise in morbidity and mortality rates (Lillestolen, 2018). Healthcare professionals must ensure good prescribing practice, as well as patient education regarding the utilization of antibiotics. They are at the forefront of calling for research and funding to address the complicated issues posed by HAIs and antibiotic resistance. With support for an educated patient population and adherence to antimicrobial stewardship practices, healthcare professionals are able to significantly reduce the incidence of HAIs, hence enhancing patient safety.

12.5.1. Training and Education on Infection Control

Education and training on infection control are key to diminishing the incidence of HAIs. Effective infection prevention and control (IPC) interventions are vital elements of healthcare delivery, which have a direct impact on the outcome of patients and on institutional values. Continuous education for health professionals supports a culture of safety, where clinicians possess the learning and capabilities to implement IPC interventions effectively. According to WHO guidelines, raising awareness of IPC practice and principles not only reduces the rate of HAI but also fosters trust in healthcare systems. The critical role of education is also attested to by the reality that a large proportion of HAIs are avoidable through standardized IPC practices, testifying to the need for formal training programs in all healthcare settings, from nursing to hospital administrative personnel, and thus addressing the multifaceted dynamics of patient safety and care successfully (Storr et al., 2017). Moreover, developing a good training model involves a strategy with theory and practice. Simulation training and practical sessions are crucial in developing competency in infection control practices by healthcare workers. These practices provide instant feedback and the development of areas that need improvement, thus creating a culture of constant improvement. Educative programs should also involve evaluation to ascertain the effect of training interventions to continue equipping healthcare staff with the latest evidence-based standards. Continuing education credits that include healthcare providers' involvement in ongoing professional development will help ensure high practice standards. As shown in various studies, including the ones presented in the European Federation of Nurses Associations, stimulation of a safety culture by rigorous training can significantly minimize the risk of HAIs and patient safety in general (Smith et al., 2008). Further, the integration of IPC education in curricula for nursing and medical students is crucial to help maintain infection control improvement. By embedding these principles into fundamental training, future healthcare practitioners will be more likely to prioritize infection prevention over the course of their careers.

Forward thinking of this type is essential to encouraging an aware workforce that understands the implications of HAIs as well as the necessity of successful IPC practice. An interprofessional format for education programs — where healthcare professions learn together as a unit — can also more effectively facilitate understanding and implementation of best practices. Such training benefits not only the individual but also brings together teams to have a more cohesive reaction to patient safety. Lastly, an investment in quality training and education programs is an investment in quality and safety in healthcare, which is essential to reduce the burden of HAIs in healthcare settings (Storr et al., 2017) (Figure 12.14).

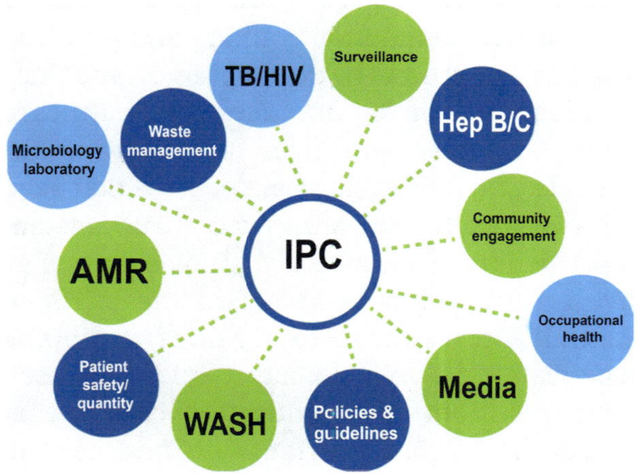

Figure 12.14. Infection prevention and control (IPC).

Source: https://d3f1iyfxxz8i1e.cloudfront.net/courses/course_image/b195c88b17a8.jpg.

12.5.2. Multidisciplinary Approach to Infection Prevention

Multidisciplinarity in infection prevention is paramount in the effort to contain hospital-acquired infection (HAI). By integrating expertise from all disciplines — nursing, epidemiology, microbiology, and public health — the healthcare facility is able to formulate a robust plan that factors in the multidimensional aspect of HAI. The interdisciplinarity of different professionals ensures that the complexities of infection control are addressed in an all-encompassing fashion, allowing out-of-the-box solutions that transcend traditional bounds. Such collaboration not only enhances communication among health care teams but also encourages the utilization of evidence-based, best practices stemming from critical research that is integral to enhancing patient safety and outcomes. Furthermore, research on high-reliability organization culture recognizes that the coming together of disparate professional perspectives can lead to significant enhancements in risk understanding and prevention from HAIs (Smith et al., 2008). Effective infection prevention strategies also require clinical staff who learn from real implementation and adapt effective practices to function in their particular environment. Case studies from various health institutions provide vital details on interventions applied to reduce HAIs, results of the interventions, and valuable lessons learned along the way (McCarthy & Blumenthal, 2006). By analyzing such case studies, multidisciplinary teams will be in a position to find reproducible and feasible best practices within their own settings. Such evidence-based problem-solving will make it possible to customize infection control measures to address institutional goals and patient needs. Secondly, cultivating a learning culture among health care workers yields successive improvements, ultimately leading to more effective infection prevention activities. In addition to the benefits of inter-professional collaboration on the part of healthcare professionals, multidisciplinary practice emphasizes stakeholder involvement, including administrative assistance. Administrative involvement by hospital administration and policymakers is essential to enable the successful distribution of resources, facilitate interdisciplinary communication, and adopt innovative infection control practices. Administrative professionals' involvement ensures infection control practices are supported by the finances and institutional influence necessary for successful implementation. As discussed in patient safety culture topics, concerted collaboration among frontline health care providers and organizational leaders builds an environment that promotes accountability and transparency. Eventually, an interdisciplinary approach develops an overall framework for combating HAIs, enhancing the overall effectiveness of infection control and prevention in the healthcare environment (Smith et al., 2008).

12.5.3. Reporting and Monitoring HAIs

Improper reporting and monitoring of HAIs are of extreme importance to enhancing patient safety and healthcare practice. Through transparency and culture, infection reporting and early notification of related incidents may be encouraged within healthcare organizations. This active role allows infection patterns to be identified early and targeted intervention to be implemented immediately. According to the European Federation of Nurses Associations (EFN), building an open culture emphasizing early reporting of errors is critical to ensure maximum patient safety (Smith et al., 2008). In addition, dissemination of findings and best practices is crucial for maintaining high standards across healthcare settings. When hospitals pursue excellence, mechanisms for routine monitoring and reporting can significantly reduce the incidence of HAIs, hence patient outcomes and workers' confidence in regard to reporting systems. Evidence-based guidelines must be applied for effective monitoring of HAIs. Studies have demonstrated that application of standardized procedures has the potential to reduce infection rates to a great extent, particularly for those procedures with a higher risk, such as central line insertions. Expert personnel who deliver these procedures are essential in order to implement prescribed protocols, as well as ongoing education for healthcare staff. Being active with cooperative networks also provides monitoring of outcomes and sharing of helpful information between institutions. By implementing such measures, hospitals can establish a strong foundation for infection control activities aligned with the most current evidence and clinical guidelines (Reilly et al., 2008). These methodologies ultimately enhance patient care as well as strengthen the overall credibility of healthcare systems. The surveillance of HAIs does not just involve the accumulation of data but also using these data effectively to promote change. Use of sophisticated data analysis software can enable real-time tracking of infection rates so hospitals can respond promptly in the event of potential outbreaks. Furthermore, engaging frontline staff in data collection and analysis can enhance ownership and accountability for patient safety. Integration of clinical teams and administrative organizations is required for data interpretation into effective strategies that reduce HAIs. Considering this field of infection control enhances the reporting process, with results having direct bearing on improvement efforts, resulting in a process of continuous improvement in patient care. From various studies, it has been observed that comprehensive reporting and monitoring of HAIs are crucial to develop a culture of patient safety as well as effective infection control practices (Figure 12.15).

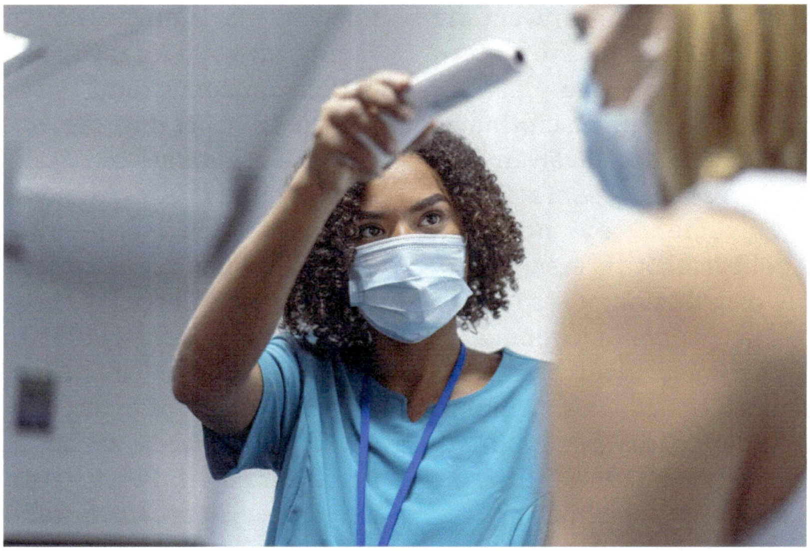

Figure 12.15. Monitoring of hospital-acquired infections (HAIs).

Source: https://www.coordinare.org.au/assets/Uploads/CTA/GettyImages-1319877948__FitWzE5MjAsMTA4MF0.jpg.

12.6. Challenges in Infection Control

Hospitals in infection control have been confronted by numerous problems in making HAIs prevention easier. One of them is adherence to evidence-based practice among the health staff, which is central to preventing infections. In that guidelines have been provided, inconsistency in application makes it hard for there to be effectiveness. High turnover rates and inadequate training can be contributory factors to the neglect of already provided procedures. In addition, the patient case types can create environments in which procedure adherence is difficult, thereby facilitating HAIs development. By embracing this challenge, emphasis on education and accountability in healthcare teams must be established, highlighting the need for safety culture that supports frequent practice and frequent surveillance of compliance with infection prevention practices. Moreover, multidisciplinary team positions cannot be emphasized enough in counteracting infection control challenges. Units that foster teamwork among different healthcare staff can better detect, screen, and address factors leading to HAIs. This is particularly critical for interventions like the prevention of central line-associated bloodstream infections, which have been shown to improve considerably with the management of dedicated teams and engagement in collaboratives. By establishing infection control teams that work together, hospitals are able to bring collective expertise together to put and enforce strong infection control procedures in place. Better communication between team members could also make it easier to react quickly to developing infection threats, ultimately leading to better patient outcomes and less prevalence of HAIs, as evidenced through effective infection control in high-reliability organizations (Reilly et al., 2008). Furthermore, the creation of an organizational safety culture where voluntary error reporting and formal best practice sharing are encouraged is key to promoting infection control. A safety culture has been shown to significantly lower the rate of HAIs by providing a setting where mistakes can be identified and they can be learned from. There is a requirement for dedicated efforts to provide transparency and realistic training in reporting processes and the prevention of infections. The European Federation of Nurses Associations highlights that safety commitment can integrate healthcare services towards a shared goal of patient health while continuously improving practices based on continuous research and feedback (Smith et al., 2008). By embracing this safety culture, healthcare units can not only combat the issue of HAIs but also establish a system that ensures ongoing improvement in infection management practices.

12.6.1. Antibiotic Resistance and Its Implications

Antibiotic resistance is increasingly being recognized as a significant public health challenge, more particularly in the case of HAIs. Antibiotics are being overused and misused, resulting in the evolution of resistant bacterial strains, and infection control is becoming harder in healthcare institutions. Hospitals being war zones for a variety of pathogens, infection control with effective steps more than ever before is the need of the hour. For example, the once-promised cure-alls, broad-spectrum antibiotics, have accidentally developed conditions favorable to resistance, creating a need for immediate education and awareness among healthcare professionals about prescribing practices. If not addressed, such knowledge gaps in education, the vicious cycle of resistance will continue to perpetuate itself, resulting in increased morbidity and mortality attributed to HAIs, particularly among vulnerable patient populations.

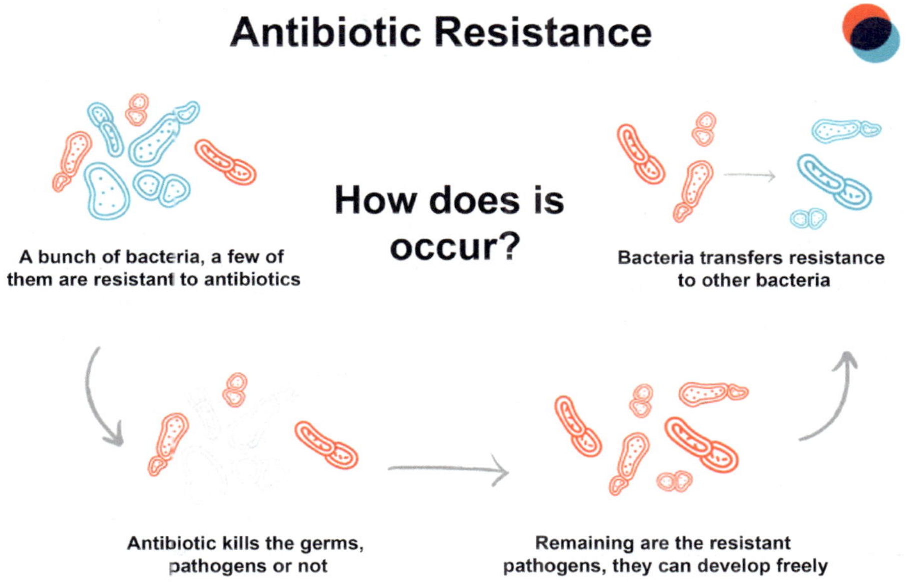

Figure 12.16. Antibiotic resistance.

Source: https://www.labtoo.com/hs-fs/hubfs/Antibiotic%20resistance%20680x482.png?width=680&height=482&name=Antibiotic%20resistance%20680x482.png.

The consequences of antibiotic resistance extend beyond personal health outcomes to its impact on healthcare systems and society. Among the significant concerns is the threat of added healthcare costs in terms of prolonged hospitalization, additional diagnostic testing, and the need for more expensive, often toxic alternative therapy. The relationship between inappropriate initial antimicrobial therapy and poor patient outcomes necessitates an aggressive approach to antibiotic stewardship. Through the case of intra-abdominal infections (IAIs), the urgency and effective source control with appropriate antimicrobial therapy are highlighted. Inadequate control of such infection is evidenced by growing resistance and mortality rates. Hence, the integration of strong antibiotic stewardship programs in hospitals is crucial in preventing such effects and improving patient care, fundamentally transforming how HAIs are managed. Moreover, the global nature of antibiotic resistance works to underscore the necessity for an overall approach to addressing this problem. Initiatives like AGORA strive to optimize the rational use of antimicrobials in treating complicated IAIs, in getting various international players into sync within this fight. The emergence of multidrug-resistant pathogens, particularly among gram-negative bacteria, is an insurmountable challenge that crosses borders, requiring a collective assault. The growing worry with bacterial resistance is then also compounded by a plateau in the development of new antibiotics, and therefore unity becomes crucial. By forging an environment of open knowledge and best practices, healthcare professionals are equipped to enhance patient outcomes and ultimately reimpose the efficacy of antibiotics against HAIs, demonstrating not just commitment to care of the individual, but to global community health (Figure 12.16).

12.6.2. Compliance with Infection Control Protocols

Excellent compliance with infection control protocols is critical in avoiding HAIs, a quality issue in healthcare. By executing established guidelines, healthcare professionals provide a safer patient experience as the risk of infections associated with invasive procedures, such as central line insertions, is reduced. Evidence points towards the importance of evidence-based practice, the cornerstone of such guidelines. For instance, specialty teams to oversee central line insertions and ongoing monitoring of the incidence of infection have been identified as important components of successful infection control programs (Reilly et al., 2008). With this systematic approach, not only increasing compliance but also instilling an atmosphere of responsibility among the healthcare providers, the sentiment reinforces the perception that it is everyone's responsibility to comply with these guidelines. The role of an organizational culture that puts a great emphasis on patient safety cannot be overstated when the matter at hand is compliance with infection control procedures. A robust culture of safety allows open communication, where workers feel comfortable reporting even perceived breaches without fear of retribution. Such a culture corresponds to the European Federation of Nurses Associations' values of fostering a culture where mistakes are reported and best practices exchanged (Smith et al., 2008). With such integration of the values, hospitals can enhance their infection control procedures so that not only are personnel compliant with guidelines but also actively engaged in improving safety procedures. Such participation is important as it sustains a culture of continuous learning and improvement, ultimately reducing the prevalence of HAIs. Training and education are fundamental in ensuring that the infection control practices are well understood by all healthcare personnel. Continuing education courses to update employees to current evidence-based infection prevention practices play an essential role in the maintenance of compliance. These courses may encompass simulation drills on proper techniques, hand hygiene workshops, and infection control rule refresher courses. The efficacy of training programs is essential, as the acquired knowledge has a direct impact on day-to-day practice and, in turn, patient outcomes.

Institutions should also ensure monitoring and measuring compliance on a regular basis through audits and feedback mechanisms because not only does this compel conformity, but it also identifies areas of improvement. Such systematic training in combination with the culture of safety within the organization places hospitals at an advantage in addressing HAIs (Figure 12.17).

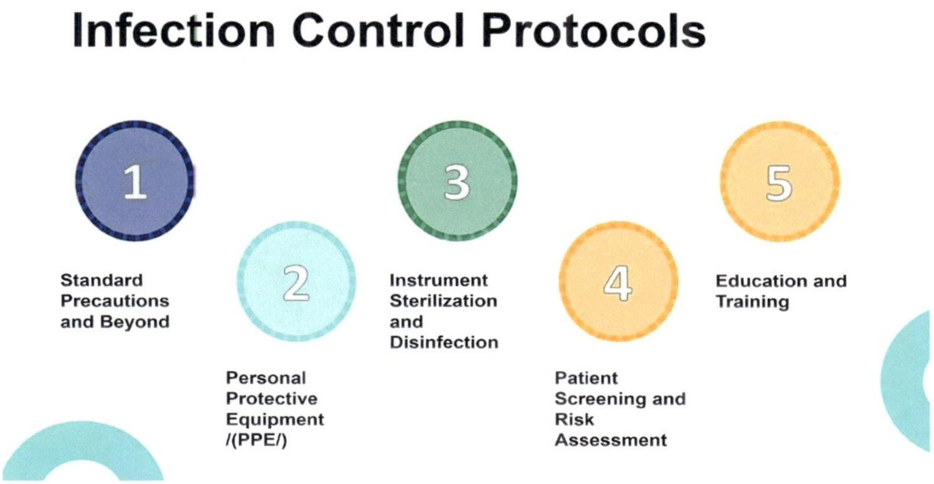

Figure 12.17. Infection control protocols.

Source: https://fastercapital.co/i/Dental-regulation-and-compliance-Navigating-Dental-Regulations--A-Guide-for-Entrepreneurs--Infection-Control-Protocols.webp.

12.6.3. Resource Limitations in Healthcare Facilities

Limited material in healthcare institutions mainly hinders hospital-acquired infection (HAI) control. Inadequate numbers of staff remain a common issue that interferes with having effective infection control measures. Evidence indicates that most health institutions have inconsistencies when it comes to the reporting of infection control indicators, an issue intensified by understaffing. In light of the outcomes of a nationwide and local review, hospitals are more likely to adopt a reactive approach towards managing staffing-linked indicators instead of a proactive one necessary to boost infection prevention practice (Iwami et al., 2017). Not only do these disadvantages erode patient safety, but they are also reflective of a cycle of poor reactions to infection outbreaks, once again calling for a shake-up of operational competencies within healthcare systems. The culture of the facility also plays a pivotal part in addressing resource shortcomings. Effective prevention of infection is not merely about compliance with guidelines, but an error-free culture of safety that gives free flow of information and early reporting of mistakes. According to the European Federation of Nurses Associations, it is possible to ensure better patient safety and HAI results by building such a culture (Smith et al., 2008). But during times of resource constraint, engaging staff in open discussions about safety becomes increasingly challenging. Such disengagement can compromise the building and sustaining of collaborative relationships required for proactive infection control of HAIs. Interdependence between organizational culture and resource allocation indicates that healthcare leaders need to invest in human and system aspects behind effective infection control. Finally, coordinating resources with infection control policies at the strategic level is necessary for improved healthcare outcomes. The gap between national policy and hospital practice at local levels typically stems from limited access to resources. Systematic reviews of regulatory settings indicate that guidance on how to improve infection prevention is available, but the capability of hospitals to utilize such indicators is largely unequal based on a lack of resources (Iwami et al., 2017). The need for hospitals to establish capacity for routine reporting and implementation of operational procedures cannot be overstated. The hospital infrastructure and resource deployment should be bolstered because it not only makes standards compliance easier but also assists in establishing a congenial environment for the systematic prevention of HAIs. Thus, addressing the challenge of resource limitations becomes the central focus in the greater fight against HAIs in health centers.

SUMMARY

The conclusion drawn from HAIs research focuses on the necessity for effective infection control interventions in healthcare facilities. The prevalence of HAIs indicates not just the exposure of the patient but also organizational defects of current healthcare protocols. For instance, the interaction between HAIs and sepsis in intensive care units reveals the devastating outcome of ineffective infection control measures; ICU-acquired sepsis patients have significantly higher mortality and extended hospital stays, foreshadowing the need for enhanced intervention and monitoring strategies. Though the data from the SPIN-UTI clearly illustrate the relationship between HAIs and resultant healthcare pressures, each institution will require a holistic strategy to maximize patient outcomes. Systematic measures that focus on firm adherence to hygiene procedures, sterilization, and environmental cleaning are also required. The full HAIs review reports that hospital environments are reservoirs of cross-transmission, necessitating the practice of effective cleaning and disinfection. With information that a variety of hand hygiene practices are able to reduce the risk of infections effectively, healthcare institutions ought to prioritize training health workers on the importance of such protocols. As evidenced in the literature, adherence to standard guidelines, for example, those that are Spaulding's classification-derived, is a key stone in combating HAIs. Promoting a safety and accountability culture in healthcare institutions will not only reduce the prevalence of infection but also improve the quality of healthcare provision. Lastly, the reduction of HAIs requires an intersectoral approach from all actors involved in the healthcare sector, for example, administrators, clinicians, and ancillary personnel. As the findings indicate, integrated practice bundles of bundled preventive strategies have been successful in restricting HAIs. Therefore, it is of extreme significance to foster an environment for the facilitation of continuous education, watchfulness, and adherence to research-demonstrated practice. Emphasizing a research agenda in favor of the reinforcement of successful preventive processes will be critical. This unified model ensures that healthcare systems are well-equipped to address not only the immediate problems that HAIs cause but also the drivers behind their persistence, hence leading to safer patient care and improved health outcomes in settings (Agodi et al., 2018; Protano et al., 2019).

A thorough comprehension of HAIs requires an investigation of important prevention measures and their enforcement in healthcare facilities. Critical areas noted in recent research highlight the significance of evidence-based infection control protocols. For example, having specific teams assigned to manage procedures, like central line insertions, has been identified as an effective measure to curb the risk of infection events. These teams play a crucial role in the sustenance of compliance with best practice and in fomenting a culture of safety within healthcare environments. Further, collective working between health facilities can lead to mutual learning and benchmarking based on infection rates, as well as further encouraging the measures used in HAI control. Ongoing monitoring and evaluation of infection rates are necessary to revise and enhance these strategies continuously, ultimately yielding improved patient outcomes through integrative infection control measures (Reilly et al., 2008). Additionally, greater utilization of antibiotics has been a major contributing factor in both curing and continuing the challenges of HAIs. Penicillin revolutionized the practice of medicine; subsequent overreliance on broad-spectrum antibiotics, however, has created mass hysteria regarding antibiotic resistance. Misuse of these powerful medicines without a thorough understanding of their biochemical mechanisms has provided the door for resistant bacterial forms to multiply, complicating infection control in hospitals. The appalling reality is that antibiotic resistance causes over a thousand fatalities per annum in the United States alone, and in poverty-stricken settings, it impacts those settings even more severely. It demands ongoing study and spending directed at comprehending the specific genetic mechanisms for resistance and the underlying cause, so that medicine can combat effectively against HAIs (Lillestolen, 2018). Essentially, a multifaceted approach to infection control in healthcare settings is the cornerstone of reducing HAIs. This includes the integration of evidence-based standards, specialist monitoring teams, and persistent infection rate monitoring, as these factors consolidate the foundation for effective infection management. At the same time, the antibiotic resistance forces remind medical professionals of the delicate balance in antimicrobial use and the necessity to create new treatment regimens. In the midst of the war against resistant infection, healthcare settings are in a special position to emphasize prevention as well as research initiatives to protect patient health. Ongoing transformation of HAIs and resistance patterns requires transformation responses that integrate clinical practice with innovative study, offering improved care and shielding in hospitals in the future.

CLOSER LOOK

HAIS IN RADIOLOGY DEPARTMENTS

In radiology departments, the risk of HAIs keeps on rising due to the rising number of patients and the opening the role of medical imaging to more interventions. Indeed, radiology departments have experienced huge revolutionary changes during recent decades with breathtaking increases in diagnostic medical imaging volumes. These advances were linked to novel cross-sectional imaging modalities such as CT and MRI, which expanded radiology's central role in the treatment of patients. There are an estimated 88 million CT scans and 42 million MRI scans performed in the US alone annually. Besides increasing the patient population, use of these new and innovative imaging modalities has also increased healthcare workers' patient-contact time within radiology departments, consequently increasing the risk of HAI infection (Figure 12.18).

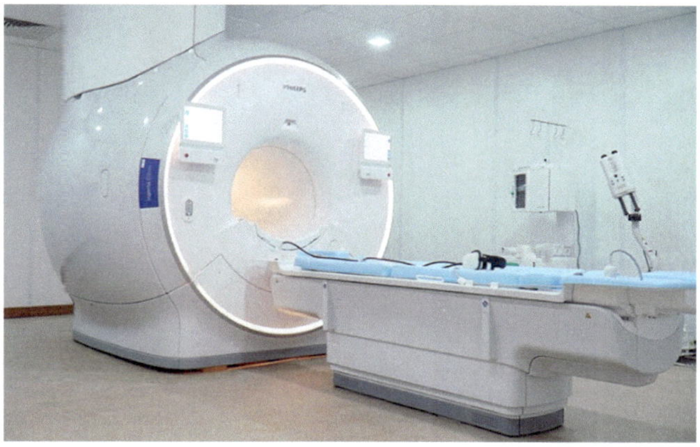

Figure 12.18. A modern magnetic resonance imaging (MRI) scanner used for noninvasive diagnostic imaging, providing high-resolution anatomical and functional insights.

Source: https://media.licdn.com/dms/image/v2/D5612AQHhkCUfT0SQXg/article-cover_image-shrink_600_2000/article-cover_image-shrink_600_2000/0/1691127475634?e=2147483647&v=beta&t=-WDC7Mqlj3VHPZvGa34Kj_ukGfXO-oCDn-cthA5V3Qs.

Besides, interventional radiologic interventions have added burden and potentially greater risk for HAIs because of the invasive nature of the procedure and direct patient contact. Percutaneous approaches to diagnostic and therapeutic endovascular interventional radiology are on the rise, and with this comes the potential for rising adverse outcomes like HAIs. Over seven million patients globally are treated with percutaneous interventional vascular procedures each year, and it is estimated that their numbers will increase even more in the next few years. Despite that, there have been limited attempts to estimate the incidence of HAIs following radiological interventional procedures. The data were variable and multifarious, and they likely were affected by a wide range of influences, such as the monocentric character of the study and the character of the procedure. As an example, due to the fact that biliary drainage is defined as "clean/contaminated" procedure, the risk of infection complications following transhepatic cholangiogram is likely the highest of any interventional procedure, 40%. On the contrary, the overall incidence of procedure-related infection is only 0.1% following the less invasive ultrasound-guided procedures such as fine-needle aspiration and referral ultrasound-guided biopsy.

During the Coronavirus disease 2019 (COVID-19) pandemic, radiology departments were at the forefront of managing the pandemic, diagnosing patients, and isolating patients who would need intensive care. Medical imaging has a very crucial role in making clinical decisions during the diagnosis, treatment, and follow-up of COVID-19 patients. During the COVID-19 pandemic, the radiology department was a "high-risk area" because it was a transit area for infected patients, non-infected patients, and healthcare workers. Infections can be contracted from infected patients through direct contact, indirect contact, droplet and/or airborne transmission. Infections can be contracted in waiting areas generally used by patients, examination rooms used for examination, procedure holding areas, and procedure rooms. According to this, the risk of infection exposure is not just exclusive to nurses, technologists, and radiologists but also includes receptionists, transporters, monitoring personnel, and even patients.

References

1. Agodi, A., Arrigoni, C., Auxilia, F., Barchitta, M., Brusaferro, S., D'Errico, M. M., Fabiani, L., et al. (2018). *Epidemiology of intensive care unit-acquired sepsis in Italy: Results of the SPIN-UTI network*. https://core.ac.uk/download/227029141.pdf (accessed on 16th July 2025).
2. Iwami, M., Ahmad, R., Castro-Sánchez, E., Birgand, G., Johnson, A. P., & Holmes, A. (2017). Capacity of English NHS hospitals to monitor quality in infection prevention and control using a new European framework: a multilevel qualitative analysis. *BMJ open*, *7*(1), e012520. https://doi.org/10.1136/bmjopen-2016-012520(accessed on 16th July 2025).
3. Singh, M., & Alam, M. (2024). A clinical review on importance of sanitizing the operating room. *International Journal of Research in Medical Sciences*, *12*(7), 2713–2717. https://doi.org/10.18203/2320-6012.ijrms20241939(accessed on 16th July 2025).
4. Ali, Y. (2018). *Decreasing CAUTI rates by educating staff on reinforcing the CAUTI bundle*. https://core.ac.uk/download/217228547.pdf (accessed on 16th July 2025).
5. Reilly, J., Stewart, S., Allardice, G. A., Noone, A., Robertson, C., Walker, A., & Coubrough, S. (2008). Results from the Scottish National HAI Prevalence Survey. *The Journal of hospital infection*, *69*(1), 62–68. https://doi.org/10.1016/j.jhin.2008.02.019(accessed on 16th July 2025).
6. Okello, T. R et al (2017). *Barriers and factors affecting personal protective equipment usage in St. Mary's Hospital Lacor in Northern Uganda*. COSECSA/ASEA Publication --East & Central African Journal of Surgery 2017; Vol. 22 (1) https://core.ac.uk/download/188828828.pdf (accessed on 16th July 2025).
7. Donà, D., Barbieri, E., Daverio, M., Lundin, R., Giaquinto, C., Zaoutis, T., & Sharland, M. (2020). Implementation and impact of pediatric antimicrobial stewardship programs: a systematic scoping review. *Antimicrobial resistance and infection control*, *9*(1), 3. https://doi.org/10.1186/s13756-019-0659-3 (accessed on 16th July 2025).
8. Rinaldi, A., Marani, A., Montesano, M., Berdini, S., Petruccioli, M. C., Di Ninno, F., Orioli, R., Ferretti, F., Tarsitani, G., Napoli, C., De Luca, A., & Orsi, G. B. (2016). Healthcare Associated Infections: educational intervention by "Adult Learning" in an Italian teaching hospital. *Annali di igiene : medicina preventiva e di comunita*, *28*(6), 441–449. https://doi.org/10.7416/ai.2016.2126 (accessed on 16th July 2025).
9. Bernard, D. (2014). *Public transportation: Perceptions of Filth Contributing to Poor Health*. https://core.ac.uk/download/56326277.pdf (accessed on 16th July 2025).
10. Douglas McCarthy and David Blumenthal (2006). *Committed to safety: Ten case studies on reducing harm to patients*. https://core.ac.uk/download/71350251.pdf (accessed on 16th July 2025).
11. Bocicor, M. I., Molnar, A. J., & Taslitchi, C. (2016). *Preventing hospital-acquired infections through a workflow-based cyber-physical system*. http://arxiv.org/abs/1702.08010 (accessed on 16th July 2025).
12. Smith, LN (Ed), Burke, J, Sveinsdóttir, H, Willman, A (2008) Patient Safety in Europe: Medication Errors and Hospital-acquired Infection. Amsterdam, Workgroup of European Nurse Researchers (accessed on 16th July 2025).

13. Cairns, S., Gibbons, C., King, H., Llano, M., et al. (2018). *Results from the third Scottish National Prevalence Survey: Is a population health approach now needed to prevent healthcare-associated infections?* https://core.ac.uk/download/293863931.pdf (accessed on 16th July 2025).

14. Callus, R., Mamo, J., Micallef, J., Montefort, S., et al. (2012). *Hospital management of community-acquired pneumonia in Malta.* https://core.ac.uk/download/46602322.pdf (accessed on 16th July 2025).

15. Protano, C., Cammalleri, V., Romano Spica, V., Valeriani, F., & Vitali, M. (2019). Hospital environment as a reservoir for cross transmission: cleaning and disinfection procedures. *Annali di igiene : medicina preventiva e di comunita, 31*(5), 436–448. https://doi.org/10.7416/ai.2019.2305(accessed on 16th July 2025).

16. Ceccarelli, G., Di Gregorio, V., Falcone, M., Farcomeni, A., et al. (2015). *The spread of multidrug-resistant infections is leading to an increase in the empirical antibiotic treatment failure in cirrhosis: A prospective survey.* https://core.ac.uk/download/54521158.pdf (accessed on 16th July 2025).

17. Madziatera, D., Msofi, K. S., Phiri, T. V., Mkandawire, S. D., & Comber, A. (2020). Availability, Accessibility and Proper Use of Personal Protective Equipment in Wards at Queen Elizabeth Central Hospital (QECH) Blantyre, Malawi: An Observational Study. *Malawi medical journal : the journal of Medical Association of Malawi, 32*(3), 124–131. https://doi.org/10.4314/mmj.v32i3.4(accessed on 16th July 2025).

18. D'Alessandro, D., Napoli, C., & Nusca, A. (2016). *Are liquids an efficient vehicle of healthcare-associated infections? A review of reported cases in Italy (2000–2014).* https://core.ac.uk/download/84928144.pdf (accessed on 16th July 2025).

19. Edwards, J. N., & Silow-Carroll, S. (2011). *Eliminating central line infections and spreading success at high-performing hospitals.* https://core.ac.uk/download/71358071.pdf (accessed on 16th July 2025).

20. Wong, C., Epstein, S. E., & Westropp, J. L. (2015). Antimicrobial Susceptibility Patterns in Urinary Tract Infections in Dogs (2010-2013). *Journal of veterinary internal medicine, 29*(4), 1045–1052. https://doi.org/10.1111/jvim.13571(accessed on 16th July 2025).

21. Gabbard, S. E. (2016). *Post Foley removal guideline process and outcome evaluation.* https://core.ac.uk/download/232575773.pdf (accessed on 16th July 2025).

22. Giraldi, G., Iachini, M., Montesano, M., Orsi, G., et al. (2019). *Excess length of hospital stay due to healthcare acquired infections: Methodologies evaluation.* https://core.ac.uk/download/227029126.pdf (accessed on 16th July 2025).

23. Katharina Hauck & Xueyan Zhao, 2010. "**A structural equation model of adverse events and length of stay in hospitals**," Monash Econometrics and Business Statistics Working Papers 4/10, Monash University, Department of Econometrics and Business Statistics.(accessed on 16th July 2025).

24. Hayward, A. C., Warren-Gash, C., Whitaker, H., Huijskens, H., Hung, T., McMenamin, J., Ren, M., et al. (2018). *Laboratory-confirmed respiratory infections as triggers for acute myocardial infarction and stroke: A self-controlled case series analysis of national linked datasets from Scotland.* https://core.ac.uk/download/153570271.pdf (accessed on 16th July 2025).

25. Ritchie, N. D., Irvine, S. C., Helps, A., Robb, F., Jones, B. L., & Seaton, R. A. (2017). Restrictive

antibiotic stewardship associated with reduced hospital mortality in gram-negative infection. *QJM : monthly journal of the Association of Physicians, 110*(3), 155–161. https://doi.org/10.1093/qjmed/hcw134(accessed on 16th July 2025).

26. Storr, J., Twyman, A., Zingg, W., Damani, N., Kilpatrick, C., Reilly, J., Price, L., Egger, M., Grayson, M. L., Kelley, E., Allegranzi, B., & WHO Guidelines Development Group (2017). Core components for effective infection prevention and control programmes: new WHO evidence-based recommendations. *Antimicrobial resistance and infection control, 6*, 6. https://doi.org/10.1186/s13756-016-0149-9(accessed on 16th July 2025).

27. Kilale, A., Pruss-Ustun, A., Reda, A. A., Doebbeling, B., Gumodoka, B., Denise, C., Kessler, C. S., et al. (2013). *Estimated risk of HIV acquisition and practice for preventing occupational exposure: A study of healthcare workers at Tumbi and Dodoma Hospitals, Tanzania.* https://core.ac.uk/download/pdf/18410863.pdf (accessed on 16th July 2025).

28. Lillestolen, D. (2018). *Infections not fought: Antibiotic resistance in underserved communities.* https://core.ac.uk/download/158970352.pdf (accessed on 16th July 2025).

29. Rosa, Elsye M., et al. "The Infection Control Risk Assessment and Strategies to Reduce HAIs at Hospital in YOGYAKARTA Indonesia." *Asian Social Work Journal*, vol. 4, no. 2, 2019.(accessed on 16th July 2025).

30. May, D., & Pitt, M. (2012). *Environmental cleaning in the NHS since the NHS Plan: A policy and evidence-based context.* https://core.ac.uk/download/157852848.pdf (accessed on 16th July 2025).

31. McCarthy, D., & Klein, S. (2011). *Keeping the commitment: A progress report on four early leaders in patient safety improvement.* https://core.ac.uk/download/71358579.pdf (accessed on 16th July 2025).

32. Mohamed, K. M., & Ali, A. M. (2023). *Hospital hygiene challenges: An overview of issues and solutions.* https://core.ac.uk/download/618379289.pdf (accessed on 16th July 2025).

33. Stewart, S., Robertson, C., Manoukian, S., Haahr, L., Mason, H., McFarland, A., Dancer, S., Cook, B., Reilly, J., Graves, N., & ECONI Steering Committee (2019). How do we evaluate the cost of nosocomial infection? The ECONI protocol: an incidence study with nested case-control evaluating cost and quality of life. *BMJ open, 9*(6), e026687. https://doi.org/10.1136/bmjopen-2018-026687(accessed on 16th July 2025).

34. Szczepura, Ala and Osipenko, Leeza (2009) Point of care tests for hospital-acquired infections (HAIs) : economic analysis report. Coventry: Warwick Medical School. (Unpublished)(accessed on 16th July 2025).

35. Sartelli, M., et al. (2016). *Antimicrobials: A global alliance for optimizing their rational use in intra-abdominal infections (AGORA).* https://core.ac.uk/download/77016212.pdf (accessed on 16th July 2025).

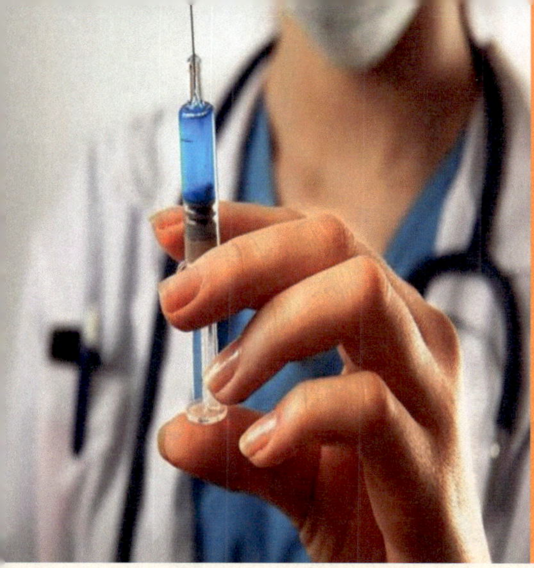

Chapter 13

VACCINES AND IMMUNO-PROPHYLAXIS

Contents

Introduction

The invention of vaccines is one of the most significant human achievements in public health history, shifting the strategy of adapting to infectious diseases. Vaccines achieve this by triggering the immune system to recognize and destroy pathogens, thereby providing a form of immunity without causing the disease. This preventive measure has not only stopped the spread of most viruses and bacteria but also achieved a spectacular decline in morbidity and mortality from the disease. Thus, vaccines and immunoprophylaxis represent a cornerstone of modern medicine, imparting not only individual protection but also herd immunity by generating community immunity. In uncovering the intricacies of vaccine development and deployment, it is evident that their purpose extends beyond prevention; they are central to supporting global health and staving off the socio-economic effects of disease. In the last few years, the range of vaccines has grown significantly, with the incorporation of new technologies and innovative methods to enhance efficacy and safety. Traditional vaccines, previously inactivated or attenuated pathogen-based, currently include subunit vaccines, mRNA technology, and vectored immunoprophylaxis (VIP) strategies. One such example is VIP technology that involves adeno-associated viruses to deliver preformed antibody genes and has demonstrated encouraging results in causing long-term immunity against malaria, a disease that kills nearly one million young children annually despite the lack of a licensed vaccine. The promise of such new approaches emphasizes the dynamic nature of immunoprophylaxis and the imperative for continued research and development to address new health issues. These developments are not only significant to combating well-established diseases but also to actively addressing prospective threats to infection. The application of vaccine practice further requires comprehensive strategies that consider various determinants of population health dynamics, socio-cultural attitudes, and access to health care. Successful immunization depends on public acceptance, education, and access, which has been dramatized by the global reaction to the COVID-19 pandemic. Failures in vaccination coverage in the face of available effective vaccines indicate the multidimensional challenge of accomplishing universal immunization and reveal deficits in public health infrastructure. Thus, it is crucial to encourage unified action by governments, health workers, and communities to facilitate vaccine acceptance and adherence to immunoprophylaxis regimes. Through scientific and societal means, the path to realizing the highest possible benefits of vaccines can be strengthened, ultimately leading to healthier populations around the world.

Definition of Vaccines

The mechanism of vaccines is really one of immune system stimulation, preparing the body to recognize and repel specific pathogens. Vaccines are really composed of antigens from disease-producing microorganisms — like viruses or bacteria — that have been inactivated or made less potent. The process is a simulation of a natural infection, which compels the immune system to respond with the activation of antibodies and memory cells. As a consequence, during actual exposure to the pathogen, the immune system responds more rapidly and optimally, of most importance in averting illness that causes significant morbidity and mortality. Secondly, these immunologic mechanisms illustrate the substantial role vaccines play in the broader public health landscape, not only personally benefiting patients but also contributing to herd immunity and disease prevention at the community level. Vaccines have been classified into various categories, and each category is designed to elicit an immune response by a different mechanism. Live-attenuated vaccines have a weakened form of the causative agent, while killed or inactivated vaccines have killed or inactivated microorganisms. Subunit, recombinant, and conjugate vaccines have various components of the pathogen, such as protein or sugar, to elicit immunity without disease. Both have their own combination of benefits; live vaccines are more likely to cause long-term immunity with fewer doses, and inactivated vaccines are more likely to be safer to use in immunocompromised individuals. Knowing the differences is essential to determine the correct vaccination strategy, particularly in vulnerable populations, as cited in recent literature on the necessity for immunoprophylaxis in patients who have impaired immune systems, such as those undergoing chemotherapy or other types of immunosuppression (Fisher et al., 2012). Vaccine importance transcends individual health; they are crucial to infection control and prevention of outbreaks. Immunization programs have previously controlled and even eradicated infectious diseases, which demonstrates the public health program's effect on population health outcomes. Notably, improvements in vaccine technology, including mRNA vaccines, have contributed to the immunoprophylaxis toolbox to combat emergent pathogens. Through continuous research and development, the capability to create vaccines at speed has been witnessed, particularly in response to global threats of viral pathogens resulting in pandemics. Effective vaccine approaches, including pre-exposure prophylaxis and other health education programs, are called for since they facilitate individual and community immunity against infectious diseases, which is critical towards securing community health and safety (Generalov et al., 2014).

Importance of Immunoprophylaxis

Immunoprophylaxis is among the pillars of preventing infectious disease, particularly among vulnerable patients such as those being treated for malignancies or undergoing hematopoietic stem cell transplants. Such patients are at added risk of morbidity from viral infections, which can be the cause of grave complications in their recovery processes. As is known from studies, pre-exposure and post-exposure prophylactic interventions, along with antiviral therapies, are crucial in minimizing such risks. Implementation of effective immunoprophylaxis into practice is not only a matter of concern for protecting patients but also of improving global health outcomes for such a high-risk population. A combined approach consisting of immunization and rigorous infection control strategies can effectively prevent serious viral infections, as well as emphasizing the imperative need for effective immunoprophylactic interventions in cancer and organ transplantation (Fisher et al., 2012). Even aside from immunocompromised patients, individuals with functional or anatomical asplenia are at significantly higher risk for infections, particularly those caused by encapsulated organisms. These patients at risk are prone to severe disease by agents like *Streptococcus pneumoniae* and *Haemophilus influenzae*, especially in the early years of life. Preventive interventions like immunoprophylaxis are particularly relevant in this group of patients and involve vaccinations for disease prevention that could lead to life-threatening illnesses. Research highlights the importance of educating asplenic patients about their levels of raised risk and the need to adhere to recommended vaccination timetables that might include more up-to-date conjugate vaccines. Regular revaccination is a central part of maintaining immunity and avoidance of overwhelming infection, and this further reinforces the utility of immunoprophylaxis in this specific population (Melles & Marie, 2004). The general influence of immunoprophylaxis has implications that extend beyond the safety of individual patients to include public health priorities. Where mass immunoprophylaxis is used, it promotes herd immunity, which has the power to effectively prevent the spread of infectious diseases among populations. Through ensuring that those who are most susceptible receive their vaccines on time, the disease burden is minimized not just on the healthcare system but on society as a whole. With this, public health programs promoting the use of immunoprophylaxis are instrumental in building community immunity against infectious diseases. Further, with still-emergent pathogens posing threats to global health, sustained support for immunization programs and recognition of the benefit of immunoprophylaxis are imperative. This multi-pronged approach ultimately fosters both individual health protection and public well-being, reminding us of the pivotal position of immunoprophylaxis in the current healthcare landscape.

13.1. History of Vaccination

The history of vaccination is a remarkable story of public health and scientific progress over centuries, emphasizing humanity's ongoing battle against infectious illness. The effective vaccine was first launched by Edward Jenner in 1796 with cowpox material to vaccinate against smallpox, a deadly disease that affected individuals globally. Jenner's pioneering efforts opened the door to the development of vaccines, establishing foundational principles of immunization that would later become the standard. Not only did this initial research prove the mechanism of utilizing a compromised or killed pathogen to induce a response in the immune system, but it also generated further interest in the subject area, paving the way for later advances in vaccine development. Jenner's work did not end with smallpox, paving the way for subsequent research that would ultimately lead to the vaccination advances we rely on today in modern medicine. Throughout the 19th century, microbiology developments began to inform the science of vaccination. Louis Pasteur was one of the dominant figures of the time and with him came the attenuated virus vaccine theories in the form of vaccinations for rabies and anthrax. Pasteur's work brought to the forefront the importance of understanding pathogens and the way they react to the immune system, significantly enhancing vaccine effectiveness. His technique also validated the necessity of scientific rigor in vaccine production, as it involved controlled laboratory investigations and clinical tests to establish safety and efficacy. These developments not only increased public confidence in vaccines but also identified the central role of preventive care activities against infectious diseases, leading to mass campaigns of immunization in urban as well as rural regions. The 20th century witnessed the dawn of a new era in vaccination with the establishment of full-immunization regimens and the development of combination vaccines. Vaccinations like the measles, mumps, and rubella (MMR) vaccine and the inactivated polio vaccine transformed global health outcomes by reducing child deaths from these diseases by a great percentage. Furthermore, new technologies like recombinant DNA and genetic engineering witnessed the emergence of innovations like the development of hepatitis B and human papillomavirus (HPV) vaccines. These innovations not only showcased the adaptability of vaccination techniques to combat various pathogens but also made vaccines more accessible to populations that were diverse, marginalized, and even distant. This chronology of development is representative of the transformation of vaccination as a mainstay in immunoprophylaxis, ultimately leading to a more developed society and shattering the hold infectious diseases had on human existence (Figure 13.1).

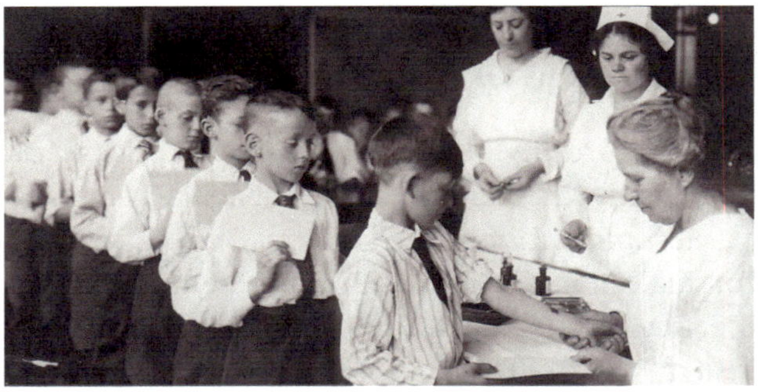

Figure 13.1. A brief history of vaccination.

Source: https://www.immunize.org/wp-content/uploads/vaccines/history-timeline-vintage-1024x512.png.

13.1.1. Early Practices and Discoveries

The history of immunoprophylaxis followed its roots back to the early applications that were the forerunners of current vaccination techniques. Variolation, for instance, was one of the first documented applications and was prevalent in the 18th century. Material from smallpox lesions was implanted in healthy persons to induce a light disease. This practice was, in turn, followed particularly in China and, later on, in Europe, where it was embraced fervently in order to combat the devastating impacts of smallpox. While variolation lowered mortality rates from epidemics, its application created the necessity for safer procedures, particularly because it failed to eliminate the risk of severe infection. This direct impact from these early experiments enabled the move to Edward Jenner's groundbreaking work with cowpox in 1796, which ultimately resulted in the production of the first ever vaccine to be successful. Edward Jenner's development of vaccination marked a fundamental turning point in immunization and public health history. By inoculating an eight-year-old boy with cowpox lesion material, Jenner demonstrated that the introduction of a less virulent pathogen initially could give protection against a more virulent disease, including smallpox. This cross-protection concept led the way to the scientific basis of vaccination and revolutionized disease prevention strategies. Jenner's work not only provoked the systematic development of vaccines against other infectious pathogens but also defined the role of immune response in managing disease. Global application of campaigns of vaccination throughout the 19th and 20th centuries resulted in spectacular declines in death rates from smallpox and other infectious diseases, demonstrating evidence of the revolutionary potential of early findings in immunoprophylaxis. As the vaccine and immunoprophylaxis science improved, so did the philosophies and methodologies guide disease prevention.

The contributions of early scientists like Louis Pasteur and Robert Koch emphasized the importance of careful laboratory inquiry complemented by epidemiologic study, a maxim that is reiterated in the development of modern vaccines. Their combined effort explained infectious disease and host immunity mechanisms that gave rise to the production of vaccines, which became the basis of vaccine production. Moreover, the intersection of epidemiologic information with laboratory research underscored the importance of aligning vaccination policy with focused populations. Now that the efficacy and safety of vaccines are well documented through solid science, historic controversy surrounding vaccine hesitancy will continue to beset vaccine efforts. While today's science struggles with these issues, understanding of early experiences' lessons remains key to the fortification of public trust in vaccination programs. This intersection of current research and historical perspective is key to the proper negotiation of the complex immunoprophylaxis in the face of globalization and shifting disease needs (Figure 13.2).

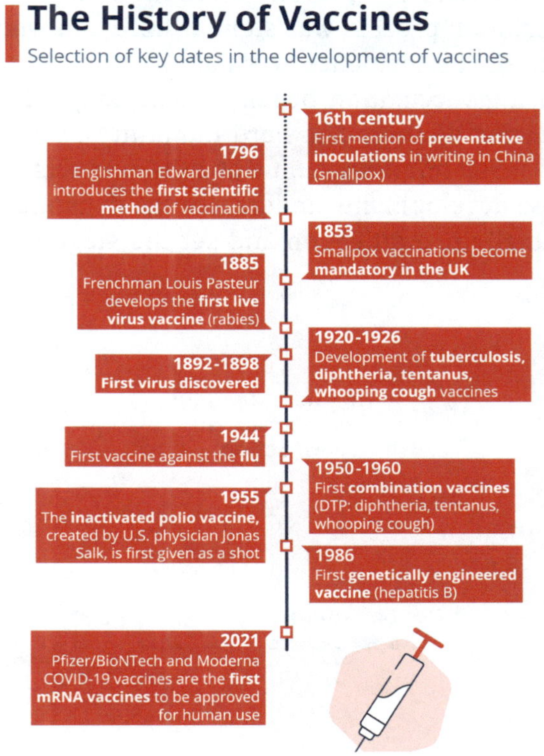

Figure 13.2. Vaccine history timeline.

Source: https://www.statista.com/chart/21725/timeline-history-of-vaccinations/.

13.1.2. Development of the Smallpox Vaccine

Smallpox vaccination marks a milestone in the history of medicine and public health. In the late 18th century, the English physician Edward Jenner made breakthroughs of revolutionary import by using cowpox, a related but milder virus, to immunize against smallpox. Observing that milkmaids who got cowpox did not get smallpox, Jenner speculated that exposure to cowpox imparted protection. Jenner tested his theory in 1796 by immunizing a boy with cowpox, followed by an exposure to smallpox without adverse consequences. This seminal work opened the door to immunization as a scientific discipline, demonstrating one disease could be used to protect against another. Jenners innovation not only initiated a tide of scientific interest but also demonstrated the practical application of vaccination, opening the door to future developments in immunoprophylaxis. The success of Jenners smallpox vaccine in the clinic fueled further research and development into the field, leading to more effective means of vaccination. In the 19th and 20th centuries, vaccination campaigns expanded with numerous different methods being employed to increase efficacy and accessibility. The inoculation process was standardized, and vaccines were mass-produced, a factor that significantly reduced the incidence of smallpox in most countries. Coupled with this, public health initiatives favoring vaccination began to take shape, highlighting how it could contribute to the control of epidemic disease. The herd immunity also became more popular during this period, illustrating that mass immunization not only protects the immunized individuals but communities as well. These developments underscore the dynamic character of immunization practice, which was critical to smallpox eradication and set the stage for integrated immunization programs (Figure 13.3).

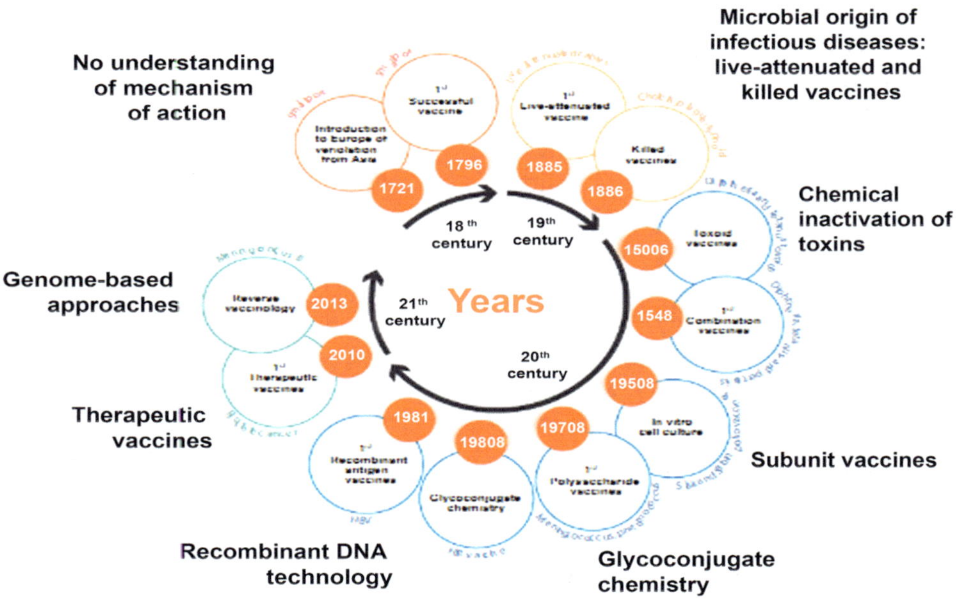

Figure 13.3. History of vaccine development.

Source: https://www.researchgate.net/publication/321127205_Vaccines_Accelerating_Innovation_and_Access_Global_Challenges_Report.

Lastly, the culmination of the various efforts to fight smallpox led to the complete elimination of the disease by the year 1980, a triumph that was recognized by the World Health Organization. The achievement is widely regarded as one of the greatest public health breakthroughs in human history, demonstrating the potential of vaccines to eliminate diseases completely. The eradication of smallpox is of particular importance for health disparities as it is the first instance of a global health disparity to be eliminated by mass vaccination efforts. As is noted, "If the definition of eradicating of a health disparity were indicated by the absence of any differences in incidence or mortality between a population's experience with a health problem, then... the only health disparity that has ever been eradicated is smallpox" (Chen, 2012). The lessons learned from this triumph continue to direct the planning of vaccines worldwide, illustrating the importance of synchronizing scientific advancements with policy formulation in resolving other health disparities effectively.

13.1.3. Milestones in Vaccine Research

The development of vaccines has been a landmark achievement in public health history, the culmination of humankind's ability to battle infectious disease through scientific means. Among the most groundbreaking achievements is the production of maternal vaccines that would immunize infants against various pathogens. One such example is the initiative known as PREPARE, which focuses on developing a platform for maternal vaccination against infection of Group B *Streptococcus* during pregnancy. GBS is one of the leading causes of life-threatening illness in infants, and maternal immunization might potentially eliminate such risks by enhancing maternal immunity and thus indirectly providing passive immunity to infants during the first vulnerable months of life. PREPARE study is aimed at the creation of protective serocorrelates against prevalent GBS serotypes, therefore uncovering the essence of combined vaccination programs that are also capable of bridging gaps in maternal and child health, particularly in low-resource settings (Berardi et al., 2020). Another landmark in the history of vaccine science is the ongoing pursuit for efficacious vaccines against Respiratory Syncytial Virus (RSV), which is a significant risk for young children worldwide. Although self-limiting, RSV infections also carry a high rate of hospitalization and the accompanying concern over misuse of antibiotics in these infections. The single option for prophylaxis, palivizumab, is sparingly utilized due to cost and the rigid criteria for its administration. This lack of effective vaccines emphasizes the necessity of new approaches to immunoprophylaxis. Researchers are already working on other monoclonal antibodies (mAbs) that provide a cheaper means of prevention for all infants, not just high-risk ones. It indicates the broader potential of vaccine research in attempting to advance the well-being of the public, but also in eliminating economic pressures brought about by frequent hospital admissions (Rocca et al., 2021). The vaccine development process continues to unfold, an indication of a more sophisticated understanding of infectious disease and immunology. With new technologies such as mRNA vaccines ushering in a new era, scientists are exploring ways to enhance efficacy as well as accessibility. While the traditional vaccine development approaches were the pillars of success of the past, new research combines novel approaches to attack new and endemic infections. Such progress is necessary, especially during times of international public health emergencies, when the simplicity of pathogen transmission can lead to such pandemics as the recent COVID-19 pandemic. Through leveraging insights from turning points in history, vaccine development nowadays strives to design an inclusive model for immunoprophylaxis that minimizes disease impact in populations and generations, an unyielding drive in advancing public health and safety.

13.2. Types of Vaccines

The development of vaccines has revolutionized public health by providing an instrument for disease prevention through stimulation of the immune system. Vaccines are categorized into a number of categories, which are designed to induce immunity through various mechanisms. Live attenuated vaccines employ weakened pathogens to elicit an immune response without causing the disease, as seen in disease prevention for conditions such as measles and mumps. Conversely, inactivated vaccines comprise killed or inactivated pathogens through chemical processes that safely stimulate an immune response without imparting the risk of infection. It is a categorization that emphasizes the diversity of techniques used in immunoprophylaxis, which is one of humankind's ongoing endeavors to prevent infectious diseases and promote health globally. The subunit vaccine is another typical type of vaccine, which employs specific components of the germ, such as proteins or carbohydrates, but not the entire germ.

This is a means that allows for a broad immune response with minimal chance of side effects from live germs. Furthermore, toxoid vaccines, which are made of inactivated bacterial toxins, are designed to inhibit toxin-induced illnesses and not the bacteria. A good example is the tetanus vaccine, which inhibits toxin production without introducing humans to live bacteria. These are some of the categories that are important in enjoying the impacts of various immunization processes, which can ensure that vaccines are optimized for use against target illnesses while keeping them safe and effective. Lastly, recombinant DNA technology has introduced new vaccine types, including recombinant vector vaccines and mRNA vaccines, which have gained importance in recent years. Recombinant vector vaccines employ a carrier empty virus to introduce DNA encoding an antigen of the target organism into host cells, which elicit an immune response. On the other hand, mRNA vaccines give the body genetic instructions to produce a target antigen and induce the immune system to recognize the pathogen. The new approaches demonstrate the dynamic nature of vaccine development and the imperative for continued research in boosting immunoprophylaxis. Combating priority public health threats, such as tuberculosis, remains important, and new vaccines will be essential in achieving global health objectives (Generalov et al., 2014; Novita, 2020).

13.2.1. Live Attenuated Vaccines

Live attenuated vaccines are of utmost significance in today's immunoprophylaxis, as they employ a weakened form of the pathogens to induce robust immune responses without causing the disease itself. The vaccines are designed to induce humoral as well as cellular immunity and offer long-term immunity to various infectious pathogens. Unlike inactivated vaccines, which require multiple doses to achieve adequate immunity, live attenuated vaccines often confer lifelong immunity following a single administration. This aspect is particularly beneficial in public health strategies for the elimination of disease. The effectiveness of live attenuated vaccines is indicative of their significance as an immunization programs globally, contributing significantly to the control and elimination of different infectious conditions.

Varicella zoster virus (VZV) is a classic example of an agent that has been brought to success through live attenuated vaccination. Chickenpox, or varicella, is a more common childhood disease, but its sequelae cause severe morbidity in immunocompromised individuals, older adults, and pregnant women. The live attenuated varicella vaccine developed has contributed significantly toward minimizing the morbidity of Varicella and its complications. As stated, although Varicella occurs most frequently in children, the potential outcome of the disease explains the importance of vaccination to safeguard susceptible individuals. Immunity programs with the varicella vaccine are now an integral component of pediatric immunization schedules in most nations, with broad immunity to the community being encouraged (Pace, 2008) (Figure 13.4).

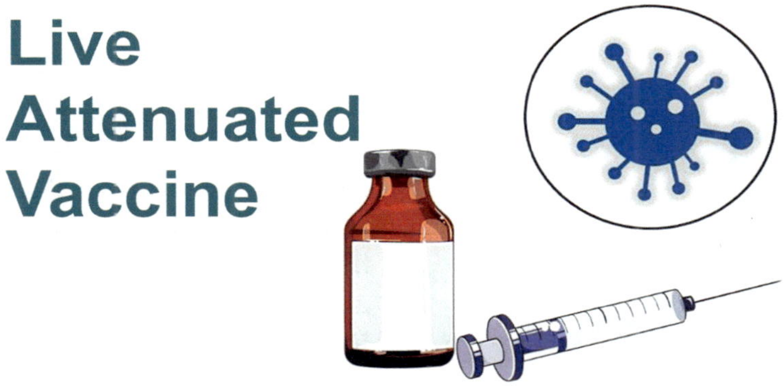

Figure 13.4. Live attenuated vaccines.

Source: https://i.ytimg.com/vi/WGfNcWyVByU/maxresdefault.jpg.

Though the advantages of live attenuated vaccines should be pointed out, their natural risks cannot be overlooked. Patients whose immune system is weakened are more likely to develop side effects from live vaccines because their bodies might not handle the weakened pathogens effectively. Through research, patients who undergo cancer treatments or those undergoing hematopoietic stem cell transplantation were highly susceptible to viral infections based on compromised immune responses. Heightened surveillance in pre- and post-exposure prophylaxis is thus essential in such groups. A combined strategy, employing live attenuated vaccines, antiviral therapy, and aggressive infection control, can effectively overcome the detrimental consequences of viral infections in high-risk patient populations (Fisher et al., 2012). This diversified strategy puts particular emphasis on the delivery of customized vaccination programs that are targeted specifically at both immunocompromised and the general populations.

13.2.2. Inactivated Vaccines

Inactivated vaccines are a valuable asset in the practice of immunoprophylaxis, giving a safe and effective method of prevention of infectious disease. Inactivated vaccines consist of killed or inactivated microorganisms, which have been physically or chemically inactivated and thus are incapable of causing disease. Through introducing the immune system to such non-viable antigens, inactivated vaccines elicit an immune response without danger of a viable infection. This characteristic renders them particularly effective for vulnerable populations, such as infants, the elderly, and individuals with compromised immunity. In addition, inactivated vaccines have fewer side effects than their live equivalents, as a result of which they become the preferred option in most public immunization programs for control of epidemics and herd immunity. The efficacy of inactivated vaccines has been demonstrated for a wide variety of pathogens, including the inactivated poliovirus vaccine and hepatitis A vaccine. Both have proven to effectively reduce the rate of their respective infections (Figure 13.5).

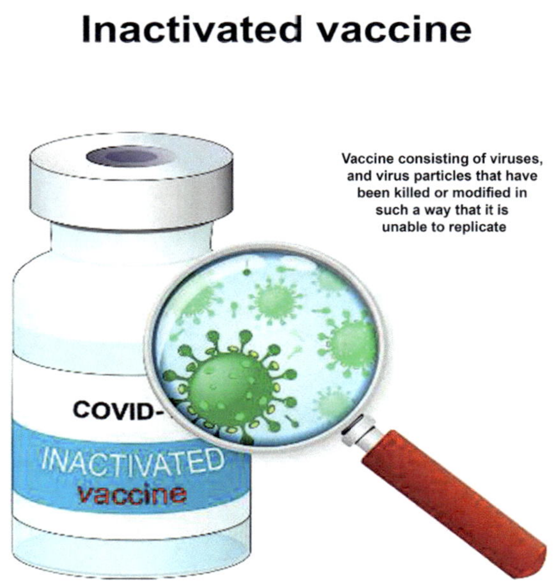

Figure 13.5. Inactivated vaccines.

Source: https://external-content.duckduckgo.com/iu/?u=https%3A%2F%2Fcdn3.vectorstock.com%2Fi%2F1000x1000%2F65%2F97%2Fcovid19-19-coronavirus-inactivated-vaccine-vaccine-vector-37336597.jpg&f=1&nofb=1&ipt=ec0bdfb797dfe041a027e13077ad46d791fa5d7d1afebc2b875f704b98900141.

However, there are limitations of inactivated vaccines that must be known. For instance, inactivated vaccines will require multiple doses to achieve full immunity and will not give long-term protection unless booster injections are repeated. Furthermore, the immunity induced by inactivated vaccines will not be of such a high intensity as that induced by live attenuated vaccines. Despite these issues, ongoing research is needed to further refine formulations and adjuvants in an effort to optimize immunity while considering the realities of vaccine delivery and administration. The value of inactivated vaccines extends beyond mere disease prevention; in diseases of augmented risk, such as pediatric oncology and recipients of hematopoietic stem cell transplantation, they are a crucial tool. In such populations, bacterial and fungal diseases is a well-known cause, but viral diseases are becoming more pronounced owing to the high risks and lack of effective treatments. Therefore, the application of inactivated vaccines could have a long way to go in diminishing cases of viral infection, for which prophylaxis is most crucial for patient protection. As reported in recent literature, coupled strategies that include vaccination, infection control, and therapeutic intervention are paramount to keeping the health of such high-risk populations (Fisher et al., 2012). Such a comprehensive strategy brings into perspective ongoing research into creating advances in inactivated vaccine technology, particularly for high-risk populations, thus creating a platform for improved prophylactic protection within the healthcare setting (Fisher et al., 2012) (Figure 13.6).

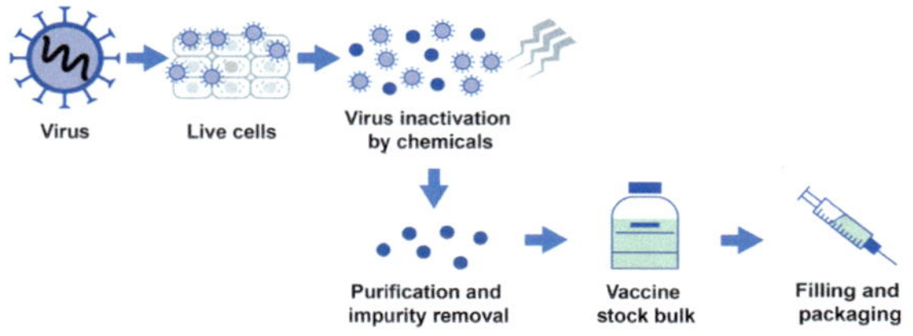

Figure 13.6. Manufacturing process of inactivated vaccines.

Source: https://external-content.duckduckgo.com/iu/?u=https%3A%2F%2Fwww.meiji.com%2Fglobal%2Fwellness-stories%2Fcommon%2Fimg%2Fcovid-19%2Fcovid-19_02.png&f=1&nofb=1&ipt=8aadd67fc84f970c57f10629665dc89dca2bba32a6c1c49f0c8da0f3f047f18e.

13.2.3. Subunit, Recombinant, and Conjugate Vaccines

The history of vaccines has improved a great deal with the introduction of subunit, recombinant, and conjugate vaccines. These vaccines utilize certain antigens in eliciting an immune response without actually introducing the entire pathogen.

Subunit vaccines have only the necessary protein components of the pathogen, without the non-essential parts that will cause unwanted side effects. This specificity is left to risks, but it still elicits the adaptive immunity of the immune system. The versatility of subunit vaccines allows them to accommodate several antigens, therefore being an ideal choice for diseases where traditional live or inactivated vaccines are dangerous. This technological advancement reinforces the position of new vaccine strategies in improving public health status. Recombinant vaccines further capitalize on immunoprophylaxis by utilizing recombinant DNA technology in the production of antigens. This method entails the insertion of the gene encoding for a target antigen in a suitable host to facilitate the large-scale production of the target proteins. The resulting proteins are isolated and applied as a component of a vaccine. Recombinant vaccines have proved effective in fighting numerous infectious diseases, including human papillomavirus (HPV) and hepatitis B. Since they can produce very specific antigens, recombinant vaccines can induce strong immune reactions without increasing the potential for side effects.

The growing amount of research incorporating recombinant vaccine technology reflects its promise of rapid development and responsiveness to emerging infectious diseases, therefore reinforcing global health security. Conjugate vaccines, on the other hand, overcome polysaccharide antigen limitations. Such antigens, typically obtained from the outer covering of bacteria, are poor stimulants of the immune system in young children. Through chemical conjugation of these polysaccharides to carrier proteins, conjugate vaccines significantly boost the immunogenicity and facilitate the induction of a strong immune response more easily. Such a process has proved highly effective in combating bacterial diseases like meningitis and pneumonia that overwhelm at-risk populations. All these improvements in vaccine conjugation techniques illustrate the power of immunological developments for surmounting limitations against traditional vaccine designs. As the environment for vaccine development changes, these techniques will serve an integral function in the continued fight against infectious diseases and bettering the health of populations around the world (Figure 13.7).

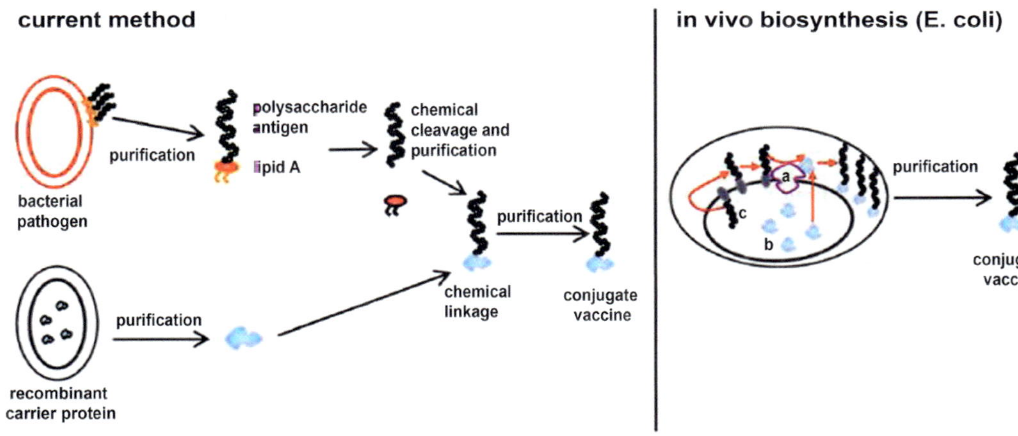

Figure 13.7. Current method for the production of conjugate vaccines and *in vivo* biosynthesis.

Source: https://www.researchgate.net/figure/Current-method-for-the-production-of-conjugate-vaccines-and-in-vivo-biosynthesis-a_fig1_45628678.

13.3. Mechanism of Action

Understanding the mode of action of vaccines is necessary for an appreciation of their role in immunoprophylaxis. Vaccines work mainly by mimicking a pathogenic infection, which provokes the immune system without causing disease. This is done by introducing antigens — substances that provoke an immune response — into the body. The immune system recognizes these antigens and develops a specific response, e.g., the production of antibodies and activation of T cells. This immune memory enables the body to respond faster and more effectively to repeated contact with the actual pathogen. The evidence has consistently demonstrated that a robust immune response not only safeguards the host but can also initiate herd immunity, suppressing transmission within populations. Consequently, this initial understanding of mechanisms highlights the efficacy of vaccines in preventing infectious diseases and the need for ongoing innovation in immunization technology. Further research into types of vaccine reveals their varied mechanisms of action, particularly for virus-like particle (VLP) vaccines. These utilize non-replicating particles that resemble the disease-inducing virus, provoking a strong immune response without risk of establishment of disease. The potential of VLP vaccines can be viewed based on their clinical applications, especially in preventing viral infections. Current studies suggest that prophylactic vaccination with VLPs has proven to be successful in clinical practice, laying a solid groundwork for their use against infection (Foerster & Molęda, 2020) (Figure 13.8).

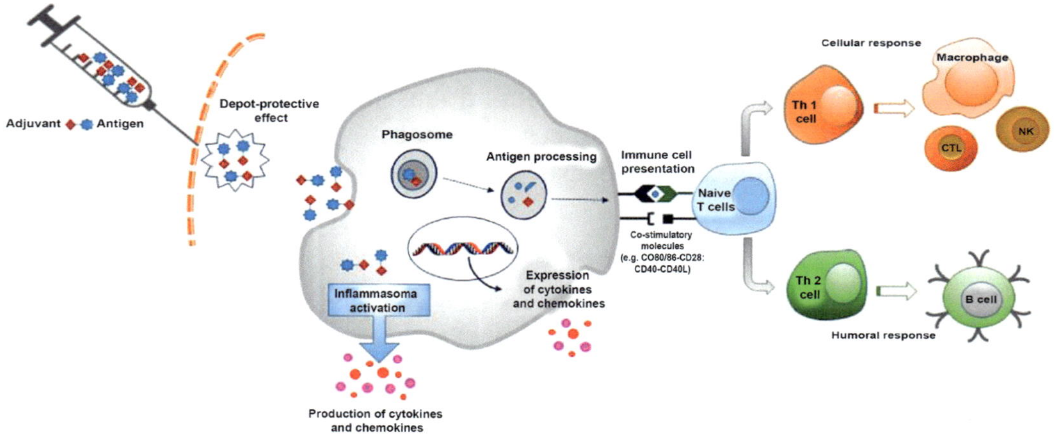

Figure 13.8. Mechanism of action of adjuvants.

Source: https://www.mdpi.com/vaccines/vaccines-10-00819/article_deploy/html/images/vaccines-10-00819-g001.png.

All the same, there are also challenges to translating these strategies to chronic infections, where therapeutic vaccine approaches are not yet established. The novel mechanism by which VLPs trigger immune responses has the potential to impact novel means of targeting specific immune pathways, ultimately leading to enhanced vaccine safety and efficacy profiles. With increased focus on novel immunotherapies, understanding specific cytokine-targeting methodologies offers new insights into mechanisms of action for vaccines. For instance, the immunization of interleukin-13 (IL-13) holds great potential for the modulation of chronic allergic disease. With the use of a vaccine that triggers the immune system to produce antibodies against this cytokine, scientists have found great potential in efficiently treating diseases like atopic dermatitis and eosinophilic esophagitis. Experiments have shown that this technique is capable of overcoming conventional monoclonal antibody therapy according to its distinct mechanism, eliciting a polyclonal response (Foerster & Molęda, 2020). This provides another advantage in precision medicine, where tailor-made immunoprophylaxis can be made to fit one's own immune fingerprint. Thus, knowledge of the mechanism of action of new vaccines not only gives access to disease prevention but also to targeted treatments at the molecular level.

13.3.1. Immune Response to Vaccination

The immune reaction to vaccination is a complex and multidimensional process that starts with the administration of an antigen into the body. This antigen, made up of inactivated or weakened pathogens or proteins, activates the immune system to become aware of the potential hazard. Upon vaccination, dendritic cells engulf the antigen and present it to T-cells, which become activated and proliferate. This stimulation leads to the production of CD4+ helper T-cells, which also enhance the immune response by stimulating B-cells to produce antibodies. These antibodies become significant in the neutralization of the causative pathogens, therefore providing a robust defense measure against future infection.

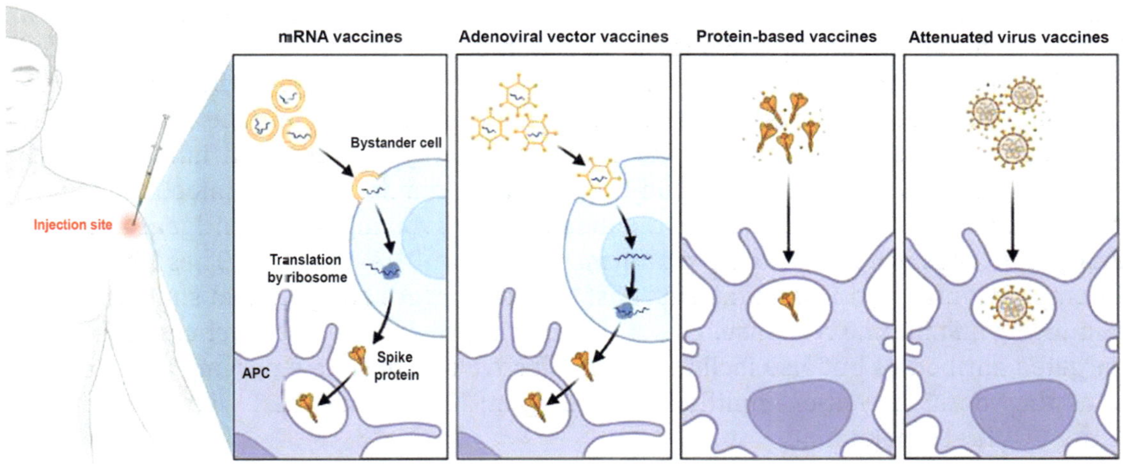

Figure 13.9. Immune responses induced by COVID-19 vaccines.

Source: https://cdn.prod.website-files.com/621e95f9ac30687a56e4297e/64a8d7ce64d21b5b0551aab3_V2_1675796277370_f819e75c-98b9-45e5-bbfa-b2c1ca5a3362.png.

The efficacy of this immune response strengthens the role of vaccines in immunoprophylaxis, thereby eliminating diseases that once were common and mostly fatal. The persistence and effectiveness of the immune response can be determined by a range of factors, including the type of vaccine used and the health and age status of the patient. Live attenuated vaccines tend to cause a more intense and longer-lasting immune response compared to inactivated vaccines because they are closer to a natural infection. Further, population studies indicate that age may influence the immune response; younger individuals are likely to have a stronger response. For example, although the immune response will gradually decline, booster doses can also restore immune memory, boosting antibody production and T-cell activation. Immune subtleties accentuate the necessity for personalized vaccination regimens, particularly in those at risk for viral infection, such as controversy surrounding efficacious immunoprophylactic measures in medical practice (Fisher et al., 2012). Ongoing research continues to examine novel vaccines that can enhance immune responses, particularly against viral infections. For instance, third-generation recombinant pre-S protein-based new-generation vaccines have been promising to protect persons at increased risk of hepatitis B virus reinfection following transplantation. These vaccines have been reported to induce a robust immune response in lamivudine prophylaxis recipients, with the response rate being up to 50% among some populations (Wong et al., 2013). This supports a root change in vaccine design, where an understanding of individual patient immunological profiles can be utilized to inform effective prevention. In addition to optimizing immunoprophylaxis, this assists in advancing knowledge of viral pathology and immune system dynamics and provides potential for further advances in vaccination (Figure 13.9).

13.3.2. Role of Antigens and Antibodies

The intricate interaction between antibodies and antigens is the foundation of immunity, particularly vaccines and immunoprophylaxis. Antigens are outside bodies, like pathogens or proteins, and they induce immunity by inducing antibody formation. The antibodies are specialized proteins that identify specific antigens and tag them for destruction or inactivation by other immune cells. This is the specificity that matters; effective vaccines must introduce antigens that are very similar to the pathogen's but that do not cause disease in order to allow the immune system to recognize and remember the threat. Such memory is crucial in conveying long-term immunity and points to the role of antigens in educating the body's defense mechanism against infection. Furthermore, advances in vaccine technology bring into the limelight the evolving role of antigens and antibodies, particularly concerning novel vaccine platforms such as mRNA vaccines. These groundbreaking vaccines employ synthetic mRNA to instruct host cells to produce antigens that simulate segments of a virus, inducing an immune response. This is not only improving the effectiveness of the generation of the targeted antibodies but also facilitating an effective response to emerging infectious diseases as soon as they occur, a well-exemplified case being mRNA vaccines that were generated to fight against the COVID-19 pandemic.

As indicated by studies, liposomal antigen application has significantly improved antigen delivery, ensuring more effective immunoprophylaxis (Grygorieva et al., 2023). This synergistic effect of antibodies and antigens in such advanced systems highlights their central role in modern medical therapies. The potential of the knowledge of antigens and antibodies in medicine extends far beyond vaccine development because they play a central role in the diagnosis of many diseases and conditions. Identification of some antibodies can serve as important biomarkers for various infectious diseases and autoimmune diseases. For instance, the occurrence of anticardiolipin antibodies has been key to the diagnosis of antiphospholipid syndrome, with insights into other complex immunological responses. Moreover, research involving liposomal antigens also suggests the potential for improving diagnostic techniques and vaccine efficiency, continuing a scientific legacy century in the making (Generalov et al., 2014). Through the demystification of antigens and antibodies, the medical community is better able to individualize immunologic interventions in favor of prevention and treatment methodologies in public health initiatives.

13.3.3. Memory Cells and Long-Term Immunity

The memory cells are one of the defining ideas of long-term immunity, and the specialized immune cells have an active role in the body's response to known pathogens. B and T cells respond to antigens through a primary immune response, producing effector cells and the development of memory cells. These cells have a long history of life following initial exposure, enabling the immune system to respond more quickly and accurately upon subsequent encounter with common pathogens. Such immunological memory is responsible for the immunizing effect of vaccines, that which condition the immune system to react against and respond to infectious agents without causing disease and providing a foundation for long-term immunity necessary for public health. The memory cell longevity is key to vaccine longevity. With the ongoing evolution of vaccination technology, with a focus on changing viral ecosystems, an assessment of how long memory responses last is necessary. It is learned that memory B cells can endure for years and are able to rapidly produce targeted antibodies upon re-exposure to target antigens. As highlighted in research, the role of specific cytokines such as interleukin-13 has been of interest because of its potential to enhance the memory response and generate long-term immunological protection. Above all, ongoing research into virus-like particle (VLP)-based vaccines is designed to take advantage of such immune responses, illustrating the critical role played by memory cells in the establishment of long-term immunity to infectious diseases more broadly, especially as the latest challenges are faced within the field of immunoprophylaxis (Foerster & Molęda, 2020). Long-term immunity not only protects individuals but also contributes to the establishment of herd immunity within populations, illustrating the broader social value of vaccination programs. Vaccines that are able to stimulate a strong memory cell response reduce the disease burden, particularly among susceptible populations such as children and the elderly. For instance, respiratory syncytial virus (RSV) remains a troublemaker among young children, highlighting the importance of efficient vaccines that can provide long-term protection (Foerster & Molęda, 2020). The mechanism of developing new vaccines is understanding the interaction between memory cells and their longevity against varied pathogens, with the mind that immunizations have to be effective for a long time. Optimizing vaccine strategies to enhance memory cell development and longevity is an important area for the development of immunoprophylaxis and safeguarding public health against existing and future infectious diseases.

13.4. Benefits of Vaccination

Vaccination is a significant public health intervention that substantially reduces the incidence of infectious diseases, thereby promoting individual and population health. Vaccines not only prevent infection, but they also play a critical role in establishing herd immunity, which is formed when a broad portion of the population becomes immune to an infectious disease. This herd immunity protects people who are unable to be vaccinated due to medical issues, such as allergies or immunosuppressive treatment. As more and more people get vaccinated, the overall disease burden reduces, resulting in fewer outbreaks along with lower healthcare costs for preventable diseases. Lastly, vaccines have previously brought about the near eradication of several diseases, so they are proven to be an asset as a preventive measure in public health strategies. The role of vaccination in child and maternal health cannot be overstated. Prevention of mother-to-child transmission (PMTCT) of disease, for instance, as in the case of hepatitis B, is a clear example of the central role that vaccination plays during pregnancy. Current guidelines promote maternal screening and early immunization of the infant, aligning with combined strategies for avoiding vertical transmission of HBV. Studies have indicated that administration of universal and regular hepatitis B birth-dose vaccines, along with post-exposure prophylaxis, lowers the risk for HBV infection in children significantly. However, there is an urgent need to address existing inequities in coverage of vaccination, specifically in high-endemic regions, in efforts to achieve global health targets. Enhancing PMTCT interventions can yield important health, social, and economic benefits in the end, forming a condition of improved maternal and child health outcomes, as noted by recent public health discussions (Restrepo et al., 2023). In addition to protecting vulnerable groups, vaccines also play a key role in reducing the number of serious respiratory illnesses among young children. New monoclonal antibodies, such as Nirsevimab, have created a new avenue for immunoprophylaxis against respiratory syncytial virus (RSV), which has its greatest impact on infants under the age of 24 months. Such vaccinations' efficiency in real-world implementations has proven wide-ranging hospitalization and ICU admission decrements for RSV, presenting the promise of vaccination in enhancing pediatric outcomes significantly. As further research continues to validate the safety and efficacy of such newer methods of immunization, the importance of funding for vaccine programs becomes increasingly clear in the prevention of the burden of child disease. Fortifying vaccination coverage not only increases the community immunity but is able to ultimately safeguards the health of the most vulnerable groups (Baldo et al., 2024) (Figure 13.10).

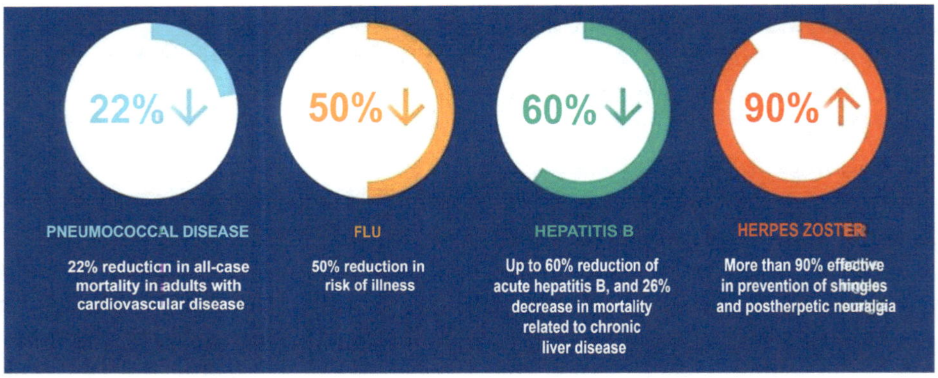

Figure 13.10. Benefits of vaccination in reducing diseases burden.

Source: https://external-content.duckduckgo.com/iu/?u=https%3A%2F%2Fwww.nfid.org%2Fwp-content%2Fuploads%2F2024%2F09%2FFigure-1-1200x600.jpg&f=1&nofb=1&ipt=eab117a21fe969b7684787910c99481d3a043ee867f86a36e3b42f3c683688b7.

13.4.1. Prevention of Infectious Diseases

Control of infectious disease has largely evolved with the expansion of medical investigation and public health intervention. Vaccines have also emerged as among the most effective weapons, conferring immunity against a broad spectrum of pathogens. By inducing the immune system to recognize particular antigens, vaccines protect against diseases such as measles, mumps, and rubella, once of predominant health importance. In addition, their role in achieving herd immunity should be emphasized; if a significant percentage of the population is vaccinated, the disease spread is lowered and by so doing, they help shield the unimmunized or immunocompromised individuals. Therefore, emphasis on vaccination as an overarching preventive measure is critical in combating infectious diseases and calls for both individual and collective responsibility for public health. Where vaccines are partially effective or not available, adjunctive strategies such as immunoprophylaxis play a key role in disease prevention. Immunoprophylaxis is utilized as the administration of particular antibodies or antigens to prevent infection, primarily in high-risk groups. In malignancy patients or in patients undergoing hematopoietic stem cell transplantation, viral infection has been the primary cause of morbidity and death. It has been noted in research that the partial efficacy of antiviral therapy merits aggressive preventive measures, for example, pre-exposure and post-exposure prophylaxis and, in addition, strict infection control procedures. The integrated strategy highlights the role of targeted interventions among high-risk groups as a means to limit the effect of infectious diseases effectively (Fisher et al., 2012). Moreover, new measures such as chemoprophylaxis and immunoprophylaxis together highlight the evolving nature of infectious disease prevention. A recent study that has considered single-dose rifampicin (SDR) with BCG immunization for leprosy contacts is a classic illustration of this approach. By the treatment of SDR among individuals closely related to new cases, the research aims to significantly reduce the rate of *M. leprae* transmission. The potential for such dual strategies to enhance preventive impacts on infectious diseases is enormous, especially when host immune responses and genetic profiles are factored in. Not only does this twin intervention try to interrupt the cycle of transmission, but it also tries to identify biomarkers that would underlie more efficacious prophylactic interventions in the future (Alam et al., 2013). Hence, the integration of chemoprophylaxis and immunoprophylaxis can be a revolutionary approach in the area of public health interventions for controlling infectious diseases (Figure 13.11).

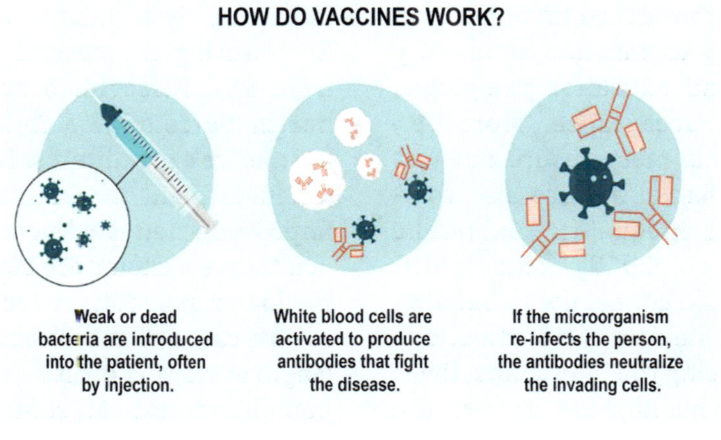

Figure 13.11. Work process of vaccines.

Source: https://i0.wp.com/post.healthline.com/wp-content/uploads/2023/04/2072254-Everything-You-Need-to-Know-About-Vaccinations-1296x728-header-body.png?w=1155&h=1843.

13.4.2. Herd Immunity and Community Protection

The theory of herd immunity is key to the success of vaccination campaigns and immunity of communities. Herd immunity is obtained when a high percentage of individuals in a population are immunized against a contagious disease, thereby restricting its overall spread, and rescuing those who are vulnerable. This indirect immunity is crucial for vulnerable populations, such as infants, the elderly, and those with compromised immune systems, who are not suitable candidates for certain vaccines. Successful vaccination campaigns that achieve herd immunity can lead to the eradication or complete elimination of disease incidence, revolutionizing public health achievement. For instance, the mass vaccination against measles in the majority of developed countries has led to a drastic reduction in cases and underscores the efficacy of mass immunization in guaranteed community health (Nair et al., 2011). Achieving herd immunity does, however, require concerted effort in vaccination and public health work, typically reflecting society's attitudes to immunization. Vaccine uptake is determined by public awareness, availability, and cultural attitudes towards vaccines. Hesitancy towards vaccines can undermine herd immunity, resulting in outbreaks of vaccine-preventable disease, such as the re-emergence of measles among populations with reduced immunization coverage. As a strategy to enhance community protection, policies and education campaigns must foster vaccine acceptance. Moreover, the health care systems must ensure not just that vaccines are available, but are also cost-effective to eliminate inequalities in public health (Beaudry et al., 2017). This multi-pronged approach would contribute to building a robust community immunity to infectious diseases, hence enhancing the interconnectivity of public and personal health. Furthermore, the application of herd immunity measures relies on international collaboration and responsive health policy. Infectious diseases are not localized, and one outbreak in one region can become a threat to others; and therefore, there needs to be coordinated deployment of vaccines as well as disease surveillance across the globe. International agencies play an important role in ensuring that this partnership is made available, as they help track disease trends and sponsor vaccine campaigns worldwide. More importantly, new vaccine technologies and immunization strategies must become a priority, namely for high-burden diseases in low-resource settings, to prevent morbidity and mortality worldwide. For instance, innovation in Vaccines and Immunoprophylaxis against diseases RSV will enable the protection of vulnerable populations and support herd immunity in general, and this will ultimately increase community resilience to infectious diseases (Nair et al., 2011).

13.4.3. Economic Impact and Healthcare Savings

The economic impact of immunization extends far beyond the direct cost of vaccine production and distribution; it redefines the nature of healthcare spending altogether. Vaccines significantly reduce the incidence of infectious illness, consequently lowering hospitalization and associated healthcare expenditures. For instance, Nirsevimab has been shown to be effective in preventing RSV hospitalization, most notably in infants who are most at risk. By lowering the cost of health complications from RSV, Nirsevimab not only improves the health outcomes of children but also saves healthcare expenditures. The economic rationale for investment in vaccines like Nirsevimab is improved when long-term healthcare savings to healthcare systems are considered, considering the lower expenditure incurred in dealing with severe cases of the disease and increasing the length of stay in hospitals, resulting in a healthier population that can contribute productively to society. Additionally, cost-effectiveness analysis demonstrates that there is a multifaceted relationship between clinical benefits and healthcare spending. For palivizumab, studies demonstrate that although it does prevent RSV hospitalizations among high-risk infants effectively, its overall cost-effectiveness seems to be limited if used indiscriminately. Cost-effectiveness analysis finds that palivizumab's

ICERs are quite disparate, indicating that although it might be warranted for certain high-risk groups, universal vaccination is not economically feasible. These findings highlight the critical aspect of healthcare economics: that immunoprophylaxis activity needs to be targeted towards those most in need to achieve the greatest economic and health returns. In doing so, the exact vaccine deployment strategy is not only to optimize resource use but also to make health systems economically viable while improving patient outcomes. An analysis of the broader economic value of vaccination illustrates great promise for the saving of healthcare systems globally. Minimization of hospitalization and healthcare costs through successful immunization programs can provide huge net savings in the long term, thus maximizing budget efficiency. Notably, the economic benefit of the programs is optimized using combinations of pharmaceutical advances, such as Nirsevimab and palivizumab, and properly designed public health campaigns. For instance, vaccinating high-risk children prevents costly severe illness and limits the long-term financial burden of chronic disease. Savings in healthcare due to successful immunization programs can then be invested in strengthening other facets of public health so that they, in turn, create a cycle of improved health, lower expenditure, and enhanced quality of life in populations (Figure 13.12).

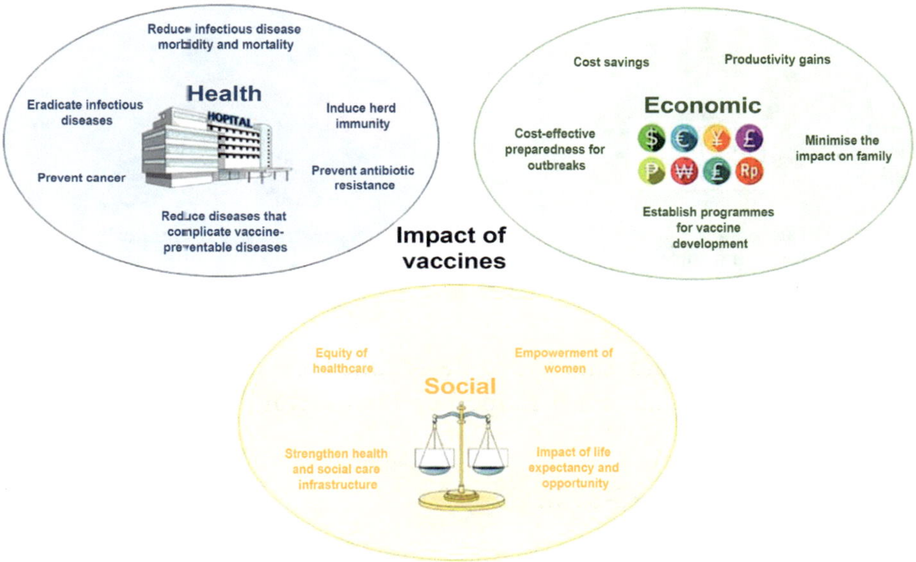

Figure 13.12. The impact of vaccines according to their health, economic or social benefit.

Source: https://www.frontiersin.org/files/Articles/550510/fmicb-11-01526-HTML/image_m/fmicb-11-01526-g001.jpg.

13.5. Vaccine Safety and Efficacy

Vaccine safety and efficacy are foremost in public health and immunoprophylaxis. Thorough preparation and rigorous testing of vaccines aim to establish their safety profiles and elicit robust immune responses to infectious pathogens. Evidence-based assessments, like clinical trials and post-marketing surveillance, play pivotal roles in screening adverse effects and overall efficacy. Understanding the risk-benefit profile of vaccines is paramount in decision-making among healthcare professionals and patients. For example, in children, the risk of bacterial and fungal infection while in fever and neutropenia has been extensively studied. Current evidence illustrates that viral pathogens are increasingly significant causes of morbidity and mortality, underlining the importance of vaccines in pre-exposure and post-exposure (Fisher et al., 2012). The comprehensive approach to vaccine safety involves not just efficacy but also the ongoing surveillance that is required to respond to new viral threats.

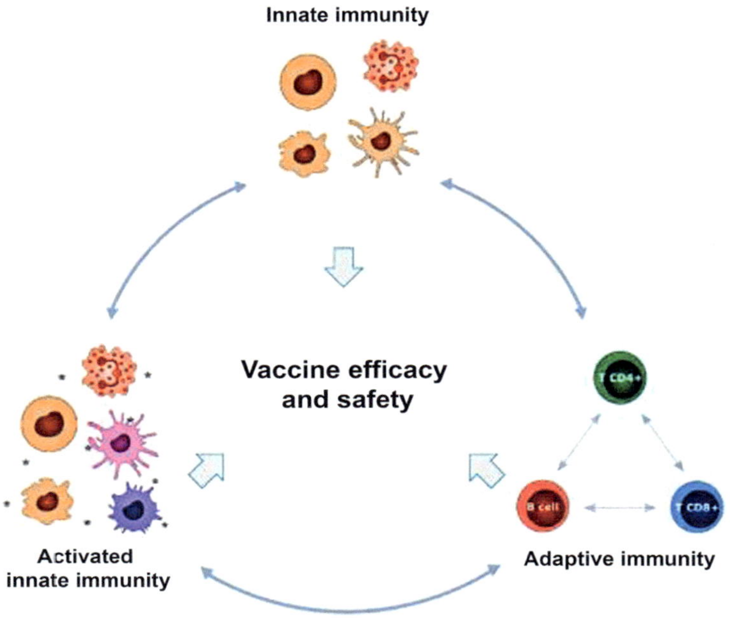

Figure 13.13. Vaccine efficacy and safety are determined by interactions between innate and adaptive immunity. These interactions are shaped by host factors and can be oriented by vaccine properties.

Source: https://www.mdpi.com/2076-393X/9/6/579.

This innovation in new vaccination techniques parallels shifting trends in immunoprophylaxis, with emphasis on vaccine efficacy and safety. VLP-based vaccination, for instance, has shown promise in the clinic, emphasizing the potential as an effective prophylactic treatment. Although these strategies have not yet provided licensed therapeutic vaccines for chronic diseases, the underlying science provides valuable lessons in immune modulation. More current studies indicate that modulation of specific interleukins, like IL-13, in vaccine regimens can be therapeutic for conditions like atopic dermatitis and eosinophilic esophagitis. This cytokine modulation focus establishes new paradigms for vaccine development, with the idea that methods that are aimed at inducing immune stimulation without causing marked adverse effects might be more effective than more conventional strategies (Foerster & Molęda, 2020). Therefore, as vaccination technologies keep improving, so does the potential to increase both safety and efficacy in public health systems. Enhancing the dialogue regarding vaccine safety and efficacy is a priority in addressing public fear and resistance to vaccines. Informed consent must be founded on honest communication about vaccine benefits and risks. Education programs for healthcare providers and the population regarding vaccine function, associated information, and best practices for surveillance of safety are crucial. Particularly in such high-risk patients as hematopoietic stem cell transplant recipients, effective prevention strategies against viral infection are crucial, that as, mass vaccination as one of the stringent infection control strategies (Fisher et al., 2012). Further, instilling confidence in vaccine programs through community outreach activities is critical in increasing public confidence in vaccines. By reducing gaps in knowledge and increasing awareness, public health officials can heighten the general perception of vaccine safety and efficacy, ultimately to improve population health outcomes and a stronger public health response (Figure 13.13).

13.5.1. Clinical Trials and Regulatory Approval

The vaccine and immunoprophylaxis clinical trial landscape is multifaceted and critical to support ensuring that safe and effective products reach the marketplace. Through the various stages of vaccine development, the significance of specified clinical trials becomes critical. The process typically begins with preclinical work, where candidates for vaccines undergo extensive laboratory testing. Following this stage, potential candidates with desirable safety and efficacy characteristics proceed to human clinical trials. The trials usually pass through Phase I, II, and III stages, each performing various test types, such as dosing, immunogenicity, and efficacy in increasing groups. By the use of these rigorous protocols, researchers are in a position to conclude that the vaccines possess the necessary safety requirements before being approved by authorities. Vaccine regulatory approval is also a major component in the model of immunoprophylaxis. Agencies such as the United States Food and Drug Administration (FDA) and the European Medicines Agency (EMA) play a pivotal role in determining whether vaccine candidates are eligible to be licensed for public use. The agencies scrutinize the data that is emanating from clinical trials to ensure the vaccines not only prove to be efficacious but also mitigate potential risks. Besides, the higher the demand for new vaccines — echoing faster progress for respiratory syncytial virus (RSV) — the more important it becomes to develop guidelines for clinical endpoints and licensure pathways. This is crucial to speed up access to lifesaving vaccines while holding strict safety standards, finally, for the public good. Coordination and concurrence among researchers, regulative bodies, and global health organizations are necessary to render the vaccine development process less bumpy in the context of clinical trials and approval processes. The World Health Organization's recent consultations regarding RSV vaccines are an indicator of the necessity for coordination in determining candidate case definitions, clinical efficacy outcomes, and trial progress paths. These discussions are particularly significant because they address not only high-income regions but also consider the unique issues confronted by low- and middle-income countries in vaccine deployment. With multiple candidates in clinical development in an expedited schedule, such as novel design of immunogens and extensive global demand, encouraging these collaborations will increase the likelihood of timely and efficacious immunization regimens for prevention of RSV and other infectious conditions, as cited in recent literature (Modjarrad et al., 2015, 2016).

13.5.2. Common Side Effects and Misconceptions

Vaccination is one of the most important public health measures for immunity against infectious diseases. Despite the enormous benefits, side effects are the frequent cause of misconceptions that deter people from taking. Side effects of the vaccination, such as mild fever, pain at the site of injection, and tiredness, are typically indicative responses in which the immune system is reacting against the vaccine. The fact that such reactions are usually temporary and a normal immune system response can be reassuring and may dispel fear of vaccination. Additionally, the incidence and severity of side effects vary between people and vaccines, though serious adverse events are very rare. It is absolutely essential to be cognizant of this fact because it will make people take healthy decisions about vaccination and it will disprove the prevalent myths that vaccines are too dangerous. Probably the most common myth that has been linked to vaccination is the misconception that vaccines can lead to the development of the diseases they are supposed to prevent. This misconception is especially harmful, as it could encourage people to avoid vaccination altogether. The reality is that most vaccines employ inactivated or weakened pathogens, or even fragments of the pathogen, which cannot infect individuals and lead to the disease they were meant to prevent. For instance, the flu vaccine is made of inactivated virus or components of the virus and, therefore, cannot induce influenza. Further, infrequent mild reactions following vaccination can occasionally be mistaken for demonstration of the disease, leading to even greater misconceptions. Public education within wider public health becomes critical in removing these myths because it educates people about the safety and efficacy of vaccines. In addition, disinformation regarding vaccine safety will lead to hesitation and, eventually, lower rates of vaccination and, by default, epidemics of vaccine-preventable diseases. Seeking clarification, there is a need to dispel myths surrounding side effects with an emphasis on balancing the benefits of immunization versus the risk of potential adverse effects. For instance, while some individuals may experience momentary discomfort from a vaccine, say soreness or fever, such side effects are minimal compared to the severe complications of the disease vaccines are meant to avert. Furthermore, it has been established that vaccines significantly reduce hospitalization and mortality rates from such infections. Public education strategies on such aspects will boost faith in immunization plans and result in enhanced health outcomes among populations as a whole, ultimately allowing immunoprophylaxis to be a generally accepted and implemented phenomenon (Wong et al., 2013).

13.5.3. Monitoring and Surveillance Post-Licensure

The surveillance and monitoring of vaccines following licensure are integral aspects in ensuring public health security as well as the efficiency of the vaccines. Even after approval of a vaccine, there is always the risk of unexpected side effects and adverse reactions that require robust surveillance mechanisms. Through this kind of effort, unusual reactions that fell through the initial clinical trials due to the constraints of sample sizes or trial lengths are picked up. Hence, public health institutions everywhere adopt various systems, such as the Vaccine Adverse Event Reporting System (VAERS) in the United States of America, to capture signals of risk from vaccines and rapidly respond to any new problems as they emerge. An effective post-licensure surveillance system enhances trust in immunization programs and results in better health outcomes in the long term, since it provides a tool to evaluate the actual-world safety and efficacy of vaccines against diseases. Apart from monitoring for safety, post-licensure surveillance also entails continued observation of the vaccine efficiency and trends in pathogen evolution. Strains of the virus in the community over a period of time might change, influencing the performance of vaccines against diseases. As such, health organizations must analyze evidence on disease immunity from vaccination in various groups and geographic regions and respond accordingly. This ongoing monitoring is particularly important for vaccines that shield against very volatile diseases, such as influenza, for which formulation revision might be necessary annually. Through active surveillance, health authorities can issue timely data on vaccine advice to medical staff and the public, ensuring optimal immunization policy based on changing epidemiological patterns . Furthermore, post-licensure monitoring forms the foundation for vaccine policy and research programs and informs decisions regarding booster doses, new product development, and extended vaccination programs. Policy decisions are made by public health authorities using data gathered through surveillance systems, balancing the necessity of attaining high vaccination coverage with the need to reduce risk. This data can also lead to further research on new vaccines or improved formulations through trends of side effects or efficacy variations seen. With the area of vaccine development being constantly in progress, continued monitoring shall be an important part to guide the way of immunoprophylaxis strategies in the world. Sustaining systematic post-licensure surveillance programs must thus be ensured in order to save lives as well as consolidate public health activities at large (Modjarrad et al., 2016).

SUMMARY

The summary on the role of vaccines and immunoprophylaxis points to the central place that these interventions hold in guaranteeing public health. While infectious diseases continue to pose a significant threat to population health, the role that can be played by vaccines in reducing mortality and morbidity cannot be overstated. By activating the immune system to detect and fight pathogens, vaccines not only safeguard individuals but also play a role in community immunity, lowering transmission rates among populations. The overall effect of immunization is indicated by the sharp reduction in the incidence of diseases that previously resulted in rampant outbreaks, thus establishing the need for immunoprophylaxis in contemporary healthcare systems. Consequently, sustained promotion of vaccination coverage is essential to ensure that such advances in public health are sustained. Further, the investigation of ethical and organizational dimensions of immunization also points to the complexity of vaccine use within complex societies. Public acceptance, access, and equity are important factors influencing vaccine distribution and acceptance. Inequity in access to healthcare can undermine vaccination, particularly among marginalized populations, and therefore demand targeted educational outreach and distributive equity. Moreover, debunking myths regarding the safety and effectiveness of vaccines is also important in fostering confidence among the public. In line with experts' point of view, effective communication must reach communities by emphasizing the importance of immunization not just for individual protection but for communal health as well (Generalov et al., 2014). Therefore, a wide-scale approach to promoting vaccines is important as we navigate the ever-changing landscape of global health. Overall, international commitment to immunoprophylaxis and vaccination must extend beyond policy-making alone; it must be joined by collaboration between health professionals, policymakers, and communities. Continuous research, innovation, and response to new infectious threats are imperative conditions for vaccine effectiveness. Global initiatives toward vaccine development should similarly optimize equitable access so that all segments gain from improvements in immunization. By eradicating the social determinants of health and removing obstacles to vaccination, the idealistic dream of achieving herd immunity becomes a reality. In the broader health promotion landscape, the function of vaccinations remains an underpinning of preventive medicine, protecting future generations from being bogged down by the burden of avoidable disease (Croubels et al., 2007).

In public health, immunoprophylaxis and vaccination are critical measures of both preventing and controlling disease. Whole-cell bacterial immunotherapy, particularly using products like MV140 and autovaccines, has proven efficacy in the case of recurrent urinary tract infections (RUTI) among susceptible elderly individuals. A 200-patient trial demonstrated a considerable reduction in the prevalence of UTIs, from seven to forty-fold, during a twelve-month period. Improvements in patients' quality of life were also noted, noting numerous advantages of such immunoprophylactic techniques. These reports highlight the importance of integrating new therapeutic strategies in clinical practice for enhancing health benefits among vulnerable populations, particularly in the context of antibiotic resistance that continues to be a strong challenge in managing recurrent infections (Lorenzo-Gómez et al., 2021). Also, the importance of safe measles immunoprophylaxis is a key area of concern, particularly in the context of the revival of diseases among certain populations. Vaccines developed for active immunization against respiratory syncytial virus (RSV) reflect the world's urgent concern to safeguard pediatric populations from serious acute lower respiratory illness. Research has unveiled the potential of several vaccine candidates, and with it, a tempered optimism among scientists regarding their efficacy and potential to lower childhood morbidity attributable to RSV. However, evidence exists that cost and affordability may constrain the extensive use of these vaccines in resource-poor environments. Prioritizing low-cost available vaccine interventions, however, could effectively reverse the health inequities experienced by children in poor populations (Nair et al., 2011). In general, inclusion of vaccines and immunoprophylaxis in public health systems does have some evidence-based potential to address significant health issues. By emphasizing research and development in effective immunization methods, particularly on priority populations such as the elderly and children aged five and below, tremendous steps can be achieved in reducing disease burdens. Advances in bacterial immunotherapy and RSV vaccine development reinforce the ongoing commitment to improving public health through preventive interventions. Lastly, collaborative effort among policymakers, medical professionals, and researchers will be essential to be able to generalize these findings into practice towards equitable health outcomes among populations (Nair et al., 2011; Lorenzo-Gómez et al., 2021).

CLOSER LOOK

CHALLENGES IN VACCINE DEVELOPMENT

One critical aspect to take into account in vaccine design is the induction of antibody-dependent enhancement (ADE) disease after immunization. While this has not been adequately characterized yet, virus-specific antibody responses can, under certain circumstances, increase the viral infection rate or cause immunopathology. Cases of pulmonary immunopathology elicited by Th2 response were also previously shown in SARS-CoV and Middle East respiratory syndrome (MERS-CoV) vaccine studies in mouse models. Although clinical trials of COVID-19 vaccine candidates have yet to provide evidence of ADE, the issue remains puzzling in this case and needs an effective T-cell response as a key parameter for successful SARS-CoV-2 vaccine development. Frequent mutations and genetic recombination resulting in variants with increased virulence and capacity to evade immune recognition are another major challenge that arises with vaccine development against viruses. With the ongoing COVID-19 pandemic, SARS-CoV-2 spike (S) protein mutations have occurred to reduce virus neutralization effectiveness. On top of this, the vaccine's ability to show efficacy against more virulent/incipient viral strains is also the highlighted concern. Further, there is still very limited knowledge on the duration of vaccine-acquired immunity, particularly the short-term and long-term safety and efficacy of most COVID-19 vaccines. It was originally anticipated that infection-induced undetectable levels of antibodies against SARS-CoV-2 will be reached within a few months following disease. Recently, however, serologic studies have reported a consistent level of neutralizing antibodies (nAbs) against the S protein receptor-binding domain (RBD) and S2 subunit between 5 and 7 months post-infection versus the quick decline of nAbs titers against the nucleocapsid (N) protein. Excluding men, frail older adults, and comorbid patients, vaccine effectiveness against serious diseases of the disease was shown to be maintained for almost 9 months but in varying rates depending on the vaccine type. Conversely, in previous such trials with SARS-CoV, measurable nAbs titers were observed up to 12–17 years after infection, with long-term reactive memory T-cells to the N protein for 17 years after infection. Amongst these studies, numerous cases of viral reactivation or reinfection have occurred in many countries, and the second infection has indeed turned out to be more severe than the first in numerous instances, especially those in Ecuador and the United States. Fortunately, and as verified by released World Health Organization (WHO) reports and recent study findings, at least portions of the developed COVID-19 vaccines are still poised to provide some level of protection against the new variant emerging strains, particularly those capable of eliciting a broad immune response. Nevertheless, the resulting nAb titers are relatively lower than the one elicited against the original strain. Also, and to date, the tested vaccines against all of these variants have not been all the approved vaccines, making the ultimate evaluation of the effectiveness of candidate vaccines difficult at this juncture. As has been speculated, in the case of low vaccine efficacy in the new variants, approaches with an added booster dose or a form of the vaccine with variant-specific proteins could provide better potency. In July 2021, Pfizer announced a booster shot plan for its COVID-19 vaccine to provide increased protection against new variants like the delta variant, which was lower in sensitive to antibody neutralization. The proposed plan was, however, contained since insufficient evidence supported the implementation of a third dose of the vaccine in the population, especially since half of the US population at the time was unvaccinated. Administration of a third dose of the Pfizer-BioNTech vaccine was, however, endorsed in individuals over the age of 65 years or those at high risk of severe disease. Likewise, Moderna also announced a third booster dose and candidates as a booster vaccine, particularly as a counter to variants strategy, after noting a six-fold decline in nAb titers against the South African variant. Extended to the implementation stage, a booster dose of the Moderna vaccine for those above 65 years of age and high-risk individuals, such as healthcare workers, has been scheduled. As in the case that has been embraced by Pfizer, however, Moderna's booster will be half a dose (50 micrograms) at least six months after the second dose. The reasoning behind this reduction in dose is motivated by a desire to reduce the risk of potential side effects that are introduced by vaccination. In the event that the COVID-19 pandemic is not controlled, booster doses for all vaccinated individuals might be back on the table (Figure 13.14).

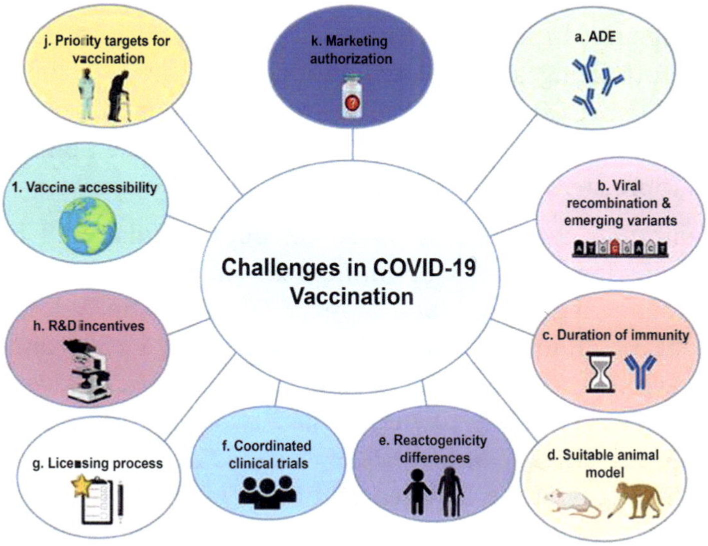

Figure 13.14. Overview of key challenges in COVID-19 vaccination, including scientific, logistical, and regulatory hurdles such as viral variants, vaccine accessibility, licensing, and immune response variability.

Source: https://www.mdpi.com/2076-393X/9/12/1474.

Interestingly, newer data on the majority of currently approved COVID-19 vaccine candidates for emergency use show that the majority of these vaccines not only protect against COVID-19 but also against other deadly diseases. In light of this, and with a quest to gain sterilizing immunity, every effort is presently being made to ensure that the majority of the population is vaccinated. Experiments in non-human primates, reported that most COVID-19 vaccine candidates have complete or partial protection against viral challenge in the lower respiratory tract and upper respiratory tracts. Similarly, experiments with recently developed vaccines revealed that there is a protective effect in the upper respiratory tract when the vaccines are administered at higher dosages. Sterilizing immunity in the upper respiratory tract may be needed in order to prevent the transmission of the virus. Thus, intranasal vaccine platforms designed to induce an intense mucosal immune response of the upper respiratory system are being explored. In May 2021, in a new study, it was stated that a single dose of an intranasal candidate COVID-19 vaccine(AdCOVID) can induce sterilizing immunity in lung tissue in vaccinated animals. This was also evident in the induction of vigorous serum-nAb responses, T cell responses, and vigorous mucosal immunity induction in vaccinated mice. Unfortunately, however, recent information from the AdCOVID phase 1 clinical trial indicated that there was no adequate stimulated immune response in healthy volunteers and thus prompted the closure of this intranasal vaccine development process. With these discouraging updates in mind, intranasal vaccines remain promising due to their ability to generate mucosal immunity on the linings of the nose and lungs, such that they not only protect against infection but also transmission. Certain other attributes advocating for the development of such new vaccine platforms with greater acceptance of vaccines among individuals are that they are needle-free, thermostable, and given in a single dose. Apart from its ability to induce robust and protective immunity against SARS-CoV-2 infection safely, one good measure of the effectiveness of a vaccine is the induction of memory cells that are able to recognize the pathogen and quickly neutralize it upon re-exposure. In most vaccine trials, efficacy is assessed based on the binding capacity and titers of neutralizing antibodies, although they provide limited information about the protective immunity against COVID-19. It needs to be mentioned here that our understanding of the protective role of nAbs against SARS-CoV-2 infection and the ability of the newly licensed COVID-19 vaccines to suppress viral transmission is primitive.

Typically, several immune mechanisms based on both cellular and humoral immunity are activated in a person following infection or immunization. During SARS-CoV-2 infection, it has been shown through evidence that robust and durable T-cell immunity to a wide range of protein targets (or epitopes) with a high level of alpha (B.1.1.7), beta (B.1.351), and gamma (P.1) variants recognition is generated. But a recent Public Health England report revealed that 34.9% of the hospitalized delta virus cases from July to August had two doses of the COVID-19 vaccine. This raises concerns regarding the efficacy of COVID-19 vaccines in conferring sterilizing immunity or, at least, adequate immunity against the delta variant or any future possible variant. Moreover, due to the high heterogeneity between reported data, the immune responses mounted after SARS-CoV-2 infection and immunization, particularly referring to the status of the adaptive immune response and how this could be exploited to develop COVID-19 vaccines capable of inducing sterilizing immunity, should be better elucidated.

A suitable animal model to investigate the pathogenesis of viral infection in human beings and the safety and efficacy of the SARS-CoV-2 vaccine is also a gigantic challenge that faces vaccine development. In current COVID-19 studies and vaccination clinical trials, many of the animal models used do not mimic the human immune response to the virus appropriately, nor do they possess the receptor needed on human cells for virus entry. Thus, the mode of action, efficacy of the vaccine, and antibody production have to be evaluated in humans for accurate estimation of risks and benefits of the vaccine; an entail provided by attainment of necessary authorization and by human subjects agreeing to participate in current studies and clinical trials. With such scarcity of conducted in vivo studies, differences in reactogenicity between the age groups following vaccine injection and immunization also become a top priority. This is largely due to the reason that most of the vaccine clinical trials have been conducted on vulnerable adults aged between 18 and 55 years, while there were only a few trials (in late stages) conducted among volunteers above 55 years of age. Minor children under 18 years of age were also not recruited into clinical trials initially.

Additionally, performing coordinated and genuine clinical trials at a previously unheard speed is another challenge kept in mind in the COVID-19 vaccine development process, with some aspects to be taken into consideration in such an 'endeavor against time' process. Apart from the importance of methodology and communication in the process of performing effective clinical trials, sample management appears to be one of the cornerstones. Given the fact that the effect of COVID-19 is disproportionately affecting the elderly and the minority ethnic group, and those patients who have co-morbidities, it is also vital that the vaccine clinical trials constitute all categories of the general population that will be vaccinated upon successful development, approval, and licensing in the marketplace. Backlash, in this case, pertaining to low age, racial, and ethnic diversity of participants in trials, has made many vaccine platforms clinical trials familiar with the risk of eroded trust in the resulting vaccines. Rationalized and harmonized regulatory licensing processes, as demanded by accelerated approval of vaccines, are also cited among the other relevant issues arising during vaccine manufacturing.

References

1. Abiodun, O., Onibonoje, O., Ola, O., & Ishola, S. (2021). Effectiveness of recombinant hepatitis B vaccine with/without the passive hepatitis B immunoglobulin vaccine in babies whose mothers are hepatitis B surface antigen positive in a private missionary hospital. *International Journal of Reproduction, Contraception, Obstetrics and Gynecology*, *10*(6), 2383–2389. https://doi.org/10.18203/2320- (accessed on 16th July 2025).
2. Alam, K. (Khorshed), Feenstra-Gols, S. G. (Sabiena G.), Geluk, A. (Annemieke), Pahan, D., et al. (2013). *The combined effect of chemoprophylaxis with single dose rifampicin and immunoprophylaxis with BCG to prevent leprosy in contacts of newly diagnosed leprosy cases: A cluster randomized controlled trial (MALTALEP study)*. https://core.ac.uk/download/43290298.pdf (accessed on 16th July 2025).
3. Ale, A., Aryal, A., Declercq, A., Depraz, M., et al. (2016). *Epidemiology, impact and control of rabies in Nepal: A systematic review*. https://core.ac.uk/download/55803198.pdf (accessed on 16th July 2025).
4. Berardi, A., Cassetti, T., Creti, R., Vocale, C., Ambretti, S., Sarti, M., Facchinetti, F., Cose, S., Prepare Network, Heath, P., & Le Doare, K. (2020). The Italian arm of the PREPARE study: an international project to evaluate and license a maternal vaccine against group B streptococcus. *Italian journal of pediatrics*, *46*(1), 160. https://doi.org/10.1186/s13052-020-00923-3(accessed on 16th July 2025).
5. Fisher, B. T., Alexander, S., Dvorak, C. C., Zaoutis, T. E., Zerr, D. M., & Sung, L. (2012). Epidemiology and potential preventative measures for viral infections in children with malignancy and those undergoing hematopoietic cell transplantation. *Pediatric blood & cancer*, *59*(1), 11–15. https://doi.org/10.1002/pbc.23417(accessed on 16th July 2025).
6. Apostolopoulos, V. (2016). *Vaccine Delivery Methods into the Future*. https://core.ac.uk/download/33478288.pdf (accessed on 16th July 2025).
7. Hoffmann, M., Baggio, M. and Krawczyk, M.W., Vaccination demand and acceptance: a literature review of key behavioural insights, EUR 31432 EN, Publications Office of the European Union, Luxembourg, 2023, ISBN 978-92-68-00276-6, doi:10.2760/420996, JRC124542.(accessed on 16th July 2025).
8. Balazs, A. B., Baltimore, D., Deal, C., Espinosa, D. A., et al. (2014). *Vectored antibody gene delivery protects against Plasmodium falciparum sporozoite challenge in mice*. https://core.ac.uk/download/33112692.pdf (accessed on 16th July 2025).
9. Baldo, V., Barbone, F., Chironna, M., Giuffrida, S., et al. (2024). *First real-world data on universal respiratory syncytial virus prophylaxis with Nirsevimab in infants*. https://core.ac.uk/download/616987295.pdf (accessed on 16th July 2025).
10. Bayliss, S., Burls, A., Cummins, C., Sandercock, J., et al. (2008). *Immunoprophylaxis against respiratory syncytial virus (RSV) with palivizumab in children: A systematic review and economic evaluation*. https://core.ac.uk/download/20540172.pdf (accessed on 16th July 2025).
11. Beaudry, F., Fairbrother, J. M., Letellier, A., Rhouma, M., et al. (2017). *Post weaning diarrhea in pigs: Risk factors and noncolistinbased control strategies*. http://hdl.handle.net/1866/18991 (accessed on 16th July 2025).
12. Rocca, A., Biagi, C., Scarpini, S., Dondi, A., Vandini, S., Pierantoni, L., & Lanari, M. (2021).

Passive Immunoprophylaxis against Respiratory Syncytial Virus in Children: Where Are We Now?. *International journal of molecular sciences, 22*(7), 3703. https://doi.org/10.3390/ijms22073703(accessed on 16th July 2025).

13. Lorenzo-Gómez, M. F., Padilla-Fernández, B., Flores-Fraile, J., Valverde-Martínez, S., González-Casado, I., Hernández, J. D., Sánchez-Escudero, A., Vicente Arroyo, M. J., Martínez-Huélamo, M., Criado, F. H., Blanco-Tarrío, E., Márquez-Sánchez, M., Flores-Fraile, M. C., Saz-Leal, P., Mirón-Canelo, J. A., García-Perdomo, H. A., & García-Cenador, M. B. (2021). Impact of whole-cell bacterial immunoprophylaxis in the management of recurrent urinary tract infections in the frail elderly. *Vaccine, 39*(42), 6308–6314. https://doi.org/10.1016/j.vaccine.2021.08.093 (accessed on 16th July 2025).
14. Blyth, C. C., Hogan, A. E., Jacoby, P., Mercer, G. N., et al. (2015). *Modelling the seasonal epidemics of respiratory syncytial virus in young children.*
15. Nair, H., Verma, V. R., Theodoratou, E., Zgaga, L., Huda, T., Simões, E. A., Wright, P. F., Rudan, I., & Campbell, H. (2011). An evaluation of the emerging interventions against Respiratory Syncytial Virus (RSV)-associated acute lower respiratory infections in children. *BMC public health, 11 Suppl 3*(Suppl 3), S30. https://doi.org/10.1186/1471-2458-11-S3-S30 (accessed on 16th July 2025).
16. Wong et al (2013) Pharmaceutical Services of Elderly Patients in Hong Kong: Scoping study to identify and analyse the nature of pharmaceutical services provided to the elderly in Hong Kong . Report to the Pharmaceutical Society of Hong Kong. https://www.pshk.hk/uploads/files/HKPJ/v20n1.pdf on 16th July 2025).
17. Chen, M. S., Jr. (2012). *Preventing hepatitis B-induced liver cancer: Implications for eliminating health disparities.* https://digitalscholarship.unlv.edu/cgi/viewcontent.cgi?article=1027&context=jhdrp (accessed on 16th July 2025).
18. Croubels, S., De Backer, P., Garré, B., Nauwynck, H., et al. (2007). *In vitro susceptibility of six isolates of equine herpesvirus 1 to acyclovir, ganciclovir, cidofovir, adefovir, PMEDAP and foscarnet.* https://core.ac.uk/download/55834721.pdf (accessed on 16th July 2025).
19. De La Hoz Restrepo, F. P., Dusheiko, G., El-Sayed, M., Ford, N., et al. (2023). *Enhancing interventions for prevention-of-mother-to-child-transmission (PMTCT) of hepatitis B virus (HBV).* https://core.ac.uk/download/564422569.pdf (accessed on 16th July 2025).
20. Melles, D. C., & de Marie, S. (2004). Prevention of infections in hyposplenic and asplenic patients: an update. *The Netherlands journal of medicine, 62*(2), 45–52.(accessed on 16th July 2025).
21. Esteghamati, A., Gouya, M. M., Keshtkar, A. A., Nadjafi, L., et al. (2011). *Hepatitis B vaccination coverage among Iranian children aged 15–26 months in 2006.* https://core.ac.uk/download/52204889.pdf (accessed on 16th July 2025).
22. Foerster, J., & Molęda, A. (2020). Virus-Like Particle-Mediated Vaccination against Interleukin-13 May Harbour General Anti-Allergic Potential beyond Atopic Dermatitis. *Viruses, 12*(4), 438. https://doi.org/10.3390/v12040438(accessed on 16th July 2025).
23. Generalov, I. I., Sencovich, S. A., & Zheleznyak, N. V. (2014). *Instructions for laboratory training in general microbiology & immunology.* https://core.ac.uk/download/80150439.pdf (accessed on 16th July 2025).

24. Modjarrad, K., Giersing, B., Kaslow, D. C., Smith, P. G., Moorthy, V. S., & WHO RSV Vaccine Consultation Expert Group (2016). WHO consultation on Respiratory Syncytial Virus Vaccine Development Report from a World Health Organization Meeting held on 23-24 March 2015. *Vaccine, 34*(2), 190–197. https://doi.org/10.1016/j.vaccine.2015.05.093(accessed on 16th July 2025).

25. Giersing, B., Kaslow, D. C., Modjarrad, K., Moorthy, V., et al. (2015). *WHO consultation on respiratory syncytial virus vaccine development: Report from a World Health Organization Meeting held on 23–24 March 2015.* https://core.ac.uk/download/42633342.pdf (accessed on 16th July 2025).

26. Grygorieva, G., Krasnopolsky, Y., & Pylypenko, D. (2023). *Liposomes: From August Wassermann to vaccines against COVID-19.* https://core.ac.uk/download/590723547.pdf (accessed on 16th July 2025).

27. Murphy, F. A. (1985). *The Epidemiology of Infectious Diseases of Livestock.* https://core.ac.uk/download/80908152.pdf (accessed on 16th July 2025).

28. Novita, B. D. (2020). *Chemoprophylaxis versus immunoprophylaxis in tuberculosis and leprosy infection.* https://core.ac.uk/download/327992363.pdf (accessed on 16th July 2025).

29. Pace, D. (2008). *Review of Varicella Zoster Virus: From Epidemiology to Prevention.* https://core.ac.uk/download/46602191.pdf (accessed on 16th July 2025).

30. Shapiro, Y. (2016). *Vaccinations: Weighing the Risks and Benefits.* https://core.ac.uk/download/217329163.pdf (accessed on 16th July 2025).

31. Jiang, H., & Wei, C. (2024). How to address vaccine hesitancy? Lessons from National Hepatitis B Immunization Program in China. *Frontiers in public health, 12*, 1286801. https://doi.org/10.3389/fpubh.2024.1286801 (accessed on 16th July 2025).

INDEX

D

E

F

G

I

K

L

M

N

O

P

W

Z